Health Behavior Change in Populations

Health Behavior Change in Populations

edited by

Scott Kahan, MD, MPH
Andrea C. Gielen, ScD, ScM
Peter J. Fagan, PhD
Lawrence W. Green, DrPH

JOHNS HOPKINS UNIVERSITY PRESS
Baltimore

Johns Hopkins University Press
2715 North Charles Street
Baltimore, Maryland 21218-4363
www.press.jhu.edu

Library of Congress Cataloging-in-Publication Data

Health behavior change in populations / [edited by] Scott Kahan, Andrea C.
Gielen, Peter J. Fagan, and Lawrence W. Green.
         p. ; cm.
     Includes bibliographical references and index.
     ISBN 978-1-4214-1455-3 (pbk. : alk. paper) — ISBN 1-4214-1455-4 (pbk. : alk.
paper) — ISBN 978-1-4214-1456-0 (electronic) — ISBN 1-4214-1456-2 (electronic)
     I. Kahan, Scott, editor of compilation.   II. Gielen, A. C. (Andrea Carlson),
editor of compilation.   III. Fagan, Peter Jerome, editor of compilation.
IV. Green, Lawrence W., editor of compilation.
     [DNLM: 1. Health Behavior.   2. Behavior Control—methods.   3. Health
Promotion—methods.   4. Public Health Practice. W 85]
     RA427.8
     362.1—dc23   2013046573

A catalog record for this book is available from the British Library.

Special discounts are available for bulk purchases of this book. For more information,
please contact Special Sales at 410-516-6936 or specialsales@press.jhu.edu.

Johns Hopkins University Press uses environmentally friendly book
materials, including recycled text paper that is composed of at least 30 percent
postconsumer waste, whenever possible.

For Meri and Cole

For Judith

For Price

For Gail

Contents

Foreword

In the 20th century, chronic diseases, such as cardiovascular disease, diabetes, and cancers, displaced acute diseases as the leading causes of death and disability. Obesity alone now accounts for more than 10% of the national disease care budget. A recent study reported that the leading risk factors for disability were tobacco smoking, high body mass index, high blood pressure, high fasting plasma glucose, and physical inactivity.*

The physical, economic, social, clinical, and communication environments constitute key modifiable determinants of these behaviors and conditions. For example, the prevalence of adults with obesity increased rapidly between 1970 and 1999, accompanied by rapid changes in the food supply that increased the availability and taste of food and simultaneously reduced its price. Estimates suggest that the energy costs of occupational physical activity decreased by more than 100 calories per day between 1960-62 and 2003-6[†] and physical activity required for housework by unemployed women decreased by more than 300 calories per day.

The debate about whether the responsibility for the health behaviors rests with the individual or the environments is at the heart of the approach to health promotion. Both individual behaviors and the environments that shape those behaviors must be addressed. An individual cannot be expected to make a healthful choice unless there are healthful choices to make. A wide array of strategies can be used to make healthier choices the default choice. In the case of tobacco, enforcement of bans on sales to minors, policies to eliminate exposure to secondhand smoke, and taxes to raise the price to make tobacco products more expensive represent strategies to discourage tobacco use and promote the more healthful choice. Strategies for smoking cessation also rely

* U.S. Burden of Disease Collaborators, The state of US health, 1990-2010: Burden of diseases, injuries, and risk factors *JAMA* 3 (10) (2013): 591-608.
† TS Church, DM Thomas, C Tudor-Locke, et al., Trends over 5 decades in U.S. occupation-related physical activity and their associations with obesity, *PLoS One* 6 (5) (2011): e19657.

on individual supports and environmental measures. The decision to stop smoking is an individual decision, but one that can be prompted or reinforced by media campaigns or images on cigarette packages that convey the adverse health effects of tobacco use, and by financial incentives for quitting provided by work sites or health plans.

As the authors point out, medical approaches have had a limited impact on the deaths and disabilities associated with chronic diseases, despite the high costs associated with the delivery of medical care. Nonetheless, the health promotion efforts that are so effective at addressing the environmental determinants of disease are less likely to have a significant impact on those already affected by chronic diseases that are driving the disease care budget. Providers increasingly recognize that they have limited capacity to address the environmental determinants of obesity and the environmental barriers to weight loss. The Affordable Care Act offers opportunities for new paradigms for clinical interventions and public health collaborations, as does the recognition that environments that support the healthful choices necessary for obesity prevention are also likely to prevent relapse after weight loss.

Baseline and outcome data are critical to assess progress, but they are often the hardest measures to institute. Survey data, such as CDC's Behavioral Risk Factor Surveillance System or the National Health and Nutrition Examination Surveys, assess health-related behaviors at the state or national level, but not their determinants. Communities that institute innovative initiatives around tobacco, nutrition, or physical activity are often challenged by the lack of expertise or resources to collect the baseline and outcome data critical to evaluate behavioral and disease outcomes. The absence of such data poses a serious barrier to progress and the spread of innovation, and the collection of such data is essential to assess progress at all levels.

Health promotion has become the discipline critical to identifying and reducing the broad determinants of chronic disease. *Health Behavior Change in Populations* will help inform and educate the next generation of practitioners and investigators, and it also provides a useful resource for those already in the field. Successful control and reduction of the chronic diseases that constitute the major cause of death and disability in the United States and other countries will require the successful application of the knowledge and strategies described herein.

William H. Dietz, MD, PhD

Acknowledgments

A textbook of this breadth and depth requires the ongoing and passionate involvement of a range of contributors, champions, and supporters.

First and foremost, we are grateful to each of the chapter authors who contributed to this text. The inspiration of their previous work and their knowledge, insights, hard work, and responsiveness to peer and editorial review were essential to making the book come to life.

We especially thank each of the editors, consultants, and others at Johns Hopkins University Press for their commitment and hard work. We appreciate their initial vision for seeing this as a valuable contribution to the public health literature, and especially their ongoing encouragement, participation, dedication, and many nudges to move the project along to culmination and publication. Special thanks go to Kelley Squazzo and Lois Crum.

We would also like to acknowledge the support received from Johns Hopkins HealthCare to enable us to convene the expert conference on health behavior change in populations that gave us the idea for this textbook.

Finally, we thank our families, friends, mentors, colleagues, students, and fellows, who directly and indirectly have played roles in our work and ultimately in this textbook.

About the Editors

SCOTT KAHAN

Dr. Scott Kahan received his undergraduate degree in bioengineering from Columbia University, his medical degree from the Medical College of Pennsylvania, and his Master of Public Health degree from the Johns Hopkins School of Public Health. He trained in Internal Medicine at Franklin Square Hospital Center and in Preventive Medicine at Johns Hopkins University, where he served as Chief Resident. He is board certified in Preventive Medicine, Obesity Medicine, and clinical nutrition.

Dr. Kahan is the director of the Strategies to Overcome and Prevent (STOP) Obesity Alliance, a George Washington University–based research and policy institute, and the founder and director of the National Center for Weight and Wellness in Washington, DC, a multidisciplinary obesity treatment center. He is editor-in-chief of a series of twelve medical textbooks published by Lippincott, Williams & Wilkins and a text on nutrition published by the PCRM foundation. He serves on the editorial review boards of more than 30 scientific journals, and he has advised the White House, the U.S. House of Representatives, the U.S. Food and Drug Administration, and numerous nongovernmental organizations on matters of obesity, nutrition, and chronic disease.

Dr. Kahan serves on the faculty of the Department of Health, Behavior, and Society, the Department of Health Policy and Management, and the Preventive Medicine Residency Program at Johns Hopkins Bloomberg School of Public Health. He also serves on the faculty of the George Washington University School of Public Health and Health Services. He was formerly the medical director of the George Washington University Weight Management Program and the associate director of the Johns Hopkins Weight Management Center. He teaches several courses at Hopkins, including Introduction to Public Health, Problem Solving in Public Health, and The Obesity Epidemic. He created and teaches one of the nation's first medical school courses exclusively focused on obesity at the George Washington University School of Medicine.

ANDREA C. GIELEN

Dr. Andrea Gielen is a professor in the Department of Health, Behavior, and Society at the Johns Hopkins Bloomberg School of Public Health and director of the Center for Injury Research and Policy in the Department of Health Policy and Management.

Dr. Gielen is the author of more than 100 scientific articles and a textbook on injury and violence prevention published by Jossey-Bass. She teaches several courses at Hopkins, including Fundamentals of Health Education and Health Promotion, Program Planning for Health Behavior Change, Behavioral Sciences and Injury Prevention, and other seminars and institutes.

Her research interests are in the development and evaluation of community and clinic-based programs that address health behavior problems affecting women and children, primarily among low-income families in urban areas. Special areas of focus are conducting intervention trials to reduce childhood injuries and domestic violence, and applying behavioral science theories and methods to understanding injury problems. Dr. Gielen was awarded the 2013 APHA Award for Excellence.

PETER J. FAGAN

Dr. Peter Fagan served as director of research at Johns Hopkins Health-Care and is an associate professor in medical psychology at the Johns Hopkins University School of Medicine, where he was director of the Sexual Behaviors Consultation Unit from 1985 to 2004.

He began his work in managed care in 1994, when he was appointed director of clinical services for TRICARE/USFHP mental health and substance abuse at Johns Hopkins Bayview Physicians, P.A. In that role he developed the administrative databases and research operations for the behavioral health services program.

Dr. Fagan's research focus is on the integration of behavioral and medical care management services and the coordination of care of individuals with medical and behavioral disorders, especially among Medicaid recipients. He is the author of the textbook *Sexual Disorders: Perspectives on Diagnosis and Treatment,* published by Johns Hopkins University Press.

Dr. Fagan received a Master of Arts degree in education from the University of Notre Dame and his doctoral degree in clinical psychology from George Washington University. He also completed a postdoctoral fellowship in the Department of Health Policy and Management at Johns Hopkins.

LAWRENCE W. GREEN

Dr. Lawrence W. Green is a professor in the Department of Epidemiology and Biostatistics, University of California–San Francisco and UCSF Comprehensive Cancer Center. As Distinguished Fellow–Visiting Scientist at the Centers for Disease Control from 1999 to 2004, he served as director of CDC's World Health Organization Collaborating Center on Global Tobacco Control, acting director of the Office on Smoking and Health, director of CDC's Office of Science and Extramural Research, and associate director for prevention research and academic partnerships in the Public Health Practice Program Office. He has recently been elected to the Institute of Medicine, National Academies.

In the 1990s Dr. Green was director of the Institute of Health Promotion Research and professor and head of the Division of Preventive Medicine and Health Promotion, Department of Health Care, University of British Columbia. He served as the first director of the U.S. Office of Health Information and Health Promotion in the Office of the Assistant Secretary for Health under the Carter administration and as vice president of the Kaiser Family Foundation. He has held full-time positions on the public health faculties at the University of California–Berkeley, Johns Hopkins University, Harvard University, and the University of Texas. Dr. Green is also past president and distinguished fellow of the Society for Public Health Education, recipient of the American Public Health Association's highest awards, and recipient of the American Academy of Health Behavior's first Research Laureate Medal. He is an associate editor of *Annual Review of Public Health* and currently serves on the editorial boards of 13 other journals. His textbooks have been widely adopted: in particular, *Community and Population Health* is in its eighth edition and *Health Program Planning: An Educational and Ecological Approach* is in its fourth edition. The latter text has been the repository for adaptation of his social-environmental PRECEDE-PROCEED model; more than 1,000 applications of that model have been reported in published case studies, research, evaluations, and other textbooks.

Contributors

JANE BERTRAND, PHD
Professor, Department of Health, Behavior, and Society
Director, Johns Hopkins Center for Communication Programs
Johns Hopkins Bloomberg School of Public Health
Baltimore, Maryland

ALLAN BEST, PHD
Director, InSource Research Group
Associate Scientist, Centre for Clinical Epidemiology and Evaluation
Vancouver Coastal Health Research Institute
Clinical Professor, School of Population and Public Health,
    University of British Columbia
Vancouver, British Columbia

MARIA BULZACCHELLI, PHD
Assistant Professor, Department of Public Health
University of Massachusetts-Amherst
Amherst, Massachusetts

MATTHEW BUMAN, PHD
Assistant Professor, School of Nutrition and Health Promotion
Exercise and Wellness Program
College of Health Solutions
Arizona State University
Phoenix, Arizona

LAWRENCE J. CHESKIN, MD
Associate Professor, Department of Health, Behavior, and Society
Director, Johns Hopkins Weight Management Center
Johns Hopkins Bloomberg School of Public Health
Baltimore, Maryland

AMY R. CONFAIR, MPH
Community Research and Policy Associate, Office for Research
Drexel University School of Public Health
Philadelphia, Pennsylvania

CAROLYN J. CUMPSTY-FOWLER, PHD, MPH
Assistant Professor and Evaluation Coordinator
Johns Hopkins University School of Nursing
Assistant Professor, Johns Hopkins Bloomberg School of Public Health
Baltimore, Maryland

GAIL DAUMIT, MD, MHS
Associate Professor of Medicine
Core Faculty, Welch Center for Prevention, Epidemiology, and
    Clinical Research
Johns Hopkins University School of Medicine
Baltimore, Maryland

MELISSA DAVEY-ROTHWELL, PHD, MPH
Associate Scientist, Department of Health, Behavior, and Society
Johns Hopkins Bloomberg School of Public Health
Baltimore, Maryland

PENNY B. DECK
PhD Student, Department of Biomedical Physiology and Kinesiology
Simon Fraser University
Burnaby, British Columbia

ELAINE DOHERTY, PHD
Associate Professor-Adjunct, Department of Health, Behavior,
    and Society
Johns Hopkins Bloomberg School of Public Health
Baltimore, Maryland

LINDA DUNBAR, PHD, RN
Vice President of Care Management
Johns Hopkins HealthCare
Glen Burnie, Maryland

WILLIAM W. EATON, PHD
Sylvia and Harold Halpert Professor and Chair, Department
    of Mental Health
Johns Hopkins Bloomberg School of Public Health
Baltimore, Maryland

MARGARET ENSMINGER, PHD
Professor and Associate Chair, Department of Health, Behavior,
    and Society
Johns Hopkins Bloomberg School of Public Health
Baltimore, Maryland

REBECCA EVANS-POLCE, BS
Predoctoral Student, Department of Health, Behavior, and Society
Johns Hopkins Bloomberg School of Public Health
Baltimore, Maryland

ANITA S. EVERETT, MD
Section Director, Community and General Psychiatry
Johns Hopkins Bayview Medical Center
Baltimore, Maryland

PETER J. FAGAN, PHD
Associate Professor, Johns Hopkins University School of Medicine
Baltimore, Maryland
Director of Research, Johns Hopkins HealthCare LLC
Glen Burnie, Maryland

DIANE T. FINEGOOD, PHD
Professor, Department of Biomedical Physiology and Kinesiology
Simon Fraser University
President and CEO, Michael Smith Foundation for Health Research
Vancouver, British Columbia

STEPHANIE FITZPATRICK, PHD
Assistant Professor, Department of Preventive Medicine
Rush University Medical Center
Chicago, Illinois

ANDREA C. GIELEN, SCD, SCM
Professor, Department of Health, Behavior, and Society
Director, Center for Injury Research and Policy
Johns Hopkins Bloomberg School of Public Health
Baltimore, Maryland

KAREN GLANZ, PHD, MPH
Professor, Department of Medicine
University of Pennsylvania
Philadelphia, Pennsylvania

LAWRENCE W. GREEN, DRPH
Professor, Department of Epidemiology and Biostatistics
Helen Diller Family Comprehensive Cancer Center
University of California–San Francisco
San Francisco, California

AYSE P. GURSES, PHD
Associate Professor
Johns Hopkins University School of Medicine
Baltimore, Maryland

ERIC HEKLER, PHD
Assistant Professor, School of Nutrition and Health Promotion
Arizona State University
Phoenix, Arizona

JUDITH HIBBARD, PHD, MPH
Professor, Department of Health Policy
University of Oregon
Eugene, Oregon

FELICIA HILL-BRIGGS, PHD
Associate Professor of Medicine
Core Faculty, Welch Center for Prevention, Epidemiology, and
    Clinical Research
Director, Cognition and Behavior Sub-Core, Diabetes Research and
    Training Center
Johns Hopkins University School of Medicine
Baltimore, Maryland

HAROLD HOLDER, PHD
Senior Research Scientist and Former Director
Pacific Institute for Research and Evaluation
Oakland, California

DAVID HOLTGRAVE, PHD
Professor and Chairman, Department of Health, Behavior, and Society
Johns Hopkins Bloomberg School of Public Health
Baltimore, Maryland

YEA-JEN HSU
Senior Research Assistant, Department of Health Policy and
    Management
Johns Hopkins Bloomberg School of Public Health
Baltimore, Maryland

LEE M. JOHNSTON
Simon Fraser University
Burnaby, British Columbia

SCOTT KAHAN, MD, MPH
Faculty, Department of Health Policy and Management
Johns Hopkins Bloomberg School of Public Health
Baltimore, Maryland
Director, Strategies to Overcome and Prevent (STOP) Obesity Alliance
George Washington University School of Public Health and
    Health Services
Washington, DC
Director, National Center for Weight and Wellness
Washington, DC

ABBY C. KING, PHD
Professor, Departments of Health Research and Policy and of Medicine
Stanford University School of Medicine
Stanford, California

ANN KLASSEN, PHD
Professor, Department of Community Health and Prevention
Associate Dean for Research
Drexel University School of Public Health
Philadelphia, Pennsylvania

HELEN C. KOENIG, MD, MPH
Physician, Jonathan Lax Treatment Center Philadelphia FIGHT
Assistant Professor, Division of Infectious Diseases, Hospital of the
    University of Pennsylvania

CARL LATKIN, PHD
Professor, Department of Health, Behavior, and Society
Johns Hopkins Bloomberg School of Public Health
Baltimore, Maryland

GEORGE LOEWENSTEIN, PHD
Professor of Economics and Psychology
Carnegie Mellon University
Pittsburgh, Pennsylvania

RYAN MACDONALD, PHD
Biostatistician, Prevention and Research Center
Mercy Medical Center
Baltimore, Maryland

JILL MARSTELLER, PHD, MPP
Assistant Professor, Department of Health Policy and Management
Johns Hopkins Bloomberg School of Public Health
Baltimore, Maryland

CARRIE L. MATTESON, PHD
School of Kinesiology
Simon Fraser University
Vancouver, British Columbia

BRIANA M. MEZUK, PHD
Assistant Professor, Department of Family Medicine and
    Population Health
Division of Epidemiology
Virginia Commonwealth University
Richmond, Virginia

ARNAB MUKHERJEA, DRPH
Postdoctoral Scholar, University of California, San Francisco
Assistant Professor, California State University, East Bay

ROBYN OSBORN, PHD
Assistant Director
National Center for Weight and Wellness
Washington, DC

A. ANT OZOK, PHD
Associate Professor, Department of Information Systems
University of Maryland-Baltimore County
Baltimore, Maryland

ELIZABETH M. PARKER, PHD, MHS
Postdoctoral Fellow, Department of Mental Health
Johns Hopkins Bloomberg School of Public Health
Baltimore, Maryland

KESHIA POLLACK, PHD, MPH
Associate Professor, Department of Health Policy and Management
Director, Occupational Injury Epidemiology and Prevention
    Training Program
Johns Hopkins Bloomberg School of Public Health
Baltimore, Maryland

PETER J. PRONOVOST, MD, PHD
Professor, Departments of Anesthesiology and of Critical Care
    Medicine and Surgery
Johns Hopkins University School of Medicine
Professor, Johns Hopkins Carey Business School
Baltimore, Maryland

BARBARA RILEY, PHD
Director, Strategy and Capacity Development
Senior Scientist, Propel Centre for Population Health Impact
University of Waterloo
Waterloo, Ontario

DEBRA ROTER, DRPH, MPH
Professor, Department of Health, Behavior, and Society
Johns Hopkins Bloomberg School of Public Health
Baltimore, Maryland

DANNY SCHIEFFLER JR., MSW
Senior Administrator
Tulane University School of Medicine
New Orleans, Louisiana

DAVID A. SLEET, PHD
Associate Director for Science, Division of Unintentional Injury
   Prevention
National Center for Injury Prevention and Control
Centers for Disease Control and Prevention
Atlanta, Georgia

MARLA STEINBERG
Adjunct Professor, School of Population and Public Health
University of British Columbia
Evaluation Consultant, Marla Steinberg and Associate
Vancouver, British Columbia

ERIC C. STRAIN, MD
Professor, Department of Psychiatry and Behavioral Sciences
Medical Director, Behavioral Pharmacology Research Unit
Johns Hopkins University School of Medicine
Baltimore, Maryland

AMBER C. SUMMERS, MHS, RD
PhD Student, Department of Health Behavior and Society
Johns Hopkins Bloomberg School of Public Health
Baltimore, Maryland

MARTHA SYLVIA, PHD, RN
Director of Outcomes and Evaluation
Johns Hopkins HealthCare
Glen Burnie, Maryland

D. ANDREW TOMPKINS, MD, MHS
Assistant Professor, Department of Psychiatry and Behavioral Sciences
Johns Hopkins University School of Medicine
Baltimore, MD

KARIN E. TOBIN, PHD, MHS
Associate Scientist, Department of Health, Behavior, and Society
Johns Hopkins Bloomberg School of Public Health
Baltimore, Maryland

INES VIGIL, MD, MPH
Medical Director
Johns Hopkins HealthCare
Glen Burnie, Maryland

KEVIN G. VOLPP, MD, PHD
Professor, School of Medicine
Professor, Wharton School
Director, Center for Health Incentives
University of Pennsylvania
Philadelphia, Pennsylvania

Reviewers

STEVEN M. ALBERT, PHD
Professor and Chair
Department of Behavioral and Community Health Sciences
Pitt Public Health
University of Pittsburgh
Pittsburgh, Pennsylvania

LISA FOLDA, MHS
Assistant Director, Undergraduate Program in Public Health Studies
Johns Hopkins University
Baltimore, Maryland

MARGARET A. HANDLEY, PHD, MPH
Assistant Professor, Department of Epidemiology and Biostatistics
Division of Preventive Medicine and Public Health
Department of Medicine, Division of General Internal Medicine
University of California-San Francisco
San Francisco, California

DONALD E. MORISKY, SCD, MSPH, SCM
Professor and former Chair
Department of Community Health Sciences
UCLA Fielding School of Public Health
University of California-Los Angeles
Los Angeles, California

Health Behavior Change
in Populations

Introduction

SCOTT KAHAN, LAWRENCE W. GREEN,
ANDREA C. GIELEN, AND PETER J. FAGAN

Health is influenced by five broad categories of factors, or *determinants:*[1] genetics, social circumstances, environmental exposures, behavioral patterns, and medical care. Public health research consistently reveals that the single greatest opportunity to improve health and the quality of life and reduce premature deaths is by addressing health behaviors, which account for nearly 50% of all deaths in the United States (Schroeder 2007). Health behaviors and the social conditions that influence them play a central role in the risk for, development of, and treatment and management of the most common causes of disease, disability, death, and health care costs in the modern world (Green and Hiatt 2009, 120-38). Surprisingly for some, medical care has only a relatively minor role in preventing premature death and improving quality of life compared with these other determinants of health, notwithstanding the much greater expenditures on medical care than on public health measures.

As difficult as it is to change personal behaviors, there is little debate about the need to do so from a societal perspective and through societal means. In addition to the death and disability attributable to behavior-associated health problems—such as heart disease, diabetes, obesity, cancer, chronic obstructive pulmonary disease, unintentional and violent injuries, many infectious diseases, and addictions—the economic costs are staggering. Three-quarters of the United States' $1.5 *trillion* in health care costs is spent on chronic diseases, the majority of which are driven by unhealthful and risky behaviors. Indeed, when taking into account other costs, such as absenteeism and lost productivity, the economic burden of just tobacco use, poor diet, physical inactivity, alcohol abuse, and unintentional injuries, alone, exceeds $500 billion yearly (Anderson 2004).

The responsibilities for health behaviors clearly extend beyond the individual. Although the individual is perhaps the "final common pathway" (i.e., lighting the cigarette, reaching for the apple, putting on the gym shoes, clicking the seat belt), our choices and behaviors rest on a multitude of influences that range from our family influences and social networks all the way to societal policies and norms. Consider the example of cigarette use. Children of smokers are much more likely to become smokers themselves. Having close friends who smoke increases the likelihood of being a smoker. Working in a blue-collar occupation and living in a poor neighborhood similarly correlate with smoking. When local or national policies are enacted to increase taxation of tobacco products, smoking rates go down (Grossman 1989). When antismoking campaigns are initiated, smoking rates and accompanying levels of smoking-associated diseases decline, sometimes precipitously.[2] When smokers have access to effective self-management skills training and smoking cessation programs, they are far more likely to quit smoking—and studies have shown that such programs can be linked to reduced mortality rates. These are just a few of the myriad determinants that influence the initiation, propagation, cessation, or adaptation of tobacco use and numerous other health behaviors. A reasonable approach to health behavior change, then, must consider individual factors, environmental and societal factors, and everything in between.

This volume comes at a time of contentious debate on health and health care and unprecedented national and international discourse on health behaviors, especially tobacco use, diet, and physical activity. The 19th century has been called the Century of Hygiene because of vast improvements in understanding of microbes and prevention of infectious disease and reforms in housing, sewage, and water supplies that transmitted them. The 20th century has been called the Century of Medicine because of the vast improvements in antibiotics, vaccines, clinical care, and treatment options, although the last half of that century also clearly demonstrated the responsiveness of public behavior to efforts to increase the public's use of these advances, such as immunizations and birth control, and the last third of that century pointed the way to successful behavioral interventions in HIV/AIDS prevention, tobacco use, injury and violence prevention, and other behavioral determinants of health.

We are now in a Century of Behavior Change, because of the huge public health burden of behavior-related disease and the difficulty society has had enforcing or even supporting health behavior changes. Many ongoing attempts by cities, states, communities, and organizations seek to make inroads on numerous behavior-related diseases, such as diabetes, obesity, cancers, heart disease, and injuries, such as those resulting from gun violence, motor vehicles, and prescription drug use. By instituting wide-ranging interventions, including policies and incentives to promote more healthful behaviors—for example, bans on indoor smoking in public places, increased taxes on tobacco products, commercial bans on trans fats, restaurant menu labeling regulations, bans on cell phone use while driving, and so forth—these initiatives and others go beyond simply educating individuals about the need to change. Although advances in health communication and education have yielded more sophisticated and effective persuasive messaging targeting individuals, societal level interventions are also needed to make healthful or safe behaviors easier and unhealthful or dangerous behaviors less so. Strategies of the future must mold the familial, social, cultural, economic, and political norms that influence what we do.

It is vitally important that we avoid the tendency for an "either-or" approach (either individual-focused or societal-focused) to behavior change intervention, but rather build approaches that include both individually and environmentally focused pieces. Before the 1970s, public health education emphasized a broad view of social determinants of health, and community organization skills were central to training programs (Glanz et al. 2008). During the next two decades, health educators and clinicians primarily focused more on intra-individual factors, such as a person's beliefs, knowledge, and skills. As discussed in Chapter 2, behavior interventions should operate at multiple levels of influence in order to achieve maximal effect. If population health interventions are based only on individual-level factors (such as increasing knowledge), or if interventions address only the environment, but not the individual, optimum results cannot be expected. For example, after schoolchildren learn in a health education lesson that they should avoid getting too much sun exposure, they might be sent outside for recess where there is no natural shade or shade structure on the playground. Clearly, this setting does not support the health education that was provided in class. Another example is that community programs might encourage residents to walk more to improve health, but if there are no sidewalks on the roads they would take, or if those roads are unsafe for walking, the messages will likely be ineffective. Similarly, building a sidewalk to make walking possible or putting up an awning alongside the playground to provide shade from the sun, by themselves, may change behavior very little without coexisting educational messages.

The idea for this textbook took root at a conference at Johns Hopkins University that was organized and led by Drs. Scott Kahan and Peter Fagan. The invitation-only conference was primarily for Hopkins faculty, health care and human resources personnel, selected research experts and key opinion leaders in behavior change science, and several community and public leaders. The speakers were all renowned experts, both from the Hopkins community and beyond, and many adapted and extended their presentations as chapters in this textbook. Particularly notable owing to the complex and multidisciplinary aspects of behavior and behavior change, this conference was jointly sponsored by Johns Hopkins HealthCare and the Johns Hopkins Bloomberg School of Public Health, School of Medicine, School of Nursing, and Department of Psychiatry and Behavioral Science.

The goal of the conference was twofold: first, to examine the evidence for changing health behaviors on a large scale; second, to delineate potential roles in supporting health behavior change on a population scale for key societal stakeholders, including health plans, employers, clinicians, researchers, policymakers, and others. This textbook begins where the conference ended and takes readers more systematically into the science and practice of health behavior change. Our primary objective is to help readers appreciate the importance of health behaviors and behavior change and to build an understanding of the principles and methods for supporting healthful behaviors on a population level. We do this by collecting and building on what has been learned from research on the multiple individual and societal determinants of health behavior, and evaluating the policies, programs, and practices in several key fields of health behavior.

In this book we present a stepwise framework encompassing various models for changing behaviors. It spans the continuum from informing the individual to modifying the surroundings and circumstances that drive decision-making and behaviors. This large-scale approach addresses not only the individual, but also the familial, interpersonal, cultural, social, political, and community influences on behavior and behavior change. The framework is then applied to health behaviors that account for the largest public health burdens. The book's emphasis on the application of theory and research to practice makes for a generalizable treatment of the subject matter, while emphasizing community-wide evaluation of policies, programs, and practices that assure cultural and situational applicability and appropriateness. It is intended to be a core textbook for intermediate or advanced courses on behavior change in public health undergraduate programs as well as introductory courses in graduate-level public health, public policy, behavioral sciences, health sciences, and other courses of study encompassing health behaviors. Additionally, we believe the text will be a welcome resource for many practicing public health professionals.

This textbook is organized into three general parts:

I. *State of the Field: Key Concepts in Health Behavior Change.* This section launches the book by presenting the current practice, process, and theories of health behavior change. Insofar as this book focuses on behavior rather than specific health problems, a firm grounding in the theories related to how best to support behavior change is valuable. Health behavior change programs grounded in theory, evidence, and assessment of local conditions can more readily encompass previous knowledge, research, and experience than programs that merely replicate a particular program that worked somewhere else. The theoretical linchpin of our presentation is the ecological model of health behavior change in which multiple determinants across the broad levels of influence are considered in any behavior change intervention. Accordingly, this first part looks at the ecological model in depth as well as at specific theories, then moves through behavior change at specific levels, and finally considers how to evaluate behavior change programs.

II. *State of the Science and Roles for Key Health Behaviors.* This section, the heart of the book, applies part I theory to practice. It deals with behavior change related to specific public health issues. This focus on the health behaviors implicated in the downstream health problems they cause—that is, heart disease, cancer, injury, and so on—is one of the components that make the book most relevant for future prevention practitioners. Arranged roughly in descending order of the magnitude of the public health burdens the behaviors present, the chapters treat key determinants and conceptual frameworks for behavior change for the specific health topics; current evidence-based interventions and best practices of planning and combining them into programs; considerations for program implementation, evaluation, and translation; roles for key stakeholders; and a roadmap for the future.

III. *Cross-Cutting Issues in Behavior Change.* Recognizing that we have moved beyond the Century of Hygiene (the 1800s) and the Century of Medicine (the 1900s) to the current Century of Behavior Change, this section considers the optimization of managing chronic disease through behavior change. Thus, as part I lays a foundation of behavior change theory and part II applies that thinking to key health behavioral problem areas, this section "cuts across" the preceding chapters with emerging important and relevant public health and policy topics.

Each chapter includes a list of sources for reference and further study. Be aware that in many cases one can gain access to those scientific articles through searching by the article's title on the Internet.

At the end of the book is a glossary with specialized terms; bold type in the text calls attention to the glossary entries.

NOTES

1. Although these factors do not uniformly determine health outcomes in the same deterministic sense that "determinants" in physics or chemistry determine changes, the term has gained currency in public health in consideration of the factors' pervasive and strong influence on health outcomes as assessed largely by correlational rather than experimental evidence.

2. See the Community Guide website, http://the communityguide.org/tobacco/RRmassreach.html.

REFERENCES

Anderson G. 2004. *Chronic Conditions: Making the Case for Ongoing Care.* Baltimore: Johns Hopkins University.

Glanz K, Rimer BK, Viswanath K, eds. 2008. *Health Behavior and Health Education: Theory, Research, and Practice.* 4th ed. San Francisco: Jossey-Bass.

Green LW, Hiatt RA. 2009. Behavioural determinants of health and disease. In *Oxford Textbook of Public Health,* ed. R Detels, R Beaglehole, MA Lansang, et al. 5th ed. Oxford: Oxford University Press.

Grossman M. 1989. Health benefits of increases in alcohol and cigarette taxes. *Br J Addict* 84 (10): 1193-1204.

Schroeder SA. 2007. We can do better—improving the health of the American people. *N Engl J Med* 357:1221-28.

Part I

STATE OF THE FIELD
Key Concepts in
Health Behavior Change

Conceptual Framework for Behavior Change

KAREN GLANZ AND SCOTT KAHAN

LEARNING OBJECTIVES

After completing the chapter, the reader will be able to

* Appreciate the importance of ecological models in the approach to health behavior change.
* Describe five general levels of influence included in ecological models.
* Define *theory* and describe several key aspects of behavior change theories.
* Describe several categorizations of health behaviors.
* Recognize several key roles for stakeholders in an ecological approach to health behavior change.

Introduction

The leading causes of death in the United States and globally are chronic, often behavior-related, diseases, including heart disease, cancer, lung diseases, diabetes, and injuries (Yach et al. 2004). Behavioral factors, particularly tobacco use, diet and activity patterns, alcohol consumption, sexual behavior, and behaviors that lead to unintentional and violent injuries, are among the most prominent contributors to mortality (Schroeder 2007). Infectious and chronic diseases, as well as injuries, are affected by behavior, and their impact may be influenced by the application of effective health behavior interventions. Substantial suffering, premature mortality, and medical costs can be avoided by positive changes in behavior.

During the past 20 years, public, private, and professional interest in preventing disease and injury, disability, and death through changes in lifestyle and participation in screening programs has dramatically increased. Health behavior interventions are being conducted not only in health care settings, but also in nonclinical community sites such as work sites, churches, and community centers (Glanz et al. 2008). Multicomponent programs to prevent chronic disease have demonstrated modest improvements in disease risk across large populations (Pennant et al. 2010), which can ultimately reduce sickness and save lives.

Interventions to improve health behavior in populations can be best designed with an understanding of relevant theories of behavior change (Glanz et al. 2008). (Interventions are broadly defined here to include environment and policy changes as well as more traditional education and communication programs for individuals and groups.) A growing body of evidence suggests that interventions developed with an explicit theoretical foundation are more effective to promote behavior change and improve health, compared with those lacking a theoretical base; strategies that combine multiple **social** and behavioral **theories** and concepts may also have larger effects than those that use a single theory or concept (Ammerman et al. 2002; Legler et al. 2002; Noar et al. 2007). The science and art of using health behavior theories reflect a combination of approaches, methods, and strategies from the social and health sciences. This broad range of perspectives from health, social, and behavioral sciences constitutes the building blocks of a multilevel "conceptual framework" for positive health behavior change. A **conceptual framework** is a set of assumptions and principles that outline and attempt to connect the factors, variables, beliefs, or actions that influence an outcome of interest. In this sense, a conceptual framework is like a map that guides researchers and practitioners to understand how to approach a certain health behavior and health problem. Conceptual frameworks contribute to successful program **planning** and **program evaluation**, and they can advance research to test innovative intervention strategies (Glanz et al. 2008).

This chapter provides an overview of contemporary behavioral science theory for development and implementation of health behavior and health promotion interventions and offers a broad conceptual framework for behavior change. The first sections describe an ecological approach to health behavior, which addresses the multiple determinants and levels of determinants that influence health and health behavior. Various types of behavior change are discussed with reference to how theoretical concepts may help to understand them. Next, selected often-used theories and their key concepts are described along with applications of their use in health behavior interventions. A later section of the chapter discusses roles for clinicians and health educators or counselors who work primarily with individuals and the roles for organizations and public health experts whose constituencies are populations. Examples of the application of theories in large public health programs illustrate the feasibility, utility, and challenges of using conceptual frameworks to understand and encourage health-promoting behavior change in populations. Finally, this chapter emphasizes the importance of **partnerships** for applying an ecological perspective in practice.

The Ecological Approach to Health Behavior

Successful public health programs and initiatives are based on an understanding of **health behaviors** and the **context** in which they occur (Glanz et al. 2008).

An **ecological approach** broadly describes the **complex** relationships and interplay between individuals and their environments (physical environment, social and cultural environment, etc). An **ecological model** of health behavior addresses the interconnectedness between behavior, biology, and environment. Four prominent Institute of Medicine (IOM) reports, one on health and behavior (IOM 2001), one on health

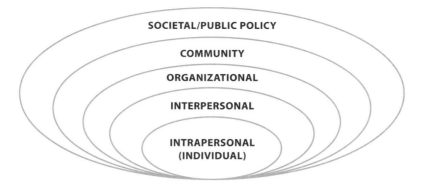

FIGURE 2.1. Basic ecological model

promotion interventions (Smedley and Syme 2000), one on educating the public health workforce (IOM 2003), and one on preventing childhood obesity (IOM 2005), were consistent in emphasizing the importance of an ecological framework to guide research and intervention.

The basic tenets of an ecological model are that

1. health and well-being are affected by a dynamic interaction among biology, behavior, and the environment; and that
2. this interaction changes over the life course of individuals, families, and communities. (Kaplan et al. 2000)

This description conveys the notion of multiple **levels of influence** on health and health-related behaviors and a "**reciprocal determinism**" between these environments and behavior. *Reciprocal determinism* refers to the theory that one's behavior both influences and is influenced by both personal-individual factors and the surrounding environment, and that the environment both influences and is influenced by the individuals within it (Gielen and Sleet 2003; Green and Kreuter 2005; Green et al. 1996; Kaplan et al. 2000; McLeroy et al. 1988; Richard et al. 1996; Sallis and Owen 1997; Simons-Morton et al. 1989; Stokols 1996).

Although many types of ecological models have been proposed, each of them fundamentally describes multiple levels of influence classified according to degrees of organizational **complexity**. In this book, we primarily refer to the following "levels" of an ecological framework (fig. 2.1):

- **Intrapersonal level**: the individual characteristics that influence behavior. These include knowledge, **attitudes**, and beliefs, which are accumulated and conditioned through a life history of exposures to the other levels. Personality traits, biology, race, **socioeconomic status**, and situational factors (e.g., personal history, substance abuse) may also be included. Strategies to address behaviors at the intrapersonal level include education sessions and **social marketing** campaigns.
- **Interpersonal level**: interactions and relationships that provide social identity, support, and role definition. These include family, friends, co-workers, peers, and **social networks**. Strategies to address interpersonal contributors to behaviors include mentoring programs and family education or counseling.
- Organizational/institutional level: the rules, regulations, policies, **expectations**, **norms**, and cultures of the institutions in which people spend their time. These factors can promote, or constrain, healthful behaviors. Such behavioral settings

include schools, workplaces, health care settings, and social institutions. Strategies to address organizational contributors to behaviors include advocating changes to company policies.

- Community level: the norms and relationships among organizations, groups, and individuals. Strategies to address community contributors to behaviors include **media advocacy** programs.
- Societal/public policy level: national, state, and local laws, policies, and structures that regulate or support healthful actions and practices for behaviors and disease detection, prevention, and treatment. Strategies to address societal contributors to behaviors include advocacy efforts addressed to public officials.

Intervention strategies are different for the various levels of influence. For example, at the more "downstream" levels, or inner concentric circles, near the individual level, the typical interventions are a variety of educational and training methods. Innovative new technologies such as computer **tailoring** and web-based learning opportunities are promising to strengthen the impact of these intervention methods. At the more "upstream" levels, where interventions focus on outer concentric circles, such as organizations, communities, and policies, media and media advocacy become important, as do **coalition** building and community organizing (Orleans et al. 1999). At the most distal levels of concentric circles, state and national policies are the points of intervention. The multiple levels of intervention are mutually reinforcing and complementary in their total effect.

A central lesson of ecological models is that, because behavior is *influenced* at multiple levels, the most effective interventions should *operate* at multiple levels. However, many population health interventions have attempted to build knowledge, **motivation**, and behavior change

skills in individuals without changing the environments that individuals live in and vice versa. In the former case, such interventions are based on individual-level theories of health promotion that emphasize the importance of **individual-level factors** (e.g., knowledge) on health behaviors and health behavior change. For example, after a health education lesson in class that encourages students to avoid getting too much sun exposure, they might be sent outside for recess where there is no natural shade or shade structure on the playground. Community programs might encourage residents to walk to shops to do errands, but those messages will be ineffective if they do not also address the lack of sidewalks or the speed of cars on roads between the residents' homes and the shops. Thus, environments and policies that do not support healthful behaviors or make unhealthful behaviors less likely can make it difficult, dangerous, or impossible to use knowledge, motivation, and skills. Similarly, interventions that address only the environment, but not the individual, may not be sufficient to lead to substantial behavior change. Building a sidewalk to make walking possible or putting up an awning alongside the playground to provide shade from the sun, by themselves, may change behavior very little.

Multiple Determinants and Multiple Levels of Health Behavior

Many social, cultural, and economic factors contribute to the development, maintenance, and change of health behavior patterns (Smedley and Syme 2000). No single factor or set of factors can adequately account for healthful or unhealthful eating or activity patterns, tobacco use, or other behaviors. Knowledge, attitudes, reactions to stress, and motivation are important individual determinants of health behavior. Families, social relationships, socioeconomic status, culture, and geography are among many other important **influences**. A broad understanding of the key factors and models for understanding behaviors and behavior change can provide a foundation for well-informed public health programs, help identify the most influential factors for a particular person or population, and enable program developers to focus on the most salient issues.

Public health and health promotion interventions are now generally recognized to most likely be effective if they embrace an *ecological perspective* (McLeroy et al. 1988; Sallis et al. 2008). That is, they should target the multiple levels of influence that affect behavior, including individual, interpersonal, organizational, and environmental factors, as can be seen in the context of groups of employees purchasing food and eating during the workday. Employees may bring their food with them from home or buy food from workplace cafeterias and vending machines. Their choices are influenced by personal preferences and **habits**; nutrition information; the availability, cost, and placement of food; friends' choices; and numerous other factors. The process is complex and is determined not only by multiple factors, but also by factors at multiple *levels*.

Before the 1970s, public health education emphasized a broad view of social determinants of health, and community organization skills were central to training programs (Glanz et al. 2008). During the next two decades, health educators and clinicians focused more on intra-individual factors, such as a person's beliefs, knowledge, and skills (except in tobacco control and injury control, in which environmental and policy initiatives were most effectively pursued and implemented). Many behavior change programs for reducing risk factors continue to have these emphases (Kok et al. 2008). In public health, we are now returning to earlier thinking, beyond the individual to the social milieu and environment, to enhance the **effectiveness** of health promotion (Sallis et al. 2008). Program planners should work toward understanding the various levels of influence that affect indi-

viduals' and populations' behaviors and health status.

The Role of Conceptual Frameworks and Theories

Increasingly, evidence supports the idea that interventions developed with an explicit theoretical foundation are more effective than those without a theoretical base (Ammerman et al. 2002; Glanz and Bishop 2010; Legler et al. 2002; Noar et al. 2007). Influential work draws on the theoretical perspectives, research, and practice tools of several disciplines, including psychology, sociology, social psychology, anthropology, education, communications, nursing, economics, and marketing (Glanz et al. 2008).

A **theory** is a set of interrelated concepts, definitions, and propositions that present a *systematic* view of events or situations by specifying relations among variables, in order to *explain* and *predict* the events or situations. Theories are by their nature *abstract:* that is, they do not have a specified content or topic area. The notion of *generality,* or broad application, is important, as is *testability* (Van Ryn and Heaney 1992). **Generality** means that the theory can be applied to a range of issues and populations and is not highly specific to one group or behavior. **Testability** means that the theory can be used to generate hypotheses that can be supported or fail to be supported through empirical research.

Theories are useful during the various stages of planning, implementing, and evaluating interventions. Program planners can use theories to shape the pursuit of answers to *why? what? how?* In other words, theories can be used to guide the search for *why* people are not following public health and medical advice or not caring for themselves in healthful ways; they can help pinpoint *what* one needs to know before developing and organizing an intervention program; they can provide insight into *how* to shape program strategies to reach people and organizations and to make an impact on them; and they also help to identify *what* should be monitored, measured, or compared in a program evaluation (Glanz et al. 2008). Behavior change programs and policies that are based on well-studied theories of behavior and behavior change are more likely to be effective.

EXPLANATORY AND CHANGE THEORIES

Theories and models can be used both to *explain* behavior and to suggest ways to achieve behavior *change.* An **explanatory theory**, often called a **theory of the problem**, helps describe and identify why a problem exists. Such theories also predict behaviors under defined conditions. They guide the search for modifiable factors that contribute to the problem, such as insufficient knowledge, **self-efficacy**, attitudes, **social support** resources, and so on. Examples of explanatory theories include the **Health Belief Model**, the **Theory of Planned Behavior**, and the **Precaution Adoption Process Model** (see chapter 6 for further discussions of individual-level health behavior change theories). In contrast, change theories, or *theories of action,* guide the development of interventions. Whereas explanatory theories *describe* why a problem exists and what can be changed, **change theories** *define* concepts and principles that can form the basis of interventions and health messages. They suggest which strategies or messages are likely to work and provide assumptions about how an intervention would be effective. They also form the basis for **evaluation**, pushing evaluators to make explicit their assumptions about how a program should work. Examples of change theories include **Diffusion of Innovations** (see chapter 7).

TYPES OF HEALTH BEHAVIORS

There are several health behavior characteristics that have important implications for understanding their determinants and the relevant conceptual framework(s) for behavior change. They include whether a behavior is one-time, episodic, or habitual; whether the recommended changes are restrictive or additive; whether to attempt change in a gradual or strict manner; and whether to focus on single or multiple behaviors.

Episodic versus Lifestyle Behaviors. A useful distinction can be made between one-time and **episodic behaviors** versus **lifestyle behaviors (habits)**. Health behavior can be something that is done once, or periodically, such as getting immunizations or a flu shot. Other health behaviors are actions that are performed over a long period of time, such as eating a healthful diet, getting regular physical activity, and avoiding tobacco use. The latter types of behaviors, which are patterns of behavior that must be sustained, are usually considered lifestyle behaviors or health habits. The process of changing habitual behavior is often more complex and requires more points of contact over time to reinforce the positive changes made, compared with changing a one-time or episodic behavior. Habitual behaviors are also inherently more difficult to define and measure because people may vary in their practices over time (e.g., eating behaviors), and more questioning may be necessary to elicit those variations in response to situations.

Sustained health behavior change involves multiple actions and **adaptations** over time. Some people may not be ready to attempt changes, some may be thinking about attempting change, and others may have already begun implementing behavioral modifications. One central issue that has gained wide acceptance in recent years is the simple notion that *behavior change is a process, not an event.* It is important to think of the change process as one that occurs in stages. It is not a question of someone deciding one day to stop smoking and the next day becoming an ex-smoker. The idea that behavior change occurs in a number of steps is not particularly new, but it has gained wider recognition in the past few years (Lippke and Ziegelmann 2008). Indeed, various multistage theories of behavior change date back more than 50 years to the work of Lewin, McGuire, Weinstein, Marlatt and Gordon, and others (Glanz et al. 2008). Although it is possible to conceptualize one-time or episodic behaviors using stage-based models, these models fit best with sustained habits or lifestyle behaviors.

Restrictive versus Additive Behaviors. Many behavior change recommendations focus on advice to restrict, limit, or stop certain behaviors such as overeating, smoking, or drinking in excess. For example, the emphasis of nutrition counseling is often to restrict intake of certain foods or nutrients, such as reducing fat and saturated fat intake, limiting calorie intake, and limiting sodium. Yet the most often-mentioned obstacle to achieving a healthful diet is that we do not want to give up the foods we like. Basic psychological principles hold that when people are faced with a restriction or loss of choice, the restricted entity becomes more attractive.

In contrast, emphasizing additive recommendations, such as increasing intake of fruits and vegetables and becoming more active, often appeals to people because the emphasis is positive rather than negative (i.e., they can do more of something rather than do less). However, research suggests that it is not necessarily easy to get people to take up a new habit, either—and some health risk behaviors (e.g., drinking and driving) need to first be stopped before new positive or substitute behaviors can take their place. Further, the general idea of "positive change" is sometimes combined with giving something else up (e.g., eat fruit *instead of* baked sweet desserts), so the "positive" message may not stand alone in the mind of the receiver.

Gradual versus Abrupt Change. A generally held view is that the chances of successful health behavior change are greater when efforts to change occur in a gradual, stepwise manner (Bandura 1986; McAlister et al. 2008). This might involve reducing **cues** to a maladaptive behavior (such as smoking) or making small dietary changes each week as the total diet approaches

recommendations. A basic principle involved is that small successes ("**successive approximations**") increase confidence and motivation for each successive change (Bandura 1986; McAlister et al. 2008). That is, recognition of each successful behavior change, even if very small, increases a person's confidence ("self-efficacy") to make a further change. For example, for a sedentary individual, attempting to exercise regularly may seem overwhelming. However, initial, smaller **goals** that ultimately lead to regular exercise, such as identifying some exercises that are enjoyable or convenient for the individual, finding an exercise partner, purchasing necessary exercise equipment (e.g., running sneakers) or joining a gym, or starting with just one day of exercise per week, may provide a more achievable path to the ultimate desirable behavior.

Although this approach is effective for many people, others become impatient or even lose their enthusiasm for changes that are only minimally recognizable. (There are also some types of behaviors for which gradual change does not work well.) An alternative is to begin with a highly restrictive change—such as quitting smoking "cold turkey" or following a very-low-calorie diet for the first two weeks of a weight loss effort. These types of programs may be useful for people who are highly motivated and "ready" to change, like newly diagnosed diabetics, survivors of a heart attack, or those who have not been successful in making gradual changes. In some cases, an abrupt or dramatic change will help someone get over withdrawal symptoms or will yield highly motivating visible or clinical changes. Such behavior changes often require careful medical supervision and may not work for everyone.

Single versus Multiple Behaviors. Much research and practice focuses on change processes for discrete behaviors, such as eating patterns, smoking, sexual risk-taking, and so on. In the ideal, the person who practices a variety of behaviors in a health-enhancing manner can be described as having a healthful lifestyle. More realistically, many people practice *some,* but not all, lifestyle behaviors in a healthful manner. Moreover, most people do not practice all healthful or risky behaviors consistently— for instance, someone might get regular, health-promoting exercise several times a week but be a cigarette smoker or seldom floss his teeth. Or someone might quit smoking, only to begin overeating as a substitute. The complex interplay between health behaviors presents important challenges, whether a given intervention addresses a single behavior or multiple behaviors, that is, any of these examples practiced in combination. More conceptual and empirical development around changes in **interdependent** behaviors is needed.

Important Theories and Constructs Guiding Intervention Approaches

As discussed earlier in this chapter, health behaviors are shaped through a complex interplay of determinants at different levels of influence. For example, physical activity is influenced by self-efficacy at the individual level, social support from family and friends at the interpersonal level, and rates of crime or police presence producing perceptions of safety at the community level. A core principle of ecological models suggests that these multiple levels of influence *interact* across levels. For example, social support for exercise from co-workers may interact with the availability of exercise equipment at the work site to facilitate increased physical activity.

Even though various theoretical models of health behavior may reflect the same general ideas, each theory employs a unique vocabulary to articulate the specific factors considered important. Also, different theories are better suited to addressing certain types of health behavior issues than others. Theories that gain recognition in a discipline shape the field, help define the scope of practice, and influence the training and **socialization** of its professionals.

Today, no single theory or conceptual framework dominates research or practice in health promotion and education. However, reviews of journal articles published in the past two decades across a broad range of health behavior topics reveal that the four most-often-used theories have been the Health Belief Model, the **Transtheoretical Model** (or **"Stages of Change"**), the **Social Cognitive Theory**, and the **Social Ecological Model** (Painter et al. 2008). These theories mainly address the intrapersonal level (Health Belief Model, Transtheoretical Model) or the interpersonal level (Social Cognitive Theory). This section briefly describes the core constructs and central elements of these four theoretical models of health behavior. Program planning frameworks, such as the **PRECEDE-PROCEED** model, typically integrate concepts from single and multiple theories to guide the development of comprehensive programs; see chapter 5 for more information.

The Health Belief Model

The **Health Belief Model** (**HBM**) was one of the first theories of health behavior and remains one of the most widely recognized. It was developed to help understand why people did or did not use preventive services offered by public health departments in the 1950s (Hochbaum 1958) and has evolved to address new concerns in prevention and detection (e.g., mammography screening, influenza vaccines) as well as lifestyle behaviors such as sexual risk behaviors and injury prevention (Champion and Skinner 2008).

The HBM theorizes that people's beliefs about whether they are at risk for a disease or health problem and their perceptions of the benefits of taking action to avoid it, influence their readiness to take action (Champion and Skinner 2008; Glanz and Rimer 2005; Rosenstock 1974). **Perceived susceptibility** and **perceived severity**, **perceived benefits** and **perceived barriers**, cues to action, and self-efficacy (discussed below)

(Rosenstock et al. 1988) are the core constructs of the HBM. The HBM has been most often applied for health concerns that are prevention related and asymptomatic, such as early cancer detection, hypertension screening, and risk reduction for cardiovascular disease—where beliefs may be as important (or more important) than overt symptoms (Will et al. 2004).

The Transtheoretical Model and Stages of Change

Long-term changes in health behavior involve multiple actions and adaptations over time. Some people may not be ready to attempt changes, whereas others may have already begun implementing changes in their smoking, diet, activity levels, and so on. The construct of "stage of change" is a key element of the **Transtheoretical Model (TTM)** of behavior change. It proposes that people are at different stages of readiness to adopt healthful behaviors (Prochaska et al. 2008). The notion of readiness to change, or stage of change, has been examined in health behavior research and found useful in explaining and predicting changes for a variety of behaviors including smoking, physical activity, and eating habits (Dijkstra et al. 1999; Glanz et al. 1998; Marcus et al. 1998). The TTM has also been applied in many settings (Prochaska et al. 2008).

Stages of Change is a model that describes a sequence of five steps in successful behavior change:

1. **Precontemplation.** No recognition of need for or interest in change
2. **Contemplation.** Thinking about changing
3. **Preparation.** Planning for change
4. **Action.** Adopting new habits
5. **Maintenance.** Ongoing practice of new, healthier behavior (Prochaska et al. 2008)

People do not always move through the stages of change in a linear manner. They often recycle and repeat certain stages; for example, indi-

viduals may relapse and go back to an earlier stage, depending on their level of motivation and self-efficacy.

The Stages of Change model can be used to help understand why people at high risk for diabetes might not be ready to attempt behavior change; it also may help to improve the success of health counseling. Another application of the Stages of Change model in organizations and communities involves conceptualizing organizations along the Stages-of-Change continuum according to their leaders' and members' (i.e., employees') **readiness** for change (Prochaska et al. 2008).

The Social Cognitive Theory

The **Social Cognitive Theory (SCT)**, the cognitive formulation of **Social Learning Theory** that has been best articulated by Bandura (1986), explains human behavior in terms of a three-way, dynamic, reciprocal model in which personal factors, environmental influences, and behavior continually interact (McAlister et al. 2008). SCT synthesizes concepts and processes from cognitive, behavioristic, and emotional models of behavior change so it can be readily applied to behavior change interventions for disease prevention and management. A basic premise of SCT is that people learn not only through their own experiences but also by observing the actions of others and the results of those actions (Bandura 1986; McAlister et al. 2008). Key constructs of Social Cognitive Theory that are relevant to health behavior change interventions include observational learning, **reinforcement**, self-control, and self-efficacy (Will et al. 2004). Some elements of behavior modification based on SCT constructs include **goal-setting**, self-monitoring, and **behavioral contracting**. Goal-setting and self-monitoring seem to be particularly useful components of effective counseling interventions.

Self-efficacy, or a person's confidence in her ability to take action and to persist in that action despite obstacles or challenges, is especially important for influencing health behavior change efforts. Health providers can make deliberate efforts to increase patients' self-efficacy using three types of strategies: (1) setting small, incremental and achievable goals; (2) using formalized behavioral contracting to establish goals and specify rewards; and (3) monitoring and reinforcement, including patient self-monitoring by keeping records (Bandura 1986).

The key SCT construct of reciprocal determinism means that a person can be both an agent for change and a responder to change. Thus, changes in the environment, the examples of role models, and reinforcements can be used to promote more healthful behavior. This core construct, which is also central to social ecological models, is more important today than ever before.

The Social Ecological Model

The **Social Ecological Model** helps in understanding factors affecting behavior and also provides guidance for developing successful programs through **social environments**. Social ecological models emphasize multiple levels of influence (such as individual, interpersonal, organizational, community, and public policy) and the core concept that behaviors both shape and are shaped by the social environment (McLeroy et al. 1988; Sallis et al. 2008). The principles of social ecological models (several have been proposed) are consistent with SCT concepts that suggest that creating an environment conducive to change is important to making it easier to adopt healthful behaviors (Bandura 1986). For example, given the growing epidemic of obesity in the United States and other developed countries, more attention is being focused on examining and improving the health-promoting features of communities and neighborhoods and reducing the ubiquity of high-calorie, high-fat food choices (Story et al. 2008).

Roles for Key Stakeholders

As part of a multilevel, ecological approach to changing health behaviors, there are roles for various individuals and groups and numerous strategies that can be accomplished at each level of influence. Here we introduce some of the roles and strategies for clinical professionals, organizations, and public health experts and discuss the importance of strategic partnerships among **stakeholders**. These topics and concepts are further addressed throughout the book.

Roles for Clinicians, Health Educators, Counselors, and Coaches

Deciding on the best intervention approach starts with understanding the population of interest and identifying the most important and most changeable determinants of the selected behavior. There are several broadly applicable and widely used theories and models for **targeting** behavioral determinants at various levels; therefore, understanding the uses, strengths, and weaknesses of available options is important (Glanz et al. 2008).

INDIVIDUAL-LEVEL STRATEGIES

Traditionally, and especially in clinical settings, strategies to change health behaviors have focused on individual-level factors such as knowledge, beliefs, and skills. The premise underlying these interventions is that the mechanisms for changing behavior lie within an individual (McLeroy et al. 1988). Health educators, counselors, and coaches can apply individual-level theories such as the HBM, which concerns an individual's beliefs regarding his susceptibility to a health problem and the severity of the problem, as well as what he sees as the benefits and barriers of taking action (Champion and Skinner 2008).

Behavior change intervention strategies directed at individuals often include goal-setting and behavioral contracting, tailored health communication, and targeting. These strategies most typically draw upon SCT (Bandura 1986) and the Stages-of-Change construct from TTM (Prochaska et al. 2008).

Goal-Setting and Behavioral Contracting. **Goal-setting** and **behavioral contracting** involve setting achievable and incremental goals, committing to achieving the goals through a behavioral contract, monitoring and documenting progress, and reinforcing goal achievement through rewards. This approach has been used to help people quit smoking, manage asthma, eat more healthfully, and exercise more (McAlister et al. 2008). Goal-setting and behavioral contracting interventions are informed by two major constructs from SCT: reinforcement and self-regulation. According to SCT, self-regulation is achieved through (1) goal-setting, or identifying achievable incremental and long-term goals, (2) systematic observation of one's own behavior, or self-monitoring, (3) feedback about the performance of the behavior and suggestions for improvement, (4) self-instruction, or active cognitive engagement with oneself during the planning and performance of the behavior, (5) reinforcement with tangible or intangible self-rewards, and (6) obtaining social support from others to encourage self-control efforts.

Goal-setting interventions must consider goal properties such as the difficulty of the goal (e.g., run a marathon versus jog for 20 minutes three times a week), proximity or time frame (e.g., lose 1 pound a week or lose 40 pounds in a year), and type of goal-setting. Types of goal-setting include *self-set, assigned, prescribed, participatory/collaborative, guided,* and *group-set* goals. Interestingly, self-set goals are not necessarily more effective than assigned goals, perhaps because self-set goals can be poorly defined or overly ambitious. Additional tenets of goal-setting as an intervention strategy are that specific goals linked with performance feedback are more effective than vague goals and that

more challenging goals often can lead to higher performance. Goal-setting is believed to work by motivating effort, persistence, and concentration. Feedback is central to goal-setting interventions, as are rewards, to reinforce the behavior as it develops.

Tailoring. **Tailoring** refers to a process of individualizing health messages to a particular person's unique needs with respect to a specific health outcome, based on an individualized assessment. Tailoring begins with an individualized assessment that typically measures theory-based determinants such as Stage of Change from the TTM and perceived barriers from the HBM. Health messages are then customized to address a person's unique combination of beliefs and circumstances. For example, a woman may be thinking about getting a mammogram but is worried about the cost. A tailored message might reinforce her interest in getting a mammogram and provide her a list of low-cost mammography services in her community. Tailoring has the potential to increase the relevance and salience of information and thereby increase the motivation to process health information. Tailoring is believed to motivate greater information processing by matching content to an individual's unique needs and interests, by contextualizing information in a meaningful way, and by packaging information to appeal to an individual's design and delivery preferences as well as her preferences for quantity and type of information (Rimer and Kreuter 2006).

Many tailoring interventions rely on the Stages-of-Change construct from the TTM (Rimer and Kreuter 2006). As described earlier in this chapter, the TTM posits that people are at different stages of readiness to adopt a behavior (Prochaska et al. 2008). For tailoring purposes, individuals are classified by stage with a few questions to assess whether they are interested in changing a specific behavior, thinking about a change, preparing to change, have already changed, or are trying to maintain a change. Following classification by stage, motivational messages can be tailored to move an individual from one stage to another. Using flu shots as the health behavior of interest, if a man is unaware of the need for a flu shot, he would be classified in the precontemplation stage. Communication strategies tailored for this stage would attempt to capture his attention through an interesting narrative or a compelling image (Rimer and Kreuter 2006). If the person was vaguely aware of flu shots but did not feel they applied to him, a tailored message might present data about his risk and how a serious case of the flu would affect him and his family. If he was already thinking about getting a flu shot but had not yet decided, a list of the pros and cons of getting a shot might help him to move toward action. A list of nearby locations of flu shots might also facilitate action. Movement to the maintenance stage could be facilitated through annual reminders.

Alternatively, communication strategies beyond health messages can be employed at each stage. According to Prochaska and colleagues (Rimer and Kreuter 2006), consciousness-raising in the form of messages about the causes and **consequences** of a behavior would be appropriate at the precontemplation change, whereas self-reevaluation through assessing and clarifying values would help move people from the contemplation to the preparation stage. Encouraging individuals to seek social support, in contrast, would be appropriate at the maintenance stage.

Early tailoring efforts often focused on written materials such as newsletters (Prochaska et al. 2008). There is now an extensive scientific literature on the impact of tailored print health behavior change interventions, and there are many examples of features contributing to their greater or lesser rates of success (Noar et al. 2007). Tailoring has also been used in print materials such as calendars; in telephone and face-to-face counseling; and, more recently, through interactive web-based programs. Puff City was a web-based program that focused on asthma management among urban African American adolescents (Joseph et al. 2007). The tailoring, delivered through four consecutive computer sessions, was based on constructs from the TTM and the HBM. Participation in the intervention had a positive impact on both behavioral and health outcomes. A tailored Colon Cancer Risk Counseling intervention for relatives of colorectal cancer patients combined face-to-face meetings with print materials and follow-up phone calls. That tailored strategy, which drew on the Precaution Adoption Process Model and the HBM, was effective at increasing screening adherence among those who received the intervention (Glanz et al. 2007). Computer tailoring has also been used successfully to promote parents' child safety behaviors in both emergency department and primary care settings (Gielen et al. 2007; McDonald et al. 2005; Nansel et al. 2002).

Targeting. Ideally, each person should be treated as an individual with unique circumstances and health history. Still, epidemiological research indicates that certain demographic subgroups differ in terms of risk factors and health behaviors. Understanding these population trends can help prepare a provider to work with various types of patients. This approach, often called **"targeting,"** is distinct from tailoring in that it uses information about a person's characteristics but without detailed individualized assessment. For example, younger persons may feel invulnerable to coronary events, and older adults may be managing multiple chronic conditions. An active middle-aged professional may place returning to his previous level of activity above important health precautions. These are just a few examples of how population subgroups may differ, and they serve as a reminder to be sensitive to group patterns but to avoid stereotyping because any individual may not fit the pattern. Within this general context, various theories and models can guide the search for effective ways to reach and positively motivate clients and patients.

INTERPERSONAL STRATEGIES

Importantly, as discussed above and throughout this text, to be most effective, behavior change programs at the individual level must consider and when necessary incorporate broader interventions that address the environments and contexts within which individuals make health behavior decisions. Although, traditionally, patient educators focus mainly on intra-individual factors, thinking beyond the individual to the social milieu can improve the chance of successful health behavior change efforts. Health providers can and should work toward understanding the various levels of influence that affect the patient's behavior and health status.

Thus, interpersonal-level strategies also may be important and useful for health counseling and patient education. Commonly used strategies at the interpersonal level include lay health advisers and social support programs, such as patient self-help or mutual support groups. Underlying theoretical constructs for these types of strategies include social support, **social norms**, and social networks (Heaney and Israel 2008).

Roles for Organizations and Public Health Experts

As ecological thinking has gained currency, intervention strategies have broadened to target factors at other levels of influence, such as organizational policies and the **built environment**. This recognition of the complex range of factors that shape health behaviors can make the **selection** of intervention strategies daunting.

Organizations and communities influence health behaviors in a variety of ways. Organizations provide goods and services and act as the primary mechanisms through which people engage with their community. Moreover, people spend a considerable amount of time in organizational settings, such as schools and work sites. Consequently, the social environments (e.g., organizational climate), built environments (e.g., ergonomics and safety from occupational hazards), and organizational policies and practices (e.g., healthful foods at meetings) contribute to shaping health behavior. Organization-level change strategies are often informed by organizational development theory (Butterfoss et al. 2008). Other **organizational interventions** are based on long-held understandings of how organizations are structured. Provider reminders and feedback in health care settings are typical of this type of strategy, and they can be considered to use prompts similar to those based on SCT, but at the organizational level.

PROVIDER REMINDERS AND FEEDBACK

Interventions that focus on changing office systems to support preventive services are increasingly common in health care settings. The use of assessment and feedback and provider reminders of various types has been found to be particularly successful in promoting cancer screening and smoking cessation. Based on a review of 20 research findings of provider assessment and feedback to increase delivery of appropriate cancer screening services, there was a median increase of 9 to 14 percentage points in the proportion of study participants completing mammography, Pap tests, or fecal occult blood tests. Provider reminders have also been found effective for increasing adherence to cancer screening **guidelines**, with an 8.8 percentage point median increase across the same three tests (Sabatino et al. 2008). A systematic review of published studies of the effectiveness of reminders to providers to discuss the importance of quitting smoking with their patients who smoke also found that various types of reminders (e.g., stickers, flow sheets, checklists, etc.) were effective in causing health care providers to strengthen their advice to patients to quit (Hopkins et al. 2001).

Community-level interventions aim to improve population health by creating healthful environments and increasing a community's capacity for problem solving through systems changes, improved public policies, and more integrated and effective collaboration between community residents and institutions (McLeroy et al. 2003).

Community **coalitions** are one form of collaborative structure that enable individuals and organizations to combine their human and material resources in working together toward a common goal. Coalitions facilitate multilevel **ecological interventions** that acknowledge that health behaviors are deeply rooted in social and cultural contexts. They provide a vehicle for consensus building and involving diverse constituencies in solving a problem. By facilitating community participation, coalitions also help to ensure that resulting interventions meet real community needs, are culturally appropriate, and are more likely to be sustained (Butterfoss and Kegler 2009).

Coalition approaches have been widely embraced by practitioners and funders in recent years. As a result, coalitions have been formed to address a long list of health issues, ranging from tobacco control to immunizations to violence prevention (Butterfoss and Kegler 2009). Coalitions have been particularly effective in tobacco control. Comprehensive state tobacco control programs, which include community coalitions, as described by the Centers for Disease Control and Prevention's Best Practices (CDC 2007), contributed to a decline in adult smoking prevalence from 29.5% in 1985 to 18.6% in 2003 (Farrelly et al. 2008). Coalitions helped to change social norms, educate the public about tobacco use and the dangers of secondhand smoke, and advocate for policies to create smoke-free environments. Community coalitions have also been useful for improving service delivery systems (Rosenthal et al. 2006), improving child vaccination rates (Findley et al. 2008), and in-creasing community capacity for collaborative problem-solving (Kegler et al. 2008).

Bringing the Ecological Model to Life

The most successful public health programs and initiatives are based on an understanding of health behaviors and the contexts in which they occur (Glanz et al. 2008). Health education and promotion theories, or conceptual frameworks, can contribute to program planning and evaluation and advance research to test innovative intervention strategies. A central lesson of ecological models is that, because behavior is influenced at multiple levels, the most effective interventions should operate at multiple levels. See chapter 3 for detailed discussion of the application of ecological thinking to tobacco control and motor vehicle safety.

Based on ecological models, we expect the strategies that most effectively improve population health behaviors to be those that create environments that make it easy to make healthful and safe choices (e.g., renovate the park, stock skim milk in stores, install bike lanes) and harder to make the unhealthful choices (e.g., slower elevators, fewer unhealthful food options), enhance social norms and social support for healthier options (e.g., with a media campaign), educate and motivate individuals to take advantage of the opportunities for healthful behaviors, and use policy (e.g., reduce prices for healthful foods, zone for more mixed land use, require bike helmet use) to also enhance health and safety. Planning models like the PRECEDE-PROCEED Model (see chapter 5) (Green and Kreuter 2005) can be used to apply these concepts to the planning of programs.

Different theoretical concepts will be required to understand different types of behavior change and shape successful change strategies. The roles and strategies will also be different for clinicians and health educators or counselors, who work primarily with individuals, than for organizations and public health experts, whose constituencies are populations. Different professionals and diverse populations will benefit from familiarity with and appreciation for all levels of determinants and solutions, and in fact, they often must work together to build comprehensive approaches to solving health behavior problems. For instance, clinicians often have access to some of the most important data on a health problem, and by working closely with public health experts who can help analyze the data and community coalitions who can use the data to advocate for policy changes, they can be powerful allies in facilitating population level health improvements.

REFERENCES

Ammerman AS, Lindquist CH, Lohr KN, Hersey J. 2002. The efficacy of behavioral interventions to modify dietary fat and fruit and vegetable intake: A review of the evidence. *Prev Med* 35 (1): 25-41.

Bandura A. 1986. *Social Foundations of Thought and Action: A Social Cognitive Theory.* Englewood Cliffs, NJ: Prentice-Hall.

Butterfoss F, Kegler M. 2009. The community coalition action theory. In *Emerging Theories in Health Promotion Practice and Research,* ed. R DiClemente, R Crosby, M Kegler. 2nd ed. San Francisco, CA: Jossey-Bass.

Butterfoss FD, Kegler MC, Francisco VT. 2008. Mobilizing organizations for health promotion: Theories of organizational change. In *Health Behavior and Health Education: Theory, Research, and Practice,* ed. K Glanz, BK Rimer, K Viswanath. 4th ed. San Francisco: Jossey-Bass.

Centers for Disease Control and Prevention (CDC). 2007. *Best Practices for Comprehensive Tobacco Control Programs—2007.* National Center for Chronic Disease Prevention and Health Promotion, Office on Smoking and Health. Atlanta, GA: CDC.

Champion VL, Skinner CS. 2008. The health belief model. In *Health Behavior and Health Education: Theory, Research, and Practice,* ed. K Glanz, BK Rimer, K Viswanath, 45-65. 4th ed. San Francisco: Jossey-Bass.

Dijkstra A, DeVries H, Roijackers J. 1999. Targeting smokers with low readiness to change with tailored and non-tailored self-help materials. *Prev Med* 28:203-11.

Farrelly MC, Pechacek TF, Thomas KY, Nelson D. 2008. The impact of tobacco control programs on adult smoking. *Am J Public Health* 98:304-9.

Findley S, Irigoyen M, Sanchez M, et al. 2008. Effectiveness of a community coalition for improving child vaccination rates in New York City. *Am J Public Health* 98:1959-61.

Gielen AC, Sleet D. 2003. Application of behavior-change theories and methods to injury prevention. *Rev Epidemiol* 25:65-67.

Gielen AC, Trifiletti L, McDonald EM, et al. 2007. Using a computer kiosk to promote child safety: Results of a randomized, controlled trial in an urban pediatric emergency department. *Pediatrics* 120:330-39.

Glanz K, Rimer BK. 2005. *Theory at a Glance: A Guide to Health Promotion Practice.* NIH Publ. 05-3896. 2nd ed. Bethesda, MD: National Cancer Institute.

Glanz K, Bishop D. 2010. The role of behavioral science theory in development and implementation of public health interventions. *Annu Rev Public Health* 31:399-418.

Glanz K, Patterson RE, Kristal AR, et al. 1998. Impact of work site health promotion on stages of dietary change: The Working Well Trial. *Health Educ Behav* 25:448-63.

Glanz K, Rimer BK, Viswanath K, eds. 2008. *Health Behavior and Health Education: Theory, Research, and Practice.* 4th ed. San Francisco: Jossey-Bass.

Glanz K, Steffen AD, Taglialatela LA. 2007. Effects of colon cancer risk counseling for first-degree relatives. *Cancer Epidem Biomarkers Prev* 16:1485-91.

Green LW, Kreuter MW. 2005. *Health Program Planning: An Educational and Ecological Approach.* 4th ed. New York: McGraw-Hill.

Green LW, Richard L, Potvin L. 1996. Ecological foundations of health promotion. Am J Health Promot 10 (4) (March–April): 270-81.

Heaney CA, Israel BA. 2008. Social networks and social support. In *Health Behavior and Health Education: Theory, Research, and Practice,* ed. K Glanz, BK Rimer, K Viswanath, 189-210. 4th ed. San Francisco: Jossey-Bass.

Hochbaum G. 1958. *Public Participation in Medical Screening Programs: A Socio-Psychological Study.* Washington, DC: US Department of Health, Education, and Welfare.

Hopkins DP, Briss PA, Ricard CJ, et al. 2001. Reviews of evidence regarding interventions to reduce tobacco use and exposure to environmental tobacco smoke. *Am J Prev Med* 20 (suppl. 2): 16-66.

Institute of Medicine (IOM). 2001. *Health and Behavior: The Interplay of Biological, Behavioral, and Social Influences.* Committee on Health and Behavior. Washington, DC: National Academy Press.

———. 2003. *The Future of Public Health in the 21st Century.* Washington, DC: National Academy Press.

———. 2005. *Preventing Childhood Obesity: Health in the Balance.* Washington, DC: National Academy Press.

Joseph C, Peterson E, Havstad S, et al. 2007. A web-based, tailored asthma management program for urban African American high school students. *Am J Respir Crit Care Med* 175:888-95.

Kaplan GA, Everson SA, Lynch JW. 2000. The contribution of social and behavioral research to an understanding of the distribution of disease: A multi-level approach. In *Promoting Health: Intervention Strategies from Social and Behavioral Research,* ed. BD Smedley, SL Syme, 37-80. Washington, DC: National Academy Press.

Kegler M, Norton B, Aronson R. 2008. Achieving organizational change: Findings from case studies of 20 California healthy cities and communities coalitions. *Health Promot Int* 23:109-18.

Kok G, Gottlieb NH, Commers M, Smerecnik C. 2008. The ecological approach in health promotion programs: A decade later. *Am J Health Promot* 22:437-42.

Legler J, Meissner HI, Coyne C, Breen N, Chollette V, Rimer BK. 2002. The effectiveness of interventions to promote mammography among women with historically lower rates of screening. *Cancer Epidem Biomarkers Prev* 11:59-71.

Lippke S, Ziegelmann JP. 2008. Theory-based health behavior change: Developing, testing, and applying theories for evidence-based interventions. *Applied Psychol* 57: 698-716.

Marcus BH, Bock BC, Pinto BM, Forsyth LH, Roberts MB, Traficante RM. 1998. Efficacy of an individualized, motivationally-tailored physical activity intervention. *Ann Behav Med* 20:174-80.

McAlister AL, Perry CL, Parcel GS. 2008. How individuals, environments, and health behaviors interact: Social Cognitive Theory. In *Health Behavior and Health Education: Theory, Research, and Practice,* ed. K Glanz, BK Rimer, K Viswanath, 167-88. 4th ed. San Francisco: Jossey-Bass.

McDonald EM, Solomon B, Shields W, et al. 2005. Evaluation of kiosk-based tailoring to promote household safety behaviors in an urban pediatric primary care practice. *Patient Educ Couns* 58:168-81.

McLeroy KR, Bibeau D, Steckler A, Glanz K. 1988. An ecological perspective on health promotion programs. *Health Educ Q* 15:351-77.

McLeroy K, Norton B, Kegler M, Burdine J, Sumaya C. 2003. Editorial: Community-based interventions. *Am J Publ Health* 93:529-33.

Nansel TR, Weaver N, Donlin M, Jacobsen H, Kreuter MW, Simons-Morton B. 2002. Baby, be safe: The effect of tailored communications for pediatric injury prevention provided in a primary care setting. *Patient Educ Couns* 46 (3): 175-90.

Noar SM, Benac CN, Harris MS. 2007. Does tailoring matter? Meta-analytic review of tailored print health behavior change interventions. *Psychol Bull* 133:673-93.

Orleans CT, Gruman J, Ulmer C, et al. 1999. Rating our progress in population health promotion: Report card on six behaviors. *Am J Health Promot* 14:75-82.

Painter JE, Borba CP, Hynes M, Mays D, Glanz K. 2008. The use of theory in health behavior research from 2000 to 2005: A systematic review. *Ann Behav Med* 35:358-62.

Pennant M, Davenport C, Bayliss S, Greenheld W, Marshall T, Hyde C. 2010. Community programs for the prevention of cardiovascular disease: A systematic review. *Am J Epidemiol* 172 (5): 501-16.

Prochaska JO, Redding CA, Evers KE. 2008. The transtheoretical model and stages of change. In *Health Behavior and Health Education: Theory, Research, and Practice,* ed. K Glanz, BK Rimer, K Viswanath, 97-121. 4th ed. San Francisco: Jossey-Bass.

Richard L, Potvin L, Kischuk N, Prlic H, Green LW. 1996. Assessment of the integration of the ecological approach in health promotion programs. *Am J Health Promot* 10:318-28.

Rimer BK, Kreuter MW. 2006. Advancing tailored health communication: A persuasion and message effects perspective. *J Commun* 56 (suppl. 1): S184-S201.

Rosenstock IM. 1974. The Health Belief Model and preventive health behavior. *Health Educ Monogr* 2:354-86.

Rosenstock IM, Strecher VJ, Becker MH. 1988. Social learning theory and the Health Belief Model. *Health Educ Q* 15:175-83.

Rosenthal M, Butterfoss F, Doctor L, et al. 2006. The coalition process at work: Building care coordination models to control chronic disease. *Health Promot Practice* 7:117S-126S.

Sabatino SA, Habarta N, Baron RC. 2008. Interventions to increase recommendation and delivery of screening for breast, cervical, and colorectal cancers by healthcare providers. *Am J Prev Med* 35 (suppl. 1): 67-74.

Sallis, JF, Owen N. 1997. Ecological models. In *Health Behavior and Health Education: Theory, Research, and Practice,* ed. K Glanz, FM Lewis, BK Rimer, 403-24. 2nd ed. San Francisco: Jossey-Bass.

Sallis JF, Owen N, Fisher EB. 2008. Ecological models of health behavior. In *Health Behavior and Health Education: Theory, Research, and Practice,* ed. K Glanz,

BK Rimer, K Viswanath, 464–85. 4th ed. San Francisco: Jossey-Bass.

Schroeder SA. 2007. We can do better—improving the health of the American people. *N Engl J Med* 357:1221-28.

Simons-Morton BG, Brink SG, Simons-Morton DG, et al. 1989. An ecological approach to the prevention of injuries due to drinking and driving. *Health Educ Q* 16 (3): 397–411.

Smedley BD, Syme SL, eds. 2000. *Promoting Health: Intervention Strategies from Social and Behavioral Research.* Washington, DC: National Academy Press.

Stokols D. 1996. Translating social ecological theory into guidelines for community health promotion. *Am J Health Promot* 10:282-98.

Story M, Kaphingst KM, Robinson-O'Brien R, Glanz K. 2008. Creating healthy food and eating environments: Policy and environmental approaches. *Annu Rev Public Health* 29:253-72.

Van Ryn M, Heaney CA. 1992. What's the use of theory? *Health Educ Q* 19:315-30.

Will JC, Farris RP, Sanders CG, Stockmyer CK, Finkelstein EA. 2004. Health promotion interventions for disadvantaged women: Overview of the WISE-WOMAN projects. *J Womens Health (Larchmt)* 13:484–502.

Yach D, Hawkes C, Gould CL, Hofman K J. 2004. The global burden of chronic diseases: Overcoming impediments to prevention and control. *JAMA* 291:2616-22.

CHAPTER 3

Evidence and Ecological Theory in Two Public Health Successes for Health Behavior Change

LAWRENCE W. GREEN AND ANDREA C. GIELEN

LEARNING OBJECTIVES

After completing the chapter, the reader will be able to

* Appreciate the public health triumphs of motor vehicle safety and tobacco control during the 20th century.
* Understand the importance of an ecological framework when addressing complex health behavioral issues, including motor vehicle safety and tobacco use.
* Describe the multiple levels of influence that play roles in health behaviors and health behavior change.

Introduction

Western cultures became increasingly dependent on the automobile and tobacco during the first half of the 20th century. The early days of motorized traffic were accompanied by extraordinarily high injury rates. Ensuring safety while facilitating mobility challenged transportation and public health professionals. Although the number of miles traveled multiplied 10 times—*1,000%*—from the 1920s to the 1990s, the annual death rate decreased by 90% (CDC 1999), thanks largely to numerous **interventions** enacted during the second half of the 20th century. Similarly, tobacco-related deaths were rapidly mounting over the 20th century. Tobacco consumption rose inexorably during the first two-thirds of the century, contributing to the rise of tobacco-related chronic diseases (such as heart disease and cancer) overtaking infectious diseases as the leading causes of death in the United States. Then, in the last third of the century, tobacco consumption decreased by more than 50%, and rates of heart disease and stroke deaths declined similarly.

This chapter explores the scientific and theoretical foundations of these successes. It illustrates how evidence generated in particular from real-time **evaluations** of policies and programs at state and local levels was disseminated and adopted across other states and communities. It illustrates also how **theory** and research helped in adapting policies and programs to the varied populations and circumstances across nations, states, and communities.

The Centers for Disease Control and Prevention (CDC) declared that improvements in motor vehicle safety and recognition of tobacco use as a health hazard were two of the ten greatest public health achievements of the 20th century in the United States (CDC 1999; Ward and Warren 2007). Notably, the reduction in motor vehicle injuries and deaths and the changes in **attitudes** toward smoking and resultant decreased rates of smoking and tobacco-related health **consequences** were the two most prominent *behaviorally related* successes among the top 10 public health accomplishments identified by the CDC.

No single intervention caused these dramatic improvements. They occurred as a result of a combination of numerous interventions, policies, programs, methods, strategies, and other factors that spanned multiple **levels of influence** and behavioral settings and addressed multiple components of, and contributors to, behavior. As described in chapter 2, an **ecological approach** to **health behavior** change, which addresses the multiple **determinants** and levels of determinants that influence health and health behavior, along with the **reciprocal determinism** of behavior and environment, produces the necessary **synergy** and comprehensiveness to address the **complex** public health and behavior-related problems of today. As we will show in this chapter, a range of initiatives and occurrences that addressed both individual

health behavior decisions and the **context** in which they occurred collectively accomplished the successes in motor vehicle safety and tobacco control. Individual knowledge, attitudes, skills, and **motivation** were ultimately addressed in concert with essential changes in the physical and **social environment** largely through important policy changes.

Studies have shown that the comprehensive, multidisciplinary approach taken to addressing motor vehicle injury and tobacco use accounts for much of the success (Allegrante et al. 2006; Economos et al. 2001; Eriksen 2005; Eriksen and Green 2009; Eriksen et al. 2007; Gielen and Sleet 2003; Green et al. 2000; Green et al. 2001; Mercer et al. 2003; OSH 2007; Sleet and Gielen 2006; Zaza et al. 2001a). Though some argue that it was not the behavioral or educational approaches at the intra- and **interpersonal levels** that accounted for such successes, but rather policy or environmental changes alone (Frieden 2010; cf. Green and Kreuter 2010), we offer here a case for the necessity of a combination of strategies that make up a comprehensive approach. Indeed, population-level changes require a sustained commitment to scientific research; **evidence-based practice** at multiple levels; government leadership; public advocacy and support; an informed and educated electorate to provide the public understanding and support for policy changes; and the engagement of varied **stakeholders** to formulate, advocate, implement, and evaluate policies and programs (Green and Kreuter 2005; Mercer et al. 2003).

Although the successes in motor vehicle safety and tobacco control were not systematically orchestrated by a group of public health professionals applying a specific theoretical model of social change, examining the confluence of these elements through the lens of an **ecological model** helps us understand the change process and reveals some order in seemingly disparate actions. As a result of this analysis, public health professionals may be better positioned to apply this model proactively to future public health problems and perhaps speed the process of change (Martin et al. 2007). We will provide insights into these formidable achievements and demonstrate separately how these population-level success stories illustrate the power of an ecological approach to public health problems. We will describe evidence of the **"reciprocal determinism"** (see chapter 2) of behavior and its environments—a fundamental tenet of ecology in which behavior of human and other organisms both influence and are influenced by their environments (Green et al. 1996). The chapter concludes with a few generalizable lessons of potential use in other areas of public health. These case studies and their evidence will be instructive for interpreting the experience, evidence, and strategies suggested for other public health problems in part III of this book, noting that the ecological approach encompasses both "top-down" structural, environmental, and policy change approaches and "bottom-up" organizational, peer, family, and individual behavior change and participatory approaches.

Public Health Success Story: Motor Vehicle Safety

The Institute of Medicine (IOM) report *Reducing the Burden of Injury* (Bonnie et al. 1999; Friere and Runyan 2006) and the CDC's "Ten Great Public Health Achievements" (CDC 1999) suggest that the comprehensive, multidisciplinary approach taken to addressing the motor vehicle injury problem is responsible for the successes that have been achieved. The motor vehicle safety experience highlights the importance of the interaction between behavior and environment in influencing a health outcome (Sleet and Gielen 2006). Death rates have gone down because both the environment (e.g., safer roadways, improved signage, increased availability of vehicles capable of withstanding crashes) and human behavior (e.g., using car seats, seat belts, and designated drivers instead of drink-

ing and driving) have changed. In other words, change happened at the confluence of individual, organizational, government, and societal levels.

Modifications to roadways and vehicles are the most commonly cited environmental determinants of success, while increased use of seat belts and child safety seats and decreased rates of drunk driving are the most frequently mentioned behavioral contributors to the sharp decline in motor vehicle fatality rates (Bonnie et al. 1999; CDC 1999; NHTSA 2003; Nichols 1994; Rivara and MacKenzie 1999; Waller 2001; Zwerling and Jones 1999). Much of the success can be understood with William Haddon's analysis of motor vehicle injuries as a function of the **classical epidemiological triad** of **host** (the driver and occupants), agent (the energy that is abruptly transferred to vehicle occupants during a crash), and environment (the roadway design, traffic signs, traffic laws, etc.). His now famous **"Haddon matrix"** combined this epidemiological framework with a time sequence, which included pre-event (factors present before the crash), event (during the crash), and post-event (after the crash) (Bonnie et al. 1999; Freire and Runyan 2006). This framework describes both the type of factors and time sequence that influence the likelihood and severity of injury, offering numerous intervention opportunities to prevent the crash and/or the injury. This type of comprehensive analysis sets the stage for an ecological approach to preventing motor vehicle crashes (MVCs), injuries, and fatalities. Here we describe several pieces that encompassed this ecological approach.

Scientific Research and Evidence-Based Practice at Multiple Levels of Influence

In addition to the scientific advances guided by the Haddon Matrix, myriad **surveillance** systems and research initiatives have provided new knowledge about risk factors and effective interventions. For example, the National Vital

Statistics System compiles death data, and the Fatality Analysis Reporting System provides detailed information on fatal MVCs (Bonnie et al. 1999; NHTSA 2000), and these have been invaluable in understanding where, when, why, and how crashes occur, to inform ideas about how to prevent them. Surveillance, together with monitoring of policy and enforcement practices across jurisdictions, provides a form of practice-based or evaluation evidence that has been influential in the diffusion of effective policies and practices and the repeal or amendment of ineffective ones.

Research and evaluation have also identified effective interventions at multiple levels for addressing the determinants of motor vehicle injuries (Rivara and MacKenzie 1999; USPSTF 1996; Zaza et al. 2001a). There is ample evidence from crash rates and arrest, injury, and death rates that certain interventions increase occupant protection and reduce alcohol-impaired driving. These evidence-based practices have included community information campaigns, education programs, **incentives**, child-seat safety laws, seat belt laws, enforcement programs, minimum legal drinking age laws, blood-alcohol-level laws, sobriety checkpoints, and others. These have been accomplished in part through the ability to trace the effects of education programs (delivered via clinicians, media, **social marketing**, etc.), policies, enforcement efforts in various jurisdictions, public support and advocacy, and changes in what constitute **"social norms,"** thanks to the availability of surveillance and monitoring systems of data collection (e.g., the National Vital Statistics System and the Fatality Analysis Reporting System).

EDUCATION AND INDIVIDUAL-LEVEL INTERVENTIONS

Educating communities and individuals has been essential to generate support for policy interventions as well as to promote safer behaviors in both the presence and absence of legislated and police-enforced behavior. For instance, the passage of car seat legislation was facilitated by community education delivered by pediatricians and others to convince parents of the safety benefits of using car seats (Eriksen and Gielen 1983). Although car seat use is now mandatory throughout the United States, the complexity of car seat installations has created an entirely new set of training needs for parents and others. There is now a National Child Passenger Safety Certification Training Program (cert.safekids.org) to prepare car seat technicians who provide personalized education to families to ensure that car seats are being used correctly to provide maximum protection.

With regard to reducing alcohol's contribution to MVC deaths, an example of the role for education can be seen in responsible beverage service training programs. These programs give those who serve alcohol the knowledge and skills to serve it responsibly and to fulfill their legal requirements (e.g., checking driver's licenses for patrons' ages), thereby helping to reduce alcohol consumption and the harms associated with excessive consumption. Holder and colleagues (2000) found significant reductions in single-vehicle nighttime crashes and violence related injuries when such measures were used as part of a comprehensive, environmentally oriented alcohol control program. However, the Community Preventive Services Task Force concluded from systematic reviews that there was insufficient evidence to support the use of beverage service training programs as single interventions.[1] This assessment further illustrates the need for ecological approaches to solving health behavior problems insofar as it speaks to the need for additional interventions, such as policy changes, to reinforce education and training of individuals.

GOVERNMENT POLICIES

Although the first federal agency specifically charged with coordinating a national highway safety program (the National Highway Safety Bureau) was not established until 1966, the federal government's leadership was apparent as early as 1935 when President Franklin D. Roosevelt called for uniform state legislation, organization of agencies for administration and enforcement, and public safety education (Zaza et al. 2001b). The Institute of Medicine (Bonnie et al. 1999) pointed out that as a result of the federal regulatory program, U.S. automakers developed a vehicle fleet that was substantially more crashworthy at the end of the century than 30 years earlier. Many policies are determined at the state and local levels (though there is considerable variation across jurisdictions), such as requirements for using safety equipment, driver licensing requirements, Driving Under the Influence (DUI) and Driving While Intoxicated (DWI) standards, and speed limits. The federal government has provided leadership in reducing some of the disparities in preventive policies through the use of incentives and disincentives. For example, states were to receive reduced federal funding if they did not pass certain laws (e.g., making it illegal to drive with a blood alcohol level [BAC] of more than .08%). The federal Highway Safety Act of 1966 also established a highway safety grant program that coordinates highway safety programmatic and research efforts across local, state, and federal levels. Through Governor's Highway Safety Representatives located in each state, this funding program has been effectively used for a variety of projects, such as evaluating motorcycle helmet laws and implementing innovative media and social marketing programs to increase the use of seat belts and child safety seats (Bonnie et al. 1999).

One controversial example of how government policy and educational intervention might work at odds with each other was the lowering in the 1960s and 1970s in many states of the age at which young drivers can obtain a driver's license if they have taken driver's education. Robertson and Fodor (1978, 959) showed that "among 16- to 17-year-olds, driver education was associated with a great increase in the number of licensed drivers, without a decrease in the fatal crash involvement per 10,000 licensed drivers." This left open the question of whether "to educate or not to educate" (Green 1980) (i.e., whether the cause of the fatal crash involvement was merely the age of the younger licensed drivers rather than the comparative competency of the young drivers who had taken driver's education). Robertson was able to carry out a later study in Connecticut, where some schools had ended their driver's education programs. He found that "substantial reductions in the numbers of 16- to 17-year-olds who became licensed occurred in the communities that dropped the course. As a result, the numbers of crashes involving 16- to 17-year-old residents in such communities were also substantially reduced" (1980, 599). This still left unresolved the question of whether a state should raise its legal licensing age and keep its driver's education programs. The combined effect of these policy and educational interventions could be greater than merely delaying eligibility for licensing or merely terminating driver's education (Green and Lewis 1986).

In the end, evidence supported a combination of skill development with restrictions on driving privileges known as graduated driver licensing (GDL) policies. These include extended, supervised practice at the learning level, restrictions on nighttime driving and passengers at the intermediate level, and eventually full privileges. An evaluation of the first two years of Michigan's GDL program implementation showed substantial crash reductions among 16-year-olds (Shope et al. 2001). A subsequent national evaluation of all 16-year-old drivers involved in fatal crashes from 1994 to 2004 found an almost 20% reduction in fatal crash involvement from comprehensive GDL programs (Chen et al. 2006). Today, all 50 states and the District of Columbia have some form of a three-stage GDL system, and in some states, completing a driver's education program allows students to meet their supervised-driving requirement (IIHS 2012).

An example of policy initiatives getting too far ahead of education of the public was the passage by state legislators of motorcyclist helmet laws in the late 1960s. The legislation was a response to federal incentives with highway-building funds and was supported by evidence that the use of helmets had resulted in substantial reductions in motorcyclists' expensive head injuries. By the early 1970s, virtually all states had universal motorcycle helmet laws. By 1976, however, states were successful in getting Congress to stop the Department of Transportation incentive program, and strong advocacy by motorcyclists who opposed such legislation resulted in a pattern of repeal, reenactment, and amendment of these state laws throughout the country, despite compelling evidence of the association between the laws and motorcycle deaths and injuries and despite general public support for such laws (NHTSA 2005). Between 1976 and 1980, 28 state legislatures repealed or weakened their motorcycle-helmet-use laws, with a consequent $180 million in costs to the states (Hartunian et al. 1983). Today, 47 states have some type of motorcycle-helmet-use laws, but the laws are continually under discussion in state legislatures, evidencing the need for constituency education and advocacy if the public health goal of saving lives and reducing injuries among motorcyclists is to be achieved.

MEDIA AND SOCIAL MARKETING

By the 1980s, the National Highway Traffic Safety Administration (NHTSA) and many states were conducting various large-scale public educational programs that helped to change safety behavior and public opinion among some individuals and, in turn, garner support for policy changes. This combination of interventional levels—education via social marketing with legislation—has succeeded dramatically. Today's public is supportive of seat belt legislation and enforcement and recognizes the **effectiveness** of seat belts (Girasek and Gielen 2003; NHTSA 2003). In 1984, seat belt usage rates were at 15%

nationally (Nichols 1994); they were up to 82% in 2007 (NHTSA, 2008). NHTSA continues to keep media attention on motor vehicle safety through public education campaigns, such as "Buckle Up America" week and "Click It or Ticket." With regard to alcohol-related MVCs (described in more detail below), the media coverage of drunk driving spurred by the founder of Mothers Against Drunk Driving (MADD) had remarkable success in both conveying information and garnering public support—changing the social norm, as we will see later.

PUBLIC SUPPORT AND ADVOCACY

Advocacy to develop public support for policy change has been an essential lever in the multifaceted path to improved motor vehicle safety. Isaacs and Schroeder (2001) highlight the adversarial and political roots of the "auto-safety crusade." They describe Ralph Nader's public hero status as a result of his landmark book *Unsafe at Any Speed* (Nader 1965) and his testimony at congressional hearings. Evolving motor vehicle product liability law and public outrage during the late 1960s also influenced automobile manufacturers to improve the crashworthiness of cars (Christoffel and Teret 1993). Acrimonious debates between industry, government, scientists, and advocates dealt with such issues as whether active (manual seat belts) versus passive (air bags and other automatic restraints) protection should be available and whether seat belt use should be voluntary or mandatory. According to Graham (1993), the adversarial relationship between the public and **private sectors** served to slow the rate of progress in reducing motor vehicle crashes. Others have argued that the public debates and **media advocacy** were precisely what gave the injury control movement newsworthiness and, consequently, impetus, public interest, public understanding, and public support for policy initiatives and industry reforms (Finnegan and Viswanath 2002).[2] In any case, the ultimate outcome was a transformation of the social norms related to motor vehicle occupant safety. Gone were the days of children riding freely in the front seat of the car, of drivers and their passengers completely unrestrained, and of intoxication being an acceptable state for a driver. Such **denormalization** of previously accepted behavior and acceptance of an industry's practices will appear again as a central element of the change in smoking behavior.

CHANGING SOCIAL NORMS

Today's high rate of child car seat use—99% in the first year of life and 92% in children ages 1 to 3 (NHTSA 2009) is testimony to the fact that a new social norm has been established concerning the safe transport of young children. This public health success in increasing the use of child restraint devices was initially stimulated by a visible champion, Dr. Robert Sanders, a pediatrician in Tennessee. It provoked far less controversy and was implemented more quickly than policies to require seat belt use. Such is the experience in many public health initiatives where protection of children is far more readily tolerated and even promoted by the public than similar restraints on or requirement of adult behavior. In 1978 Dr. Sanders succeeded in getting the first law passed requiring the use of car safety seats (Graham 1993). Spurred by his advocacy and the research evidence that infants were at significantly elevated risk of death as motor vehicle occupants (Baker, 1979), a seemingly spontaneous social movement erupted. State and local government representatives from health, transportation, and law enforcement, along with community advocates (e.g., pediatricians, childbirth educators, women's clubs), rallied to support not just legislation but also a variety of educational activities and low-cost car seat rental programs (Eriksen and Gielen 1983). NHTSA facilitated the process by training potential local advocates in states throughout the country. Illustrating the efficacy of a multilevel approach that combines education and support at the individual level with legisla-

tion at the government level and support or advocacy at the community level, by 1985 all 50 states (and the District of Columbia) had laws requiring the use of car safety seats (Nichols 1994).

Changed social norms are even more notable in the issue of drunk driving. Again, there were champions and a strong grassroots movement. Doris Aiken started Remove Intoxicated Drivers (RID) in 1978 and Candy Lightner started MADD in 1980, after tragic drunk-driving crashes that killed a daughter of each woman (Isaacs and Schroeder 2001). Stories about victims of drunk drivers and their families were widely reported in all major media, and new chapters of the organizations sprang up all over the country. By elevating the visibility of the families of victims and influencing the public agenda, these groups brought pressure to bear on policymakers (Bonnie et al. 1999). Isaacs and Schroeder (2001) called the effect of this movement on public policy "stunning," noting that between 1981 and 1985 state legislatures passed *478 laws* to deter drunk driving. In 1984 Congress required states to pass a law increasing the minimum drinking age to 21 years or risk losing a portion of their federal highway safety funds. Most recently, Congress used the same approach to encourage states to lower their BAC levels for drunk driving from 0.10 to 0.08. As Graham describes it, "changes in social norms, in part spurred by such citizen activist groups as MADD, have apparently achieved what many traffic safety professionals believed was virtually impossible: a meaningful change in driver attitudes and behaviors resulting in a reduction of traffic fatalities" (1993, 524). Like the change in social norms affecting smoking in public places (described in more detail below), the shift came when multifaceted efforts consistent with an ecological approach were in place. In this instance, advocacy to change public opinion by reframing the individual-level behavior of drinking and driving from a matter of personal risk to one of imposing risks on others was accompanied by society providing support for the policy-level interventions that reduce risky individual behavior and protect entire communities.

Summary

As a result of this broad, ecological approach to injury prevention, countless lives and dollars have been saved. This is a classic description of the utility of an ecological approach to changing health behaviors that involves individual education, the media, outreach, policy advocacy, community changes, and policy interventions. Multilevel approaches came into favor in recent decades because the evidence was clear that "single-shot" interventions, even when done on a mass scale, as in media campaigns, were ineffective across a wide array of health-related behaviors. Theory-testing research and practice-based evaluations also demonstrated the importance of contextual effects on health-related behaviors. Safety behaviors are no exception. While engineering solutions such as improved roadway designs and safer cars were an essential part of the motor vehicle success story, so too were behavior change interventions based on science that operated at multiple levels and were responsive to the contextual influences on individual behavior.

Public Health Success Story: Tobacco Control

Tobacco use and tobacco-related health problems, such as heart disease, cancer, stroke, and chronic lung disease, have been declining, thanks to a combination of medical and public health developments in the last third of the 20th century. The success in health behavior change, as with motor vehicle safety, was achieved primarily by a comprehensive ecological approach—a combination of research, education, public health policy, regulations of industry marketing, mass media, legal challenges to the industry, environmental control, and evaluations of comprehensive statewide programs.

Of all chronic disease prevention and health promotion efforts, tobacco control is the one most cited as a great success story of health behavior change on a population scale. Ironically, at least in North America, Europe, Australia, and New Zealand, this success, at least initially, was not the result of direct application of the hundreds of controlled clinical trials, though the effectiveness of smoking cessation inched up with intervention trials that demonstrated marginal improvements in counseling and pharmaceutical techniques. It was much more the consequence of a series of planned media and educational events, popular media, and policy initiatives to control advertising and restrict smoking in public places, and the environmental changes associated with them. These were supported by evidence from evaluation of their impact through yearly measures of tobacco consumption, gathered in comparable forms across jurisdictions that were demonstrating alternative policy initiatives. The mass media acted to "soften" public opinion (the denormalization of smoking in public places and of tobacco industry promotions), assisting policy changes favoring smoking cessation, as seen in the history of events shown in figure 3.1.

The story of this social experiment in many countries is told most vividly in the connections between events and tobacco use seen in figure 3.1. We will use these associations to draw potential "lessons" or hypotheses from tobacco control regarding ways to control many chronic diseases at the population level. This analysis will demonstrate the necessity of changing risk conditions in the social and physical environment as both a precursor to and an accompaniment of behavior change.

Research and evaluation have shown that the results of denormalization strategies can be enhanced by other policies and programs that can have an additive or multiplicative effect on reducing both tobacco consumption and the

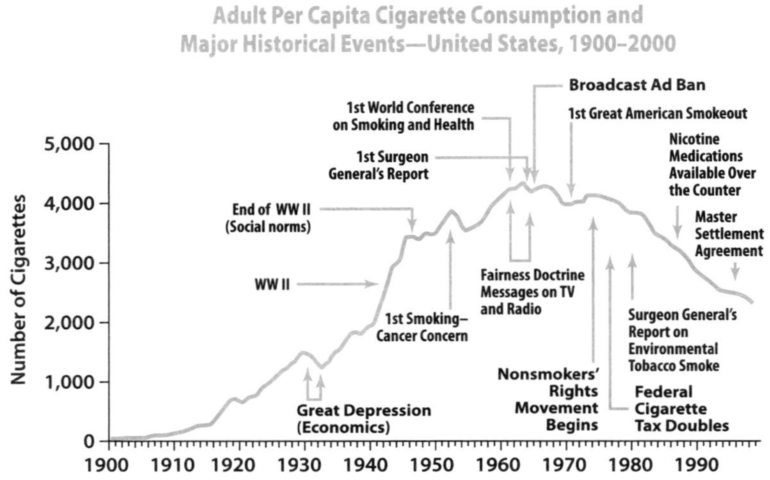

FIGURE 3.1. The association of movements in the trend line for tobacco consumption with historical events in the social, economic, and policy environments.
Source: Adapted from 1986 to 2000 series of Surgeon General Reports (Eriksen et al. 2007).

premature mortality it causes. The strategies with the greatest impact include tobacco price increases, high-intensity media campaigns, comprehensive cessation treatment programs, strong health warnings, stricter smoke-free air regulations, advertising bans, and youth access laws (e.g., Levy et al. 2012). Although price increases appear to have an independent effect, the smoke-free air regulations, advertising bans, and youth access laws depend on both the laws and their enforcement. These, in turn, have depended on building an informed and activated electorate through community-level organization and communications, because community policies controlling tobacco promotions and smoking in public places could be passed at local levels when they could not overcome industry lobbying and resistance at state and national levels.

Scientific Research and Evidence-Based Practice at Multiple Levels of Influence

The emergence of the 20th century anti-tobacco movement as the century approached the apex of tobacco consumption shown in figure 3.1 can be traced to the publication of three key research studies in 1950 that strongly linked tobacco smoking and lung cancer (Doll and Hill 1950; Levin 1950; Wynder and Graham 1950). Though suspicion had long abounded that tobacco adversely affected health, this research and its combination with a wide range of other evidence reviewed for the first Surgeon General's Report on Smoking and Health (USDHEW 1964) provided substantial and authoritatively reviewed scientific evidence that spurred the anti-tobacco movement and helped it gain traction.

Scientific research linking environmental tobacco smoke ("passive" or "secondhand" smoke) to cancer played a key role in the second anti-tobacco push during the last decades of the century. Although the negative health effects of tobacco smoke on nonsmokers had been suspected for several decades, research reviewed by the U.S. Environmental Protection Agency (1992) led that agency to declare secondhand smoke a carcinogen. A World Health Organization study confirmed a consistent 20–30% increased risk of lung cancer in spouses of smokers (IARC 2004). Further, laboratory research showed that secondhand smoke may be more toxic than primary smoke (Schick and Glantz 2007).

EDUCATION AND INDIVIDUAL-LEVEL INTERVENTIONS

A steep reduction in tobacco consumption followed the first Surgeon General's Report on Smoking and Health in January 1964 (USDHEW 1964). Former surgeon general Luther Terry led the committee of experts that examined the evidence for the 1964 report, which clearly implicated cigarette smoking as a cause of lung cancer and other health problems and called for public health action. The evidence was compelling for some, although the tobacco industry rebounded repeatedly with marketing strategies that recruited new smokers and reassured continuing smokers. With each new tobacco marketing strategy and design of the nicotine delivery device (e.g., filters, menthol), smoking prevention and cessation research stimulated policy and program responses, which produced, in turn, evaluations of policies and programs that inspired other jurisdictions to try similar policy and program strategies.

Several medical programs also contributed to the decreased rate of tobacco use and mitigation of tobacco-related health problems. These included implementing screening programs to detect risk factors or early signs of tobacco-related disease, prescribing pharmaceutical agents to treat tobacco-related diseases (e.g., chemotherapies and bronchitis medications) or assist in tobacco quitting attempts (e.g., Chantix, Zyban, and the nicotine patch), and counseling by physicians and health professionals. The efficacy of individually tailored programs of behavior change and pharmacotherapy to reduce nicotine dependence, however, was only marginal until the nicotine replacement therapies became available without prescription, and telephone hotlines became more widely available (Shiffman et al. 1998).

Thus, the evidence became clear that education and counseling increasingly empowered individuals, organizations, and communities to self-manage health-related behavior change outside the health care system (Daynard 2003; Eriksen 2005; Green et al. 2001; Green et al. 2003; Mercer et al. 2003). The public had to come to an understanding through education that medical intervention alone would not save them from the harms of tobacco, that other levels of influence were at work—powerful commercial forces were trying to entice them to consume products that were addictive and harmful to their health—and that multiple attempts and multifaceted approaches to quit smoking would be required for most people seeking to rid themselves of the **habit**.

GOVERNMENT POLICIES

Numerous policy-level influences contributed to the progressive reduction in tobacco use. In particular, the tobacco control story highlights the role of the states as agents of and laboratories for effective policy change (OSH 2007). For example, reductions in nonsmokers' exposure to secondhand smoke followed the widespread passage of local clean-air ordinances and implementation of statewide, comprehensive tobacco control programs and policies in California, Massachusetts, Florida, Arizona, Oregon, and Mississippi (Eriksen et al. 2007). The evidence demonstrated that the prevalence of smoking declined for most age groups and all race/ethnicity groups in California, and both youth smoking and aggregate cigarette sales have declined significantly and independently in proportion to tobacco control program expenditures in states that followed California's lead (Farreley et al. 2003; Farreley et al. 2008; Taurus et al. 2005). Heart attack death rates improved swiftly after smoking prevalence declined and rebounded when the California program support was cut back (Fichtenberg and Glantz 2000). Rates of chronic lung disease and bronchial cancer responded as well, although with greater lag times. These improvements were especially noticeable in California, where lung cancer rate declines were four times greater than in the rest of the United States (CDHS 2006).

The other set of government policies that significantly affected smoking rates was increasing the cost of smoking via taxation of tobacco products (Dorfman et al. 2005). In some states, tobacco taxes were dedicated in part to support comprehensive, statewide tobacco control programs that included mass media **counter-advertising**, school-based programs and policies, smoking cessation supports, and others. Evidence from systematic evaluations showed that each of these components contributed synergistically to the overall effectiveness of the state programs, but none except the increased price of cigarettes could be shown by itself to reduce smoking rates. The synergistic effects of combining interventions, and the selective effects of some interventions for some populations, accounted for the growing recognition of the importance of multicomponent, **multilevel interventions**.

Policies that restrained and countered the marketing of tobacco were also essential. Laws were passed that increased the penalty for the sale of cigarettes to minors, removed cigarette vending machines from public places where minors could have access to them, and restricted advertising in media that reached youth (including bans on broadcast media advertising of tobacco). None of these policy-level interventions would have been as effective as they were without the support and advocacy of individuals, influential organizations, and ad hoc anti-tobacco groups.

PUBLIC SUPPORT AND ADVOCACY

As with motor vehicle injury control, tobacco control depended on public support for most of the governmental initiatives, legislative acts, and regulatory controls on tobacco marketing and consumption. The clean air initiatives for smoke-free schools, then airlines, then other workplaces, then restaurants, then public buildings, then even bars, and now some open spaces such as parks, beaches, and areas near entryways, was prompted by public concern and advocacy. These were directed initially at protecting children from secondhand smoke exposure and **modeling** of smoking behavior (e.g., by teachers at schools). Public concern then shifted to include protecting adults and asserting clean air as a right, especially as evidence emerged that implicated secondhand smoke as a first-class carcinogen (USEPA 1992). Key to the effectiveness of these advocacy efforts was a drumbeat of mass media messages that "denormalized" smoking and the tobacco industry's glamorization of smoking.

MEDIA AND SOCIAL MARKETING

The earliest intervention following the first Surgeon General's Report on Smoking and Health in the mid-1960s was a ruling that for every minute of tobacco advertising on broadcast media, the radio or television companies were required to provide equal time for counter-advertising (public service advertisements) by anti-tobacco organizations. These counter-advertising messages were so successful, and sufficiently threatening to the tobacco industry, that the tobacco industry voluntarily backed off from advertising in the broadcast media. (Unfortunately, the savings in their advertising budgets was used to diversify to more targeted and arguably more effective advertising in specific magazines and other print and billboard outlets.)

The counter-advertising was synergistic with other mass media efforts, especially news that contributed to the growing discomfort with secondhand smoke and to outrage at the marketing practices of the tobacco industry. As with the motor vehicle safety experience, this growing public concern and outrage fueled litigation and the threat of litigation against the industry and a sense among the public that they had been deceived by the industry.

The anti-tobacco push led by mayor Michael Bloomberg and health commissioner Thomas

Frieden in New York City provides an example of the effectiveness of media campaigns as part of a larger ecological approach. In January 2006, New York City launched its largest-ever media campaign to combat tobacco use. Public education messages in print and online, targeted ad campaigns (e.g., "Everybody Loves a Quitter," "Every Cigarette Is Doing Damage," "Secondhand Smoke Kills"), and commercials showing testimonials by sick and dying smokers were effective in increasing quit rates. Evaluation studies showed that calls to dedicated telephone assistance lines (which were mentioned in all ads—"Quit Smoking Today. Call 311") quadrupled in the first six months after the start of the media campaign (January–June 2006), compared with the same period the year before (January–June 2005).

These accomplishments—changing the media environment with regard to advertising cigarettes and using the media to engage smokers in quitting—which focus on the individual, when combined with policy changes focused on populations, created a new landscape, one in which society's **norms** about the acceptability of smoking clearly changed.

CHANGING SOCIAL NORMS

The public health approach generally produced successful behavior change across boundaries of age, sex, race, and ethnicity (although disparities in smoking prevalence persist across socioeconomic strata, and the industry continues to target some advertising and product appeals to specific groups, as with menthol to the African American population). Conscious efforts were made in the statewide and community campaigns to employ methods, messages, and channels appropriate to different socioeconomic, age, sex, and ethnic groups. With these messages came a gradual shift in social norms: what the public perceived as acceptable public behavior. The changing social norms, in turn, fueled public support for increased restrictions on tobacco advertising and higher taxes on to-

bacco, which in turn helped finance counter-advertising campaigns and tobacco education programs. The growing public support was particularly notable in the passage of the smoke-free ordinances at local levels, where the tobacco industry could not lobby as effectively as it could in state legislatures and Congress.

Summary

The tobacco control experience provides another model of an ecological approach to health behavior change. The success in reducing rates of smoking resulted from interventions at the inner spheres of influence (e.g., smoking cessation programs in clinical settings), community support for cessation (e.g., community- and state-organized telephone quit-lines), environmental change (e.g., organizational and state/local smoke-free indoor area policies), and national policies (e.g., state and federal taxation of tobacco that make smoking more expensive and less attractive, national policies restricting advertising and requiring cigarette labeling that further support the closer-to-home interventions).

Conclusions

As the motor vehicle safety and tobacco control examples illustrate, interventions on health behavior problems should link multiple levels of influence by building comprehensive efforts across levels and assuring that they are coordinated in a mutually supportive way (Gielen and Sleet 2003; Green and Kreuter 2005). Comparing an educational approach to a policy approach, for example, builds a false dichotomy; rather, it is essential to *combine* strategies at all levels to produce synergy. Research on interventions and the factors that influence behavior change is necessary to determine which combinations of interventions, provided in what order, are needed for a specific population, situation, and problem. However, a sufficient evidence base supports the notion that intra- and interpersonal interventions often need to come first, so that the electorate will be informed about, receptive to, and ready to support subsequent policy-level interventions (Green and Kreuter 2005). This issue is particularly salient for potentially controversial policy interventions—traffic safety and tobacco control are examples—as in most areas of health involving human behavior and having overtones of pleasure, privacy, freedom, convenience, or cost. The complexity of the change process provides further rationale for taking comprehensive, multilevel approaches. There is still much to learn, however, about how interventions at these multiple levels interact with one another to produce the desired outcomes, both from a practical perspective and a theoretical one.

We conclude with a few generalizable lessons of potential use in other areas of public health. What accounts most notably for the successes in motor vehicle safety and tobacco control are the following five factors.

1. *Research.* Without the underpinning of good science, neither success story would have been possible. Basic science research, applied science research, surveillance research, and evaluation processes were essential for progress in these areas. Having various sources of continuously monitored behavior, crash incidents, circumstances of the crashes, and consequences of the crashes enabled a systematic reconstruction of causal (and potentially modifiable) factors for motor vehicle injuries. Having comparable measures of tobacco consumption over time and between jurisdictions enabled the policies and programs of states and localities to be compared and made it possible for the more successful ones to be emulated by other jurisdictions. This was a synergistic and reciprocal building of evidence-based practices and practice-based evidence. Using scientific research methods to understand the risk and protective factors led to the identification of effective countermeasures to prevent motor vehicle

injuries (e.g., seat belts, helmets) and to reduce tobacco consumption through the constraints on industry practices, environmental controls on smoking in public, and ultimately the changing of social norms.

2. *Ecologically comprehensive interventions.* Rather than putting all of the effort into one level of change (e.g., policy or education), motor vehicle injury control and tobacco control have maintained synergistic, mutually reinforcing, multidisciplinary, multilevel (local, state, national), multisectoral (health, education, law enforcement, education, manufacturing, and commercial marketing) approaches to bringing down injury rates and tobacco consumption. Clearly, ecologically comprehensive approaches require participation by diverse stakeholders and a considerable investment of time and other resources for success.

3. *Environmental factors.* With the recognition that multiple levels of factors influence health-related behaviors, the importance of the environment has taken on enhanced meaning in public health intervention research and practice. These higher-level factors, sometimes referred to as contextual factors or structural factors, and their interactive effect with behavior on health outcomes is apparent in motor vehicle safety and tobacco control. The physical environment shapes exposure to risks such as dangerous highways and readily accessible tobacco products, and part of the success in addressing these two public problems is attributable to minimizing such risks. The social environment shapes norms through media and policy exposures, and again, changing norms such as smoking in the movies or implementing seat belt use laws underlie some of the successes in the story of motor vehicle safety and tobacco control.

4. *Public support and advocacy.* Challenging government and industry leadership to improve upon roads and crashworthiness of vehicles; to support laws regulating drinking while driving and seat belt and car seat usage; and to augment

tobacco taxes and restrain smoking in public places, the public has played a powerful role as an informed electorate, thanks to advocacy and educational efforts. These same advocacy and educational efforts may influence social norms about motor vehicle safety and smoking more generally and could yield other positive voluntary changes in safety behaviors and in other health-related behaviors. Because of the controversial nature of many of the interventions with motor vehicles and tobacco control, public support is essential. Finding ways to garner that support is likewise essential, and the building of stakeholder **partnerships** and **coalitions** is crucially important. Equally important is the availability of solid evidence to inform both the electorate and the decision makers. Thus, the lessons learned from tobacco and motor vehicle safety not only provide useful examples of ecological approaches, but also reinforce the value of the current emphasis in public health on translation and dissemination from science to policy and practice (Green, Glasgow, et al. 2009; Green, Ottoson, et al. 2009; Pollack et al. 2010).

5. *Reciprocal determinism.* We also emphasize the importance of reciprocal determinism. This central tenet of ecological theory and science holds that organisms are influenced by their environment and in turn influence their environment. As applied to the human species, it claims that as people are influenced by their home, school, recreational, work, social, economic, physical, and media environments, they also can exert agency, will, and effort in changing, resisting and adapting to these environments through their behavior. They do this as individuals, collaboratively as partners with others, as families, as advocacy groups, as organizations, and as political parties. Policies influence peoples' behavior, but people create those policies.

Despite the dramatic successes achieved in reducing motor vehicle injuries and fatalities and smoking-related diseases and deaths, much remains to accomplish. There are high risk groups that require special attention. For example, American Indians and Alaskan Natives have higher smoking rates and experience motor vehicle death rates and smoking-related disease rates that far exceed those of other ethnic groups (Pollack et al. 2012; Thorne et al. 2007). Youth in general are at higher risk for unsafe behaviors of all types, including driving-related risks and beginning tobacco use. Although we have made strides in addressing this age group through graduated driver licensing and restricted access to products, much remains to be done. Applying an ecological model to build comprehensive, multilevel interventions focused on the needs of these special populations and others should yield effective strategies.

A significant advantage for ensuring future success is that public opinion and social norms appear to be supportive of motor vehicle safety and tobacco control initiatives, including policy and legislative interventions. Historically, in the injury control and substance abuse fields, we tended to treat the public simply as recipients of professional admonitions to behave safely, to comply with the law (Gielen and Girasek 2001), and to exercise personal restraint. Public information campaigns and school health programs with those **objectives** were the mainstay of safety education and tobacco control. As shown in this chapter, the evidence for an ecological approach highlights the need to incorporate other levels and targets of intervention. What the evidence from the motor vehicle safety and tobacco control experiences has shown, as with some of the other great public health achievements of the 20th century, is that an active and engaged public can promote significant and sustained changes in both public policy and personal safety and health behavior. Emerging health and safety problems such as obesity, emergency preparedness, and prescription drug overdose, to name just a few, may benefit from these lessons. Meaningful partnerships with the intended recipients of our interventions and adherence to a multilevel, comprehensive approach should help us meet the future challenges of addressing health and safety problems of the 21st century.

Although these evidence-based "lessons" have served as guides, if not inspiration, in other public health initiatives, their generalizations to other health behavior issues in public health, such as physical activity and nutrition, must acknowledge that there may be unique issues in changing these pervasive behaviors and associated lifestyles. The commercial interests and contemporary environmental and media influences will likely bring new and perhaps even more complex issues into play than those successfully dealt with in the motor vehicle and tobacco control experience (Green et al. 2003; TFCPS 2005). Applying the frameworks, theories, and strategic approaches described throughout this text should well prepare the next generation of public health **change agents** to meet such challenges.

NOTES

1. The Community Guide website (www.the communityguide.org) is CDC's website to summarize the systematic reviews, recommendations, and other deliberations of the Community Preventive Services Task Force. The www.thecommunityguide.org/alcohol /beverage_service.html web page summarizes the specific review and recommendation of the Task Force on server training interventions. For updates to systematic reviews of evidence-based preventive interventions to promote population health, see www.thecommunity guide.org.

2. For an annotated bibliography on media advocacy, see L Dorfman, P Gonzalez, Media advocacy, in *Oxford Bibliographies Online Public Health,* ed. L. Green (New York: Oxford University Press, 2010).

REFERENCES

Allegrante JP, Mark R, Hanson DW. 2006. Ecological models for the prevention and control of unintentional injury. In *Injury and Violence Prevention: Behavioral Science Theories, Methods, and Applications,* ed. AC Gielen, D Sleet, R DiClemente, 105-26. San Francisco: Jossey-Bass.

Baker SP. 1979. Motor vehicle occupant deaths in young children. *Pediatrics* 64:860-61.

Bonnie RJ, Fulco CE, Liverman CT, eds. 1999. *Reducing the Burden of Injury: Advancing Prevention and Treatment.* Institute of Medicine. Washington DC: National Academy Press.

California Department of Health Services (CDHS). 2006. *California Tobacco Control Update 2006: The Social Norm Change Approach.* Sacramento: California Department of Health Services.

Centers for Disease Control and Prevention (CDC). 1999. Ten greatest public health achievements—United States, 1900-1999. *MMWR* 48:241-43.

Chen L-H, Baker SP, Li G. 2006. Graduated driver licensing programs and fatal crashes of 16-year-old drivers: A national evaluation. *Pediatrics* 118 (1) (July): 56-62.

Christoffel T, Teret SP. 1993. *Protecting the Public: Legal Issues in Injury Prevention.* New York: Oxford University Press.

Daynard RA. 2003. Lessons from tobacco control for the obesity control movement. *J Public Health* Policy 24:291-95.

Doll R, Hill A. 1950. Smoking and carcinoma of the lung: Preliminary report. *Br Med J* 2:739-48.

Dorfman L, Gonzalez P. 2010. Media advocacy. In *Oxford Bibliographies: Online Public Health,* ed. L. Green. New York: Oxford University Press.

Dorfman L, Wilbur P, Lingas EO, Woodruff K, Wallack L. 2005. Accelerating policy on nutrition: Lessons from tobacco, alcohol, firearms, and traffic safety. Berkeley Media Studies Group, Berkeley, CA.

Economos CD, Brownson RC, DeAngelis MA, et al. 2001. What lessons have been learned from other attempts to guide social change? *Nutr Rev* 59 (3): S40-S56.

Eriksen MP. 2005. Lessons learned from public health efforts and their relevance to preventing childhood obesity. In *Preventing Childhood Obesity: Health in the Balance,* ed. Committee on Prevention of Obesity in Children and Youth, Food and Nutrition Board, Board on Health Promotion and Disease Prevention, JP Koplan, CT Liverman, VI Kraak, Appendix D, 343-75. Washington, DC: National Academy Press.

Eriksen MP, Gielen AC. 1983. The application of health education principles of automobile child restraint programs. *Health Educ Q* 10 (1): 30-55.

Eriksen MP, Green LW. 2009. Reducing tobacco use. In *Principles of Public Health Practice,* ed. FD Scutchfield, CW Keck. 3rd ed. Clifton Park, NY: Thomson/Delmar Learning.

Eriksen MP, Green LW, Husten CG, Pederson LL, Pechacek TF. 2007. Thank you for not smoking: The public health response to tobacco-related mortality in the United States. In *Silent Victories: The History and Practice of Public Health in Twentieth-Century America,* ed. JW Ward, C Warren, 423-36. Oxford: Oxford University Press.

Farrelly MC, Pechacek TP, Chaloupka FJ. 2003. The impact of tobacco control program expenditure on aggregate cigarette sales: 1981-2000. *J Health Econ* 22:843-59.

Farrelly MC, Pechacek TF, Thomas KY, Nelson D. 2008. The impact of tobacco control programs on adult smoking. *Am J Public Health* 98:304-9.

Fichtenberg CM, Glantz SA. 2000. Association of the California Tobacco Control Program with declines in cigarette consumption and mortality from heart disease. *N Engl J Med* 343 (24): 1772-77.

Finnegan JR Jr., Viswanath K. 2002. Communication theory and health behavior change: The media studies framework. In *Health Behavior and Health Education: Theory, Research, and Practice,* ed. K Glanz, BK Rimer, FM Lewis, 361-88. 3rd ed. San Francisco: Jossey-Bass.

Freire K, Runyan CW. 2006. Planning Models: PRECEDE-PROCEED and Haddon Matrix. In *Injury and Violence Prevention: Behavioral Science Theories, Methods, and Applications,* ed. AC Gielen, DA Sleet, RJ DiClemente, 127-58. San Francisco: Jossey-Bass.

Frieden TR. 2010. A framework for public health action: The health impact pyramid. *Am J Public Health* 100 (4): 590-95.

Gielen AC, Girasek D. 2001. Integrating perspectives on the prevention of unintentional injuries. In *Integrating Behavioral and Social Sciences with Public Health,* ed. N Schneiderman, J Gentry, JM deSilva, M Speers, H Fomes. Washington, DC: APA Books.

Gielen AC, Sleet D. 2003. Application of behavior-change theories and methods to injury prevention. *Epidemiol Rev* 25:65-67.

Girasek DC, Gielen AC. 2003. The effectiveness of injury prevention strategies: What does the public believe? *Health Educ Behav* 30 (3): 287-304.

Graham JD. 1993. Injuries from traffic crashes: Meeting the challenge. *Ann Rev Public Health* 40:515-43.

Green, LW. 1980. To educate or not to educate: Is that the question? *Am J Public Health* 70 (6) (June): 625-26.

Green LW, Eriksen MP, Bailey L, Husten C. 2000. Achieving the implausible in the next decade: Tobacco control objectives. *Am J Public Health* 90:337-39.

Green LW, Glasgow RE, Atkins D, Stange K. 2009. Making evidence from research more relevant, useful, and actionable in policy, program planning, and practice: Slips "twixt cup and lip." *Am J Prev Med* 37 (6S1): S187-S191.

Green LW, Kreuter MW. 2005. *Health Program Planning: An Educational and Ecological Approach.* 4th ed. New York: McGraw-Hill.

——. 2010. Evidence hierarchies versus synergistic interventions. *Am J Public Health* 100 (10) (Oct.): 1824-25, http://ajph.aphapublications.org/doi/pdf/10 .2105/AJPH.2010.197798.

Green LW, Lewis FM. 1986. *Measurement and Evaluation in Health Education and Health Promotion.* Palo Alto, CA: Mayfield.

Green LW, Mercer SL, Rosenthal AC, Dietz WH, Husten CG. 2003. Possible lessons for physician counselling on obesity from the progress in smoking cessation in primary care. In *Modern Aspects of Nutrition: Present Knowledge and Future Perspectives,* ed. L Elmadfa, E Anklam, JS Konig, 191-94. Vol. 56. Basel, Switzerland: Karger.

Green LW, Nathan R, Mercer SL. 2001. The health of health promotion in public policy: Drawing inspiration from the tobacco control movement. *Health Promot J Aus* 12 (2): 12-18.

Green LW, Ottoson JM, Garcia C, Hiatt R. 2009. Diffusion theory and knowledge dissemination, utilization, and integration in public health. *Annu Rev Public Health* 30:151-74.

Green LW, Richard L, Potvin L. 1996. Ecological foundations of health promotion. *Am J Health Promot* 10 (4): 270-81.

Hartunian NS, Smart CN, Willemain TR, Zador PL. 1983. The economics of safety deregulation: Lives and dollars lost due to repeal of motorcycle helmet laws. *J Health Polit Policy Law* 8 (1) (Spring): 76-98.

Holder HD, Gruenewald PJ, Ponicki WR, et al. 2000. Effect of community-based interventions on high-risk drinking and alcohol-related injuries. *JAMA* 284:2341-47.

Insurance Institute for Highway Safety (IIHS). 2012. How to make young driver laws even better. *Status Report* 47 (4) (May 31).

International Agency for Research on Cancer (IARC). 2004. *Tobacco Smoke and Involuntary Smoking.* IARC Monographs on the Evaluation of Carcinogenic Risks to Humans, vol. 83, http://monographs.iarc.fr/ENG /Monographs/vol83/index.php.

Isaacs SL, Schroeder SA. 2001. Where the public good prevailed: Lessons from success stories in health. *Am Prospect* 12 (10) (June): 26-30.

Levin M. 1950. Tobacco smoking and cancer. *JAMA* 144 (9): 782.

Levy D, Gallus S, Blackman K, et al. 2012. Italy SimSmoke: The effect of tobacco control policies on smoking prevalence and smoking-attributable deaths in Italy. *BMC Public Health* 12 (Aug 29): 709.

Martin JB, Green LW, Gielen AC. 2007. Potential lessons from public health and health promotion for the prevention of child abuse. *J Prev Interv Community* 34 (1-2): 205-22.

Mercer SL, Green LW, Rosenthal AC, Husten CG, Khan LK, Dietz WH. 2003. Possible lessons from the tobacco experience for obesity control. *Am J Clin Nutr* 77 (4 suppl.): 1073S-1082S.

Nader R. 1965. *Unsafe at Any Speed: The Designed-in Dangers of the American Automobile.* New York: Grossman.

National Highway Traffic Safety Administration (NHTSA). 2000. *Traffic Safety Facts, 1999: A Compilation of Motor Vehicle Crash Data from the Fatality Analysis Reporting System and the General Estimates System.* DOT HS 809 100. Washington, DC: U.S. Department of Transportation, National Highway Traffic Safety Administration.

———. 2003. Trends in occupant restraint use and fatalities. Available at National Highway Traffic Safety Administration, www.nhtsa.dot.gov/people/injury /research/BuckleUp/ii__trends.htm.

———. 2005. Traffic safety facts, motorcycle helmet use laws, March, NHTSA. Available at National Highway Traffic Safety Administration, www.nhtsa.gov.

———. 2008. Traffic safety facts: Seat belt use in 2007—demographic results. Available at www-nrd .nhtsa.dot.gov/pubs/810932.pdf.

———. 2009. Child restraint use in 2008—demographic results. Available at www-nrd.nhtsa.dot.gov/Pubs /811148.pdf.

Nichols JL. 1994. Changing public behavior for better health: Is education enough? *Am J Prev Med* 10 (suppl. 1): 19-22.

Office on Smoking and Health (OSH). 2007. *Best Practices for Comprehensive Tobacco Control Programs—2007.* 2nd ed. Atlanta, GA: National Center for Chronic Disease Prevention and Health Promotion, Centers for Disease Control and Prevention. Available at www .cdc.gov/tobacco (accessed Aug. 4, 2008).

Pollack KM, Frattaroli S, Young JL, Dana-Sacco G, Gielen AC. 2012. Motor vehicle deaths among American Indian and Alaska Native populations. *Epidemiol Rev* 34 (1): 73-88.

Pollack KM, Samuels A, Frattaroli, Gielen AC. 2010. The translation imperative: Moving research into policy. *Inj Prev* 16:141-42.

Rivara FP, and MacKenzie EJ, eds. 1999. Systematic reviews of strategies to prevent motor vehicle injuries. *Am J Prev Med* 16 (suppl. 1): 1-90.

Robertson LS. 1980. Crash involvement of teenaged drivers when driver education is eliminated from high school. *Am J Public Health* 70 (6) (June): 599-603.

Robertson LS, Zador PL. 1978. Driver education and fatal crash involvement of teenaged drivers. *Am J Public Health* 68 (10) (Oct.): 959-65.

Schick SF, Glantz S. 2007. Concentrations of the carcinogen 4-(methylnitrosamino)-1-(3-pyridyl)-1-butanone in sidestream cigarette smoke increase after release into indoor air: Results from unpublished tobacco industry research. *Cancer Epidem Biomarkers Prev* 16 (8): 1547-53.

Shiffman S, Mason KM, Henningfield JE. 1998. Tobacco dependence treatments: Review and prospectus. *Ann Rev Public* Health 19:335-58.

Shope JT, Molnar LJ, Elliott MR, Waller PF. 2001. Graduated driver licensing in Michigan: Early impact on motor vehicle crashes among 16-year-old drivers. *JAMA* 286 (13): 1593-98.

Sleet DA, Gielen AC. 2006. Injury Prevention. In *Health Promotion in Practice,* ed. SS Gorin, J Arnold, 361-91. San Francisco: Jossey-Bass.

Task Force on Community Preventive Services (TFCPS). 2005. *The Guide to Community Preventive Services: What Works to Promote Health?* Oxford: Oxford University Press.

Tauras JA, Chaloupka FJ, Farrelly MC, et al. 2005. State tobacco control spending and youth smoking. *Am J Public Health* 95:338-44.

Thorne SL, Malarcher A, Maurice E, Caraballo, R. 2007. Cigarette smoking among adults, United States. *MMWR* 57 (45): 1221-26.

U.S. Department of Health, Education, and Welfare (USDHEW). 1964. *Smoking and Health: Report of the Advisory Committee to the Surgeon General of the Public Health Service.* PHS publication no. 1103. Washington, DC: USDHEW, Public Health Service, Centers for Disease Control.

U.S. Environmental Protection Agency (USEPA). 1992. *Respiratory Health Effects of Passive Smoking: Lung Cancer and Other Disorders.* Publ. no. EPA/600/6-90 /006F. Washington, DC: USEPA, Office of Research and Development, Office of Air and Radiation.

U.S. Preventive Services Task Force (USPSTF). 1996. *Guide to Clinical Preventive Services.* 2nd ed. Baltimore: Williams & Wilkins.

Waller PF. 2001. Public health's contribution to motor vehicle injury prevention. *Am J Prev Med* 21 (4) (suppl.): 1-2.

Ward JW, Warren C, eds. 2007. *Silent Victories: The History and Practice of Public Health in Twentieth Century America.* New York: Oxford University Press.

Wynder EL, Graham EA. 1950. Tobacco smoking as a possible etiologic factor in bronchiogenic carcinoma. *JAMA* 143:329-36.

Zaza S, Briss PA, Harris KW, eds. 2005. *The Guide to Community Preventive Services: What Works to Promote Health?* New York: Oxford University Press.

Zaza S, Thompson RS, and Harris KW, eds. 2001a. The guide to community preventive services, reducing injuries to motor vehicle occupants, systematic reviews of evidence, recommendations from the task force on community preventive services, and expert commentary. *Am J Prev Med* 21 (4) (suppl.): 1-90.

Zaza S, Thomspon RS, and Harris KW, eds. 2001b. Letter from Franklin D. Roosevelt. In The guide to community preventive services, reducing injuries to motor vehicle occupants, systematic reviews of evidence, recommendations from the task force on community preventive services, and expert commentary. *Am J Prev Med* 21 (4) (suppl.): inside front cover.

Zwerling C, Jones MP. 1999. Evaluation of the effectiveness of low blood alcohol concentration laws for younger drivers. *Am J Prev Med* 16 (suppl. 1): 76-80.

CHAPTER 4

Extending the Ecological Model

Key Stakeholders and Organizational Partnerships

BARBARA RILEY AND ALLAN BEST

LEARNING OBJECTIVES

After completing the chapter, the reader will be able to

* Explore the role of various stakeholders in influencing population behavior change.
* Position organizational partnerships temporally and substantively within the field of population-based prevention.
* Critically examine diverse forms of organizational partnerships and their strengths and limitations.
* Identify critical success factors for organizational partnerships.
* Describe promising future directions for organizational partnerships to support behavior change in populations.

Introduction

Most health behaviors are influenced by a complex array of factors operating at multiple levels of influence within an ecological system; as described in chapter 2, these include individual, interpersonal, family, organizational, community, and societal levels. This well-accepted view of health behavior provides a rationale for the importance of strategic partnerships between stakeholders and concerted organizational action, including organizations working together in partnerships of many varieties. We use the term **partnerships** broadly to include many types of collaborative arrangements (e.g., alliance, network, coalition, consortium), consisting of stakeholders working together to achieve common goals.

Although **ecological approaches** have usefully reinforced the need for multiple levels of influence and multiple strategies (e.g., education, policy, media), they have been less effective in focusing attention on the interrelationships within and across levels and how **interventions** need to take these relationships into account in their design and implementation (Golden and Earp 2012; Kok et al. 2008). Instead, each layer of influence has typically been targeted and examined on its own, often carefully documenting the setting within which interventions are implemented, but without information about how the setting or **context** at one level (e.g., a family physician's office, a community support program, a national **social marketing** campaign) interacts with settings at other levels (Richard et al. 1996). In the past decade, the limits to this approach have been increasingly recognized as programs within organizations and settings have foundered from lack of support or **reinforcement** from other settings and organizations to which their patients, clients, students, or workers relate. More focus is needed on partnerships that *link* organizations and promote health behavior change at a population level (e.g., Crilly et al. 2009).

At the core of this chapter is the importance of strategically involving the individuals and groups—that is, **stakeholders**—who are affected by a given problem. This chapter focuses on ways that a diverse and complementary range of stakeholders (private and public sectors; research, practice, and policy; etc.) can best organize and complement each other to promote and support behavior change in populations. On the assumption that relevant individuals and groups will have a greater influence together than they can have on their own, understanding what types of organizational partnerships to form and how partnerships can function effectively to produce desired results are essential skills for facilitating behavior change in broad populations. Many of the organizational forms discussed in this chapter are ways to ensure meaningful input from relevant stakeholders.

The initial sections of this chapter will discuss types and categories of **key stakeholders** and make a case for the importance of organizational partnerships, including a brief overview of partnership drivers. Then we will outline functions of organizational partnerships—what they must accomplish to advance health behavior change at a population level—and summarize critical success factors for organizational partnerships. We then provide three examples of different types of organizational partnerships and their successes, challenges, and lessons. Finally, we conclude the chapter by summarizing key issues and lessons and making recommendations for organizational partnerships designed to enhance population-based prevention through health behavior change.

Key Stakeholders

Other chapters in this book (especially in part III) describe specific stakeholders that are relevant to influencing specific health behaviors and outcomes. In this section, we provide a brief overview of some key stakeholder groups, including government, health services, **nongovernmental organizations**, and the **private sector**, and describe some traditional and emerging roles that may be relevant for population behavior change efforts.

Planned approaches to behavior change on a population level are influenced by a wide range of factors; for example, content knowledge (e.g., **planning** and **evaluation** models for population behavior change; understanding of local context, **norms** and practices), skills (e.g., negotiation, program and policy development, communications and media relations), resources, political will, and public support. Many stakeholders contribute directly to, or influence, these factors. No "ideal" recipe exists for roles and contributions of particular organizations. Nevertheless, different categories of stakeholders have overarching goals and policy frameworks that help to define a range of possible roles. In the area of population and public health, we have seen organizations embrace a wide range of roles, only some of which may be considered "traditional," according to their goals and structures.

Government

The traditional role of government is to promote the health and well-being of its population (Blackburn and Walker 2005). Complex population health problems require broad governmental action. Government roles must consider all levels of government: federal, state/provincial, and local.

Government actions relevant to health behavior change at a population level include establishing regulatory frameworks (e.g., for food and drug companies), enforcing laws and regulatory codes (especially at the federal level where these involve interstate or interprovincial commerce), developing action plans (e.g., for chronic disease prevention, such as obesity, diabetes, and cardiovascular disease) and conceptual/policy frameworks, monitoring and **surveillance** activities, conducting research and evaluation, and coordinating efforts across sectors in specific topic areas.

Health Services

By *health services* we mean the full range of health care and prevention services in the "formal" health system, including physicians and supplementary health care practitioners, laboratory services and diagnostic procedures, emergency and hospital care, home care, and public health, as distinct from "informal" or complementary health services, such as those offered by social services, education, nongovernment organizations, and private sectors.

The role of health services in population behavior change is evolving, especially with the transition from infectious to chronic disease concerns over the past generation. Over the past 20 years, there have been calls for a greater focus on prevention in health services to be accomplished in part through restructuring health systems so that they are more focused around individual, family, and population needs rather than the preferences and convenience of the practitioners and managers who deliver services (Crampton and Starfield 2004; Forster and Gabe 2008; Green 1994; Stewart 2001).

Nongovernmental Organizations and Advocates

Although definitions of **nongovernmental organizations** (NGOs) vary, here we use the term to refer to any professional, nonprofit, or public interest organization or association that is neither under the direction of, nor affiliated with, a government (adapted from Lohmann 1992). NGOs can provide services directly; however, they tend to focus on **capacity building** within communities, grassroots empowerment, policy influence, and funding research. Some examples of NGOs in the arena of health behavior change include disease-oriented groups (e.g., cancer, heart disease, diabetes), community service groups (e.g., YMCAs), citizen advocacy groups, and so forth.

The Private Sector

Consensus is rapidly growing that key public health challenges can only be addressed through broad partnerships that include both public and private sector organizations. For example, there now is general agreement that food growers, manufacturers, retailers, and others in the production and distribution chain need to be meaningfully engaged to address the increased prevalence of obesity. Private sector fitness facilities play a key role in population strategies to increase activity. Affordable infectious disease strategy in developing countries requires active partnership with the private sector pharmaceutical industry. However, there has heretofore been insufficient trust and investment in public-private collaboration to support population-wide behavior change, perhaps in part because profit, rather than health, is the main driver in the private sector (e.g., the food industry makes healthful products as long as they make a profit). Public-private partnerships may be enhanced by organizations with expertise and experience building bridges across sectors, such as academic health sciences centers, state public health departments, and some consulting firms.

Research Organizations

Universities, research funders, health service organizations, and independent researchers and evaluators all have important roles to play in producing and using relevant evidence to support population health behavior change. While some trends are promising, such as a growing emphasis on population health intervention research, many systemic factors, such as tenure and promotion policies and procedures for academic researchers, university support for applied and interdisciplinary research, and funding opportunities for evaluation and other community practice-based research (cf. Institute of Medicine 2010), need to catch up to better support relevant and rigorous solution-oriented science.

Technical Assistance Organizations

The importance of strengthening knowledge and skills among a variety of professionals and citizens for developing partnerships (Butterfoss 2004; Roberts 2004) and for population-based behavior change (Catford 2009) is now widely recognized. Often referred to as **capacity building** and accomplished through technical assistance, it normally includes training, consultation, and networking services. If requisite expertise and skills are not present within an organizational partnership, then capacity building may be needed, or some short-term services to assist with some of the tasks in the problem-solving process (e.g., evaluation).

The Case for Organizational Partnerships

One of the core differences between individual-focused behavior change and population-level behavior change is the use of community approaches, including building partnerships. Community approaches attempt to tackle community problems, such as substance abuse (e.g., Hallfors et al. 2002) and childhood obesity (e.g., Institute of Medicine 2012), by organizing the community to bring about change. We will look at the history of such organizational partnerships and at what drives them today, including what we call the **complexity** imperative, and differing perspectives on **knowledge translation**—that is, processes for enabling application of research to policy and practice.

A History of Organizational Partnerships in Public Health

Community mobilization has a long and honorable history in public health, including the immunization campaigns of the 1950s and 1960s, the international family planning programs of the 1960s, and some of the earlier hygiene campaigns of the first half of the 20th century (Rosen 1993). Community mobilization was a deeply rooted component of the World Health Organization and other bilateral and multilateral community development programs in developing countries (e.g., for clean water) and in the United States, such as for welfare reform, which produced most of the early (1950s and 1960s) textbooks on community organizing. John F. Kennedy's (New Frontier) and Lyndon Johnson's (New Society, War on Poverty) legislative initiatives in the 1960s also are important, with each act of legislation containing the words "maximum feasible participation" (Moynihan 1969). There were also the "Community Chest" and "United Way" partnerships to raise and distribute donations to community charities and NGOs.

Building on this foundation, the community-based cardiovascular disease prevention studies that began in the 1970s were pioneers in moving prevention and health risk behavior from the clinic (or individual) to the community. Widely referred to as *community trials,* such efforts in Europe (e.g., Finland, Wales), the United States (e.g., Stanford, Pawtucket, Minnesota), and elsewhere generated considerable interest in working with and through community systems (e.g., schools, local government, media) (Bracht 1990) to promote population health behavior change. In their reflections on realistic outcome goals for community-based heart health programs, Mittelmark and colleagues (1993) conclude that the most enduring lessons are about community mobilization. This is a significant insight for many who were steeped in the tradition of controlled research studies that limited the degree to which communities could deviate from predetermined, scientific protocols for the interventions.

Based at least in part on these early experiences, a strong trend emerged in the 1980s and 1990s to form multisector community partnerships (including health service organizations, but also social service agencies, schools, local government, etc.) as a means to develop and implement comprehensive, health promotion strategies. A strong **"wisdom literature"** (a body of knowledge that captures the experiences of practitioners) emerged on ways to engage various community champions and organizations, such as through advisory boards, steering committees, and working groups, and ways to ensure that practices were tailored and adapted to local context. Toward the end of the millennium, consensus emerged on empirical and theoretical foundations for community partnerships (Butterfoss and Kegler 2002), often referred to as *community coalitions.*

A first step was to specify the niche occupied by community partnerships. They tend to be characterized as a specific type of structured collaboration consisting of individuals representing diverse organizations, groups, or constituencies within the community who agree to work together to achieve common goals (Butterfoss and Kegler 2002). In contrast to short-term grassroots partnerships that form for a specific purpose (e.g., support for or opposition against a proposed policy), community partnerships are characterized as formal, multipurpose, and enduring. The theoretical foundations for the development and maintenance of community partnerships borrow from many fields of practice and study, including community development and empowerment, interorganizational relations, adult education, and political science.

For a time, community partnerships were viewed as somewhat of a panacea for population behavior change. For example, the 1990s saw increasing requirements on the part of federal government (in the United States and Canada) and other granting agencies (e.g., foundations) for partnerships and coalitions even to qualify to apply for and receive community health grants. Although the possible contributions and benefits of community coalitions are still widely acknowledged, since the first decade of the 2000s, more attention is being directed to other types of partnerships (such as **networks**, communities of practice) that may help to achieve the complex goals and actions in dynamic environments for behavior change at a population level. For example, more emphasis is being placed on the need for multilevel initiatives that go beyond local communities. This requires a broader understanding of partnerships, including relationships within and across different jurisdictional levels.

Partnership Drivers Today

We have shown that organizational partnerships have a long history. Nevertheless, the main factors driving partnerships have changed over time. Most recent drivers include a deeper understanding of complexity and models of knowledge translation.

THE COMPLEXITY IMPERATIVE

Population and public health problems, such as obesity and tobacco use, are now consistently described as complex problems or "wicked problems," deeply embedded within the fabric of society (Kreuter et al. 2004). As such, both the factors underlying health behaviors and behavior change and the solutions required to promote healthful behaviors are complex. Early models of health behavior change tended to focus on the individual and often suggested simple direct relationships between knowledge and behavior (cf. Green 2006). However, such a **reductionist** approach that addresses single factors or **determinants** is unlikely to be effective for creating sustained behavior change; integrated, systems-level interventions provide a more appropriately complex approach to addressing the complex problems of poor health behaviors in populations (see also chapter 21). Such **ecological interventions** should approach both individuals and their environments (social, physical, economic, organizational, etc.), considering the relationships among these multiple **influences** on behavior and the reciprocal influences of individual and collective behavior on environments.

A classic metaphor to reveal the differences between simple and **complex systems** is a machine versus a living system. Machines, no matter how sophisticated and intricate, can be understood by looking at the individual parts. A living system, on the other hand, can only be understood as an integrated whole: "A complex system is not constituted merely by the sum of its components, but also by the intricate and interacting relationships between these components" (Cilliers 1998, 2, in Anderson et al. 2005).

Viewing the world as such a complex living system has implications for organizational partnerships. One implication, as we have discussed, is the need to consider the roles and interplay of many organizational forms that extend well beyond community partnerships.

For example, complexity requires a blending of shared practice among individuals (e.g., communities of practice, exchange networks), organizational partnerships (e.g., alliances, joint ventures, public-private partnerships), legislative and regulatory alignment (e.g., international, national, and state policy), and stakeholder engagement (e.g., advocacy, citizen participation).

Another implication of complexity for organizational partnerships is shared accountability and credit. If the world operates as a living system, then the actions of many organizations are interdependent and dynamic and influence each other in multiple ways. As part of a living system, no single organization can be responsible for health outcomes, nor can any one of them claim full credit for positive outcomes; instead, accountability and credit must be shared. This can make it difficult to attribute credit to individual organizations, especially small organizations that need to show their contributions / returns on investment to constituents or donors. This is true whether organizations choose to work alone or with others. Partnering explicitly acknowledges the **interdependence** of actions and thereby has the potential to create **synergy** across organizational efforts. Nevertheless, especially in a climate of limited resources and increased accountability, frameworks for shared accountability need to be developed that also allow the contributions of individual organizations to be profiled.

A related challenge is the need to demonstrate outcomes (e.g., on population health), usually in a short period of time. These expectations are unrealistic, especially for complex problems, insofar as population-level outcomes are typically produced through multiple pathways, delayed, and difficult to measure. Given the perceived urgency to produce outcomes, organizations may be hesitant to partner when building consensus with other organizations would typically increase the time needed for planning. On the other hand, partnerships may also help to create the necessary synergy across organizational efforts to optimize successful results over the long term. Evaluation strategies need to take these tensions into account by identifying meaningful short-term markers of progress, defining and measuring outcomes at an appropriate level of aggregation, and making contributions of different organizations visible.

EVOLVING MODELS OF KNOWLEDGE TRANSLATION

The evolution of conceptual models for **knowledge translation** provides a useful parallel to the shift from emphasis on individual behavior change to population perspectives as well as the shift from an emphasis on principles of evidence-based medicine (e.g., reliance on tightly controlled study designs and internal validity) to a stronger focus on intervention **theory** (including organizational strategies), external **validity** of studies (including participatory methods [see Green 2001; Van de Ven and Johnston 2006]), and learning from practice (Best et al. 2003; Davies et al. 2008; Glasgow and Emmons 2007; Green and Glasgow 2006; Green, Glasgow, et al. 2009; Green, Ottoson, et al. 2009; Rychetnik et al. 2002; Truman et al. 2000).

The emerging systems models illustrate both the specific challenges of complex systems and the key role of organizational partnerships (Best et al. 2009; Best and Holmes 2010).

Linear versus Relationship Models. Thinking about knowledge translation has evolved from linear to relationship and systems models. In the *linear model,* knowledge is seen as a product whose use depends on effective transmission and packaging (Best, Hiatt, and Norman 2008; Best et al. 2009). In contrast, though *relationship models* take the linear model principles for dissemination and diffusion into account, they focus on the interactions among people who use the knowledge. The emphasis is on the sharing of knowledge, the development of partnerships, and the fostering of networks among

stakeholders with common interests (Graham et al. 2006; Lomas 2007). In the relationship model, knowledge is seen to come from multiple sources (research, theory, practice, policy), not just from the researcher. Its use depends on effective relationships and processes (Best, Hiatt, and Norman 2008). This view begins to counter the perspective that research is worth disseminating just because it passed peer review. Instead, other considerations such as external validity, relevance, and adaptability come to the fore as equally important considerations that require a different perspective on the one-way research-to-policy-and-practice assumption of linear models.

The Systems Model. Further, a *systems model* builds on linear and relationship thinking and allows us to build a more robust **conceptual framework** of knowledge to action. It recognizes that diffusion and dissemination processes and relationships themselves are shaped, embedded, and organized through organizational structures that influence the types of interactions that occur among multiple stakeholders with unique worldviews, priorities, languages, means of communication, and **expectations** (Frenck 1992). These stakeholders are tied together by a system (which, in turn, is shaped by culture, structures, priorities, and capacities [Best et al. 2009]) that requires explicit processes to activate systems change if its various parts are to be linked together. Consequently, a systems way of thinking is needed to bring about that activation for the purposes of moving from knowledge to action (Best and Holmes 2010; Best, Trochim, et al. 2008; Holmes et al. 2012).

While these models refer to the progression of knowledge to action and the required individual and organizational changes, the same principles link the roles of individuals, practitioners, organizations, and systems in population health behavior change (Best et al. 2003). Some key issues surface around roles in the production and implementation of evidence and in the strengthening of leadership, networks, and capacity (Best and Holmes 2010).

Types of Organizational Partnerships

The language used to describe a relationship between two or more organizations continues to expand; the terms *partnerships, joint ventures, consolidations, networks, coalitions, collaboratives, alliances, consortiums, associations, conglomerates, councils, task forces,* and *groups* have all been used. A common typology does not exist. Our goal in this chapter is to reveal a range of possibilities and to link these to specific purposes and functions. We start this section by discussing a community of practice as a "pre-partnership" and then profile a few other types of partnerships that may be effective to influence population behavior change.

A **community of practice (CoP)** can be conceptualized as an early or informal form of partnership that operates in parallel with, and in support of, more formal configurations. While the term often is used loosely as a synonym for network, when it is more specifically and narrowly defined, the key features of a CoP are these (Wenger et al. 2002): It is a group of individuals with a common concern or passion that engages in an interactive process for sharing knowledge, planning, and learning; the interaction typically emerges naturally—the true CoP is emergent, self-governing, and dynamic. A CoP is especially important to capture the tacit knowledge and wisdom of individuals in action (Nonaka et al. 2000).

Organizations can enable and support CoPs as a key mechanism for sharing tacit knowledge and learning that is central to organizational **objectives** and strategy. However, if organizational partnerships formalize a CoP as a purposeful structure to be managed by the partnership (Barwick et al. 2008), it is better seen as a network than a CoP. A network normally takes a more structured approach to development

and support of the interaction (Garcia and Dorohovich 2007).

More structured approaches are what we refer to as *partnerships* (also called by many other names, as noted above). Partnerships represent some arrangement involving two or more organizations that has (1) come together for a common purpose and (2) become semi-autonomous but maintains accountability and feedback loops to its organizations of origin. Organizational forms are structures of human relationships designed to achieve shared goals. Organizational forms have clear boundaries and well-defined roles, and individuals or subgroups have authority (by assumption or delegation) to lead the activities of the organization (Roberts 2004).

Most collaboration theorists contend that partnership efforts fall across a continuum of low to high **integration** (Gajda 2004). The level of integration is determined by the intensity of the partnership's process, structure, and purpose. For example, integration is *low* if the process and structure are limited to communicating information and exploring interests. Integration is considered *medium* if the group plans together to achieve mutual goals while maintaining separate identities. Integration is *highest* if the group merges to form a single identity. Note that this does not imply that the highest integration is always the best—more focused and coordinated sharing of functions and resources may be more optimal in some circumstances than in others.

The levels of integration are often described on a continuum, with points defined variably by different collaboration theorists (Bailey and Koney 2000; Hogue 1993; Peterson 1991). A low level of integration is typically referred to as *networking* or *cooperation,* whereby fully independent groups share information that supports each other's organizational outcomes. A moderate level of integration is often described as *coordination,* whereby independent parties align activities or cosponsor events or services that support mutually beneficial goals. High integration is typically referred to as *collaboration,* in which individual entities give up some degree of independence in an effort to reach a shared goal.

In the past decade, substantial interest and work on networks has occurred, which goes well beyond the characterization above as a low level of partnership integration. As for other types of organizational relationships, no consistent definition of organizational networks exists in the literature. Based on an extensive review of organizational networks, Provan, Fish and Sydow propose the concept of **whole networks**, defined as follows, which may provide useful guidance.

> [A whole network is] a group of three or more organizations connected in ways that facilitate achievement of a common goal. That is, the networks we discuss are often formally established and governed and goal directed rather than occurring serendipitously. . . . Relationships among network members are primarily nonhierarchical, and participants often have substantial operating autonomy. Network members can be linked by many types of connections and flows, such as information, materials, financial resources, services, and social support. Connections may be informal and totally trust based or more formalized, as through a contract. Examination and analysis of a whole interorganizational network includes organizations (nodes) and their relationships (ties), the absence of relationships, and the implications of both for achieving outcomes. However, unlike traditional network research, the focus here is on the structures and processes of the entire network rather than on the organizations that compose the network. (Provan et al. 2007, 482)

While networks can be an effective organizational form to advance public health strategy (Riley et al. 2012), developing an evidence base

to examine the influence of organizational networks on population health outcomes presents many challenges. The field has moved from citing limited evidence to demonstrate a positive influence to acknowledging the complexity of the influence and the inappropriateness of research questions and designs that examine only causal relationships (Green and Kreuter 2002). New conceptual frameworks and expectations for organizational networks are needed to correct this mismatch and to understand what it takes to create effective partnerships.

In this chapter, we approach the dilemma of creating effective partnerships by starting with what a partnership is intended to achieve (i.e., functions for population behavior change) and then providing an overview of relevant stakeholders and principles of organizing and operating that will contribute to achieving partnership goals.

Functions of Partnerships to Enhance Population-Level Behavior Change

A significant focus in population behavior change has been on "what works" and, more recently, what results can be achieved under varying circumstances. Comparatively less emphasis has been placed on *how* change happens in communities and other settings. We suggest that *what* and *how* must work in unison in an intentional process of change.

There are many models of planned approaches to change. We present a process with five interacting milestones, which is informed by various theories (e.g., **diffusion of innovations**, **organizational learning**) (Greenhalgh et al. 2004; Greenhalgh et al. 2005; Sanson-Fisher 2004) and procedural models for planning and evaluation (e.g., **RE-AIM** in Glasgow et al. 1999; **PRECEDE-PROCEED** in Green and Kreuter 2005). A fuller description of this process appears elsewhere (Riley et al. 2007).

While the milestones may seem discrete, they typically occur in a nonlinear way, with feedback loops and ongoing **adaptations**. Cutting across all milestones is the importance of involving stakeholders who are affected by the problem or possible solutions. Many of the organizational forms discussed in this chapter are ways to ensure meaningful input from relevant stakeholders.

Milestone 1: Identify Needs and Opportunities

This milestone is about defining the problem and understanding the determinants of the problem. Needs for health behavior change at a population level are most often informed by surveillance data that shows trends over time and in particular populations. This is typically the work of public health epidemiologists. Health problems can also be defined by concerned individuals or groups, who may draw on any combination of information, experience, values, and a deep understanding of the local context. Common **triggers** to initiate action on health problems are health-related events (e.g., heart attack) of an opinion leader or a person who is influential in some way, such as a politician or a school board trustee.

What contributes to the population behavior problem must also be examined, so that interventions are appropriately targeted to issues that require change. This understanding is developed for many health issues in other chapters, along with solutions that are considered most promising to move population behaviors in a positive direction.

There are growing numbers of new partnerships between academics and practitioners in the form of community-based participatory research, or practice-based research networks that are instrumental in assessing needs and opportunities. These partnerships also achieve subsequent milestones, including evaluating programs and services at key stages along the research-to-action or action-to-research continua.

Milestone 2: Scan and Select Intervention Options

Major achievements in this milestone are developing criteria for selecting intervention options and identifying and evaluating intervention options with respect to these criteria.

Processes for scanning and selecting interventions are the subject of considerable reflection in public health (Anderson et al. 2005; Briss et al. 2004). It is now widely acknowledged that the concepts and tools of evidence-based medicine are not appropriate for public health interventions that are more deeply embedded within social, political, economic, organizational, and other contexts. Thus, it is generally accepted that to optimize the impact on desired population behavior change, a wide range of the best available evidence should be considered. To this end, other chapters provide the evidence base for interventions to address specific issues. Existing interventions are a useful starting point, preferably those with demonstrated **effectiveness**, or at least feasibility, **scalability**, and acceptability for particular audiences and settings. New and promising ideas can also emerge.

Partly because of limitations of research (notably, efficacy and effectiveness studies) and the context-**sensitivity** of public health interventions, the debate has broadened regarding factors to consider when selecting interventions. A set of more inclusive criteria includes and goes beyond effectiveness to include plausibility and practicality (Cameron et al. 1998; Swinburn et al. 2005). **Effectiveness** typically assesses through some empirical study whether the intervention did or did not work under real world conditions. **Plausibility** assesses whether an intervention will likely be effective based on its attributes (e.g., content, processes, cultural fit), the probable **reach** of the intervention, and the presence of other complementary interventions or conditions for success. **Practicality** assesses the readiness of the organizational setting and the availability of the necessary technical, financial, and human resources to implement the intervention.

Milestone 3: Build Capacity for Implementation

Building capacity involves mobilizing and developing necessary skills, resources, and conditions for change that include individual capacities, organizational capacities, and a supportive environment (McLean et al. 2005).

Efforts to enhance evidence-based public health have mainly focused on collating, synthesizing, and disseminating evidence (Speller et al. 2005). For the evidence to be used appropriately, various capacities must be present at individual, organizational, and environmental levels. Such capacities have been the topic of considerable research in the last 15 years (e.g., Germann and Wilson 2004; Joffres et al. 2004; NSW Health 2001; Riley et al. 2001). Capacity at the individual level usually refers to knowledge and skills of those individuals responsible for implementation. Capacity at an organizational level typically includes domains such as organizational commitment, culture, structures, processes, and resources. Capacity at the environmental level most often refers to factors such as public opinion, political will, networks, and available information and resources.

Milestone 4: Implement the Interventions

Early and sustained implementation includes **tailoring**, implementing, and adapting interventions and developing organizational routines that support these activities.

Implementing one or more interventions that already exist covers a wide spectrum from straightforward borrowing or adoption of the intervention to substantial **adaptation** so that interventions developed and implemented elsewhere will fit organizational goals and circumstances. By far, adaptation is most common, and it is consistent with the need for interventions to fit local context to have a positive influence (Green 2001; Smedley et al. 2001). A dynamic tension exists, however, between the need for adaptation and the traditional scientific requirement for implementation "fidelity"—or implementing interventions as initially designed. Adaptation typically continues over time as implementation is sustained.

Milestone 5: Monitor and Evaluate

This milestone is grounded in a commitment to learning, and to the obligation to assure that the adaptations that deviate from previously tested evidence-based interventions made to fit the local circumstances still work. It involves relevant **monitoring** and selective **evaluation** studies to improve the implementation and impact of interventions over time. Feedback has a powerful influence on behavior, including behaviors related to implementation of interventions and decisions about sustainability (Bandura 1986; Green and Kreuter 2005). Monitoring and evaluation are well-established tools to provide feedback on circumstances and results. The most useful evaluations will be relevant to intervention decisions; they will be informed by an evidence-informed intervention theory (i.e., assumptions about the change process); they will be guided by all three **selection** criteria for interventions (i.e., effectiveness, plausibility, practicality); and studies will include strong assessments of the implementation process and its interplay with a dynamic context.

Making Partnerships Work

Several factors are critical for making partnerships work (Best and Hall 2006).

Clear, common aims. It often takes time and cycling through direction-setting, action, and trust-building to develop the overarching partnership-level goal, common language, and aims to enable and sustain productive partnership, but investment in good convergence of interests and coordination of goals is essential (Drath et al. 2008; Huxham 2000; Kreuter et al. 2000; Lasker et al. 2001; Provan et al. 2007). Developing shared vision, readiness, and sufficient capacity before launching major initiatives is important (Best and Holmes 2010; Provan et al. 2003), and these call upon participatory planning among the partner organizations (e.g., Best et al. 2003).

Trust. This essential foundation builds on itself over time with success, often starting with modest, low-risk initiatives (Vangen and Huxham 2003).

Collaborative leadership. Effective interorganizational partnership requires sustained, engaged, distributed leadership and accountability and a shift in leadership style from "command and control" leading and managing to facilitating and empowering—from delegation to participation (Best and Holmes 2010; Huxham 2003; Iles and Sutherland 2001; Lomas 1993; Provan and Milward 1995; Provan, Fish, and Sydow 2007; Snowden and Boone 2007; Trochim et al. 2007).

Sensitivity to power issues. In an interorganizational partnership, each partner brings different resources to the table. Effective collaboration requires careful negotiation of expectations and ground rules for decision making (Best and Hall 2006; Butterfoss and Kegler 2002; Greenhalgh et al. 2004; Huxham 2003; Provan and Milward 2001).

Membership structures. Shared understanding about what the collaboration involves and formalized rules, roles, and structures enable participation and strengthen relationships (Butterfoss and Kegler 2002; Huxham 2003; Lipparini and Lomi 1999; Provan et al. 2007). Both governance and task structures are important. The evidence shows the need for effective coordination infrastructure with agreed action strategies and sufficient resources, capacity, and role clarity to support good communication and management functions (Provan and Milward 2001; Provan et al. 2007; Synder and Wenger 2003).

At the same time, increased levels of integration (and conversely, decreased levels of fragmentation) (Provan et al. 2004), coupled with local clustering into dense subnetworks ("small world networks") can be a particularly effective way to organize health systems (Baum et al. 2003; Best and Holmes 2010; Provan and Sebastian 1998). Granovetter's (1985) concept of strength in multiple weak ties highlights the potential value of local clustering into dense subnetworks with short paths and relatively few ties; that can be a particularly effective way to organize. Green (2000) summarized several caveats with regard to coalitions and concluded that a "Noah's Ark Principle of Partnering" (go forth two-by-two after agreement on mission and strategy by the larger coalition) is likely to be a more effective action-stage model than trying to micromanage implementation by large multi-organizational coalitions, insofar as smaller, more flexible groupings are better positioned for action.

Because membership often is dynamic and changing, continuing work is essential to sustain the shared understanding and common focus (Huxham and Vangen 2000). Effective coordination structures speed uptake of **innovations**.

Action learning. Effective collaborations continuously improve through feedback loops and reflective, shared learning (Greenhalgh et al. 2004; Schön 1983; Senge 1990).

Realistic expectations. The mere presence of organizational partnerships cannot be causally linked to changes in health improvements they seek to attain, and partnerships sometimes produce dysfunctional behavior in the planning and implementation process, such as ignoring evidence-based interventions in favor of home-grown interventions without evidence or evaluation (Green and Kreuter 2002; Hallfors et al. 2002). The partners must understand and commit to the need for coordinated and effective interventions across multiple levels of change (e.g., individual, organizational, community) (Best and Holmes 2010), and they must understand, communicate, and evaluate meaningful markers of progress over time.

Understanding of a change process. Organizational partnerships exist to change the status quo. In order to support population behavior change, members must understand and embrace a collective problem-solving process that allows for enhancing evidence-informed practice in one or more topic areas of interest. Robust strategic communication is needed to catalyze, coordinate, and support change (Best and Holmes 2010).

Examples of Partnerships

We now illustrate some of the concepts we have presented, with three examples of organizational partnerships. All of them go beyond the individual issue areas tackled in other chapters and address more comprehensive strategies. They share an objective to link action and science. All illustrations have publicly available evaluations or one or both authors of this chapter were directly involved. Selections also include different types of partnerships, various strengths and challenges, and main lessons that relate to concepts discussed in this chapter.

"Fighting Back" Community Substance Abuse Coalitions

This example is of community-initiated/community-based partnerships. A main contribution from this example is potentially faulty assumptions about community coalitions.

Fighting Back was the largest demonstration program ever of the Robert Wood Johnson Foundation (RWJF); it ran through much of the 1990s (Green and Kreuter 2002; Hallfors et al. 2002). The goal was to reduce the demand for drugs through community coalitions. Local political, business, and grassroots leaders were to come together to assess the substance abuse problems in their respective communities and to develop a comprehensive, coordinated re-

sponse. A comprehensive response was to include public awareness, prevention, **targeting** especially children and youth, early identification and intervention, environmental improvement, treatment, and relapse prevention. Taken together, the strategies were intended to change community norms, organizational policies, and individual behaviors. They were to be designed based on local context and needs.

Fourteen communities, all midsized (ranging from 100,000 to 250,000 residents) and both urban and rural, participated in Fighting Back. An extensive evaluation involving 12 of the communities examined the extent to which coalitions attained selected substance abuse goals. The evaluation used a prospective design with two to three demographically similar comparison communities for each Fighting Back community and extensive quantitative and qualitative methods. None of the three hypotheses were supported: strategy outcomes were not shown to correlate positively with specific targets, sites that had more comprehensive programs were not shown to have better outcomes, and sites with higher dose strategies did not have better outcomes. The overall conclusion from the evaluation was that "comprehensive community coalitions are intuitively attractive and politically unpopular, but the potential for adverse effects must be considered" (Hallfors et al. 2002, 237).

In their review of the Fighting Back evaluation, Green and Kreuter (2002) suggest significant cautions about **quasi-experimental** designs that make erroneous or at least untested assumptions about coalitions. For example, coalitions were used as the independent variable and were expected to result in community-wide changes in substance use and abuse. Starting in the 1980s, the literature began to suggest that such inflated expectations of community coalitions were faulty. It was increasingly recognized that much more needed to be learned about the forms of partnerships and coalitions that may be most useful for different purposes.

Another challenge noted by Green and Kreuter (2002) was the relative absence of a research utilization focus within the Fighting Back coalitions that would help to blend practice-based and academic research-based evidence with decision making about local priorities and strategies. The communities generally preferred homegrown interventions to evidence-based interventions, rather than starting with the evidence-based interventions and adapting them to the local situation. The next illustration gives much more emphasis to the research focus.

Prevention Research Centers

This illustration is an example of university-based research centers intended to focus on practice-based research in partnership with communities. The promise of this approach is a high potential for research that is relevant to practice and linking innovative approaches across centers from different jurisdictions with diverse contexts.

In 1986, the Centers for Disease Control and Prevention (CDC) funded the first three university-based Centers for Research and Demonstration of Health Promotion and Disease Prevention, later known as Prevention Research Centers (PRCs) (Green 2007; Green and Stoto 1997; Stoto et al. 1997). Ten years later, the number of centers had grown to 14. PRCs were intended to be the public health equivalent of Practice-Based Research Networks in primary care. The mandate of PRCs included providing the public health community with workable strategies to address major public health problems.

One of the early **consequences** of the PRCs was what was referred to as "academic drift," which was at least in part due to **incentives** for academics (Green and Stoto 1997; Stoto et al. 1997). As funder, the CDC intervened to ensure a sustained focus on practical solutions. An important and enduring role for the CDC is to pro-vide strong influence by steering and coordinating functions, especially given academic reward structures that bias toward academic goals rather than practical solutions.

As the numbers of PRCs continued to grow, an intentional learning agenda with more emphasis from the CDC on participatory research helped inform and facilitate university-community partnerships that hold promise for more practical purposes.

Canadian Heart Health Initiative

The Canadian Heart Health Initiative (CHHI) (Naylor et al. 2002; Riley et al. 2009) is an example of multilevel, multisectoral partnerships. The CHHI was initiated by the federal government, in partnership with provincial governments through negotiated federal-provincial agreements. The CHHI illustrates the interdependence of partnerships at different levels—local, provincial, national, and international—and the complementary contributions from each level.

The purpose of the CHHI was to develop and disseminate programs and policies that would improve health at a population level. Building capacity to better link research and evaluation with public health policy and practice was central to the CHHI. The initiative was pan-Canadian, and it involved both health and nonhealth sectors. An international community of countrywide initiatives to prevent and reduce noncommunicable disease focused on policy development. Across Canada, a national coalition brought together provincial investigators from research, policy, and practice sectors. These cross-sector partnerships were mirrored at provincial and local levels.

The CHHI provided many lessons related to organizational partnerships and coalitions, including formation, operations, and outcomes. Lessons included the importance of government commitment to coalitions, champions at multiple levels within the public health system, and facilitative leadership. The CHHI informed dialogue about realistic expectations and the importance of capacity building at organizational and system levels. The initiative also revealed many barriers to sustaining activity and "**scaling up**" without systemic changes within the public health system.

Conclusion

This chapter reveals many key issues and lessons related to stakeholders and organizational relationships for population health behavior change:

- Along with a shift in focus from individual behavior change to population behavior change, the program emphasizes collective action.
- Collective action, primarily in the form of community mobilization, has a very long and rich history in public health, including campaigns for hygiene (pre-1950s), immunization and family planning (1950s and 1960s), and community-based programs to address widespread problems, such as tobacco, injury, cardiovascular disease and substance abuse (1970s and on).
- An ecological view of health behavior provides a rationale for the importance of organizational action, including organizational partnerships.
- Application of ecological approaches has usefully reinforced the need for multiple levels of influence (e.g., individual, organization, community, state/province) and multiple strategies (e.g., education, policy, media). Little attention has been focused on the relationships of interventions within and across levels and implications for organizational partnerships, although such relationships fall within the scope of **ecological models**.
- Complexity and other forms of **systems thinking** help to address the limited ways in

which ecological intervention models have been applied, and these are major drivers for organizational partnerships today.
- This "complexity imperative" understands population and public health problems (e.g., obesity, tobacco) as complex, with multiple influences operating in dynamic, nonlinear ways. Solutions also need to be understood and advanced using principles and practices of complexity.
- Some implications of a complex worldview for organizational partnerships include shared accountability, interplay of many organizational forms (e.g., communities of practice, joint ventures, citizen participation), and challenges with attribution of outcomes to, accountability of, and visibility of individual organizations.
- Another main partnership driver today is evolving models of knowledge translation (Brownson et al. 2012; Meissner et al. 2013). Thinking about knowledge translation has evolved from linear to relationship to systems models. The latter are particularly relevant to population health behavior change and emphasize considerations such as external validity, relevance, and adaptability.
- Historical developments and present-day drivers have resulted in many types of organizational forms (e.g., communities of practice, networks, coalitions, alliances, task forces, etc). Different forms are sometimes distinguished by the strength of ties among organizations, often referred to as levels of integration (e.g., from networking to collaboration). The learning agenda needs to include improved understanding of levels of integration that best serve varied purposes (e.g., educational and advocacy or policy change objectives) and that best serve organizational goals.
- The goal of population health behavior change is best achieved using a collaborative, planned approach, co-designed by

partnership members, that (1) identifies needs and opportunities; (2) scans and selects intervention options; (3) builds capacity for implementation; (4) initiates and sustains implementation; and (5) monitors, evaluates, and incorporates feedback.

- This change process requires a wide array of content knowledge, skills, and resources. These contributions may be provided by a range of stakeholders, defined by sector (i.e., government, nongovernment, private) or by function (e.g., research, technical assistance, public health services).
- Based on results from an extensive review, critical success factors for partnerships include the following:
  - Clear common aims
  - Trust
  - Collaborative leadership
  - Sensitivity to power issues
  - Membership structures
  - Action learning
  - Realistic expectations
  - Understanding of a change process

Many experiential and empirical lessons continue to enrich our understanding of the character, functions, and consequences of organizational partnerships. For example, we learned about unrealistic expectations of community coalitions, corresponding ill-suited approaches to evaluation, and limits to community-driven coalitions through the RWJF Fighting Back community substance abuse coalitions. We learned about the potential "academic drift" and strategies to support more practical science through the CDC PRCs. And we learned about the practice of multilevel and multisectoral partnerships and the importance of capacity building and change at organizational and system levels through the CHHI.

To apply state-of-the-evidence in specific areas of health behavior, we must also apply state-of-the-evidence in organizational partnerships. An eclectic evidence base, including theory, empirical studies, and experience, suggests some promising directions for advancing the science and practice of organizational partnerships for population health behavior change. We describe three directions.

A first direction is to *develop a robust action learning agenda* for organizational partnerships that support population health behavior change. Even within the very modest amount of research that focuses on population health interventions, most studies explore the effectiveness of educational or environmental change initiatives. Useful complementary research would examine the interorganizational forms that enable appropriate design, implementation, evaluation, and adaptation of initiatives over time. Future studies should also aim to build a deeper and more nuanced understanding of benefits and drawbacks for different organizational partners and desired and unintended consequences of organizational partnerships. The context or circumstances under which various consequences are experienced must be a central focus, consistent with the complexity imperative.

Second, *conceptual models for organizational partnerships specific to population health behavior change need to be strengthened*. Butterfoss and Kegler (2002) provide one example, with a synthesis of theoretical and empirical work on community coalitions. This chapter provides another example, emphasizing the many and varied organizational forms that need to be considered. It also highlights concepts such as collaborative governance, shared accountability, and organizational identity that need to be more prominent in guiding research and practice in organizational design. The evolution of conceptual models for knowledge translation over the past 15 years provides a useful parallel to how work on organizational design could unfold, with a similar emphasis on complexity and other schools of systems thinking (see chapter 21; Brownson et al. 2012; Meissner et al. 2013).

A third direction is to *ensure a systemic approach to change that spans research, policy, and practice institutions.* Practice to date has typically been to provide relatively short-term (up to five years) incentives to form partnerships that are expected to address complex and widespread health problems. These efforts will be quicker to launch and more enduring if incentives (e.g., mandates and reward structures) encourage collective action that effectively links evidence and action. For the research community, relevant, practical, and solution-oriented science needs to be rewarded. For the policy and practice community, evidence-informed action and learning need to be rewarded.

An orientation toward systemic approaches or system transformation has currency internationally. Within Canada, one example is the Population Health Intervention Research Initiative for Canada (PHIRIC). In 2006, PHIRIC was conceived as a 10-year initiative to increase the quantity, quality, and use of population health intervention science. Colleagues from research, policy, and practice organizations meet regularly to strategize levers and priorities for change, such as academic reward structures, research funding mechanisms, and graduate student training.

If the goal is to apply the best available evidence to achieve population-level impact, more emphasis needs to be directed to the science and practice of organizational partnerships. Complexity and other forms of systems thinking are providing impetus and insight for next-generation approaches.

REFERENCES

Anderson LM, Brownson RC, Fullilove MT, et al. 2005. Evidence-based public health policy and practice: Promises and limits. *Am J Prev Med* 28 (suppl. 5): 226–30.

Bailey D, Koney K. 2000. *Strategic Alliances among Health and Human Services Organizations: From Affiliations to Consolidations.* Abridged. Thousand Oaks, CA: Sage.

Bandura A. 1986. *Social Foundations of Thought and Action: A Social Cognition Theory.* Englewood Cliffs, NJ: Prentice-Hall.

Barwick MA, Boydell KM, Stasiulis E, Ferguson HB, Blase K, Fixsen D. 2008. Research utilization among children's mental health providers. *Implement Sci* 3:19.

Baum JAC, Shipilov A, Rowley T. 2003. Where do small worlds come from? *Ind Corp Change* 12 (4): 697–725.

Best A, Hall N. 2006. *Rapid Review on Interorganizational Partnerships.* Vancouver, BC: HealthShares.

Best A, Hiatt RA, Norman CD. 2008. Knowledge integration: Conceptualizing communications in cancer control systems. *Patient Educ Couns* 71:319–27.

Best A, Holmes B. 2010. Systems thinking, knowledge, and action: Towards better models and methods. *Evidence and Policy* 6 (2): 145–59.

Best A, Stokols D, Green LW, Leischow S, Holmes B, Buchholz K. 2003. Health promotion and community partnering: Translating theory into effective strategy. *Am J Health Promot* 18 (2): 168–76.

Best A, Terpstra JL, Moor G, Riley B, Norman CD, Glasgow RE. 2009. Building knowledge integration systems for evidence-informed decisions. *J Health Org Man* 23 (6): 627–41.

Best A, Trochim W, Moor G, Haggerty J, Norman C. 2008. Systems thinking for knowledge integration: New models for policy-research collaboration. In *Organizing and Reorganizing: Power and Change in Health Care Organizations,* ed. E Ferlie, P Hyde, L McKee. London: Routledge.

Blackburn GL, Walker WA. 2005. Science-based solutions to obesity: What are the roles of academia, government, industry, and health care? *Am J Clin Nutr* 82 (suppl. 1): 207S–210S.

Bracht N. 1990. *Health Promotion at the Community Level.* Newbury Park, CA: Sage.

Briss PA, Brownson RC, Fielding JE, Zaza S. 2004. Developing and using the Guide to Community Preventive Services: Lessons learned about evidence-based public health. *Annu Rev Public Health* 25: 281–302.

Brownson R, Colditz G, Parker E, eds. 2012. *Dissemination and Implementation Research: Translating Science to Practice.* New York: Oxford University Press.

Butterfoss FD. 2004. The coalition technical assistance and training framework: Helping community coalitions help themselves. *Health Promot Pract* 5 (2): 118–26.

Butterfoss F, Kegler M. 2002. Towards a comprehensive understanding of community coalitions: Moving from practice to theory. In *Emerging Theories in Health Promotion Practice and Research,* ed. R DiClemente, R Crosby, M Kegler, 194–227. San Francisco: Jossey-Bass.

Cameron R, Walker R, Jolin MA. 1998. *International Best Practices in Heart Health.* Toronto: Ontario Public Health Association.

Catford J. 2009. Advancing the "science of delivery" of health promotion: Not just the "science of discovery." *Health Promot Int* 24 (1): 1-5.

Cilliers P. 1998. *Complexity and Post Modernism: Understanding Complex Systems*. New York: Routledge.

Crampton P, Starfield B. 2004. A case for government ownership of primary care services in New Zealand: Weighing the arguments. *Int J Health Serv* 34 (4): 709-27.

Crilly T, Jashapara A, Ferlie E. 2009. Research utilisation and knowledge mobilisation: A scoping review of the literature. National Institute for Health Research Service Delivery and Organisation, London.

Davies H, Nutley S, Walter I. 2008. Why "knowledge transfer" is misconceived for applied social research. *J Health Serv Res Policy* 13:188-90.

Drath W, McCauley CD, Pauls J, Van Velsor E, O'Connor PMG, McGuire JB. 2008. Direction, alignment, commitment: Toward a more integrative ontology of leadership. *Leadership Quart* 19:635-53.

Forster R, Gabe J. 2008. Voice or choice? Patient and public involvement in the National Health Service in England under New Labour. *Int J Health Serv* 38 (2): 333-56.

Frenck J. 1992. Balancing relevance and excellence: Organizational responses to link research with decision-making. *Soc Sci Med* 35:1397-1404.

Gajda R. 2004. Utilizing collaboration theory to evaluate strategic alliances. *Am J Eval* 25 (1): 65-77.

Garcia J, Dorohovich M. 2007. The truth about building and maintaining successful communities of practice. *Defense Acq Rev J* 12 (1): 19-33.

Germann K, Wilson D. 2004. Organizational capacity for community development in regional health authorities: A conceptual model. *Health Promot Int* 19 (3): 289-98.

Glasgow RE, Emmons KM. 2007. How can we increase translation of research into practice? Types of evidence needed. *Annu Rev Public Health* 28:413-33.

Glasgow RE, Vogt TM, Boles SM. 1999. Evaluating the public health impact of health promotion interventions: The RE-AIM framework. *Am J Public Health* 89 (9): 1322-27.

Golden SD, Earp JA. 2012. Social ecological approaches to individuals and their contexts: Twenty years of *Health Education and Behavior* Health Promotion Interventions. *Health Educ Behav* 39 (3): 364-72.

Graham ID, Logan J, Harrison MB, et al. 2006. Lost in knowledge translation: Time for a map? *J Contin Educ Health Prof* 26: 13-24.

Granovetter M. 1985. Economic action and social structure: The problem of embeddedness. *Am J Soc* 91 (3): 481-510.

Green LW. 1994. Refocusing health care systems to address both individual care and population health. *Clin Invest Med* 17 (2): 133-41.

———. 2000. Commentary: Caveats on coalitions: In praise of partnerships. *Health Promot Practice* 1:64-65.

———. 2001. From research to "best practices" in other settings and populations. *Am J Health Behav* 25 (3): 165-78.

———. 2006. Public health asks of systems science: To advance our evidence-based practice, can you help us get more practice-based evidence? *Am J Public Health* 96 (3): 406-9.

———. 2007. The Prevention Research Centers as models of practice-based evidence: Two decades on. *Am J Prev Med* 33 (1 suppl.): S6-S8.

Green LW, Glasgow RE. 2006. Evaluating the relevance, generalization, and applicability of research: Issues in external validation and translation methodology. *Eval and Health Profess* 29 (1): 126-53.

Green LW, Glasgow RE, Atkins D, Stange K. 2009. Making evidence from research more relevant, useful, and actionable in policy, program planning, and practice: Slips "twixt cup and lip." *Am J Prev Med* 37 (6S1): S187-S191.

Green LW, Kreuter MW. 2002. Fighting back or fighting themselves? Community coalitions against substance abuse and their use of best practices? *Am J Prev Med* 23 (4): 303-6.

———. 2005. *Health Program Planning: An Educational and Ecological Approach*. 4th ed. New York: McGraw-Hill.

Green LW, Ottoson JM, Garcia C, Hiatt R. 2009. Diffusion theory and knowledge dissemination, utilization, and integration in public health. *Annu Rev Public Health* 30:151-74.

Green LW, Stoto MA. 1997. Commentary: Linking research and public health practice: A vision for health promotion and disease prevention research. In *Research Linkages between Academia and Public Health Practice*, guest ed. CG Healton, TE Novotny. Oxford: Oxford University Press. Supplement to *Am J Prev Med* 13 (6): 5-8.

Greenhalgh T, Collard A, Begum N. 2005. Sharing stories: Complex intervention for diabetes education in minority ethnic groups who do not speak English. *Br Med J* 330 (7492): 628.

Greenhalgh T, Robert G, Macfarlane F, Bate P, Kyriakidou O. 2004. Diffusion of innovations in service organizations: Systematic review and recommendations. *Milbank Q* 82: 581-629.

Hallfors D, Cho H, Livert D, Kadushin C. 2002. Fighting back against substance abuse: Are community coalitions winning? *Am J Prev Med* 23 (4): 237-45.

Hogue T. 1993. Community-based collaboration: Community wellness multiplied. Oregon Center for Community Leadership, Oregon State University, http://crs.uvm.edu/nnco/collab/wellness.html (accessed Jan. 24 2001).

Holmes BJ, Finegood DT, Riley BL, Best A. 2012. Systems thinking in dissemination and implementation research. In *Dissemination and Implementation Research in Health: Translating Science to Practice,* ed. R Brownson, G Colditz, E Proctor. New York: Oxford University Press.

Huxham C. 2000. The challenge of collaborative governance. *Pub Man* 2:337-57.

———. 2003. Theorizing collaboration practice. *Pub Man Rev* 5: 401-23.

Huxham C, Vangen S. 2000. Ambiguity, complexity, and dynamics in the membership of collaboration. *Human Rel* 53:771-806.

Iles V, Sutherland K. 2001. *Organizational Change: A Review for Health Care Managers, Professionals, and Researchers.* London: National Co-ordinating Centre for NHS Service Delivery and Organization.

Institute of Medicine. 2010. *Bridging the Evidence Gap in Obesity Prevention.* Washington, DC: National Academies Press.

———. 2012. *Accelerating Progress on Obesity Prevention.* Washington, DC: National Academies Press.

Joffres C, Heath S, Farquharson J, Barkhouse K, Latter C, MacLean DR. 2004. Facilitators and challenges to organizational capacity building in heart health promotion. *Qual Health Res* 14 (1): 39-60.

Kok G, Gottlieb NH, Commers M, Smerecnik C. 2008. The ecological approach in health promotion programs: A decade later. *Am J Health Promot* 22:437-42.

Kreuter MW, De Rosa C, Howze EH, Baldwin GT. 2004 Understanding wicked problems: A key to advancing environmental health promotion. *Health Educ Behav* 31:441-54.

Kreuter MW, Lezin N, Young L. 2000. Evaluating community based collaborative mechanisms: Implications for practitioners. *Health Promot Practice* 1:49-63.

Lasker RD, Weiss ES, Miller R, Community-Campus Partnerships for Health. 2001. Promoting collaborations that improve health. *Educ Health (Abingdon)* 14 (2): 163-72.

Lipparini A, Lomi A. 1999. Interorganizational relations in the Modena biomedical industry: A case study. In *Interfirm Networks: Organization and Industrial Competitiveness,* ed. A. Grandori. 120-50. London: Routledge.

Lohmann RA. 1992. *The Commons: New Perspectives on Nonprofit Organizations and Voluntary Action.* San Francisco: Jossey-Bass.

Lomas J. 1993. Diffusion, dissemination, and implementation: Who should do what? *Ann NY Acad Sciences* 703:226-35.

———. 2007. Decision support: A new approach to making the best healthcare management and policy choices. *Healthcare Q* 10:16-18.

McLean S, Feather J, Butler-Jones D. 2005. *Building Health Promotion Capacity: Action for Learning, Learning from Action.* 1st ed. Vancouver, Canada: UBC Press.

Meissner HI, Glasgow RE, Vinson CA, et al. 2013. The U.S. training institute for dissemination and implementation research in health. *Implement Sci* 8 (12). Available at www.implementationscience.org (accessed June 15, 2013).

Mittelmark MB, Hunt MK, Heath GW, Schmidt TL. 1993. Realistic outcomes: Lessons from community-based research and demonstration programs for the prevention of cardiovascular disease. *J Public Health Policy* 14 (4): 437-62.

Moynihan DP. 1969. *Maximum Feasible Misunderstanding: Community Action in the War on Poverty.* New York: Free Press.

Naylor P, Wharf-Higgins J, Blair L, Green LW, O'Connor B. 2002. Evaluating the participatory process in a community-based heart health project. *Soc Sci Med* 55 (7): 1173-87.

New South Wales Health Department (NSW Health). 2001. A framework for building capacity to improve health. NSW Health Department, Sydney, Australia.

Nonaka I, Toyama R, Konno N. 2000. SECI, *Ba,* and leadership: A unified model of dynamic knowledge creation. *Long Range Plan* 33:5-34.

Peterson NL. 1991. Interagency collaboration under Part H: The key to comprehensive, multidisciplinary, coordinated infant/toddler intervention services. *J Early Interven* 15:89-105.

Provan KG, Fish A, Sydow J. 2007. Interorganizational networks at the network level: A review of the empirical literature on whole networks *J Man* 33:479-516.

Provan KG, Isett KR, Milward HB. 2004. Cooperation and compromise: Conflicting institutional pressures on interorganizational collaboration. *Nonprofit Volunt Sect Q* 33 (3): 489-514.

Provan KG, Milward HB. 1995. A preliminary theory of interorganizational network effectiveness: A comparative study of four community mental health systems. *Admin Science Q* 40:1-33.

———. 2001. Do networks really work? A framework for evaluating public-sector organizational networks. *Pub Admin Rev* 61 (4): 414-23.

Provan KG, Nakama L, Veazie MA, Teufel-Shone NI, Huddleston C. 2003. Building community capacity

around chronic disease services through a collaborative interorganizational network. *Health Educ Behav*
30 (6): 646-62.

Provan KG, Sebastian JG. 1998. Networks within
networks: Service link overlap, organizational
cliques, and network effectiveness. *Acad Man J*
41:453-63.

Richard L, Potvin L, Kishchuck N, Prlic H, Green LW.
1996. Assessment of the integration of the ecological
approach in health promotion programs. *Am J Health
Promot* 10:318-28.

Riley BL, Garcia J, Edwards N. 2007. Organizational
change for obesity prevention—perspectives,
possibilities, and potential pitfalls. In *Obesity Epidemiology and Prevention: A Handbook,* ed. S Kumanyika, RC
Brownson. New York: Springer.

Riley BL, Norman CD, Best A. 2012. Knowledge
integration in public health: A rapid review using
systems thinking. *Evidence and Policy* 8 (4): 417-32.

Riley B, Stachenko S, Wilson E, et al. 2009. Can the
Canadian Heart Health Initiative inform the
population health intervention research initiative for
Canada? *Can J Publ Health* 100 (1): i20-i26.

Riley BL, Taylor SM, Elliott SJ. 2001. Determinants of
implementing heart health: Promotion activities in
Ontario public health units: A social ecological
perspective. *Health Educ Res* 16 (4): 425-41.

Roberts J. 2004. *Alliances, Coalitions, and Partnerships;
Building Collaborative Organizations.* Toronto, ON: New
Society.

Rosen G. 1993. *A History of Public Health.* Baltimore:
Johns Hopkins University Press.

Rychetnik L, Frommer M, Hawe P, Shiell A. 2002.
Criteria for evaluating evidence on public health
interventions. *J Epidemiol Commun Health* 56 (2): 119-27.

Sanson-Fisher RW. 2004. Diffusion of innovation theory
for clinical change. *Med J Aust* 180 (6): 55.

Schön D 1983. *The Reflective Practitioner.* New York: Basic
Books.

Senge PM. 1990. *The Fifth Discipline.* New York:
Doubleday.

Smedley BD, Syme SL, Committee on Capitalizing on
Social Science and Behavioral Research to Improve
the Public's Health. 2001. Promoting health:
Intervention strategies from social and behavioral
research. *Am J Health Promot* 15 (3): 149-66.

Snowden DJ, Boone ME. 2007. A leader's framework for
decision-making. *Harvard Bus Rev* 85 (11): 68-76.

Speller V, Wimbush E, Morgan A. 2005. Evidence-based
health promotion practice: How to make it work.
Promot Educ (suppl. 1), 15-20.

Stewart M. 2001. Towards a global definition of
patient centred care: The patient should be the
judge of patient centred care. *Br Med J* 322 (7284):
444-45.

Stoto MA, Green LW, Bailey LA, eds. 1997. *Linking
Research and Public Health Practice: A Review of CDC's
Program of Centers for Research and Demonstration of
Health Promotion and Disease Prevention.* Washington,
DC: National Academy Press.

Swinburn B, Gill T, Kumanyika S. 2005. Obesity
prevention: A proposed framework for translating
evidence into action. *Obesity Rev* 6 (1): 23-33.

Synder W, Wenger E. 2003. *Communities of practice in
government: The case for sponsorship.* Washington, DC:
Council of Chief Information Officers.

Trochim W, Cabrera D, Tenkasi R, et al. 2007. How we
organize: Purposeful adaptive systems. In *Transform-
ing Tobacco Control through Systems Thinking: Integrating
Research and Practice to Improve Outcomes*, ed. A Best,
P Clark, S Leischow, W Trochim. Smoking and
Tobacco Control Monograph 18, Bethesda, MD:
National Institutes of Health.

Truman BI, Smith-Akin CK, Hinman AR, et al. 2000.
Developing the guide to community preventive
services—overview and rationale. *Am J Prev Med* 18
(suppl. 1): 18-26.

Van de Ven AH, Johnson PE. 2006. Knowledge for
theory and practice. *Acad Man Rev* 31:802-21.

Vangen S, Huxham C. 2003. Nurturing collaborative
relations: Building trust in interorganizational
collaboration. *J Applied Behav Science* 39:5-31.

CHAPTER 5

Program Planning for Health Behavior Change Interventions

CAROLYN J. CUMPSTY-FOWLER AND
SCOTT KAHAN

LEARNING OBJECTIVES

After completing the chapter, the reader will be able to

* Appreciate the importance of program planning as a prerequisite for implementing health behavior change interventions.
* Recognize the ethics involved in health interventions and be familiar with the ethics framework for public health action described in this chapter.
* Understand the importance of planning models to guide the program planning process.
* Describe the PRECEDE-PROCEED planning model, which is covered in some depth in this chapter.
* Describe the phases and steps of program planning to guide the approach to health behavior change interventions.

Introduction

Planning is not a single action; it is a process. How often have we heard the Lao-Tzu quotation "A journey of a thousand miles begins with a single step"? The implied message is *Don't just stand there, do something.* Or should we? A more recent translation, "A journey of a thousand miles begins at the spot under one's feet; therefore deal with things before they happen; create order before there is confusion," encourages restraint.[1] The journey motif appears frequently in discussions of planning (Freire and Runyan 2006; Gielen et al. 2008; Green and Kreuter 2005). Successful journeys require a clear sense of purpose and destination, careful planning that considers **context** and resources, reflective travel, flexibility, and the ability to appreciate lessons and skills learned along the way. This list is important because "the actual journey rarely mirrors the imagined one" (Freire and Runyan 2006, 127). In this chapter, we will walk readers through the hypothetical program-planning journey. We posit that becoming comfortable with the inevitability of encountering something unexpected helps program planners respond thoughtfully to such surprises.

Health is a **complex** construct. While an individual's decision to adopt a healthful behavior or lifestyle is usually or mostly voluntary, it is never simple. **Health-behavior**-related choices are influenced not only by dynamic social, political, physical, and economic factors, but also by culture and history (Green and Kreuter 1999, 2005).[2] A central tenet of health promotion planning, therefore, is that behavior change requires the voluntary participation of the intended audience, whether an individual, a group, or a population (Glanz and Rimer 2005, 39–43; Green and Kreuter 1999, 506; 2005, G-4). However, given such audience diversity, the importance of audience-specific behavior change **interventions** is apparent. Why would any individual or group accustomed to determining their lifestyle and health-related practices buy into a generic behavior change program? Peter Drucker's much-quoted advice: *"The aim of marketing is to know the customer so well that the product or service fits him* [or her or them] *and sells itself"* (Drucker 1973, 64–65) is equally germane in health promotion. No problem has only one solution; one-size-fits-all interventions seldom work for populations any more than for individuals (Glanz and Rimer 2005; Green and Kreuter 2005). Abraham Maslow cautioned: "If you only have a hammer, you tend to see every problem as a nail." Similarly, Green warns of the risks of **"grab-bag" syndrome** (Green and Kreuter 1991, 25), that is, selecting nonstrategic intervention approaches because they are compatible with the program planner's previous experience, preferred approaches, or skill set.

To be successful, health promotion planning must respect the importance of context. It must also represent an active collaboration between the program and the participants. As Green explains, this is a pragmatic rather than a philosophical view: "The cumulative evidence from decades of research in education and other fields tells us that the durability of cognitive and behavioral changes depends on the degree of active rather than passive participation of the learner" (Green and Kreuter 1991, 20). Program journeys should not begin with a hasty, uninformed step by the program planner, but rather with reflection, observation, and informed, collaborative decision making.

Skeptics may dismiss planning as the preliminary busywork that delays the "real work" of program delivery; unfortunately, a rush to action may condemn a program to failure. An ounce of planning can prevent a pound of misguided action. If the only cost of program failure were our own frustration, failure to plan would be less damaging. Unfortunately, potential harm as well as waste may result from inappropriate or inadequately implemented interventions. Planning, therefore, is an ethical responsibility. "First, do no harm" is a central concept in medicine. It would be unethical if patients presenting to an emergency room received treatment uninformed by a careful assessment of the current status and history and by medical knowledge and delivered without regard for unintended risk, process, timing, or dose. Why then are inadequately informed and planned behavior change programs tolerated? In 2001, bioethicist Nancy Kass provided a six-question ethics framework for public health action:

- What are the public health **goals** of the proposed program?
- How effective is the program in achieving its stated goals?
- What are the known or potential burdens of the program?

- Can burdens be minimized? Are there alternative approaches?
- Is the program implemented fairly?
- How can the benefits and burdens of a program be fairly balanced? (Kass 2001)

The time to ask—and answer—these questions is during planning. For example, planners must question during the planning process whether a program can be effective or implemented fairly, not after implementation when the damage has already been done. Learning to ask the right questions of the right people may be the most important skill a health-behavior-change professional must learn. We cannot ask or answer questions in isolation; we must involve other people, especially our intended audience. This, together with having the persistence and humility to obtain and be informed by the answers, is essential to informed decision making. Planning must be a systematic process of inquiry that respects and engages **key stakeholders** from the very beginning (Gielen et al. 2008; Green and Kreuter 2005; see note 2 to the current chapter) and recognizes that individuals and communities deserve better than programs based on what Boorstin called "an illusion of knowledge."[3]

In this chapter, readers will discover that the quality of planning has far-reaching **consequences**, not only for achieving the desired behavior change, but also for our ability to evaluate and sustain outcomes. The challenge that every behavior change program planner faces is how to identify the questions that will correctly inform the program. The danger is that our questioning is limited. We are guided by personal opinion or assumptions and inhibited when we do not know what we do not know. Engaging with **stakeholders** during the planning process is both informative and protective. Through active listening to the community, we can become more aware not only of our assumptions, but also of the other people with whom we should be talking to gain greater

knowledge. Browne and Keeley have this to say about critical thinking: "We move forward by interacting attentively with other people; without them we are lost as learners. Critical thinking relies heavily on being able to listen with respect to what others have to say" (2011, 9). Not asking questions, asking the wrong questions, and asking questions of the wrong people are expensive errors that can be avoided with careful, thoughtful, participatory assessment. Assessment is a core public health function and a fundamental building block of program planning (Green and Kreuter 2005; IOM 2010). Community health assessment recognizes that communities (and individuals) have both needs and assets; they also have preexisting preferences and priorities (Green and Kreuter 2005; NCPHO 2010). Once again, a formative assessment is useful only if the right questions are asked and answered. Questions such as "What is the problem?" or "What must be done to change behavior?" seldom have obvious answers, and the best *possible* evidence is seldom available. Nevertheless, such questions must be answered with the best *available* evidence (IOM 2010). All behaviors—from risky to health promoting—result from a complex interaction of factors. At first glance, an overweight child, a teenager who engages in unprotected sex, a pregnant woman who continues to smoke, a busy executive who texts while driving, and an elderly man who refuses to manage his type 2 diabetes may be labeled as sharing a common trait: "This individual makes poor choices." Faced with this assumption, common responses include: "If people knew better, they would choose healthful behaviors"; "If they really wanted to change, they would"; "If they had a little willpower, they would change"; and "If they're only harming themselves, let them get on with it." If an individual's choices endanger others, society may be more willing to respond with policy and penalties, but the focus remains on the individual. Until we move our focus beyond the individual's choices and actions to include behavioral and environmental precursors, we may overlook important, modifiable risk and protective factors A similar change in focus can move our thinking from "What is going wrong?" and "What is the problem we need to change?" to "What is going right?" and "How did that happen?" This is the approach adopted by proponents of **positive deviance** (see positivedeviance.org). Jerry Sternin, a pioneer of the positive-deviance approach, describes the power of the "somersault question" that "turns circular logic on its head by looking at an issue the other way around" (Pascale et al. 2010, 29–30). In 1990 Sternin was director of a resource-challenged Save the Children program to address childhood malnutrition in poor Vietnamese villages. He explains that until the questions "somersaulted" away from questions about poverty and malnutrition, the solution was obscured. The question that led to Sternin's self-described epiphany was this: "Do you mean it's possible today for a very, very poor child in this village to be well nourished?" (30). It was. Sternin recognized that the solution to malnutrition already existed in "bright spots" within the village; it lay in the wisdom and child-feeding behaviors of the mothers of well-nourished children. He learned—and the positive-deviance approach is now based on repeated observations of this— that "in every community there are certain individuals or groups whose uncommon behaviors and strategies enable them to find better solutions to problems than their peers, *while having access to the same resources and facing similar or worse challenges.* The Positive Deviance approach is an asset-based, problem-solving, and community-driven approach that enables the community to discover these successful behaviors and strategies and develop a plan of action to promote their adoption by all concerned" (positivedeviance.org; emphasis added).

The take-home message for planners is the need to understand the full range of contextual factors: the *bright spots* as well as the challenging needs, the possible solutions as well as the problems, the resilient people and groups as well as those who are apparently defeated. The value of building strategic community **partnerships** to accomplish this understanding cannot be overstated; it is discussed fully in chapter 4. Planners who identify and understand both positive and negative social-ecological **influences** on the behaviors they wish to change will be able to make more informed diagnoses, identify potential solutions, and understand which behavior change theories are appropriate to the program. The use of **theory** in health behavior change programs is discussed in chapter 2. This applies both to problem theories (which help us understand the causal factors, or **determinants**, associated with a health behavior problem or its effects) and **causal theories** (which explain the mechanism by which a determinant influences the effect) (Green and Kreuter 2005, 199). Determinants may be biological or behavioral; they may be found in the proximal physical and **social environment** or located more distally, such as social policies and access to health care. Not all determinants are causal. **Key determinants** (or critical factors) may cause the problem; influence the recognition of the problem; or predispose, enable, or reinforce the problem or **proximal determinants**.

Planning methods vary from program to program. Indeed, planning may be recklessly unstructured or so complex that the means obscure the ends. The *quantity* of planning does not reflect the *quality* of the planning. In this chapter, quality is interpreted as the relevance, accuracy, timeliness, and utility of the information. Specifically, the quality of program planning depends on the relevance of questions asked, the accuracy and relevance of information collected, the planning team's willingness to be informed by it, and a healthy mistrust of assumptions. Expert planners need to be collaborative with other disciplines and with those who live with the problem for which a program is being planned. They need to be adaptable and know the importance of curiosity, collaboration, humility, persistence, and restraint. Above all, as emphasized previously, planners must learn to ask—and find answers for—the right questions.

But how do we know we are asking the right questions?

Using Planning Models to Guide the Planning Process

Logic models and planning models are similar but complementary. Although some see them as the same, we suggest that a logic model shows the presumed relationships between causes and effects; a planning model is a procedural model that adds steps in diagnosing or assessing the causes, guiding the information gathering and therefore improving the thinking process. This, as will be discussed later in the chapter, improves the logic model. No matter where, when, or how we begin the planning process, we will encounter uncertainty and an element of risk. The fearless (or foolish) rush ahead; the cautious, or risk-averse, may experience decision paralysis. Neither is effective. Brownson and colleagues (2011) describe the following "key elements" to guide decision making:

- Approaching the problem in a rational and systematic fashion
- Acquiring sufficient evidence on all alternatives
- Relying on experience, intuition, and judgment

Including *all* of these elements is important. Successful decision-makers question assumptions. Using a planning model supports logical decision making (and logic modeling) through making the planner aware of areas of inquiry and systematizing that inquiry. Numerous planning models have been developed, used,

and tested. Examples include **PRECEDE** and **PRECEDE-PROCEED** (Green and Kreuter 1991, 1999, 2005), MATCH (Simons-Morton et al. 1995), PATCH (Green and Kreuter 1992; Nelson et al. 1986; Wurzback 2002), MAPP (NACCHO 1997–2000), **RE-AIM** (Glasgow et al. 1999; Green and Glasgow 2006), Intervention Mapping (Bartholomew et al. 2001), Getting to Outcomes (Chinman et al. 2004), the Healthy Living and Working Model (Paton et al. 2005), the Practical, Robust Implementation and Sustainability Model (PRISM) (Feldstein and Glasgow 2008), and Settings for Health Promotion (Poland et al. 2000, 341–51; 2009). This list is not exhaustive, and interested readers are encouraged to explore these further.

In this chapter, we use PRECEDE-PROCEED to illustrate the application of a planning model during the three planning phases: preplanning, planning, and reviewing and refining the plan. We chose to use this exemplar model for various reasons: First, it is widely considered among the most, if not the most, influential and valuable model in program planning. Second, examples of its use in various populations, health problems, and settings can be searched on a website containing over a thousand published applications (www.lgreen.net). However, no model is universal; a planner's situation may be best served by combining elements of different models. Connecting themes can be identified in many planning models. These include (1) engaging partners in planning and program implementation, (2) using original data and prior evidence to guide program development and decision making, (3) employing an **ecological approach** (see chapter 2) and social-behavioral theories to analyze the varied sources and **levels of influence** on the problem and to develop a comprehensive intervention strategy, (4) identifying and mobilizing preexisting resources and building community capacity; and (5) using **evaluation** and assessment to improve program delivery and outcomes.

The PRECEDE-PROCEED Planning Model

The first iteration of the **PRECEDE-PROCEED** model was published by Dr. Lawrence W. Green in 1974 (Green 1974), although the acronym PRECEDE was first used in 1980 (Green et al. 1980). For more than 40 years, the model has been tested, refined, and applied in many contexts, populations, and health-related issues.[4]

PRECEDE-PROCEED is a multiphased planning model. Each letter of the acronym represents a construct included in the model: PRECEDE stands for Predisposing, Reinforcing, and Enabling Constructs in Educational/Environmental Diagnosis; PROCEED stands for Policy, Regulatory, and Organizational Constructs in Educational and Environmental Development.

The first four phases of the PRECEDE-PROCEED model are the formative ones. They *precede* intervention development and delivery to ensure that the program is appropriate to the needs and circumstance of those who will receive it (Green and Kreuter 2005, 245). These phases include the following:

Phase 1: Social assessment and **situation analysis**

Phase 2: Epidemiological assessment

Phase 3: Educational and ecological assessment of predisposing, reinforcing, and **enabling factors**

Phase 4: Administrative and policy assessment and administrative alignment

The relevance of using PRECEDE in the planning process is clear. How the remaining four phases of the PROCEED part of the model fit into a program's planning stages may not be immediately clear. But when viewed as a cyclical process in which evaluation feeds back continuously into **adaptations** of the ongoing program, the discovery of limitations in the implementation and monitoring of the intensity and quality of interventions offers continuous opportunities for improvement of the program plan:

Phase 5: Implementation

Phase 6: **Process evaluation**

Phases 7–8: Outcome and **impact evaluation**

The evaluations of behavioral impact (e.g., reductions in risk factors), health outcomes, and impact on social or economic indicators all produce bottom-line, practice-based evidence of the ultimate value of the combination of polices and interventions in the particular population and context. Such evidence complements the scientific evidence from more highly controlled studies of more contained interventions in more selective samples of people. It offers more of a reality testing of the scientific evidence than is provided by most controlled-trial studies (Green 2001).

Thus, PROCEED's role in planning is to ensure that the emerging and evolving program is "available, accessible, acceptable, and accountable" (Green and Kreuter 2005, 245). It also offers evidence of what works in the particular setting, population, and circumstances of the program, and by analyzing subgroup differences in the receptivity and response to the program, it can suggest ways to improve the program for specific segments of the population. Thoughtful planning guided by PRECEDE-PROCEED begins with the end in mind. The circular model starts and ends with a situational assessment of **quality-of-life**-related indicators. As shown in figure 5.1, arrows in the model always point toward the end; we use backward steps in the causal chain (from what needs to happen eventually to what needs to happen now) to complete the diagnosis and identify the interventions necessary to change ultimately the intended quality-of-life-related outcome. Phase 1 (social assessment and situation analysis), during which the desired end is identified, is located on the upper right-hand side of the graphic. The

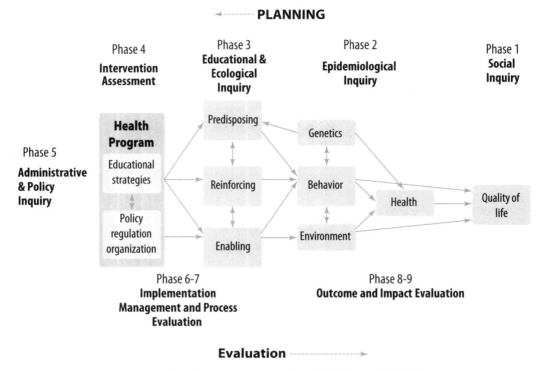

PLANNING

FIGURE 5.1. Generic representation of the PRECEDE-PROCEED Model
for health program planning and evaluation.
Source: Green and Kreuter 2005, 10. Reprinted with permission from McGraw-Hill.

diagnostic process moves from right to left through a comprehensive assessment process until we are ready to proceed with development, implementation, and evaluation of the intervention. At this point, the model moves left to right—back toward the intended outcomes. The eight phases will be described in more detail as we move through the chapter.

A discussion of planning is incomplete without consideration of evaluation. Neither can occur effectively without the other. The quantitative assessment of needs during the planning phases establishes baselines and **objectives** against which progress can be assessed in the later ("summative") evaluation. These early assessments of needs are also referred to as **formative evaluation**, insofar as they "evaluate" what prior policies and program efforts have left undone. Evaluation may appear at the end

of some planning frameworks, but in this chapter, we posit that thinking about and doing evaluation early is critical. Formative evaluation is an essential component of program development. If the goals, the objectives, and the logic model rationale underlying program development decision-making are not explicit, the utility of subsequent process and outcomes evaluation is compromised. As Carol Weiss said, "The sins of the program are often visited on the evaluation" (Weiss 1973). Evaluation that occurs early in the planning process helps us understand the context and plan program implementation protocols that can be monitored and adapted if alternative approaches are found that are more helpful, feasible, acceptable, or economical than those originally planned. Each program component should exist for a well informed and clearly articulated reason and be specifically described, acceptable, actionable, and measurable. Documentation of the planning rationale is critical. If, during planning, we do not document the formative evaluation data that inform program decisions and design, our ability to improve or alter program outcomes is limited.

The Phases and Steps of the Planning Process

Former president Dwight D. Eisenhower once observed: "Plans are useless but planning is in-dispensable." Although some who have experienced the consequences of poor planning may share this opinion, we suggest that careful, thoughtful planning can indeed produce useful plans. In this chapter, we introduce planning in three phases: preplanning, planning, and plan revision. Several steps need to be completed within each of these phases (see fig. 5.2). These are presented here as consecutive steps; however, in practice, planners may move in and out of the phases and steps as decisions are reviewed and revised. What many think of as planning (i.e., preparing an action plan to guide program

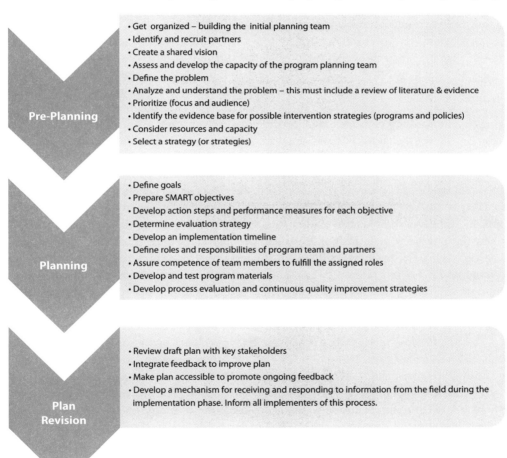

Pre-Planning
- Get organized – building the initial planning team
- Identify and recruit partners
- Create a shared vision
- Assess and develop the capacity of the program planning team
- Define the problem
- Analyze and understand the problem – this must include a review of literature & evidence
- Prioritize (focus and audience)
- Identify the evidence base for possible intervention strategies (programs and policies)
- Consider resources and capacity
- Select a strategy (or strategies)

Planning
- Define goals
- Prepare SMART objectives
- Develop action steps and performance measures for each objective
- Determine evaluation strategy
- Develop an implementation timeline
- Define roles and responsibilities of program team and partners
- Assure competence of team members to fulfill the assigned roles
- Develop and test program materials
- Develop process evaluation and continuous quality improvement strategies

Plan Revision
- Review draft plan with key stakeholders
- Integrate feedback to improve plan
- Make plan accessible to promote ongoing feedback
- Develop a mechanism for receiving and responding to information from the field during the implementation phase. Inform all implementers of this process.

FIGURE 5.2. Phases and steps of program planning. *Source:* Inspired by the North Carolina Community Health Assessment Guidebook, 2011, http://publichealth.nc.gov/lhd/cha/docs/CHA-GuideBookUpdatedDecember15-2011.pdf.

implementation) actually occurs fairly late in the planning process. Moore and Morris (2011) emphasize that "program objectives must be clearly stated before the methods to answer or achieve them are determined—not the other way around." Before stating which objectives warrant priority, one must delineate clearly the relative importance and changeability of competing needs and demands for improved quality of life, of social and health conditions, and of their behavioral and environmental determinants. These are all encompassed in the "Pre-Planning," or intervention development, phase in figure 5.2. Comprehensive planning activities are more likely to result in flexible, user-friendly plans that work—or are readily adapted to work—in changing environments.

Preplanning

During the preplanning phase, we will lay the foundation for the behavior change program plan. The scope and **complexity** of the preplanning phase is determined in part by contextual factors, our familiarity with the situation, the availability of an evidence base, resource availability, and time. An individual program planner may not always be in a position to define key issues adequately; we may not know what we do not know. For this reason, assembling a planning team for the 10 steps of the preplanning phase is critical.

STEP 1: GET ORGANIZED—BUILDING THE INITIAL PLANNING TEAM

The truism (though a cliché) "those who fail to plan, plan to fail" applies equally to planning itself. Successful program planning is planned planning. Possibly the greatest mistake planners make is to assume they are equipped to do the planning by themselves. Another error is to assume that all members of the planning team need to be trained in public health or program planning. Lay members of the community or population affected by the problem bring im-

portant insights to be included on the planning team. Engaging stakeholders and getting input from the intended audience is an often-overlooked, albeit challenging, part of planning. Indeed, "there is no better way to build support for public health interventions than to mobilize and engage residents in the process—identifying important health issues, developing strategies for addressing these issues, and initiating actions and interventions" (Thompson and Kinne 1990). The importance of investing time and, if necessary, resources in this step cannot be overemphasized. A practical solution to the problem of not knowing where to start this inclusive planning process is to convene a *small* preliminary advisory team—note the emphasis on small (Cohen et al. 2002). Rather than convening an "all-inclusive" planning team that is often nothing more than a large convenience sample of the "obvious" community, we encourage restraint. As planning needs are further defined, additional planning team members can be recruited. With a clear understanding of who is needed—people with access, connections, influence, personal experience, resources, or specific skills—identifying how to reach and recruit them becomes that much easier. Although there must always be a stable core planning team, planning team membership should not be perceived as a lifetime commitment. Busy people may hesitate to commit to a lengthy, project-long engagement. Many important contributions can be made in relatively little time. This applies at every level of planning. Once the planning team is able to approach potential team members or planning partners with specific requests and a realistic estimate of time commitment, they are more likely to recruit—and where necessary retain—the right people. The Prevention Institute has developed a brief *Collaborative Effectiveness Assessment* that can be used to reflect on the status of the collaborative planning team.[5] Readers are also encouraged to review "Reliability-Tested Guidelines for Assessing Participatory Research Projects" (Mercer et al. 2008).

STEP 2: IDENTIFY AND RECRUIT PARTNERS

Successful health behavior change programs in populations seldom occur without partnerships, but not all partnerships are effective. Partnerships are a means to an end, not an end in themselves. Without a clear understanding of the intended end, or purpose, of the partnership, the appropriate means cannot be built. Think of partnership identification and **recruitment** as an iterative developmental process; we use our increasing understanding of the context and purpose of the partnership to hone and expand our membership. With a strong core planning team, we are equipped to build out—adding layers of connection and influence as we benefit from our planning colleagues' "gifts of association." Kretzman and McKnight (1993) describe these as the numerous, diverse connections and relationships of individual community members that are so influential in resource identification and community mobilization. We are often told there is strength in numbers, yet bigger is not always better with partnerships. The Prevention Institute's eight-step coalition guide warns against overloading **coalitions** and partnerships.[6] As described in chapter 4, convening, managing, and sustaining partnerships require considerable skill (Green 2000; Green and Novick 2001).

STEP 3: CREATE A SHARED VISION

Planning teams may come together with different perceptions of what is meant by preplanning. For some it may be a simple assessment of needs; others may advocate for an assets inventory, a systematic population survey, a community-based participatory research process, or extensive focus groups. Some may prioritize numbers and quantitative data; others value stories. Most important, professionals may be too narrowly focused on a health problem (childhood obesity) or health-related need (such as increasing levels of physical activity), while the community is concerned about a broader social concern such as crime and unsafe neighborhoods. Creating a *shared vision* prevents *tunnel vision*. When health professionals view social problems through the eyes of the community, they are more likely to realize that what looks like a problem (lack of physical activity) may actually be a symptom of another bigger problem (the lack of safe environments in which children can be active). Is this visioning step a one-time short-term exercise or an ongoing process? There is no correct answer; circumstances dictate the need. What is constant is the need for diverse planning team members to agree on the vision, the purpose, and the product of the planning.

STEP 4: ASSESS AND DEVELOP PROGRAM-PLANNING TEAM CAPACITY

Program-planning capacity is a composite of skills, access, and resources. Collectively, a planning team should have the necessary interdisciplinary and intersectoral capacity. Because all professional members will bring skills from varied disciplines or sectors that they represent, and lay members will have access and experience in various segments of the community, each needs to be understood and respected. Teams will function more cohesively, and therefore effectively, if each member understands the full scope of the planning process. A graduate-school-trained epidemiologist, a local community representative, and a health educator bring very different skills to the planning table, but none should be viewed as more or less valuable than another. Even if all the necessary components are in place, developing the capacity of the team to work together may still be necessary. An often-overlooked issue is the ability of the planning team to communicate in the same language. Jargon, acronyms, and technical terminology are at best unhelpful and at worst potentially alienating.

A planning budget should be developed to ensure that resources are both available for planning and appropriately allocated. In-kind and volunteered resources should be documented to reflect the true cost of program planning and to mitigate the potential **power differential** between those who have money and those who do not. Community participants may feel more ownership of the program if their many nonmonetary contributions to the planning process are explicitly identified and reported.

STEP 5: DEFINE THE PROBLEM

With the planning team in place, we can begin the participatory situational assessment (as part of PRECEDE phase 1, Green and Kreuter 2005, 9–10, 19–21, 29–68). The first step is information gathering. **Primary data** that we gather ourselves (using methods such as community surveys, focus groups, telephone interviews, face-to-face interviews with key informants, and questionnaires administered in public places such as shopping malls) are important but may be costly. Where possible, planners should reduce data cost and redundancy by identifying and using preexisting (secondary) data. **Secondary data** are those collected for other purposes, usually by other people. Examples include census data, national surveys such as the National Health Interview Survey, the Youth Risk Behavior Survey Surveillance System, and the National Hospital Ambulatory Medical Care Survey as well as data sets, such as the CDC Web-based Injury Statistics Query and Reporting System, claims data for the Medicare and Medicaid systems, and public vital statistics records (Boslaugh 2007). Secondary data resources are becoming easier to find and use, thanks to technology. Partners in Information Access for the Public Health Workforce, a collaboration of U.S. government agencies, public health organizations, and health sciences libraries, has assembled a comprehensive set of health data tools and statistics that can be accessed through its website (http://phpartners.org/health_stats.html). The Public Health Foundation's Public Health Improvement Resource Center (www.phf.org/improvement/) is a searchable performance-improvement-focused online resource. Primary data collection can be used to validate or explain secondary data findings. If, when we present demographic and needs-assessment data, the community members' problem definition, concerns, and priorities do not align with our professional assessment, we should recognize this as protective rather than inconvenient. Our scientific assessment tools might give greater **specificity** to the objective measures of needs, but the community's subjective perceptions can prove decisive in understanding what motivates their **attitudes** and behavior toward the problems (Green and Kreuter 2005, 38–42). Programs that do not address community priorities and contexts are unlikely to be supported, accepted, or effective. Participatory research methods can often help reconcile the differing views that various parties bring to the planning process of needs assessment and priority setting.

STEP 6: ANALYZE AND UNDERSTAND THE PROBLEM

Planning models and behavior change theories are essential components of this step. Planning models direct our attention to areas that may otherwise be ignored. PRECEDE phases 2–4 are relevant here. Phase 2, epidemiological assessment, answers the question, "Which factors are most important in causing or influencing the problem outcome?" Causes are sometimes referred to as "determinants," though both terms imply a greater degree of certainty and universality of **causation** than is generally found in social and behavioral phenomena (Green and Kreuter 2005, 30–32). Causes and influences are often numerous, so planners must focus on identifying those that can be most cost-effectively influenced by an intervention. For example, although genetic factors may be present, they are unlikely to be influenced by behavior change interventions and can be disregarded for most planning purposes. Most modifiable factors can be classified as *behav-*

ioral, lifestyle, or *environmental* (Green and Kreuter 2005, 14, 30–32). Behavior, such as physical activity, is a specific, observable, often measurable action that has a specific frequency, duration and purpose, whether conscious or not. Lifestyle is more complex, comprising a collection of patterned behaviors (such as physical inactivity, hours spent watching television or playing video games, consumption of high-calorie foods and sugar-sweetened beverages) that may have health-related consequences (childhood obesity). Environmental factors can be physical (e.g., outdoor spaces, air quality, urban design, weather, access to healthful food) or social (**social norms**, reimbursement of preventive care, health- and safety-promoting policy). *Proximal* social environmental factors are those closer to the person or the community (peer and family influences, culture, social norms, etc.) or closer in time to the behavior, such as behavioral **cues** or prompts, visual stimuli in the media, or placement of products in social environments. *Distal* social environmental influences include broader political factors (such as public-safety-related laws, federal food-labeling regulations, or school policies that limit the availability of sugar-sweetened beverages in school vending machines) and socioeconomic factors (unemployment, or unhealthful food choices that are more affordable than healthful food).

Next, we must understand factors that influence the behavioral, lifestyle, or environmental issues we intend to address with the intervention. PRECEDE Phase 3 identifies three categories of factors that may be addressed with educational or **ecological interventions** (Green and Kreuter 2005). **Predisposing factors** include knowledge, perceptions, attitudes, beliefs, values, and preferences (e.g., for sweet or salty food). These are often addressed with educational strategies. **Enabling factors** are usually environmental (access to healthful foods, food labeling, portion sizes in restaurants, etc.) and are best addressed with interventions that re-

move barriers and make it easier to adopt healthful behaviors (e.g., healthful food options in school cafeterias, single-serving snack packaging). **Reinforcing factors** are the positive or negative consequences of a behavior (such as peer approval or disapproval, **social support**, enforcement of laws pertaining to drunk or distracted driving).

Once we understand the factors associated with the behavior, the planning team should strive to understand the relationships between the factors and the behaviors. Here the planning team most needs understanding of and ability to apply individual and population or community-level behavior change theories.

The utility of these analyses depends on the field of vision of the program planners. If they restrict their analysis to understanding the present situation, they may omit important historical and future considerations. It is not enough to ask "Where are we?"; planners must also ask "How did we get here?" Behaviors and their predisposing, enabling, and reinforcing influences have histories; ignoring these may blind them to critical factors or challenges that limited behavior change success previously. They must also look to the future. What emerging or other predicted factors may challenge adoption or maintenance of the new behavior? What are the threats to intervention sustainability? What are the unintended risks associated with possible program choices? Answering these questions enables planners to identify and prioritize factors that must be addressed (singly or in combination) by the interventions.

STEP 7: PRIORITIZE THE FOCUS AND THE AUDIENCE

"Less is more" applies to intervention planning. Prioritizing target behaviors enables a strategic focus on resources, thereby maximizing intervention intensity. Once potential target behaviors have been identified, they should be prioritized using two criteria: importance and

TABLE 5.1. Rankings of behaviors (or other change targets) on the two dimensions of importance and changeability

	More important	Less important
More changeable	High priority for program focus (Quadrant 1)	Low priority except to demonstrate change for political purposes (Quadrant 3)
Less changeable	Priority for innovative program; evaluation crucial (Quadrant 2)	No program (Quadrant 4)

Source: Green and Kreuter 2005, 128.

changeability (Green and Kreuter 2005, 176–78). Table 5.1 illustrates a simple decision template that yields four categories of possible action. This analysis helps the planning team select the behaviors that will be addressed in the health-behavior change program.

Criteria used to prioritize the audience to receive the intervention may vary in different contexts. Ever-present resource challenges may constrain intervention **reach** and intensity. Evenly distributing resources across the entire population may appear to be the most equitable solution, but is it? Planners must ask whether it is better to serve more people with fewer resources or less intensity, or to deliver a more robust intervention to fewer people. If widespread distribution means intervention dilution (offering part of an intervention, or offering it less frequently), successful outcomes are unlikely. Under-resourcing interventions carries the additional risk of intervention resistance. For example, readers may be aware of concerns about the increasing prevalence of antibiotic-resistant microorganisms, which the Centers for Disease Control and Prevention has attributed to the widespread use and misuse of antibiotics.[7] When the prescribed antibiotic (intervention) is not appropriate for the patient's condition (intervention need), is not given in the right dose (intervention intensity) for the correct period of time (intervention duration), or if patient adherence is low, the potential treatment failure and antibiotic resistance in-

creases. The analogy to inappropriate delivery of intervention in a health behavior change program is clear. Criteria used to prioritize may include, but are not limited to, these: level of need, vulnerability of population (more at risk or underserved), readiness to change, willingness to engage, ability to access. When planners are in doubt about the ethical implications of resource distribution decisions, requesting an ethics consult is a prudent course of action.

STEP 8: IDENTIFY THE EVIDENCE BASE FOR POSSIBLE INTERVENTION STRATEGIES (PROGRAMS AND POLICIES)

No single intervention can be labeled "the best," and single strategies seldom achieve lasting change (Mercer et al. 2004; Sleet and Gielen 1998). Intervention choice should be guided by audience and contextual factors as well as by the evidence base. Definitions of what constitutes appropriate and sufficient "evidence" vary by discipline and by the urgency or necessity of action in the absence of conclusive evidence (IOM 2010). Brownson suggests that "for a public health professional, evidence is some form of data—including epidemiological (quantitative) data, performance or outcome results of program or policy evaluations, and qualitative data—for uses in making judgments or decisions" (Brownson et al. 2009, 177). Evidence-based health promotion decisions should consider the evidence and program context as well as adaptability, feasibility, replicability, and cost-effectiveness (Farris et al. 2004). In addition to reviewing the literature, behavior change program planners are encouraged to consider preexisting health promotion resources, such as curricula and educational materials (Hill et al. 2010), **surveillance** systems (IOM 2010, 2013), and critical literature reviews, such as the Guide to Community Preventive Services (www.thecommunityguide.org). Planners may be concerned that evidence is skimpy as applied to the particular community or to specific populations within the community because the best published evidence was produced in unrepresentative populations or circumstances. Even evidence from randomized control trials (often considered the scientific gold standard) may have limited utility if derived from studies done in controlled settings and with volunteer subjects unrepresentative of the circumstances and people in the populations where the program will be implemented (Glasgow et al. 2006; Green et al. 2009; Rossi et al. 2004). *Fitting the context* is therefore critical for any evidence-based strategy to achieve desired program outcomes (Chinman et al. 2004). Participatory planning helps align theory, available evidence, expert opinion, the planning team's professional experience/judgment, and the indigenous wisdom of local residents to fill gaps in knowledge (Green and Ottoson 2004). PRECEDE Phase 4, administrative and policy assessment and intervention alignment, refers to this process as "intervention matching, mapping, pooling and patching" (Green and Kreuter 2005, 197-215). Selected interventions should *match* the ecological level of influence; be *mapped* with theory to predisposing, enabling, and reinforcing factors; and be *pooled* with evidence from prior evaluations of interventions and professional experience, as well as community-preferred interventions in order to *patch* evidence gaps (Green and Glasgow 2006; Green and Kreuter 2005, 197-215).

STEP 9: CONSIDER RESOURCES AND CAPACITY

Too often, program planning decisions are confined by the financial bottom line. Fiscal considerations are important but not paramount. Resources and capacity are the "inputs" in program logic models; some—but not all—resources are monetary. Planners should not select activities based only on cost. Resources enable them to complete the activities needed to achieve their intended outcomes and impact. Resource and capacity decisions are best approached with backward thinking. Instead of asking "What can we do with the resources we have?" and subsequently realizing that this approach is limited, planning teams should ask the following three questions to achieve a broader, more effective approach: "What resources and capacity are needed to implement this strategy?" "What resources and capacity do we have?" and "What resources and capacity could we mobilize and develop with other organizations and sectors?" Participatory planning may reveal community resources and capacity that make the previously unaffordable program feasible. (The value of community partnerships and coalitions is discussed in chapter 4).

STEP 10: SELECT STRATEGIES

Later chapters in this text provide excellent evidence to support program choices, whether individual- or population-level change strategies or specific health challenges. In these, we introduce readers to the theory and evidence that should inform program choices. Mapping interventions on theories is also the subject of a book by Bartholomew and colleagues (2011) and of chapters in a book by DiClemente and colleagues (2013). The strategy prioritization and **selection** process requires us to compare strategies. The risk associated with this step is limiting the range of considerations, or subjective decision making. An example of limited decision making is selecting interventions based only on cost (as

Intervention:	Option 1	Option 2	Option 3
Effectiveness			
Feasibility			
Cost Feasibility			
Sustainability			
Ethical Acceptability			
Political Will			
Social Will			
Potential for Unintended Benefits			
Potential to "Do No Harm" (there is little potential for unintended risks)			
Final Priority Rating			

Compare each intervention against the decision criteria (NOT against other options). Rate each *High, Medium,* or *Low*. Do NOT assign a numeric score as the criteria are not equally important. Ethical acceptability must always score high; if it does not the intervention cannot be considered.

FIGURE 5.3. The Revised Intervention Decision Matrix, v. 2010.
Source: Fowler and Dannenberg 2011.

described in Step 9); subjective decision making may consider various factors but substitutes personal opinion for evidence. Testing assumptions about appropriateness and feasibility with formative evaluation, therefore, is essential for *objective* decision making. Although the relative importance of selection criteria will vary in different contexts, several should be considered: potential **effectiveness**, feasibility, cost-feasibility, sustainability, ethical acceptability, the level of political and social will for the strategy, timeliness, and the potential for unintended outcomes (positive or negative) of the proposed actions. Once again, unless prompted, planners may not recognize evidence gaps. The Revised Intervention Decision Matrix (Fowler and Dannenberg 2011) has been used to teach intervention strategy selection in graduate injury prevention and public health problem-solving courses at Johns Hopkins Bloomberg School of Public Health since 1995.

Using this matrix has resulted in several revisions; the latest is shown in figure 5.3.

In the matrix, candidate strategies, which may also include different levels of intervention intensity (distributing free low-cost smoke alarms versus installing long-life smoke alarms), are compared against nine decision criteria. To prevent merely selecting the best of a bad bunch, strategies are not compared with each other but evaluated solely on their own merit. Criteria are rated high, medium, or low; criteria are not assigned a numeric score or weighted because the relative importance of each criterion depends on the context. Only one criterion, ethical acceptability, is nonnegotiable. Any strategy that is not rated high on ethical acceptability must be excluded from consideration.

The utility of the analysis is determined by the quality of the information that informs it. In our experience, students frequently express frustration that they cannot assign grades for all criteria because they do not know what the evidence suggests. Recognizing what we do not know is where learning begins. In the absence of scientific evidence, professional judgment and the indigenous wisdom of the community must be exercised at many points in the planning process, especially where the problem is new or the population in which it is being addressed is different from those in which previous research has been done. Invoking theory to generalize from research on similar problems or in similar populations should be done with caution. Formative evaluation can be used to answer many of these questions as well as to determine the acceptability of program components and reveal planning gaps or areas of uncertainty. Wrestling with challenging program decisions may be frustrating, but experiencing frustration during the decision-making process is certainly preferable to the consequences of implementing a poorly informed behavior change strategy. Acknowledging the necessity of turning to alternative sources of decision making in the absence of objective evidence carries with it the responsibility to evaluate the eventual program implementation and effectiveness.

Planning

Once we have agreed on behavior change strategies, we begin the **planning** phase of program implementation, which, like preplanning, comprises 10 steps. Important questions must be answered: How much of what entity will be done, how, by whom, with what resources, by when, and with what accountability indicators? The answers, when well integrated, produce the program plan.

STEP 1: DEFINE GOALS

Goals are the program's visions for change. They describe the destinations we hope to reach on the program journey. Goals can be big or small, visionary or practical, designed to inform action or mobilize organizations to great accomplishment. Which is better: the *Big Hairy Audacious Goal* (or *BHAG*) (Collins 2001; Collins and Porras 1997) or more tangible, manageable goals? Self-proclaimed "big-picture" planners may espouse the value of visionary goals, or "stretch goals." Vision, unfortunately, does not become reality without smaller, well-defined goals. We need both: visionary goals, such as Healthy People (healthypeople.gov) and more immediately achievable goals, such as "within 2 years, sugar-sweetened beverages will not be available for purchase in any Healthy County Public School" (IOM 2013). Whether big or small, goals describe destinations; they do not tell us how to get there. That is the role of objectives (Green 2011; Green and Allegrante 2011).

STEP 2: PREPARE SMART OBJECTIVES

If *goals* are the intended outcomes of our program, then **objectives** are the **change agents**. Objectives development is a critically important part of program planning because the objectives provide the framework around which we will build the rest of the program. The quality and utility of the final program plan is closely related to the quality and integrity of the program objectives. Objectives are often called the *milestones* of programs, representing important steps in the program journey. Objectives describe important impacts and interim outcomes (such as changes in knowledge, attitudes, skills, and access to resources that may be required for behavior change) but may also describe the development of the infrastructure needed to achieve behavior change outcomes. Successful programs are built step by step. Objectives are the building blocks, specifying what is to be achieved: "*Who* will attain *how much* of *what* by *when*?" (Green and Kreuter 2005, 100). Good objectives are also **SMART**: **S**pecific, **M**easurable, **A**chievable, **R**elevant, and **T**ime-bound:

- **S**pecific: Do your objectives identify a single, concrete, and unambiguous outcome?
- **M**easurable: Can you objectively measure (i.e., is it quantifiable) whether you are meeting the objectives?
- **A**chievable: Are the objectives you set realistically attainable?
- **R**elevant: Are the objectives you set specifically related to the goal(s)?
- **T**ime-bound: By when should this objective be achieved?

A frequently asked question is, How big should objectives be? The answer is determined to some extent by the planning team's needs and preferences. If we return to our analogy of a program journey with objectives as program milestones, the closer we place our milestones together, the less chance there is of getting side-tracked or lost. Multiple smaller objectives may also encourage program staff. Each represents an achievement necessary to accomplish the longer-term goals. Smaller, specific objectives may also be more easily measurable.

STEP 3: DEVELOP ACTION STEPS AND PERFORMANCE MEASURES FOR EACH OBJECTIVE

Several activities will be necessary to achieve an objective. As shown in table 5.2, these are often described and numbered to show their relationship to the objective. To facilitate process evaluation, a performance measure or indicator can be defined for each activity.

Program planning teams must also determine who will be responsible for program implementation. If implementation responsibilities will be delegated to another person or other people, or to people with a different level or type of training and supervision than those who have made it work in previous trials of the intervention, the plan's level of detail may need to be increased. Consider this scenario: if our objective is to obtain the supplies necessary to com-

TABLE 5.2. Developing action steps and performance measures

Objective 1:

Activity no.	Activity	Performance indicator
1.1		
1.2		
1.3		

plete a project, and the acquisition is being delegated to another person, how likely are we to obtain the correct supplies by issuing the instruction, "By close of business next Friday, you will have purchased the necessary supplies." Compiling an itemized list of supplies needed would increase the likelihood that the supplies purchased would be correct. Clearly defined plans, such as checklists (Gawande 2009), may save time and resources and, most importantly, may reduce errors of implementation.

STEP 4: DETERMINE EVALUATION STRATEGY

Evaluation of behavior change programs is discussed in chapter 9. The current chapter will address only the importance, with regard to subsequent evaluation, of decisions that are made during planning. PRECEDE-PROCEED phases 6–8 are process, impact, and outcomes evaluation, respectively (the terms *impact* and *outcome* are used interchangeably among professional disciplines). Process evaluation monitors the quality and quantity of implementation with questions such as, Is it happening? Is it being implemented according to plans (process fidelity)? Is the intended audience being reached? What is going well, and what is not? Process evaluation alerts us to the need for program adjustment or improvement. Impact and outcome evaluation measure the immediate and longer-term effects of the intervention: Are we achieving the intended change? How much change? Is it enough change? etc. Planning decisions determine whether an intervention is evaluable. SMART objectives are measurable, activities with clearly defined performance measures are measurable, and programs with clearly documented logic models are more evaluable (Fitzpatrick et al. 2010).

STEP 5: DEVELOP THE IMPLEMENTATION TIMELINE

Particular attention should be paid to the implementation timeline. Because certain program activities may need to be achieved within a limited time period (e.g., school semester, budget cycle, legislative session, season conducive to outdoor activities), specifying time requirements is important. A specific timeline becomes even more critical when subsequent, time-sensitive activities are dependent on earlier activities (such as obtaining permission from the school board to implement a school-based intervention). A timetable or graphic depiction of time requirements for each activity, such as a **Gantt chart**, may clarify specific implementation periods. Denoting timelines as generic blocks of time (e.g., month 1 or weeks 4–8), is an easily avoided limitation. Not all weeks are equally available for action. School vacations; competing activities (such as student achievement testing); holiday weekends; and irregular, infrequent, or overscheduled committee meetings are a few of many challenges that might present timeline restrictions. When a program component is time sensitive, such as submitting policy recommendations to a policy-making body or obtaining permission to purchase materials within a fiscal year, specifying actual dates (e.g., March or March 1–March 31) is critical for success.

STEP 6: DEFINE THE PROGRAM TEAM AND PARTNER ROLES AND RESPONSIBILITIES

Managing programs that involve multiple partners is fraught with challenges. The promise of combined resources and talents will not be realized if these are not delivered, or if they are not used effectively (Butterfoss and Francisco 2004). SMART objectives and clear documentation of the activities necessary to achieve these provide a strong foundation. Considering, delegating, and documenting roles and responsibilities during the planning process is essential to success. Delegation should be unambiguous and in writing. Developing a consensus-based accountability monitoring process permits the team to track the progress of delegated responsibilities. Assigning roles and responsibilities to partners should be a participatory process that respects the skills, resources, and time constraints of those involved.

STEP 7: ASSURE THE TEAM MEMBERS' COMPETENCE TO FULFILL ASSIGNED ROLES

Competence should not be assumed. Team members and partners who are assigned to roles for which they are not fully competent are being set up for failure. Not only does this approach compromise program success, but it will also undermine the trust relationships necessary for effective teams. Disregarding someone's limits (time, skills, knowledge, comfort level, etc.) is just as disrespectful as ignoring the person's strengths. During planning, teams should consider the competencies needed to achieve each role and responsibility. If there is any doubt about the competence of a team member, that member's performance should be monitored and the team member should be mentored. Training and supervision arrangements should be built into plans, schedules, and budgets.

STEP 8: DEVELOP AND TEST THE PROGRAM MATERIALS

Developing and pretesting or evaluating program materials is another area of program development about which much has been written and for which many resources are available.

Program materials, in many cases, will be the program messengers; therefore, they must be appropriate to the audience. Formative evaluation includes pilot testing and revision of program messages and materials, to ensure that the content, wording, grammar, and presentation are understandable and effective for the target audience. Ignoring this step in the process can mean an otherwise thoughtful intervention has limited real-world effectiveness.

STEP 9: DEVELOP PROCESS-MONITORING AND QUALITY IMPROVEMENT (QI) STRATEGIES

The important work of planning an evaluable program (described in Step 3, above) is undermined if the team does not develop a process to monitor program implementation. Some of the questions that must be answered include these:

> How will process and outcome data be collected and managed?
>
> Who will be responsible for analyzing the data (process and outcome data)?
>
> How will process data be used to improve the program, and by whom?
>
> How will program changes be monitored?
>
> What resources are needed and available for process monitoring?
>
> How will process monitoring be used to inform program quality improvement?[8]

STEP 10: INTEGRATE THE PROGRAM PLANNING COMPONENTS

A good program plan should tell a coherent, logical story and answer all of the following questions: What is the purpose of this program? What do we hope to achieve (goals) and for whom and by when? What are the main steps needed to achieve this (objectives)? How will these steps be accomplished (activities)? Who will do them (documentation of role assignment), with what resources (resource alloca-

tion), and by when (timeline)? How will we know that they have happened (process monitoring)? How will we improve activities if we learn changes are necessary (implementation of a Quality Improvement process)? How will we know if we made a difference (impact and **outcome evaluation**)?

Each component is important, but integrating them into one plan closes gaps. Each step in the planning process should inform the next. An objective and its action steps, evaluation indicators, resource allocation, and timeline, and the person responsible, should all be aligned. One suggestion for mapping out this alignment is to list the steps in columns on a table. Once aligned, objectives should be sequenced. Finally, review the plan.

Reviewing and Refining the Plan

Integrating plan components is not the end of the planning process. Our familiarity with the planning components may cause us to overlook planning gaps, unrealistic timelines, and so forth. The following four steps are key to the reviewing and refining phase of a program plan and ensuring its success.

STEP 1: REVIEW THE DRAFT PLAN WITH KEY STAKEHOLDERS

Ask an uninvolved colleague to look at the plan. She or he may be able to see errors or ambiguities that others closer to the project have not seen. As much as possible, make sure that no jargon or acronyms are contained in the planning document. If abbreviations are used, they should be explained in footnotes or a glossary. If stakeholder advisory groups have been established (as recommended previously), draft plans should be shared with them for review. This process will be much less contentious if those groups have had opportunities to review and interpret the products of earlier phases before the plan itself is promulgated.

STEP 2: INTEGRATE FEEDBACK TO IMPROVE THE PLAN

If stakeholder or external reviewer feedback is solicited, it must be *used.* Stakeholders who have been engaged from the beginning of the planning process can provide valuable contextual and programmatic insights that should be taken seriously. Even if suggested changes cannot be made, the reasons underlying the decision to forgo those changes should be shared, so that stakeholders can see that their efforts were recognized and respected. The revised draft should be circulated for comment and revised again if necessary. Without adequate documentation, the rationale for changes can be lost or forgotten. As is the case with medical documentation, if plan revision wisdom is not documented, it does not exist.

STEP 3: MAKE THE PLAN ACCESSIBLE TO PROMOTE ONGOING FEEDBACK

Plans are not carved in stone; they can and should be reviewed and adjusted as the situation changes. Soliciting ongoing feedback is important, but this can only be achieved if the plan is accessible. Plans can be distributed to stakeholders or made available on a website. When plans are shared, unexpected stakeholders may be identified. Resource challenges or gaps may be addressed only when people are made aware of them. Remember, the main reason people do not give (time, money, skills, insights, resources) is because they were never asked to contribute. Although transparency builds trust, our willingness to be informed by, and *act on,* community feedback is important. Michael Fullan explains it this way: "People believe something when they have witnessed and experienced it repeatedly—just as they can smell rhetoric and lip service a mile away. Trust is an outcome of modeling—proving yourself through your action over time. Being open is a powerful step in the right direction" (2011, 116).

STEP 4: DEVELOP A MECHANISM FOR RECEIVING AND RESPONDING TO INFORMATION DURING IMPLEMENTATION AND INFORM ALL IMPLEMENTERS OF THIS PROCESS

One potential danger of thorough planning is that planners may optimistically assume that they have anticipated all problems, eliminated uncertainties, and designed a robust intervention. Roman philosopher Pliny the Elder (who died, ironically, when the unpredictable eruption of Mount Vesuvius destroyed Pompeii), provides wise counsel for the implementation process: "In these matters the only certainty is that nothing is certain." We must establish a mechanism for identifying and responding to information on an ongoing basis.

If planning has been a truly participatory process that engages community members, developing and maintaining lines of communication will be less challenging. Even with good relationships, the ability to communicate should not be assumed. As important as communication is during the planning process, it is far more important during implementation (Fullan 2011).

Using Logic Model Development to Improve Program Planning

Because the logic model development process—especially when done collaboratively—challenges us to be critically reflective about our assumptions and decision making, it is an important program-planning tool.[9] Dialogue about differing opinions and perspectives may help make implicit assumptions more explicit; identify ambiguities, problems, and unasked or unanswered questions; and point the way to creative solutions.

Logic models are required by many funding agencies, a fact that may be intimidating to those unfamiliar with the development process. Creating logic models is a skill well worth honing. The PRECEDE-PROCEED generic model

TABLE 5.3. Essential content for a basic logic model

Inputs	Activities	Outputs	Impacts and outcomes			
			Most health behavior changes require the achievement of several outcomes. Outcomes can be divided or categorized in many ways: time-related (months, years, phases; early, late); levels of change (knowledge, attitudes, beliefs, skills, behaviors); social-ecological level (individual, family, community, . . . policy). etc. The planner will select the outcomes most useful to program stakeholders.			
			Immediate impacts	Short-term	Intermediate	Long-term
What resources are necessary to complete the activities needed to achieve outcomes?	What activities are needed to achieve intended outcomes?	How will we know that activities happen as planned?				**Start your thinking here.** What health-related outcomes are desired or planned? Examples: changes in mortality, morbidity, health-related quality of life, costs. Next, identify other outcomes that must come about in order for these longer-term outcomes to be achieved.
6	5	7	4	3	2	1
It is tempting to allow available resources to determine what the program will do. Although resources are an important consideration, begin by thinking about what activities are necessary to achieve outcomes. Then think about what resources are or may be available. Resources are much more than money or your organization's own resources. In-kind resources are often essential to success. Examples: partnerships, skills, preexisting products, stable programs into which this program can be integrated, etc.	Once intended outcomes are identified, we must specify the activities needed to achieve them. We must also recognize that some activities are needed to build infrastructure to do the project and that these do not achieve outcomes in their own right. We refer to these as *instrumental outcomes*. Activities involved in establishing and maintaining a coalition are examples of activities needed to achieve an *instrumental outcome*. Activities must always be clearly linked to the outcome(s).	Outputs are accountability measures or process indicators. These are monitored during process evaluation. Outputs indicate that an activity happened, e.g., the number of educational sessions held, but do not measure outcomes (changes in knowledge, etc.). Outputs should not be confused with, or claimed as, outcomes.	Immediate changes, such as knowledge change after training, may be necessary but not sufficient to achieve sustained behavior change. Each outcome is a step toward the final intended outcome.	Short-term changes, such as awareness, attitudes, beliefs, access to a resource (safety product, smoking cessation classes), or initiation of a health-promoting behavior change (exercise, dietary changes, smoking cessation, not texting while driving), are important steps forward but if not sustained will not result in longer-term outcomes.	Intermediate changes may take time to accomplish. Depending on circumstances, some will be challenging and are therefore longer-term outcomes. Examples include changes in policy, regulation, and legislation; organizational practices, social norms, sustained behavioral change, social and physical environmental changes, and health or safety-related product development.	

could be a starting point to flesh out each of the boxes with more specific social, health, behavioral, environmental, predisposing, enabling and reinforcing factors. Excellent free resources are available to help with developing a logic model from scratch, including the University of Wisconsin Extension's Program Development and Evaluation website[10] and the *Logic Model Development Guide* of the W. K. Kellogg Foundation (WKKF), which defines a program logic model as "a picture of how your organization does its work—the theory and assumptions underlying the program. A program logic model links outcomes (both short- and long-term) with program activities/processes and the theoretical assumptions/principles of the program" (W. K. Kellogg Foundation 2004b). An annotated list of advantages of developing a logic model can be accessed from the Community Tool Box.[11]

A logic model can be used during program planning, implementation, staff and stakeholder orientation, evaluation, and advocacy. The Community Tool Box describes eight benefits identified by experienced logic model developers:

- Logic models integrate planning, implementation, and evaluation.
- Logic models prevent mismatches between activities and effects.
- Logic models leverage the power of partnerships.
- Logic models enhance accountability by keeping stakeholders focused on outcomes.
- Logic models help planners to set priorities for allocating resources.
- Logic models reveal data needs and provide a framework for interpreting results.
- Logic models enhance learning by integrating research findings and practice wisdom.
- Logic models define a shared language and shared vision for community change.

The greatest benefit of a logic model may be the development process itself. WKKF suggests

in its *Evaluation Handbook* that "most of a logic model's value is in the process of creating, validating, and then modifying the model. In fact, an effective logic model will be refined and changed many times throughout the evaluation process as staff and stakeholders learn more about the program, how and why it works, and how it operates" (W. K. Kellogg Foundation 2004a).

Logic models can take many forms and should be structured to meet the needs of the program planners. There is no right way to build a logic model; it should be a flexible, **iterative process** informed by your needs. Essential logic model components include inputs, activities, outputs, and outcomes. The purpose and context of the health behavior change program should be included either as components of the model itself or as annotations. Any program constraints and assumptions must be clearly specified. Logic models are often read from inputs to outcomes, but the order in which we must think through program logic to *construct* the model is different. Typically, forward logic (thinking about the rationale for, and consequences of, proposed activities) and backward logic (thinking about the desired outcomes and how these are influenced and therefore will be achieved) are combined. Although both are important, we suggest beginning at the end. This follows both the scientific grounding and philosophy of PRECEDE-PROCEED (Green and Kreuter 2005) and the approach we would take when planning any journey, to bring back the analogy we proposed in the beginning of the chapter. Henry Kissinger put it this way: "If you don't know where you're going, every road will get you nowhere." Table 5.3 illustrates essential content for a basic logic model; the numbers indicate the suggested order of thinking.

Conclusions: Using Planning Methods to Improve Existing Programs

The critical thinking and planning methods used while *forming* programs may also be used to *reform* programs. Within a given behavior change program, we might well see several planning-implementation-evaluation cycles. Lessons learned at the end of one cycle inform subsequent planning activities. Indeed, we need not await the completion of an entire planning-evaluation cycle, because each phase calls into question some of the assumptions and proposed objectives, targets, or methods of the previous phases of that same cycle. Planning may also be used when increasing the scale or reach of a program or to adjust model- or **evidence-based programs** to new settings. In resource-challenged settings, *reformative* planning may be used to protect or sustain programs, either by identifying new resources or by scaling down programs in an informed and strategic way.

While most people respect the need for caution and planning in new or unfamiliar settings, many inadvertently discount the potential risk in familiar settings. There are numerous examples—from public safety, aviation, intensive care units, and so forth—that emphasize the potential dangers in routine activities (Gawande 2008). Circumstances change; implementers are fallible. What can planning strategies do about that? Planning can help programs anticipate risk and plan to avoid it, either by using protocols or checklists (Gawande 2009; Nance 2008) or through early identification of and rapid response to problems. Thorough planning integrates lessons learned through review of poor or unanticipated outcomes to protect future plans. Whenever possible, planning teams should designate time to share lessons learned.

Those who have been subjected to rigid, underinformed, unrealistic plans might be skeptical about the value of program planning. A frequent complaint about planning is that time and resources are invested in developing plans that are not subsequently implemented. The risk for developing low-utility plans increases when the level at which planning is done is too far from where the plans will be implemented or too centralized relative to the multiple local

settings with all their variations of circumstances and population mixes, and when planners are rigid and uncompromising. We hope this chapter has highlighted the difference between writing a program plan and doing thorough planning. A strategically informed program plan should be a living document: informed by and respectful of community, detailed enough to inform action, flexible enough to respond to the constantly changing implementation context, and equipped with early-detection components to alert the program team to emerging challenges and opportunities.

Even though we begin with the end in mind and should never take our eyes off the behavior change goal, the sage advice of Giordano Bruno, an Italian philosopher (1548–1600), nevertheless applies: "If the first button of one's coat is wrongly fastened, all the rest will be crooked."

NOTES

1. The quotation is from Lao-Tzu's *Book of the Way,* chapter 64a. Lao-Tzu (604–531 BC) was a Chinese philosopher and the founder of Taoism.

2. Also, LW Green, P Rabinowitz, PRECEDE-PROCEED, in the Community Tool Box (www.communitytoolbox.org). For PRECEDE-PROCEED, see http://ctb.ku.edu/en/table-contents/overview/chapter-2-other-models-promoting-community-health-and-development/section-2.

3. Daniel J. Boorstin (1914–2004) served as the twelfth librarian of the U.S. Congress from 1975 until 1987. The complete quotation is "The greatest obstacle to discovery is not ignorance, it is the illusion of knowledge."

4. A full history of the development and evolution of PRECEDE-PROCEED, a listing of published applications of the models, and related resources can be found at www.lgreen.net/precede.htm (accessed Oct. 5, 2011).

5. The *Collaborative Effectiveness Assessment* can be accessed at www.preventioninstitute.org/component/jlibrary/article/id-193/127.html.

6. You can find this guide at www.preventioninstitute.org/index.php?option=com_jlibrary&view=article&id=104&Itemid=127.

7. See Centers for Disease Control and Prevention, www.cdc.gov/drugresistance/campaigns.html.

8. Also see U.S. Dept. of Health and Human Services, www.hrsa.gov/healthit/toolbox/HealthITAdoption toolbox/QualityImprovement/whatisqi.html.

9. *The Critical Thinking Community* website, www .criticalthinking.org (accessed Oct 5, 2011), contains extensive critical thinking resources and publications.

10. See Program Development and Evaluation at www.uwex.edu/ces/pdande/evaluation/evallogicmodel .html.

11. See Community Tool Box, http://ctb.ku.edu/en /tablecontents/sub_section_main_1877.aspx (accessed Oct. 5, 2011).

REFERENCES

Bartholomew LK, Parcel GS, Kok G, Gottlieb NH, Fernández ME. 2011. *Planning Health Promotion Programs: An Intervention Mapping Approach.* 3rd ed. San Francisco: Jossey-Bass.

Boslaugh S. 2007. *Secondary Data Sources for Public Health.* New York: Cambridge University Press.

Browne MN, Keeley SM. 2011. *Asking the Right Questions: A Guide to Critical Thinking.* 10th ed. Boston: Pearson.

Brownson RC, Baker EA, Leet TL, Gillespie KN, True WR. 2011. *Evidence-Based Public Health.* 2nd ed. New York: Oxford University Press.

Brownson RC, Fielding JE, Maylahn CM. 2009. Evidence-based public health: A fundamental concept for public health practice. *Annu Rev Public Health* 30:175–201.

Butterfoss FD, Francisco VT. 2004. Evaluating community partnerships and coalitions with practitioners in mind. *Health Promot Pract* 5 (2): 108–14.

Chinman M, Imm P, Wandersman A, et al. 2004. *Getting to Outcomes 2004: Promoting Accountability through Methods and Tools for Planning, Implementation, and Evaluation.* Santa Monica, CA: Rand Corp. Report may be downloaded from www.rand.org/pubs/technical_ reports/TR101.html (accessed May 5, 2011).

Cohen L, Baer N, Satterwhite P. 2002. Developing effective coalitions: An eight step guide. In *Community Health Education and Promotion: A Guide to Program Design and Evaluation,* ed. ME Wurzbach, 144–161. 2nd ed. Gaithersburg, MD: Aspen. This document can be downloaded from www.preventioninstitute.org /component/jlibrary/article/id-104/127.html (accessed Oct. 5, 2011).

Collins J. 2001. *Good to Great: Why Some Companies Make the Leap . . . and Others Don't.* New York: Harper Collins.

Collins JC, Porras JI. 1997. *Built to Last.* New York: Harper Collins.

DiClemente RJ, Salazar LF, Crosby RA. 2013. *Health Behavior Theory for Public Health.* Burlington, MA: Jones & Bartlett Learning.

Drucker P. 1973. *Management: Tasks, Responsibilities, Practices.* New York: Harper and Row.

Farris, RP, Haney DM, Dunet DO. 2004. Expanding the evidence for health promotion: Developing best practices for WISEWOMAN. *J Women's Health* 13:634–43.

Feldstein AC, Glasgow RE. 2008. A Practical, Robust Implementation and Sustainability Model (PRISM) for integrating research findings into practice. *Jt Comm J Qual Patient Saf* 34 (4) (April): 228–43.

Fitzpatrick JL, Sanders JR, Worthen BR. 2010. *Program Evaluation: Alternative Approaches and Practical Guidelines.* 4th ed. Prentice Hall.

Fowler CJC, Dannenberg A. 2011. The Revised Intervention Decision Matrix. Johns Hopkins University, Baltimore.

Freire K, Runyan CW. 2006. PRECEDE-PROCEED and the Haddon Matrix. In *Injury and Violence Prevention: Behavioral Science Theories, Methods, and Applications,* ed. AC Gielen, DA Sleet, RJ DiClemente, 127–58. San Francisco: Jossey-Bass.

Fullan M. 2011. *Change Leader: Learning to Do What Matters Most.* San Francisco: Jossey-Bass.

Gawande A. 2008. *Better: A Surgeon's Notes on Performance.* Picador.

———. 2009. *The Checklist Manifesto: How to Get Things Right.* New York: Metropolitan Books.

Gielen AC, McDonald EM, Gary TL, Bone LR. 2008. Using the PRECEDE-PROCEED model to apply health behavior theories. In *Health Behavior and Health Education: Theory, Research, and Practice,* ed. K Glanz, B Rimer, K Viswanath, chap. 18. 4th ed. San Francisco: Jossey-Bass.

Glanz K, Rimer B. 2005. *Theory at a Glance: A Guide for Health Promotion Practice.* NIH Publication. No. 05-3896. Bethesda: National Cancer Institute, National Institutes of Health, U.S. Dept. of Health and Human Services.

Glasgow RE, Green LW, Klesges LM, et al. 2006. External validity: We need to do more. *Ann Behav Med* 31 (2) (April): 105–8.

Glasgow RE, Vogt TM, Boles SM. 1999. Evaluating the public health impact of health promotion interventions: The RE-AIM framework. *Am J Public Health* 89 (9): 1323–27.

Green LW. 1974. Toward cost-benefit evaluations of health education: Some concepts, methods, and examples. *Health Educ Monogr* 2 (supp. 2): 34–64.

———. 2000. In praise of partnerships: Caveats on coalitions. *Health Promot Practice* 1 (1): 64–65. which reflects on the experience of a Foundation grant program for community health promotion programs that required coalitions.

———. 2001. From research to "best practices" in other settings and populations. Research Laureate address at the American Academy of Health Behavior. *Am J Health Behav* 25 (3): 165-78.

——. 2011. Population health objectives and targets. In *Oxford Bibliographies Online—Public Health.* New York: Oxford University Press.

Green LW, Allegrante JP. 2011. Healthy people 1980-2020: Raising the ante decennially or just the name from public health education to health promotion to social determinants *Health Educ Behav* 38 (6): 558-62.

Green L, Daniel M, Novick L. 2001. Partnerships and coalitions for community-based research. *Public Health Rep* 116 (suppl. 1): 20-31.

Green LW, Glasgow RE. 2006. Evaluating the relevance, generalization, and applicability of research: Issues in external validation and translation methodology. *Eval and Health Profess* 29 (1): 126-53.

Green LW, Glasgow RE, Atkins D, Stange K. 2009. Making evidence from research more relevant, useful, and actionable in policy, program planning, and practice: Slips "twixt cup and lip." *Am J Prev Med* 37 (6S1): S187-S191. Full text online at http://rwjcsp.unc .edu/resources/articles/S187-S191.pdf.

Green LW, Kreuter MW. 1991. *Health Promotion Planning: An Educational and Environmental Approach.* 2nd ed. Mountain View, CA: Mayfield.

——. 1992. CDC's Planned Approach to Community Health as an application of PRECEDE and an inspiration for PROCEED. *J Health Educ* 23 (3): 140-47.

——. 1999. *Health Promotion Planning: An Educational and Ecological Approach.* 3rd ed. Mountain View, CA: Mayfield.

——. 2005. *Health Program Planning: An Educational and Ecological Approach.* 4th ed. New York: McGraw-Hill.

Green LW, Kreuter MW, Deeds S, Partridge K. 1980. *Health Education Planning: A Diagnostic Approach.* Palo Alto: Mayfield.

Green LW, Ottoson JM. 2004. From efficacy to effectiveness to community and back: Evidence-based practice vs. practice-based evidence. In *From Clinical Trials to Community: The Science of Translating Diabetes and Obesity Research,* ed. L Green, R Hiss, R. Glasgow, et al., 15-18. Bethesda, MD: National Institutes of Health.

Hill EK, Alpi KM, Auerback MA. 2010. Evidence-based practice in health education and promotion: A review and introduction to resources. *Health Promot Practice* 11 (3): 358-66.

Institute of Medicine (IOM). 2010. *Bridging the Evidence Gap in Obesity Prevention: A Framework to Inform Decision Making.* Washington, DC: National Academy Press.

——. 2013. *Evaluating Obesity Prevention Efforts: A Plan for Measuring Progress.* Washington, DC: National Academy Press.

Kass NE. 2001. An ethics framework for public health. *Am J Public Health* 91 (11): 1776-82.

Kretzman JP, McKnight JL. 1993. *Building Community from the Inside Out: A Path toward Finding and Mobilizing a Community's Assets.* Chicago: ACTA. Community assets inventory tools can be downloaded from www.abcdinstitute.org/resources/ (accessed Oct. 26, 2011).

Mercer SL, Kahn LK, Green LW, et al. 2004. Drawing possible lessons for obesity prevention and control from the tobacco control experience. In *Obesity Prevention and Public Health,* ed. D Crawford, RW Jeffrey, chap. 11, 231-64. New York: Oxford University Press.

Mercer S, Green LW, Daniel M, et al. 2008. Reliability-tested guidelines for assessing participatory research projects. In *Community-Based Participatory Research for Health: From Process to Outcomes,* ed. M Minkler, N Wallerstein, 399-406 (Appendix C). 2nd ed. San Francisco: Jossey-Bass.

Moore JB, Morris SF. 2011. Putting the technology cart before the methodological horse. *J Public Health Man Pract* 17 (3): 193-94.

Nance JJ. 2008. *Why Hospitals Should Fly: The Ultimate Flight Plan to Patient Safety and Quality Care.* Bozeman, MT: Second River Healthcare Press.

National Association of County and City Health Officials (NACCHO). 1997-2000. *Mobilizing for Action through Planning and Partnerships.* Available for download from www.naccho.org/topics/infrastruc ture/mapp/upload/MAPP_Handbook_fnl.pdf (accessed Oct 5, 2011).

Nelson C, Kreuter M, Watkins N, Stoddard R. 1986. Planned approach to community health: The PATCH program. In *Community-Oriented Primary Care: From Principles to Practice,* ed. P Nutting, 27-31. HRSA-HRS-A-PE 86-1. Washington, DC: U.S. Department of Heath and Human Services Administration.

Pascale R, Sternin J, Sternin M. 2010. *The Power of Positive Deviance: How Unlikely Innovators Solve the World's Toughest Problems.* Boston: Harvard Business Press.

Paton K, Sengupta S, Hassan L. 2005 Settings, systems, and organisation development: The Healthy Living and Working Model. *Health Promot Int* 20:81-89.

Poland B, Green LW, Rootman I, eds. 2000. *Settings for Health Promotion: Linking Theory and Practice.* Newbury Park, CA: Sage.

Poland B, Krupa G, McCall D. 2009. Settings for health promotion: An analytic framework to guide intervention design and implementation. *Health Promot Practice* 10:505-16.

Rossi PH, Lipsey MW, Freeman HE. 2004. *Evaluation: A Systematic Approach.* 7th ed. Thousand Oaks, CA: Sage.

Simons-Morton BG, Greene WH, Gottlieb NH. 1995. *Introduction to Health Education and Health Promotion.* 2nd ed. Prospect Heights, IL: Waveland.

Sleet DA, Gielen AC. 1998. Injury prevention. In *Health Promotion Handbook,* ed. Sheinfeld Gorin S, Arnold J. St. Louis, MO: Mosby.

Thompson B, Kinne S. 1990. Social change theory (application to community health). In *Health Promotion at the Community Level,* ed. N Bracht, 45–65. Newbury Park, CA: Sage.

W. K. Kellogg Foundation. 2004a. *Evaluation Handbook.* 2004 updated ed. Available for download from www.wkkf.org/knowledge-center/knowledge-center-landing.aspx (accessed May 5, 2011).

———. 2004b. *Logic Model Development Guide.* 2004 updated ed. Available for download from www.wkkf.org/knowledge-center/knowledge-center-landing.aspx (accessed May 5, 2011).

Weiss CH. 1973. Between the cup and the lip. *Evaluation* 1 (2): 54.

Wurzbach ME. 2002. *Community Health Education and Promotion: A Guide to Program Design and Evaluation.* 2nd ed. Gaithersburg, MD: Aspen.

Behavior Change at the Intrapersonal Level

ROBYN OSBORN, SCOTT KAHAN,
STEPHANIE FITZPATRICK, AND
FELICIA HILL-BRIGGS

LEARNING OBJECTIVES

After completing the chapter, the reader will be able to

* Define important terms in the study of behavior change at the intrapersonal level of influence.
* Review and explain major theories of health behavior change at the intrapersonal level of influence.
* Describe the importance of understanding antecedents and consequences of behavior change at an individual level.
* Describe how to implement health behavior change interventions with greater specificity and sensitivity for individuals, toward the ultimate goal of improving effectiveness of interventions at the population level.

Introduction

Many theories have been proposed over the years to explain human behaviors—that is, *why people do what they do.* Several important theories have been developed or applied specifically to **health behavior** and health behavior change at the individual level. These theories include key factors known to play a role in why and how people make decisions, consciously or unconsciously. Of course, as explained throughout this book, ultimately our decisions and health behaviors are a **consequence** of many factors, not only *intra*personal factors, but also the **influences** of *inter*personal, environmental, and social factors. This chapter outlines fundamental theories of health behavior at the **intrapersonal level** of influence and describes how these theories are applied. Ultimately, our goal is to highlight how individual change theories are relevant for understanding population health.

The Health Belief Model

The **Health Belief Model** (HBM) was one of the first models developed to describe health behavior, and it remains widely referenced by researchers and clinicians to explain why individuals engage (or do not engage) in health-related behaviors (Strecher and Rosenstock 1997b). Originated in the early 1950s by social psychologists who sought to explain why so many individuals did not participate in available preventive health screenings, the model has been refined over the years (Strecher and Rosenstock 1997a). In brief, it describes how an individual's perceptions affect the likelihood that he will take health-related action. These perceptions can be divided into three main categories: perceived susceptibility, perceived severity, and perceived trade-off between benefits and barriers (Glanz and Rimer 1997).

Individual perceptions interact with modifying factors, such as demographic variables and **cues** to action (e.g., a reminder from a physician or a television ad) (Glanz and Rimer 1997), to determine the likelihood of action. In this model, **perceived susceptibility** refers to an individual's belief about how likely it is that she will experience the health condition. Individuals can exhibit a wide variety of susceptibility beliefs, ranging from denial to the feeling that there is a real danger or risk of experiencing the condition. **Perceived severity** refers to the beliefs a person holds about how serious the given disease or condition is and how it would impact his life. These considerations include both the medical impact (e.g., pain or disability) and the social and emotional consequences (e.g., loss of work, difficulties with family or relationships). The combination of perceived susceptibility with perceived severity has been labeled **perceived threat** (Strecher and Rosenstock 1997a). Finally, an individual's **perceived benefits** and

barriers to taking action describe the individual's evaluation of the impact of taking action on a perceived threat. If an individual believes that taking action will reduce threat, then that action is likely to be perceived as beneficial. However, even when benefits are understood and acknowledged, if the barriers to or costs of taking action are too great or outweigh the benefits, then action may not occur. Barriers can include issues of convenience, cost, and physical or emotional pain or discomfort.

The concept of **self-efficacy** (Bandura 1977a), briefly defined as a person's sense of control or agency, is relevant to the HBM, particularly when applying the model to behavior change in which **complexity**, difficulty or uncertainty of the action is in play. In attempting behavior change, an individual must both perceive a threat to her present behavior pattern and have confidence in her ability to carry out the desired change (Strecher and Rosenstock 1997a). The amount or strength of self-efficacy a person has influences how much effort she will put forth in the process of behavior change and how long she will persist in the face of barriers (Bandura and Adams 1977). A person who is low in self-efficacy, even in the face of high perceived threat, may not take action to change her behavior. Importantly, self-efficacy is not a general trait an individual possesses. Rather, it is dynamic, both evolving and **context** specific. A person who is trying to lose weight may report high self-efficacy for skipping dessert after dinner at home but low self-efficacy for resisting dessert when dining at a favorite restaurant.

The Transtheoretical Model and Stages of Change

As the name implies, the **Transtheoretical Model** (TTM), including the **Stages of Change** (SOC) concept, was initially developed to integrate and span multiple psychological and behavior change theories (Prochaska et al. 2008). Ten processes, including consciousness raising, dramatic relief, environmental reevaluation, social liberation, self-reevaluation, stimulus control, helping relationships, counterconditioning, **reinforcement management**, and self-liberation, were identified as processes that individuals could use as they engaged in behavior change (DiClemente and Prochaska 1982; Prochaska et al. 2008). From their initial work with smokers attempting to quit, Drs. Carlo DiClemente and James Prochaska learned that individuals used these various processes in different ways and at different times during their attempts at cessation; DiClemente and Prochaska realized that behavior change occurred in stages, not as a discrete event (Prochaska and DiClemente 1983; Prochaska et al. 2008). Thus, the SOC model was developed.

The five stages of the SOC model include precontemplation, contemplation, preparation, action, and maintenance (Prochaska et al. 2008). Briefly defined, **precontemplation** is the stage at which an individual has no intention to change behavior in the near future, often considered as within the next six months. Individuals in precontemplation are unlikely to say that there is anything they would like to change about their current behavior patterns; they are not working on or thinking about change. **Contemplation** describes the stage in which an individual is aware of a problem and is considering making a change sometime soon (within the next six months). Those in the **preparation** stage intend to take action in the next month and may be doing small things to set up their environment to make change easier. For example, someone in the preparation stage may make a doctor's appointment to discuss smoking cessation strategies, but he is still an active smoker and has not yet tried to quit. Those in the **action** stage are actively modifying their behavior, experiences, or environment in order to change. A smoker may be using nicotine replacement and attending smoking cessation support groups. **Maintenance** is described as continued action and efforts to prevent relapse.

Individuals are thought to cycle through these stages, and it is assumed that change, and progression through the stages, may not be linear (Glanz and Rimer 1997). Rather, people move in and out of the various stages through periods of progression and relapse. Within the context of the SOC model, the concept of **readiness** helps explain how individuals move through the series of stages while working toward behavior change. Individuals who are in precontemplation are presumed to be low in readiness to change. However, avoid making assumptions about readiness to change (or lack thereof). Not all behavior changes are alike. Although a smoker's ultimate behavior change seems clear-cut (i.e., quitting), other changes are multidimensional (Rollnick et al. 1991). Individuals attempting to lose weight may be at varying levels of readiness for the multiple components of behavior changes required for weight loss. For example, a person may be high in readiness and in the **preparation** stage for reducing calorie intake but in precontemplation and low in readiness to start an exercise routine. Therefore, to best understand and predict an individual's likelihood to change, it is important to be specific about which behavior(s) are in question.

When applied to behavior change programs, the SOC has been used to modify treatment to meet individual needs. This type of treatment **tailoring**, based on the individual's stage, has shown some improved treatment outcomes (Perz et al. 1996). As such, providers are not restricted to working only with individuals who are "ready" to change, but have the opportunity to consider changing their message or type of support based on the individuals' needs. The practice of **motivational interviewing** (**MI**) (Rollnick et al. 1991) captures this dynamic interaction between patient and provider. MI emphasizes staying congruent with the individual's ever-changing readiness, perceptions of the importance of change, and confidence in the ability to change.

The Theory of Planned Behavior

Originating from the **Theory of Reasoned Action** (Ajzen and Fishbein 1980), the **Theory of Planned Behavior (TPB)** explains people's behavior in specific contexts (Ajzen 1991). The theory holds that people's behaviors are influenced by their beliefs about the consequences of their actions and the expectations of others (Ajzen 2001; Ferster and Culbertson 1975). Central to the TPB are the concepts of **behavioral intention** and perceived behavioral control. The TPB differs from the Theory of Reasoned Action in its addition of perceived behavioral control. **Perceived behavioral control** combines a person's actual level of control with her confidence in her ability—similar to the concept of self-efficacy. Perceived behavioral control, like self-efficacy, is context specific, rather than a generalized state (Ajzen 1991).

According to this theory, when behavioral intention is held constant, the likelihood of action is increased by increasing perceived behavioral control (Armitage and Christian 2004). The usefulness of perceived behavioral control to predicting behavioral outcomes increases as volitional control over the behavior declines. The TPB incorporates the concepts of **attitude** and **norms** with perceived behavioral control as **determinants** of an individual's intention to perform a behavior. Combining a favorable attitude and norm with greater perceived behavioral control is thought to result in a stronger intention to act (Ajzen 1991). Therefore, when a person thinks that a behavior is normative for a group of people and has a positive attitude toward the behavior, behavior change may be facilitated (or more attractive to the individual).

Social Learning Theory / Social Cognitive Theory

Originating from **Social Learning Theory (SLT)** (Bandura 1977b), **Social Cognitive Theory (SCT)**, describes how individual factors interact with environmental factors to influence behavior. SLT proposed that behavior patterns are acquired both by direct experience and by the (social) observation of others; it is more fully described in chapter 7 of this text. SCT further proposed that *environmental factors* (including both the **social environment** and the physical environment) combine with individual factors (including the cognitive, emotional, and biological components) to determine behavioral outcomes. The theory posits that behavior change is made possible by a personal sense of control. Individuals do not make behavior change in a vacuum. Rather, change occurs in a social context where individuals are constantly receiving feedback from others and from the environment, where they observe others making changes (Glanz and Rimer 1997). The very concept that observation of others making changes can be an agent for individual behavior change provides the groundwork for support groups and group therapy.

Interrelated constructs that are central to this theory include self-efficacy (discussed above), expectancies, and incentives. **Expectancies** refer to a person's opinions about how his behavior is likely to influence outcomes. In general, a person with high self-efficacy and expectancies is thought to be more likely to engage in behavior change, particularly when the **incentives** (defined as the value of a particular object or outcome to an individual) are high.

Self-efficacy can be enhanced by various mechanisms. Successfully completing a task or changing behavior in the desired way can lead to enhanced self-efficacy through a sense of personal mastery. Watching the success of peers can also be of benefit as providing role **modeling** or vicarious reinforcement (Luszcynska and Schwarzer 2005). Some self-help programs capitalize on this concept by partnering individuals in different stages of behavior change. For example, a person who has successfully engaged in a daily exercise routine may be partnered with someone who is just starting out. The hope is, of course, that by learning and watching the exerciser, the newcomer will gain self-efficacy and be more likely to continue her own program. With regard to health behavior change, these concepts work in tandem to help us understand and even predict behavior, and thereby to plan public health messaging and social organizational strategies. "Both outcome expectancies and self-efficacy beliefs play influential roles in adopting new health behaviors, eliminating detrimental habits, and maintaining what has been achieved. These constructs are seen as direct predictors of behaviors. They also operate through indirect pathways, affecting goal setting and the perception of sociostructural factors" (131).

Learning/Behavior Theories

Inherent in the concept of behavior change theories are the concepts of how people learn and how behavior results from learned associations between external stimuli in the environment (an object, another person, etc.) and internal stimuli (thoughts or feelings) (Domjan 2009). **Classical conditioning** refers to the type of conditioning first discovered by Ivan Pavlov. It explains the process of pairing a stimulus with an emotional or behavioral response. Classical conditioning describes how humans develop behavioral responses to stimuli that are not naturally occurring. If a person routinely eats a tasty ice cream cone from the ice cream truck, over time, the sound of the truck's music coming down the street can make his stomach growl and his mouth water. In other words, people make associations that cause them to generalize their response to one stimulus (the ice cream cone) onto a neutral stimulus that it is paired with (the music of the ice cream truck). Similarly, cigarettes can be paired with feelings of relaxation after repeated "smoke breaks" during which the smoker steps away from the hectic office to have a cigarette. Classical conditioning connects feelings with environmental

cues and with behaviors. Hearing a song on the radio that sparks a strong emotion is another example. The song itself does not necessarily evoke the emotion, but rather what that song has been paired with in the past, perhaps a person's first dance at her wedding. Thus, changing the environment and environmental cues can be an effective method for supporting behavior change. For example, a public communication effort could suggest that individuals try to lose weight by taking alternate routes to avoid passing by, for example, a fast food restaurant that they are accustomed to stopping at every night.

Operant conditioning can be thought of as learning that occurs as the result of rewards or punishments. How a person behaves can become conditioned to receive a reward or avoid punishment. When a person performs a certain behavior that results in a positive consequence, she is more likely to repeat that behavior in the future. **Reinforcement** describes the process of increasing or decreasing a specified behavior by using a system of consequences (Domjan 2009). When and how often a behavior is reinforced has a great impact on the strength and rate of the response. Conditioning and reinforcement are particularly relevant in terms of health behavior change. For example, using **positive reinforcement**, a system of rewards can be implemented to encourage new desirable behaviors. A person trying to quit smoking may decide to buy himself a new CD after being cigarette free for one week. Such systems of rewards, also known as positive reinforcement, can increase the likelihood of the desired behavior change. This type of behavior analysis, which examines the **antecedents** and consequences of a behavior, is a common method in behavior change work. In helping patients understand their own behavior, providers can look for the possible rewards following the behavior and work to change the patterns and schedules of reinforcements to help support the change in behavior. Such guidance to

Examples of basic science research	Descriptions	Sample public health applications
Basic behavioral science		
Communication and language	Processing of language, cognitive and social bases of speech, communication strategies, how messages are processed and understood	Formulation of public health messaging, communication strategies, and message representation
Problem solving, decision making, and judgment	Thinking and problem solving, how decisions are made, how choices are judged, risk-taking behavior	Medical decision making; differential action-taking in response to health risk status
Behavioral and cognitive neurosciences	Understanding neural mechanisms underlying emotion, behavior, self-regulation, learning, and memory	Neural processes in satiety; environmental manipulations that override biopsychological self-regulation of feeding behavior
Mechanisms of behavior	Operant and Pavlovian conditioning; behavior motivation and learning	Reward and incentive-based interventions to improve health behaviors; environmental modifications to promote health
Behavioral genetics	Contributions of both genes and environment to individual differences in behavior	Individual, family, and subgroup differences in depression, personality, and aging
Psychoneuroimmunology	Mind-body interrelationships among behavioral, neural, endocrine, and immune functions; effect of mind and personality traits on disease and health	Behavioral changes affecting immunological function; Protective effects of behavior modification, coping, and belief systems
Sensation and perception	Taste, sight, sound, smell, touch; sensory processing and interpretation of stimuli; thresholds and preferences; influence on behaviors	Health care overutilization due to symptom overperception; delay in help-seeking due to poor symptom perception
Attention, learning, and memory	Neurocognitive function, thinking behavior, aging and cognitive disorders; brain behavior relationships	Cognitive function and dementia in chronic disease; effect of cognitive impairment on disease self-management
Vulnerability and resilience	Effects of stress on psychological and physical health; biological, psychological, and social sources of vulnerability and resilience to threats	Health risk identification and protective factors

(*continued*)

TABLE 6.1. (*continued*)

Examples of basic science research	Descriptions	Sample public health applications
Basic social science		
Group behavior, social networks, and influences	Patterns of group behavior and group decision making; how social networks and groups shape individual behavior; understanding social influences of persuasion, conformity, and peer pressure	Social networking and community-building for health-promoting behaviors
Social cognition	Perception, processing, judgment, and storage of social information; understanding social interaction; behavioral and interpersonal consequences of social cognition, including processes of attribution, stereotyping, attitudes, and attitude change	Provider-patient relationships, interaction, and bias; overcoming stereotypes
Social neuroscience	Understanding neural and neurobiological mechanisms underlying human interaction and social behavior; use of neuroimaging to examine human social functioning	Health benefits of social support; health risks of loneliness, social isolation

practitioners can be taken to scale through professional education to make the primary target of behavior change that of health care professionals, and the secondary target their patients, producing through the multiplier effect a population-level change in behavior of people at health risk.

Basic Behavioral Science Applications to Health Behavior Change

While theoretical descriptions are useful for a global understanding of behavior change, empirical data are also important and contribute both to the refinement of extant theories and to the creation of new models and **adaptations** of **interventions** to varied populations and contexts.

Basic Behavioral and Social Science Research

Theories of behavior change provide proposed explanations and models of health behavior change, but the disciplines of basic behavioral and social science contribute empirically derived propositions regarding mechanisms and processes of behavior and behavior change (Ajzen 2001; Ferster and Culbertson 1975). The National Institutes of Health (NIH) has adopted a **basic Behavioral and Social Sciences Research (b-BSSR)** framework to promote incorporation of the basic sciences for more effective clinical and public health interventions.

According to the NIH framework, b-BSSR furthers understanding of fundamental mechanisms and patterns of behavioral and social functioning. These mechanisms interact with each other, biology, and the environment. The **goal** of b-BSSR is to lead to new intervention approaches for reducing risk behaviors and improving the nation's health.[1] Key areas of b-BSSR are (1) behavioral and social processes research, involving the study of human or animal functioning at the individual, small group, institution, organization, community, and population levels; (2) biopsychosocial research, involving the study of bidirectional and multi-level interactions between biological factors and behavioral or social variables; and (3) research methodologies and tools.[2] B-BSSR encompasses many content domains that are relevant to understanding and intervening on public health problems. Table 6.1 provides an overview of domains, their descriptions, and sample applications to public health.

Designing Interventions for Behavior Change in Individuals

Successful health behavior change interventions are designed in accordance with the fundamental theories described in this chapter. They consider individual factors of self-efficacy, **motivation**, and reasons for change along with social and environmental factors. Application of these theories typically follows a common model, described below.

THE A-B-C MODEL OF BEHAVIOR CHANGE

The classic model of intervention for behavior change is the **antecedent-behavior-consequence (A-B-C) model** (figure 6.1) (Bandura 1974; Malott 2008). Based on basic behavioral science of behavioral conditioning, learning, and motivation, the model emphasizes causal relationships between antecedents, consequences, and behaviors. **Antecedents** precede a specified behavior and serve as **triggers** for that behavior. Antecedents can exist in many domains; for example, triggers for unhealthful food choices may include any of the following:

- environmental: advertisements, sales on unhealthy foods, etc.
- sensory or perceptual: smell of food, appetite, etc.
- emotional: boredom, loneliness, happiness, depression, etc.
- intrapersonal: belief states, cognitive attributions, etc.
- interpersonal/social: friends going out to eat, etc. (Ajzen 2001; Bandura 1974; Ferster and Culbertson 1975; Malott 2008)

The **consequence** that follows a behavior serves as a reinforcer, which increases or maintains the behavior that it follows. Positive reinforcement presents a positive stimulus (e.g., extrinsic or intrinsic reward or incentive), which

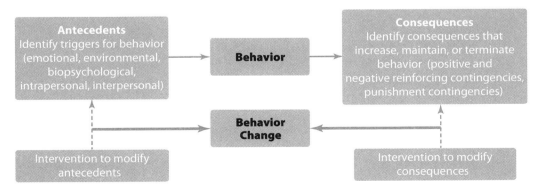

FIGURE 6.1. The classic A-B-C model for designing interventions for individual behavior change

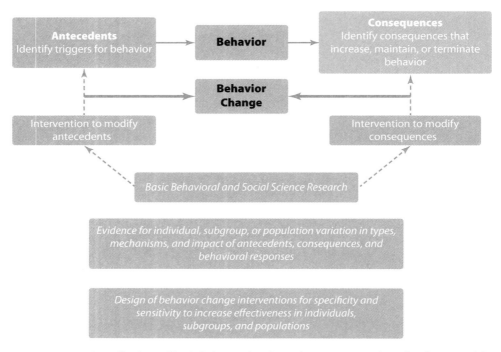

FIGURE 6.2. Contributions of basic behavioral and social science research to the classic model of intervention for behavior change

increases or maintains a behavior. **Negative reinforcement** increases or maintains a behavior through removal of an aversive stimulus (e.g., one's health insurance premium decreases after smoking cessation). In contrast to reinforcement, which increases behaviors, *punishment* is the presentation of an aversive stimulus, which decreases or terminates the behavior it follows (e.g., health insurance premium increases for failure to comply with a wellness program). To change behavior with the A-B-C model, interventions are possible on the antecedents or the consequences of the behavior (Ajzen 2001; Bandura 1974; Ferster and Culbertson 1975; Malott 2008).

SENSITIVITY AND SPECIFICITY

Owing to individual differences, no intervention applied to a population will have a uniform effect across the population. Some individuals, subgroups, or communities will benefit; some

will demonstrate a worsening of the target behavior; and others will experience no intervention effect (Cohen and Lazarus 1979). **Surveillance** and monitoring of antecedents is necessary to identify accurately the behavioral triggers within individuals or subgroups. Similarly, surveillance and identification of variance in types, salience, and impact of consequences is necessary for understanding reward and deterrent contingencies.

A particular contribution of basic behavioral and social science research is identification of variations in behavioral mechanisms and processes among individuals, subgroups, communities, and populations that provide researchers and policymakers with insight regarding intervention applicability and appropriateness (figure 6.2). Designing and implementing health behavior change interventions with greater **specificity** and **sensitivity** for individuals, subgroups, and communities leads to improved ef-

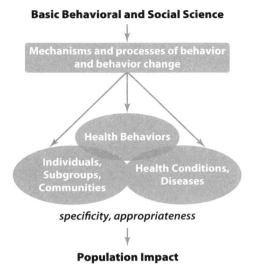

Basic Behavioral and Social Science

Mechanisms and processes of behavior and behavior change

Health Behaviors

Individuals, Subgroups, Communities

Health Conditions, Diseases

specificity, appropriateness

Population Impact

FIGURE 6.3. Pathways through which basic behavioral and social science yield population impact

fectiveness of intervention at the population level (figure 6.3).

Conclusion

This chapter has reviewed several theories of individual health behavior that have relevance for understanding population health. Explanatory factors for understanding why people take (or do not take) certain actions are useful for developing public health initiatives and for understanding the success or limitations of these initiatives. Ultimately, the most successful health behavior change programs will be developed at the intersection of individual factors and population application.

NOTES

1. NIH OppNet, NIH OppNet Basic Behavioral and Social Science Network, http://oppnet.nih.gov/index.asp.

2. Basic or fundamental research, NIH Office of Behavioral and Social Sciences Research, http://obssr.od.nih.gov/about_obssr/BSSR_CC/BSSR_definition/definition.aspx#bfr.

REFERENCES

Ajzen I. 1991. The theory of planned behavior. *Organ Behav Hum Decis Process* 50:179-211.

———. 2001. Nature and operation of attitudes. *Annu Rev Psych* 52:27-58.

Ajzen I, Fishbein M. 1980. *Understanding Attitudes and Predicting Social Behavior.* Englewood-Cliffs, NJ: Prentice-Hall.

Armitage CJ, Christian J. 2004. From attitudes to behavior: Basic and applied research on the theory of planned behavior. In *Planned Behavior: The Relationship between Human Thought and Action,* ed. CJ Armitage, J Christian. New Brunswick, NJ: Transaction.

Bandura A. 1974. Behavior theory and the models of man. *Am Psychol* 29 (12): 859-69.

———. 1977a. Self-efficacy: Toward a unifying theory of behavior change. *Psychol Rev* 84:191-215.

———. 1977b. *Social Learning Theory.* Englewood Cliffs, NJ: Prentice Hall.

Bandura A, Adams NE. 1977. Analysis of self-efficacy theory of behavioral change. *Cognit Ther Res* 1 (4): 287-310.

Cohen S, Lazarus RS. 1979. Coping with stress of illness. In *Health Psychology: A Handbook,* ed. GC Stone, F Cohen, NE Alder. San Francisco: Jossey-Bass.

DiClemente CC, Prochaska JO. 1982. Self change and therapy change of smoking behavior: A comparison of processes of change in cessation and maintenance. *Addictive Behav* 7:133-42.

Domjan M. 2009. *The Principles of Learning and Behavior.* 6th ed. Belmont, CA: Cengage Learning.

Ferster CB, Culbertson S. 1975. *Behavior Principles.* Englewood Cliffs, NJ: Prentice-Hall.

Glanz K, Rimer B. 1997. *Theory at a Glance: A Guide for Health Promotion Practice.* U.S. Department of Health and Human Services. Bethesda, MD: National Cancer Institute.

Luszcynska A, Schwarzer R. 2005. Social cognitive theory. In *Predicting Health Behaviour: Research and Practice with Social Cognition Models,* ed. M Conner, P Norman, 127-69. 2nd ed. New York: Open University Press.

Malott RW. 2008. *Principles of Behavior.* Englewood Cliffs, NJ: Prentice-Hall.

Perz CA, DiClemente CC, Carbonari JP. 1996. Doing the right thing at the right time? The interaction of stages and processes of change in successful smoking cessation. *Health Psychol* 15:462-68.

Prochaska JO, DiClemente CC. 1983. Stages and processes of self-change of smoking: Toward an integrative model of change. *J Consult Clin Psychol* 51 (3): 390-95.

Prochaska JO, Redding CA, Evers KE. 2008. The transtheoretical model and stages of change. In *Health Behavior and Health Education: Theory, Research, and Practice,* ed. K Glanz, BK Rimer, K Viswanath, 97-121. 4th ed. San Francisco: Jossey-Bass.

Rollnick S, Mason P, Butler C. 1991. *Health Behavior Change: A Guide for Practitioners.* Edinburgh: Churchill Livingstone, 1999.

Strecher VJ, Rosenstock IM. 1997a. The health belief model. In *Cambridge Handbook of Psychology, Health, and Medicine,* ed. A Baum, S Newman, J Weinman, R West, C McManus, 113-17. Cambridge: Cambridge University Press.

———. 1997b. The health belief model. In *Health Behavior and Health Education: Theory, Research, and Practice,* ed. K Glanz, FM Lewis, BK Rimer. San Francisco: Jossey-Bass.

Behavior Change at the Interpersonal Level

Social Networks

CARL LATKIN, MELISSA DAVEY-ROTHWELL,
AND KARIN E. TOBIN

LEARNING OBJECTIVES

After completing the chapter, the reader will be able to:

* Discuss theories of social influence and support.
* Describe social network function and structure terminology.
* Design a tool to collect social network data.
* Apply social network principles to the design of behavior change interventions.

Introduction

The opinions, thoughts, behaviors, advice, and support of those around us—including peers, family members, friends, coworkers, sex partners, health professionals, and others—influence our behavior and, ultimately, our health. Consider an individual who attempts to lose weight, while his spouse repeatedly purchases bags of chips and other fattening (and difficult to resist) snack foods and leaves them out in the open. Or the added difficulty of trying to quit smoking while a spouse, officemates, or friends continue to smoke. In both scenarios, temptation is heightened by proximity. Clearly, the behaviors of others in our social world influence our **health behaviors**.

Individuals are embedded within a constellation of social and contextual factors, which influence behavior and behavior change (Asch 1952; Sherif 1936). Empirical research from both social psychology and public health has convincingly demonstrated that individuals will be more inclined to adopt a given behavior if they perceive that peers are engaged in the behavior. In the case of interpersonal relationships, **social network** members influence each other's behaviors through observing others (**modeling**); by access to information, material resources, and emotional support; and by **social norms**. There is also a large and consistent body of epidemiological evidence that finds that higher levels of **social support** are linked to lower levels of mortality (Gielen et al. 2001; Klassen and Washington 2008; Knowlton et al. 2006; Lett et al. 2007).

As described in earlier chapters, the **interpersonal level** of influence resides alongside the **intrapersonal level**, the organizational level, the community level, and the policy level within an ecological framework of health behavior. Each level of influence plays a role in existing health behaviors as well as in the likelihood of adopting health behavior changes. In this chapter, we focus on the interpersonal relationships and interactions that help to shape our health behaviors. We describe several theories of social influence and support, and we discuss how they can be applied to the design of interpersonal-level behavior change **interventions**. In particular, after a general description of the interpersonal-level theories of behavior change, we concentrate on social networks and inter- and intrapersonal social interactions, which are particularly important in health behaviors and health behavior change.

Theories of Social Influence

There are numerous theories that describe interpersonal processes and the effects they have on behavior. For the purposes of this chapter, we will briefly describe those most relevant to social networks, including Social Learning Theory, Social Identities, Social Comparison Theory, Diffusion of Innovations, and Social Capital. These are key theories of social influence that are used to inform the development of behavior change interventions and programs.

Social Learning Theory and Social Cognitive Theory

Development of the **Social Learning Theory** (**SLT**) and the **Social Cognitive Theory** (**SCT**) is largely attributed to Albert Bandura (1977a, 1977b, 1994, 1997, 2004) (see also chapter 6). According to SLT, individuals learn not only from their own experiences, but also by observing and imitating others' actions and behaviors (and the rewards and repercussions of those actions) (Bandura 1977b). A classic example is Bandura's "Bobo doll" experiment, in which he observed that children exposed to videos of aggressive models behaved more aggressively, compared with children who were not exposed to the models (Bandura et al. 1961). Such modeling can occur through mass communication or via members of our social networks, such as peers and family members. The modeling by peers and family members tends to have a greater impact on our behaviors than modeling by strangers.

SCT, which evolved from SLT, posits that observing and imitating alone are not sufficient; the conscious adoption of a new behavior generally requires a measure of **self-efficacy**, the belief that one can successfully engage in the behavior (Bandura 1986). Key constructs of SCT, in addition to self-efficacy and observational learning, include behavioral capability, goals and outcome expectancies, reinforcements, and reciprocal determinism. **Behavioral capability** is the knowledge and skills necessary to perform a given behavior (i.e., one must know what to do and how to do it). **Goals, expectations** (anticipated outcomes of a given behavior), and **reinforcements** (positive or negative responses to a given behavior that may affect whether it will be repeated) also affect the likelihood of behavior change.

Reciprocal determinism describes a dynamic interaction between the individual and the environment in which they continually influence each other—adjustments in the environment cause changes in the individual and their behaviors, and the adoption of new behaviors can cause changes in the environment and the individual. For example, when a healthful eating campaign is initiated in a workplace, the work environment may be changed through the offering of subsidized healthful food options and nutrition classes. As a result of changes in the environment, individuals may begin to adopt more healthful eating habits.

Social Identities

Social identities may have powerful **influences** on behavior. Social identity theories, based on the work of Tajfel (1974) and Turner (1978), suggest that when individuals identify with a group, the collective group concept becomes part of their self-concepts. In this process, a redefinition of self emerges, and the individuals' behaviors tend to become congruent with the group's goals and actions. Social identity can motivate individuals to protect their identity or to enhance community solidarity. Enhancing a current social identity or providing new identities can motivate health promotion behaviors and advocacy among network members, or it can be used as a method of social influence. People are strongly influenced by those with whom they have a shared social identity, compared to those with whom they don't. Social identity may be linked to membership in groups, neighborhoods, professions, sports team preferences, ethnic identity, and behaviors. A classic example of social identity is a group of football fans. At football games, people identify with being a fan by dressing in the sport paraphernalia and cheering for their team. Social identity may also explain why some groups adopt certain health behaviors.

Social Comparison Theory

Hyman (1942) proposed that an individual's **attitudes** and behaviors are influenced by **refer-ence groups**, which are clusters of people that serve as reference points for behaviors and attitudes. Individuals look at other people in their **social environment** as a guide to what constitutes appropriate behavior.

Festinger's (1954) **Social Comparison Theory** refined the concept of reference groups. According to this theory, individuals not only look at the behaviors of others as a guide, they also *compare* their own behaviors to those of others, such that an individual's behavior is based on comparisons made with others, including the reference groups. Through observing others' behaviors and comparing our own actions, **norms** about which behaviors are appropriate for a given social environment may emerge. Furthermore, these observations and comparisons may be more influential if an individual perceives that members of the reference group are similar to her. Often the most important reference group for an individual is her social network. For example, research suggests that adolescents are more likely to smoke if their peers also smoke (Kelly et al. 2011). Studies have also shown that among adolescents, when an important social network member smokes, such as a best friend or a boyfriend, the likelihood of smoking is even higher (Holliday et al. 2010). Thus, by being around people with whom they identify who smoke, adolescents are influenced to smoke, too.

Diffusion of Innovations

The **Diffusion of Innovations Theory (DIT)** describes how new behaviors, ideas, programs, and innovations diffuse through social systems (Rogers 2003, 1962; Rogers and Shoemaker 1971; Wejnert 2002). In terms of health behavior, an innovation could be the use of a new safety feature in a car or making use of screening or preventive testing services. This theory suggests that **innovations** are more likely to be diffused when they are considered to have relative advantage over prior behaviors and practices, are compatible with existing practices, can be easily tried, and have observable results. Within a social system, some individuals (**innovators**, or **opinion leaders**) are the first to adopt a new behavior, and their adoption has a strong influence on others adopting the behavior. A key aspect is the structure of social networks and peer-to-peer communication as a means to diffuse the innovation. For example, utilizing **peer-educators** to diffuse information and skills and change norms has been a successful approach in both developed and developing nations. The advent and ubiquity of the Internet, social media sites, and cellular technology have made it possible for diffusion to occur faster and more broadly. According to this theory, there are five categories of individuals adopting an innovation: the innovators, the early adopters, the early majority, the late majority, and laggards. *Innovators* are a small segment of this population and are characterized as eager to try novel concepts, even if benefits of the innovation are not readily apparent. *Early adopters* join when the benefits of the innovation begin to emerge. *Early majority* individuals are characterized as more pragmatic than early adopters; they will adopt the innovation when the benefits are clear, the results are observable, and the ease of use is high. *Late majority* individuals and *laggard*s tend to be risk avoidant and are the last to adopt the innovation. Innovators and early adopters are the optimal types of individuals for initiating changes in norms and behavioral practices.

Social Capital

Social capital has been conceptualized as a phenomenon that links individuals together through their collective action and enables them to access resources through processes of trust, cooperation, bonding, and the formation and perpetuation of social norms (Coleman 1990; Fukuyama 1999; Portes 1998; Putnam 1996). Explicit at the center of Social Capital Theory is the social network and its norms of reciprocity (i.e., helping one another out) and mutual trust (i.e., trusting one another) (Bourdieu 1986). Resources flow through **networks**, based on both who is in the network and the roles that they occupy. Resources may be provided directly by close members or through secondary or tertiary members (Elgar et al. 2011). Numerous studies have demonstrated that having greater levels of social capital is linked to improved physical and mental health as well as reduction in disease and risk factors (Dean and Sharkey 2011; Elgar et al. 2011; Fujiwara and Kawachi 2008; Holtgrave and Crosby 2006; Kelly et al. 2009; Kim and Kawachi 2006; Siahpush et al. 2006; Sivaram et al. 2009).

Two dimensions of social capital have been described: bonding and bridging (Putnam 2000). **Bonding social capital** is the relationship between people who share similarities such as belonging to the same organization, family, or neighborhood. Bonding social capital reinforces the group's social identity. **Bridging social capital** is established between individuals or organizations that are not similar but have shared associations. Examples of bridging social capital are relationships between work colleagues or between individuals from different faiths or religious institutions. Both forms of capital can be leveraged to effect behavior change of the members of the groups. Another example of increasing bridging social capital is a neighborhood watch program designed to encourage individuals to engage in patrolling their neighborhood to deter criminal activity. Measures of social capital in the literature have varied. Some examples of measures include neighborhood attachment, support networks, feelings of trust and reciprocity, civic engagement, confidence in social institutions, and participation in formal groups such as neighborhood associations or labor unions.

Social Networks

Each of the theories discussed above explains how interpersonal processes can influence health and behavior. The rest of this chapter focuses specifically on social networks, which are a key interpersonal element of public health. The final section describes how diseases spread among people and populations and offers insights into how prevention messages and resources can reach a larger number of individuals.

A **social network** can be defined as a set of individuals who are connected by relationships. Relationships are the key factor in social network analyses. In the study of health behaviors, social network analyses often focus on the relationship among individuals. Social network members may be directly or indirectly linked by behaviors, emotions, group membership, social position, physical settings, or a specific type of interaction (e.g., sexual contact, drug sharing, classmates). We use a social network perspective to examine interpersonal relationships because it can simultaneously examine a wide range of relationships and their impact on different health behaviors and conditions. As a result of the rising popularity of social media sites such as Facebook, the term *social network* has become a common part of everyday vocabulary. In this chapter, we discuss why and how social networks influence our behavior in both positive and negative ways. We conclude the chapter with case studies of effective social-network-based interventions.

Social networks are often discussed in terms of structure (Who is in the social network? What types of relationships exist?) and function (What do the people in the social network do?). There are two basic types of social networks: egocentric (or personal) networks and sociometric networks. **Egocentric networks** are usually conceptualized as one individual who is the focal individual (or ego), along with his social ties. For example, egocentric networks for students may include their friends, family members, partners, neighbors, and classmates. In contrast, **sociometric networks** tend to link many individuals, or *nodes,* and may be considered bonded groups. An example of a sociometric network would be a class roster turned into a matrix, with *ones* indicating friendships and *zeros* indicating the lack of friendship between classmates. Such a matrix can be analyzed to obtain social network indicators and the relationships between network members. An example of a sociometric network can be seen in figure 7.1 (this social network is from the SHIELD study, a human immunodeficiency virus [HIV] prevention project, which we describe in detail later in the chapter). The circles are social network members and the lines indicate ties or relationships between the network members. This figure represents drug network members who reported sharing with one another injection materials, which can transmit HIV, hepatitis C, and other infectious diseases.

Social Network Structure

Social network structure refers to who is in the network and what relationships exist among members. Social network structural components include *network size* (i.e., number of network members), *direction of the relationship* (unidirectional or bidirectional), *multiplexity* (i.e., the number of relationships between the ego and a network member, which is measured by the number of network members named in two or more functional or relational network domains), **density** (i.e., the proportion of individuals within a network who are linked to each other divided by the number of possible links), and *centrality* (i.e., individuals within a network with the highest numbers of direct and indirect ties).

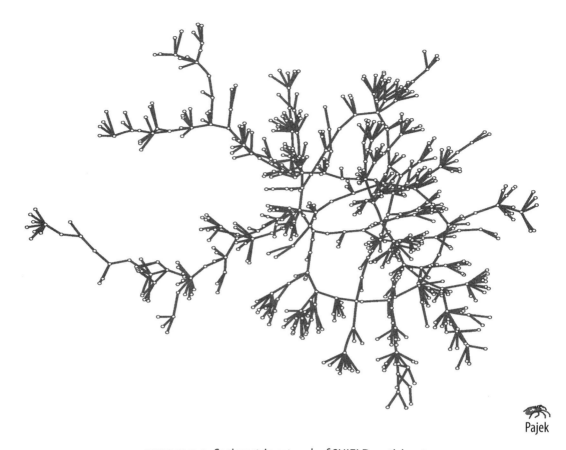

FIGURE 7.1. Sociometric network of SHIELD participants

Density of social networks, which refers to the degree of interconnectedness among the network members, has been linked to health and behaviors (Ashida and Heaney 2008; De et al. 2007; Smith et al. 2004). With personal network inventories, density may be elicited with the question "Please tell me which people on this list are friends with other people on the list" or "Please tell me which people on this list know the other people on the list." In figure 7.2, two social networks comprising four people are presented. The circles represent people and the lines indicate friendship ties between network members. Social Network A is a network with high density because all the members are connected to each other. Social Network B has low density since there are few connections between the members.

Functions of Social Networks: How Social Networks Influence Behavior

As we have explained, behavior is influenced by other individuals and our social interactions

Social Network A

Social Network B

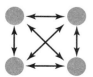 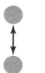 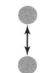

FIGURE 7.2. Density of social networks

with them (Latkin and Knowlton 2005). In this section, we will describe three processes through which social networks shape behavior:

1. As a source of social support and resources
2. As a source of interpersonal conflict (i.e., people argue or do not get along with one another) and stress
3. As a source of social norms

Identifying and **targeting** these various processes leads to more effective behavior change interventions.

Networks as Channels of Social Support and Resource Exchange

Social network members may provide one another social support, which is highly associated with health outcomes. **Social support** is intangible or tangible resources offered by one person to another. Common categories of social support include emotional, informational, financial, and material support. Furthermore, social support may be either perceived or enacted. **Perceived support** is an individual's perception of support he could potentially receive from social network members if needed. For example, Do I have someone I can talk to when I am down? Do I have someone who could lend me money when I need it? **Enacted** (or *actual*) **support** refers to support that has actually been provided by social network members. How many people have I talked to when I was upset this month? Who has given me a loan in the past?

Perceived emotional and material support has a strong influence on psychological well-being, whereas actual support (i.e., enacted support) received is often helpful for caregiving relationships. Understanding patterns of support exchange and contingencies of support exchange within a population contributes to a greater understanding of health behaviors; for

example, one may focus on a community's pattern of resource exchange in seeking to meet basic subsistence needs (e.g., food, shelter, clothing, school tuition) and how this may differ by setting.

Because it emphasizes resources and both the benefits and costs of maintaining supportive ties, **network analysis** is well suited to the study of disadvantaged populations in limited resource settings. Prior studies indicate that individuals of lower **socioeconomic status**, having fewer personal reserves of economic resources, are more likely to utilize network support (Hobfoll 2001). Those of very low socioeconomic status tend to rely on their networks for support exchange for basic subsistence needs (Stack 1974).

The Role of Interpersonal Conflict within a Network and Health Outcomes

Many studies of social network ties and health focus on the positive, supportive qualities of the connections and ignore negative or problematic qualities. However, research suggests that the latter qualities of relationships may be more consequential to health than supportive qualities (Fiore et al. 1983; Rook 1984). Conflictive compared to supportive qualities of ties have been found to have greater associations with stability and duration of relationships as well as health outcomes. Conflict among network members may lead to network instability and dissolution of these relationships (e.g., "breakups"). Practicing behaviors that violate social norms among network members may be one factor that leads to conflict and potential dissolution of relationships (Turner et al. 1998).

Norms and Social Networks

Another way that social networks influence behavior is through the creation and enforcement of norms. Several terms have been used to refer to norms, including *peer norms* (Cho et al. 2010; Wallace et al. 2008), *social norms* (Perkins and Craig 2006; Scholly et al. 2005), *perceived norms* (Barroso et al. 2010; Davey-Rothwell and Latkin 2007; Rimal et al. 2005), and **subjective norms** (Gatt and Sammut 2008; Johnson et al. 2008; Krupp et al. 2010). This wide variety of terms reflects a lack of uniformity in the conceptualization and operationalization of this construct.

Lapinski and Rimal (2005) distinguish between collective and perceived norms. **Collective norms** are those established by the group or social system (i.e., social norms). **Perceived norms** are the norms as an individual perceives them. Often there is a disconnect between collective and perceived norms. For example, Perkins and colleagues (2005) demonstrated that college students often overestimate how much their peers drink alcohol. Thus, the perceived norm for peer drinking is different from the actual norm. Perceived norms have been categorized as *descriptive* and *injunctive* (also referred to as *prescriptive* and *proscriptive norms*) (Cialdini et al. 1990). **Descriptive norms** have to do with our perception of the behaviors practiced by other people in the social environment. These norms assess the perceived prevalence of a behavior in a group. **Injunctive norms** relate to our perceptions of the behaviors, attitudes, and beliefs that are considered appropriate or acceptable in the social group. These norms consider the outcome of our behavior—approval or sanctioning by others.

The influence of norms may vary according to relationship and similarity between the individual and others. Teenagers may be more persuaded by other teens than by their parents for their clothing choices but not for political or religious affiliations. Norms may be developed and transferred through observing others' behaviors, receiving positive and **negative reinforcement** for behaviors, and verbal communication (Oostveen et al. 1996).

Social networks tend to reinforce social norms. Some networks may have more homogeneous norms about drinking, whereas others are more heterogeneous. For example, within an adolescent's social network, peer norms may promote alcohol consumption, whereas parental norms are opposed to alcohol use. Thus there can be competing and contradictory norms within the same social network. Social norms have been found to be associated with numerous health behaviors, including smoking (Buttross and Kastner 2003), alcohol consumption (Neighbors et al. 2007), exercise (Okun et al. 2003; Sorensen et al. 2007), dietary practices (Eisenberg et al. 2005), eating behaviors (Baker et al. 2003), sun protection and sunbathing (Jackson and Aiken 2000), and adolescent sexual behaviors (Buhi and Goodson 2007). Social norms play a central role in the maintenance of social behaviors and present barriers to altering social behaviors (Bettenhausen and Murnighan 1991; Coleman 1990; Myers and Bishop 1970; Newcomb 1958; Tittle 1977).

Social Networks: Their Role and Importance in Behavior and Behavior Change

In this section we describe how egocentric and sociometric networks have been used to learn how diseases spread through a social network. For example, social networks have been used to describe HIV transmission (Klovdahl et al. 1994; Latkin, Sherman, and Knowlton 2003; Wylie and Jolly A. 2001). There is a strong relationship between egocentric network factors and substance use and HIV-risk behaviors among highly impoverished populations in the United States and internationally. Network characteristics, such as network size, composition, and density (i.e., closeness among network members), have been found to be associated with HIV-risk behaviors, such as sharing injection equipment; drug use cessation (Buchanan and Latkin 2008; Davey-Rothwell et al. 2008; Latkin et al. 2010; Latkin et al. 2011; Tobin and Latkin 2008); having multiple sex partners, same sex partners, or unprotected sex; exchanging sex for money or drugs; and age mixing of sex partners (i.e., having sex with partners who are much older or younger) (Barrington et al. 2009; el-Bassel et al. 1998; Miller 2003).

A set of landmark studies using the longitudinal Framingham Heart Study data set examined sociometric (i.e., in a bonded group of people) social network factors and changes in various health issues: obesity, smoking, depression, happiness, and alcohol use. The Framingham Heart Study began in 1948 by recruiting 5,209 men and women from Framingham, Massachusetts, to identify factors over a long period that lead to cardiovascular disease (Dawber 1980; Dawber et al. 1963). Participants return to the study every two years, and several other cohorts have been enrolled. The Framingham study also included several cohorts in which the children of the original participants were used as the ego or focal individuals, enabling social networks to be constructed from the tracking sheets that identified individuals who were close to them (e.g., friends and relatives). The study recorded detailed information about all first-order relatives and at least one close friend.

Researchers in the Framingham study created a social network data set based on 5,124 participants (from the original 5,209) and their family members, friends, spouses, neighbors, and co-workers (Fowler and Christakis 2008). As an illustration of how social network characteristics relate to health-related outcomes, the researchers found that participants were substantially more likely to drink heavily if a person they were directly connected to also drank heavily. This effect was observed even within three degrees of separation within the network (e.g., friend of a friend of a friend) (Rosenquist et al. 2010). In examining the spread of happiness in a social network, the Framingham researchers found that happiness was clustered within networks (Fowler and Christakis 2008). Members of the social network who were surrounded by happy people were more likely to be happy in the future.

Collecting Egocentric Social Network Data

In order to understand how social networks influence health behavior as well as to identify who may be influential network members, information on individuals' social networks must be collected. A **social network inventory** is one such method for assessing the structure of an individual's social network. A social network inventory can identify supportive and problematic network members, and this information in turn can inform behavior change efforts. For example, for an individual trying to quit smoking, how many smokers are in her network, and who may be a source of support for the quitting efforts? Do cancer patients have people in their social network who can provide emotional or material support or who are sources of conflict or stress?

The social network inventory is divided into two sections. In the first section, the *name-generating* section, the participant is asked to list people based on different functions and roles. For sociometric network analyses, participants are usually asked to provide the full names of their network members. For the collection of egocentric network data, and in order to maintain confidentiality, participants are asked to use only the first names and last initials of their social network members. When participants are unable or unwilling to provide names, one can to use nicknames or initials to clarify who they are talking about during the inventory.

Participants may be asked to list individuals from whom they receive intimate, instrumental, social/recreational, informational, and material support. For public health studies, network analysts often include name generators such as sources of health advice and individuals with whom participants engaged in specific health behaviors during a specified time frame: used drugs, drank alcohol, ate meals, exercised, or had sex. Here are some commonly used name-generating questions:

TABLE 7.1. Social network inventory

First name	Last initial	Question 1 (advice)	Question 2 (loan)	Question 3 (argue)	Question 4 (sex)	Gender	Age
Mary	G	Yes	Yes	Yes	Yes	Female	45
Robert	T	Yes	No	No	Yes	Male	23
Butch	L	No	Yes	No	No	Male	58
Laura	G	No	Yes	No	Yes	Female	43
Larry	S	No	No	Yes	Yes	Male	49

1. Who have you gotten advice from or talked to about something personal in the past 6 months? (emotional support)
2. Who could you go to if you needed a loan of $1,000? (financial support)
3. Who on this list do you not get along with or frequently argue with? (interpersonal conflict)
4. Who have you had sex with in the past 3 months? (sex network)

The second part of the inventory is used to collect *network characteristics.* Once the network members have been listed, additional information is collected on each listed member, including age, gender, race/ethnicity, socioeconomic status, type of relationship (e.g., kin, friend, spouse), level of trust, duration of relationship, and reciprocity of the relationship.

Table 7.1 is an abridged example of a network inventory. For each network member, the person's first name and last initial (or nickname) is listed in the grid. Questions 1–4 are name generating. In the table, Mary and Robert were listed for question 1. For question 2, Mary was listed again, and Butch and Laura were added to the inventory. Larry was added to the inventory by question 3. After all network members were listed, the gender and age of each person were collected.

The data from the social network inventory provides rich information about the roles and characteristics of each network member. For example, who is Mary G. and what does she do for me? The data may also be compiled to get a comprehensive assessment of the network by totaling the number of social network members who play a specific role or share a quality. For instance, do I have people in my social network that I can turn to for advice or for a loan?

The total size of the network, or **range**, is calculated as the number of people listed. The total size in the table 7.1 example is five network members, two women and three men. The number of people who provided emotional support (e.g., advice) is two, while the number who provided financial support is three. Finally, the number of conflictual ties (e.g., argue) is two.

Social network inventories and analyses allow us to characterize social environments and determine how the structure of a network and the functions of network members influence health behaviors. Understanding the composition and function of social networks can help develop behavior interventions designed to promote health behaviors. These interventions should be tailored based on the network composition, the feasibility of different behavior change strategies, and the social norms within the networks. For example, a network that is composed of mainly family or kin may not be amenable to an intervention designed to promote sexual risk reduction but may be ideal for promoting exercise or healthful eating. Networks are often situated within geographic, social, political, technological, and political contexts. These structural factors exert influence on networks and need to be considered when developing network interventions. For example, an intervention designed for networks in a rural setting should consider the physical distance between members, which may limit face-to-face contact.

Social Networks and Social Media

There is a burgeoning literature and interest in the role of social media, such as Twitter, MySpace, and Facebook, and how they influence health behaviors. There are active online support networks for a wide range of disease and health conditions (Griffiths et al. 2009; Hong et al. 2011; Melling and Houguet-Pincham 2011; Weitzman et al. 2011). For example, social media forums have become popular for promoting tobacco use cessation (Bock et al. 2008; Cobb et al. 2010; Cunningham et al. 2006; Houston et al. 2010; Saul et al. 2007). Furthermore, these resources are utilized by a variety of people. In a recent study, Chou and colleagues (2009) found that although younger people are more likely to use social networking sites, online support groups, and blogs, there were no differences in race, education, and health care access among people who used social media for these purposes and those who did not. Many individuals log on to such health-related Internet networks. Although individuals may enter these online support networks as strangers, they often find supportive others online. Most only visit these sites a few times. A smaller proportion continue their involvement, and some become highly involved, spending hours each day sending and receiving messages from site members. As with face-to-face networks, peer leaders emerge, and individuals develop specific roles within these social networks. Sometimes the networks break into subnetworks based on similarities or conflict among the network members.

One key question for health professionals is how to utilize existing online networks and develop new online networks to promote positive health. Yet we cannot assume that such networks will necessarily influence health behaviors. Not all members of online networks influence health behaviors. It is not uncommon to have hundreds of "friends" on Facebook, yet it is unlikely that all of these individuals have a significant influence on our health behaviors. In developing online social network programs, it is important to identify the structural aspects of networks and the key individuals within the networks who can successfully promote behavior change. Another public health challenge is to address networks that may promote deleterious health behaviors, such as smoking, drug abuse, and harmful sexual behaviors.

Social-Influence-Oriented Interventions

Effective interventions that focus on the interpersonal level to target behavior change use role modeling and social comparison mechanisms to alter social norms. Social network interventions for health behavior capitalize on naturally occurring social influence processes and can also reach hidden populations and be sustained through changing social norms.

Interventions that Alter Social Norms

One type of social-network-oriented intervention focuses on changing individuals' perceptions of their referent group norms rather than altering social norms of existing groups (Latkin, Forman, et al. 2003). These interventions are often implemented on community-wide scales and may utilize multimedia campaigns including billboards, radio, and television. One appealing aspect of norm change interventions is that often norms are self-maintaining, and hence, the common problem of decay or relapse is avoided. An example of sustained change in health behavior is the transformation over the past century in spitting practices in the United States. Public spitting was socially acceptable through the mid-19th century. However, around 1880, public health campaigns and legislation introduced for tuberculosis control mandated against public spitting (Chapman 1995). Today, even in the absence of these campaigns and ordinances, antispitting norms are maintained, and public spitting is infrequent. More recently, anti-tobacco public health campaigns and legislation have helped to alter norms about public tobacco smoking in the United States. Although only a few decades ago, cigarette smoking was considered glamorous, it is now widely considered socially unacceptable.

Social norm interventions for college alcohol consumption are based on the findings that the majority of college students overestimate the prevalence of alcohol consumption on campus. The college campaign targeting alcohol consumption presents descriptive normative information to students about the actual drinking patterns on campus. The goal of providing this normative information is to reduce drinking. However, some students may perceive that the norm is lower than it actually is, which may lead them to increase their alcohol consumption. Another social norm intervention has been to provide households with both descriptive and injunctive normative information about their energy consumption. The normative information compared their consumption to that of the rest of the neighborhood households (Schultz et al. 2007). In California, this approach was found to be effective in reducing energy consumption among households that were using more than the average amount of electricity in their neighborhoods.

CASE EXAMPLES

Alcohol misuse and abuse in college settings is a public health problem. It is well established that college students overestimate the drinking frequency of other students and the amount of alcohol consumed by their peers who drink, and this has been found to increase their own consumption of alcohol (Perkins et al. 1999; Per-

kins et al. 2005). Some interventions have been developed to change the perceived norms about college student alcohol use. In the *Bling* intervention, students used wireless keypads to answer questions about their perceptions of their peers' drinking and then questions about their own drinking (LaBrie et al. 2010). Their responses were instantly displayed on an overhead screen, and the intervention was found to be effective in immediately correcting misperceptions of alcohol use. Interventions have also been tested to change norms and risky alcohol behaviors (Moreira et al. 2009). Perkins and Craig (2006) developed a media campaign on a college campus to correct misperceptions about peer drinking as well as reduce personal alcohol use among student athletes. This campaign included advertisements in campus newsletters, email communications, peer education, and posters and multimedia kiosks in popular venues. In addition to changing the misconception that student athletes drank frequently and in large quantities at social events, the intervention led to reductions in alcohol consumption, binge drinking, and blood alcohol levels.

Peer-Based Interventions

The goal of **peer-based interventions** is to use social networks as a way to disseminate information and resources about health promotion and disease prevention. Two types of peer-based interventions are the popular opinion leader model and peer education.

THE POPULAR OPINION LEADER MODEL

Individuals with high centrality (i.e., a high number of direct or indirect ties or key individuals through whom resources flow within a network), or those who are rated by many network members as sources of health information or advice, may be important targets of intervention not only because of the greater potential exposure of their ties, but also because they may be important sources of social influence on network members. Highly central individuals are termed **opinion leaders**.

The first step to develop an opinion-leader-based intervention is to identify the central and highly influential opinion leaders. This can be done by observing the **target population** to see who is popular, well-liked, or respected and by interviewing people of the target population and asking them to nominate people whom they consider trendsetters or who have a high degree of influence on others. For example, in a classroom setting you could interview or survey the class and ask, "Who do you think is the most popular of the class?" "Who do people copy?" and "Who is a trendsetter?" and see whose name is most frequently listed. Once opinion leaders are identified, they can be trained to disseminate health-related information, promote various health messages, and model health behaviors. Opinion leaders can also be identified through sociometric network analyses, which provide quantitative information on various measures of centrality.

The key components of a network-oriented peer education intervention include having identifiable networks, credible key network members, network stability, an understanding of which network members influence which behaviors, the ability to train key network members in communication methods, adequate venues for communication about the health behaviors, and sustained interactions with network members.

CASE EXAMPLES

An opinion leader approach to behavior change has been used for HIV prevention intervention in natural social environments. An opinion leader approach to educating peers on HIV and risk reduction has been successfully applied in an intervention for gay men attending bars in small towns (Kelly et al. 1992) and for family planning (Kincaid 2000). In gay bars in urban U.S. settings, bartenders were identified as popular and credible sources of information and were successfully used to promote HIV risk reduction (Kelly et al. 1992).

In a family planning intervention in Bangladesh, a network-focused intervention was compared to a field peer health worker intervention (Kincaid 2000). In the network condition, family health workers held discussion groups in homes hosted by women who had been identified as those individuals whom community members sought out for health advice. One of the goals of the meetings was to increase discussion of family planning among women, family members, and spouses. All three conditions were hypothesized to influence family planning decisions. In the comparison condition, without discussion groups, the health workers visited the women's individual homes. Results indicated that women in the network intervention were almost twice as likely to report using modern contraceptives as those in the control condition (Kincaid 2000). In both of these examples, popular individuals served as an avenue to disseminate information to other people.

THE NETWORK-ORIENTED PEER EDUCATOR MODEL

An alternative to the popular opinion leader model is the **peer educator** model, which is based on the premise that individuals in all positions in a social network can influence others in that social network and that many members of the network can be trained in leadership, communication, and social influence skill. This model is especially applicable in settings where clear opinion leaders cannot be established, where opinion leaders are not common, or where the opinion leaders may not have the time or interest to promote the behavior change. A religious leader in inner-city neighborhoods may be popular but may not want to promote HIV prevention or may not have frequent opportunities to talk about HIV prevention with high risk groups such as injection drug users and commercial sex workers.

Moreover, such a leader may not have influence on such behaviors.

Peer education programs have been developed and tested in a range of settings (e.g., developing countries, schools, communities) with a variety of populations (e.g., students, drug users, commercial sex workers) targeting several health behaviors such as smoking, weight loss, and HIV and sexually transmitted infection risk (Agha and Van Rossem 2004; Campbell and MacPhail 2002; Davey-Rothwell et al. 2011; Goldfinger et al. 2008; Starkey et al. 2009; Tobin et al. 2011). With the network-oriented peer educator model approach, identifying the motives of the peer educator to promote your health message or disseminate information is important. This can be accomplished by conducting focus groups with potential peer educators and asking them to identify motivators and barriers to conducting **outreach** to their peers. Another important component to developing a peer-educator-oriented intervention is to identify the settings where peer educators will be interacting with their peers. For instance, if a group of college-aged peer educators are being trained to talk to their peers about binge drinking, how do they plan to initiate these conversations? When you know about the range of different settings in which peer educators are conducting outreach, you can tailor the communication skills that they will need to enable the most effective and productive interaction. Another important consideration in developing a peer-educator-oriented intervention is to provide the information and skills training and practice for the peers to successfully engage in the health behavior.

Peer education programs may change the behavior of the peer educator or the recipients of the peer education. Although network approaches to peer education are powerful tools for behavior change, there are several challenges and potential negative outcomes. Challenges to peer education include life events and mobility that may alter network composition, lack of resources and competing demands that impede peer education activities, and lack of interest from individuals with high centrality or those who have influential roles. Potential negative outcomes include role conflict between members of the community and the institutional representative, lack of control over the messages of peer educators, negative reactions from network members, and issues of the role of peer educators after programs end.

CASE EXAMPLES

One of the seminal peer educator interventions in HIV/AIDS prevention (SHIELD) was developed in Baltimore, Maryland, to train current and former drug users to conduct HIV prevention outreach to people in their networks and communities (Latkin, Sherman, and Knowlton 2003). Peer educators were trained in HIV risk reduction and communication skills for talking to others about HIV prevention through peer outreach. Results from the six-month follow-up show that peer educators trained to conduct outreach reduced injection risk behaviors and increased condom use with casual partners as compared to the **control group**. This model has been tailored and implemented in a variety of other locations including Philadelphia, Pennsylvania; Vietnam; St. Petersburg, Russia; Chang Mai, Thailand; and Chennai, India. In addition to changing HIV-related health behaviors, these interventions have been found to also alter norms within the network and lead to greater endorsement of risk-reduction norms.

Peer education programs have also been conducted in clinical settings. As part of the diabetes management intervention Project DULCE, community health workers who also had diabetes were trained to be peer educators (Philis-Tsimikas et al. 2011; Philis-Tsimikas et al. 2004). The peer educators led classes on strategies for diabetes management and also shared their personal experiences with the condition. After one year in the program, participants in the peer education program reported improved health, knowledge, and self-efficacy.

Conclusion

Substantial scientific evidence exists on the role of **interpersonal factors** in health behaviors and the risk of disease and premature death. Moreover, a range of established social influence theories are available that can guide research and intervention development to target health behaviors. In this chapter, we primarily discussed the social network as a key example of interpersonal influence. Interventions that target interpersonal influence processes, especially within a social network, can have a broad impact and therefore play an important role in the field of health education and public health. Considerations of the interpersonal level of influence on health and behavior should include the geographic and political context of individuals and their social networks. With the widespread use of social media, the Internet, and cellular technology, the social network and interpersonal influence processes are even more salient.

REFERENCES

Agha S, Van Rossem R. 2004. Impact of a school-based peer sexual health intervention on normative beliefs, risk perceptions, and sexual behavior of Zambian adolescents. *J Adolesc Health* 34 (5) (May): 441-52.

Asch SE. 1952. Rules and values. In *Social Psychology,* ed. SE Asch, 350-63. Upper Saddle River, NJ: Prentice-Hall.

Ashida S, Heaney CA. 2008. Differential associations of social support and social connectedness with structural features of social networks and the health status of older adults. *J Aging Health* 20 (7) (Oct.): 872-93.

Baker CW, Little TD, Brownell KD. 2003. Predicting adolescent eating and activity behaviors: The role of social norms and personal agency. *Health Psychol* 22 (2) (March): 189-98.

Bandura A. 1977a. Self-efficacy: Toward a unifying theory of behavioral change. *Psychol Rev* 84 (2) (March): 191-215.

———. 1977b. *Social Learning Theory.* Englewood Cliffs, NJ: Prentice Hall.

———. 1986. *Social Foundations of Thought and Action: A Social Cognitive Theory.* Englewood Cliffs, NJ: Prentice-Hall.

———. 1994. Social cognitive theory and exercise of control over HIV infection. In *Preventing AIDS: Theories and Methods of Behavioral Interventions,* ed. RJ DiClemente, JL Peterson, 25-60. New York: Plenum Press.

———. 1997. *Self-Efficacy: The Exercise of Control.* New York: W. H. Freeman.

———. 2004. Health promotion by social cognitive means. *Health Educ Behav* 31 (2) (April): 143-64.

Bandura A, Ross SA, Ross D. 1961. Transmission of aggression through imitation of aggressive models. *J Abnorm Soc Psychol* 63:575-82.

Barrington C, Latkin C, Sweat MD, Moreno L, Ellen J, Kerrigan D. 2009. Talking the talk, walking the walk: Social network norms, communication patterns, and condom use among the male partners of female sex workers in La Romana, Dominican Republic. *Soc Sci Med* 68 (11) (June): 2037-44.

Barroso CS, Peters RJ, Johnson RJ, Kelder SH, Jefferson T. 2010. Beliefs and perceived norms concerning body image among African-American and Latino teenagers. *J Health Psychol* 15 (6) (Sept.): 858-70.

Bettenhausen KL, Murnighan JK. 1991. The development of an intragroup norm and the effects of interpersonal and structural challenges. *Admin Science Q* 36 (1) (March): 20-35.

Bock BC, Graham AL, Whiteley JA, Stoddard JL. 2008. A review of web-assisted tobacco interventions (WATIs). *J Med Internet Res* 10 (5) (Nov. 6): e39.

Bourdieu P. 1986. The forms of capital. In *Handbook of Theory and Research for the Sociology of Education,* ed. JG Richardson, 241-58. New York: Greenwood Press.

Buchanan AS, Latkin CA. 2008. Drug use in the social networks of heroin and cocaine users before and after drug cessation. *Drug Alcohol Depend* 96 (3) (Aug. 1): 286-89.

Buhi ER, Goodson P. 2007. Predictors of adolescent sexual behavior and intention: A theory-guided systematic review. *J Adolesc Health* 40 (1) (Jan.): 4-21.

Buttross LS, Kastner JW. 2003. A brief review of adolescents and tobacco: What we know and don't know. *Am J Med Sci* 326 (4) (Oct.): 235-37.

Campbell C, MacPhail C. 2002. Peer education, gender, and the development of critical consciousness: Participatory HIV prevention by South African youth. *Soc Sci Med* 55 (2) (July): 331-45.

Chapman S. 1995. Great expectorations! The decline of public spitting: Lessons for passive smoking? *Br Med J* 311 (7021) (Dec. 23-30): 1685-86.

Cho H, Sands LP, Wilson KM. 2010. Predictors of summer sun safety practice intentions among rural high school students. *Am J Health Behav* 34 (4) (July-Aug.): 412-19.

Chou WY, Hunt YM, Beckjord EB, Moser RP, Hesse BW. 2009. Social media use in the United States: Implications for health communication. *J Med Internet Res* 11 (4) (Nov. 27): e48.

Cialdini RB, Reno RR, Kallgren CA. 1990. A focus theory of normative conduct: Recycling the concept of norms to reduce littering in public places. *J Pers Soc Psychol* 58 (6): 1015-26.

Cobb NK, Graham AL, Abrams DB. 2010. Social network structure of a large online community for smoking cessation. *Am J Public Health* 100 (7) (July): 1282-89.

Coleman, JS. 1990. *Foundations of Social Theory.* Cambridge, MA: Harvard University Press.

Cunningham JA, Selby P, van Mierlo T. 2006. Integrated online services for smokers and drinkers? Use of the check your drinking assessment screener by participants of the stop smoking center. *Nicotine Tob Res* 8 (suppl. 1) (Dec.): S21-S25.

Davey-Rothwell MA, Kuramoto SJ, Latkin CA. 2008. Social networks, norms, and 12-step group participation. *Am J Drug Alcohol Abuse* 34 (2): 185-93.

Davey-Rothwell MA, Latkin CA. 2007. Gender differences in social network influence among injection drug users: Perceived norms and needle sharing. *J Urban Health* 84 (5) (Sept.): 691-703.

Davey-Rothwell MA, Tobin K, Yang C, Sun CJ, Latkin CA. 2011. Results of a randomized controlled trial of a peer mentor HIV/STI prevention intervention for women over an 18 month follow-up. *AIDS Behav,* April 6.

Dawber, TR. 1980. *The Framingham Study: The Epidemiology of Atherosclerotic Disease.* Cambridge, MA: Harvard University Press.

Dawber TR, Kannel WB, Lyell LP. 1963. An approach to longitudinal studies in a community: The Framingham Study. *Ann NY Acad Sci* 107:539-56.

De P, Cox J, Boivin JF, Platt RW, Jolly AM. 2007. The importance of social networks in their association to drug equipment sharing among injection drug users: A review. *Addiction* 102 (11) (Nov.): 1730-39.

Dean WR, Sharkey JR. 2011. Food insecurity, social capital, and perceived personal disparity in a predominantly rural region of Texas: An individual-level analysis. *Soc Sci Med* 72 (9) (May): 1454-62.

Eisenberg ME, Neumark-Sztainer D, Story M, Perry C. 2005. The role of social norms and friends' influences on unhealthy weight-control behaviors among adolescent girls. *Soc Sci Med* 60 (6) (March): 1165-73.

El-Bassel N, Cooper DK, Chen DR, Schilling RF. 1998. Personal social networks and HIV status among women on methadone. *AIDS Care* 10 (6) (Dec.): 735-49.

Elgar FJ, Davis CG, Wohl MJ, Trites SJ, Zelenski JM, Martin MS. 2011. Social capital, health, and life satisfaction in 50 countries. *Health Place,* July 6.

Festinger L. 1954. A theory of social comparison processes. *Human Rel* 7 (2): 117-40.

Fiore J, Becker J, Coppel DB. 1983. Social network interactions: A buffer or a stress. *Am J Commun Psych* 11 (4) (Aug.): 423-39.

Fowler JH, Christakis NA. 2008. Dynamic spread of happiness in a large social network: Longitudinal analysis over 20 years in the Framingham Heart Study. *Br Med J* 337 (a2338): 1-9.

Fujiwara T, Kawachi I. 2008. A prospective study of individual-level social capital and major depression in the United States. *J Epidemiol Commun Health* 62 (7) (July): 627-33.

Fukuyama F. 1999. *The Great Disruption: Human Nature and the Reconstitution of Social Order.* New York: Free Press.

Gatt S, Sammut R. 2008. An exploratory study of predictors of self-care behaviour in persons with type 2 diabetes. *Int J Nurs Stud* 45 (10) (Oct.): 1525-33.

Gielen AC, McDonnell KA, Wu AW, O'Campo P, Faden R. 2001. Quality of life among women living with HIV: The importance of violence, social support, and self care behaviors. *Soc Sci Med* 52 (2) (Jan.): 315-22.

Goldfinger JZ, Arniella G, Wylie-Rosett J, Horowitz CR. 2008. Project HEAL: Peer education leads to weight loss in Harlem. *J Health Care Poor Underserved* 19 (1) (Feb.): 180-92.

Griffiths KM, Calear AL, Banfield M. 2009. Systematic review on internet support groups (ISGs) and depression (1): Do ISGs reduce depressive symptoms? *J Med Internet Res* 11 (3) (Sept. 30): e40.

Hobfoll SE. 2001. The influence of culture, community, and the nested-self in the stress process: Advancing conservation of resources theory. *Applied Psychol* 50 (3): 337-421.

Holliday JC, Rothwell HA, Moore LA. 2010. The relative importance of different measures of peer smoking on adolescent smoking behavior: Cross-sectional and longitudinal analyses of a large British cohort. *J Adolesc Health* 47 (1) (July): 58-66.

Holtgrave DR, Crosby R. 2006. Is social capital a protective factor against obesity and diabetes? Findings from an exploratory study. *Ann Epidemiol* 16 (5) (May): 406-8.

Hong Y, Pena-Purcell NC, Ory MG. 2011. Outcomes of online support and resources for cancer survivors: A systematic literature review. *Patient Educ Couns,* July 26.

Houston TK, Sadasivam RS, Ford DE, Richman J, Ray MN, Allison JJ. 2010. The QUIT-PRIMO provider-patient internet-delivered smoking cessation referral intervention: A cluster-randomized comparative effectiveness trial: Study protocol. *Implement Sci* 5 (Nov. 17): 87.

Hyman HH. 1942. The psychology of status. *Arch Psychol* 269:5-91.

Jackson KM, Aiken LS. 2000. A psychosocial model of sun protection and sunbathing in young women: The impact of health beliefs, attitudes, norms, and self-efficacy for sun protection. *Health Psychol* 19 (5) (Sept): 469-78.

Johnson RM, Runyan CW, Coyne-Beasley T, Lewis MA, Bowling JM. 2008. Storage of household firearms: An examination of the attitudes and beliefs of married women with children. *Health Educ Res* 23 (4): 592-602.

Kelly AB, O'Flaherty M, Connor JP, et al. 2011. The influence of parents, siblings, and peers on pre- and early-teen smoking: A multilevel model. *Drug Alcohol Rev* 30 (4) (July): 381-87.

Kelly BD, Davoren M, Mhaolain AN, Breen EG, Casey P. 2009. Social capital and suicide in 11 European countries: An ecological analysis. *Soc Psychiatry Psychiatr Epidemiol* 44 (11) (Nov.): 971-77.

Kelly JA, St Lawrence JS, Stevenson LY, et al. 1992. Community AIDS/HIV risk reduction: The effects of endorsements by popular people in three cities. *Am J Public Health* 82 (11) (Nov.): 1483-89.

Kim D, Kawachi I. 2006. A multilevel analysis of key forms of community- and individual-level social capital as predictors of self-rated health in the United States. *J Urban Health* 83 (5) (Sept.): 813-26.

Kincaid DL. 2000. Social networks, ideation, and contraceptive behavior in Bangladesh: A longitudinal analysis. *Soc Sci Med* 50 (2) (Jan.): 215-31.

Klassen AC, Washington C. 2008. How does social integration influence breast cancer control among urban African-American women? Results from a cross-sectional survey. *BMC Womens Health* 8 (Feb. 6): 4.

Klovdahl AS, Potterat JJ, Woodhouse DE, Muth JB, Muth SQ, Darrow WW. 1994. Social networks and infectious disease: The Colorado Springs study. *Soc Sci Med* 38 (1) (Jan.): 79-88.

Knowlton A, Arnsten J, Eldred L, et al. 2006. Individual, interpersonal, and structural correlates of effective HAART use among urban active injection drug users. *J Acquir Immune Defic Syndr* 41 (4) (April 1): 486-92.

Krupp K, Marlow LA, Kielmann K, et al. 2010. Factors associated with intention-to-recommend human papillomavirus vaccination among physicians in Mysore, India. *J Adolesc Health* 46 (4) (April): 379-84.

LaBrie JW, Hummer JF, Grant S, Lac A. 2010. Immediate reductions in misperceived social norms among

high-risk college student groups. *Addictive Behav* 35 (12) (Dec.): 1094-101.

Lapinski MK, Rimal RN. 2005. An explication of social norms. *Communication Theory* 15 (2): 127-47.

Latkin CA, Forman V, Knowlton A, Sherman S. 2003. Norms, social networks, and HIV-related risk behaviors among urban disadvantaged drug users. *Soc Sci Med* 56 (3) (Feb.): 465-76.

Latkin CA, Knowlton AR. 2005. Micro-social structural approaches to HIV prevention: A social ecological perspective. *AIDS Care* 17 (suppl. 1) (June): S102-S113.

Latkin CA, Sherman S, Knowlton A. 2003. HIV prevention among drug users: Outcome of a network-oriented peer outreach intervention. *Health Psychol* 22 (4) (July): 332-39.

Latkin C, Yang C, Srikrishnan AK, et al. 2011. The relationship between social network factors, HIV, and hepatitis C among injection drug users in Chennai, India. *Drug Alcohol Depend* 117 (1) (Aug. 1): 50-54.

Latkin C, Yang C, Tobin K, Hulbert A. 2010. Factors associated with recruiting an HIV seropositive risk network member among injection drug users. *AIDS Behav*, March 6.

Lett HS, Blumenthal JA, Babyak MA, et al. 2007. Social support and prognosis in patients at increased psychosocial risk recovering from myocardial infarction. *Health Psychol* 26 (4) (July): 418-27.

Melling B, Houguet-Pincham T. 2011. Online peer support for individuals with depression: A summary of current research and future considerations. *Psychiatr Rehabil J* 34 (3) (Winter): 252-54.

Miller M. 2003. The dynamics of substance use and sex networks in HIV transmission. *J Urban Health* 80 (4) (Dec.) (suppl. 3): 88-96.

Moreira MT, Smith LA, Foxcroft D. 2009. Social norms interventions to reduce alcohol misuse in university or college students. *Cochrane Database Syst Rev* 3 (July 8): CD006748.

Myers DG, Bishop GD. 1970. Discussion effects on racial attitudes. *Science* 169 (947) (Aug. 21): 778-79.

Neighbors C, Lee CM, Lewis MA, Fossos N, Larimer ME. 2007. Are social norms the best predictor of outcomes among heavy-drinking college students? *J Stud Alcohol Drugs* 68 (4) (July): 556-65.

Newcomb TM. 1958. Attitude development as a function of reference groups: The Bennington study In *Readings in Social Psychology*, ed. EE Maccoby, TM Newcomb, EL Hartley, 265-75. New York: Holt.

Okun MA, Ruehlman L, Karoly P, Lutz R, Fairholme C, Schaub R. 2003. Social support and social norms: Do both contribute to predicting leisure-time exercise? *Am J Health Behav* 27 (5) (Sept.-Oct.): 493-507.

Oostveen T, Knibbe R, De Vries H. 1996. Social influences on young adults' alcohol consumption: Norms, modeling, pressure, socializing, and conformity. *Addictive Behav* 21 (2): 187-97.

Perkins HW, Craig DW. 2006. A successful social norms campaign to reduce alcohol misuse among college student-athletes. *J Stud Alcohol* 67 (6) (Nov.): 880-89.

Perkins HW, Haines MP, Rice R. 2005. Misperceiving the college drinking norm and related problems: A nationwide study of exposure to prevention information, perceived norms, and student alcohol misuse. *J Stud Alcohol* 66 (4) (July): 470-78.

Perkins HW, Meilman PW, Leichliter JS, Cashin JR, Presley CA. 1999. Misperceptions of the norms for the frequency of alcohol and other drug use on college campuses. *J Am Coll Health* 47 (6) (May): 253-58.

Philis-Tsimikas A, Fortmann A, Lleva-Ocana L, Walker C, Gallo LC. 2011. Peer-led diabetes education programs in high-risk Mexican Americans improve glycemic control compared with standard approaches: A Project DULCE promotora randomized trial. *Diabetes Care,* July 20.

Philis-Tsimikas A, Walker C, Rivard L, et al. 2004. Improvement in diabetes care of underinsured patients enrolled in Project DULCE: A community-based, culturally appropriate, nurse case management, and peer education diabetes care model. *Diabetes Care* 27 (1) (Jan.): 110-15.

Portes A. 1998. Social capital: Its origins and applications in modern sociology. *Ann Rev Soc,* 1-24.

Putnam RD. 1996. The strange disappearance of civic America. *Am Prospect* 24:34-48.

———. 2000. *Bowling Alone: The Collapse and Revival of American Community.* New York: Simon & Schuster.

Rimal RN, Lapinski MK, Cook RJ, Real K. 2005. Moving toward a theory of normative influences: How perceived benefits and similarity moderate the impact of descriptive norms on behaviors. *J Health Commun* 10:433-50.

Rogers, EM. 1962. *Diffusion of Innovations.* New York: Free Press.

———. 2003. *Diffusion of Innovations.* 5th ed. New York: Free Press.

Rogers, EM, Shoemaker, FF. 1971. *Communication of Innovations: A Cross-Cultural Approach.* 2nd ed. New York: Free Press.

Rook KS. 1984. The negative side of social interaction: Impact on psychological well-being. *J Pers Soc Psychol* 46:1097-1108.

Rosenquist JN, Murabito J, Fowler JH, Christakis NA. 2010. The spread of alcohol consumption behavior in a large social network. *Ann Intern Med* 152 (7) (April 6): 426-33, W141.

Saul JE, Schillo BA, Evered S, et al. 2007. Impact of a statewide internet-based tobacco cessation intervention. *J Med Internet Res* 9 (3) (Sept. 30): e28.

Scholly K, Katz AR, Gascoigne J, Holck PS. 2005. Using social norms theory to explain perceptions and sexual health behaviors of undergraduate college students: An exploratory study. *J Am Coll Health* 53 (4) (Jan.-Feb.): 159-66.

Schultz PW, Nolan JM, Cialdini RB, Goldstein NJ, Griskevicius V. 2007. The constructive, destructive, and reconstructive power of social norms. *Psychol Sci* 18 (5) (May): 429-34.

Sherif M. 1936. *The Psychology of Social Norms.* New York: Harper.

Siahpush M, Borland R, Taylor J, Singh GK, Ansari Z, Serraglio A. 2006. The association of smoking with perception of income inequality, relative material well-being, and social capital. *Soc Sci Med* 63 (11) (Dec.): 2801-12.

Sivaram S, Zelaya C, Srikrishnan AK, et al. 2009. Associations between social capital and HIV stigma in Chennai, India: Considerations for prevention intervention design. *AIDS Educ Prev* 21 (3) (June): 233-50.

Smith AM, Grierson J, Wain D, Pitts M, Pattison P. 2004. Associations between the sexual behaviour of men who have sex with men and the structure and composition of their social networks. *Sex Transm Infect* 80 (6) (Dec.): 455-58.

Sorensen G, Stoddard AM, Dubowitz T, et al. 2007. The influence of social context on changes in fruit and vegetable consumption: Results of the healthy directions studies. *Am J Public Health* 97 (7) (July): 1216-27.

Stack, CB. 1974. *All Our Kin: Strategies for Survival in a Black Community.* New York: Harper & Row.

Starkey F, Audrey S, Holliday J, Moore L, Campbell R. 2009. Identifying influential young people to undertake effective peer-led health promotion: The example of A Stop Smoking In Schools Trial (ASSIST). *Health Educ Res* 24 (6) (Dec.): 977-88.

Tajfel H. 1974. Social identity and intergroup behavior. *Soc Sci Info* 13 (2): 65-93.

Tittle CR. 1977. Sanction fear and the maintenance of social order. *Soc Forces* 55 (3) (March): 579-96.

Tobin KE, Kuramoto SJ, Davey-Rothwell MA, Latkin CA. 2011. The STEP into action study: A peer-based, personal risk network-focused HIV prevention intervention with injection drug users in Baltimore, Maryland. *Addiction* 106 (2) (Feb.): 366-75.

Tobin KE, Latkin CA. 2008. An examination of social network characteristics of men who have sex with men who use drugs. *Sex Transm Infect* 84 (6) (Nov.): 420-24.

Turner HA, Pearlin LI, Mullan JT. 1998. Sources and determinants of social support for caregivers of persons with AIDS. *J Health Soc Behav* 39 (2) (June): 137-51.

Turner JC. 1978. Social comparison and social identity: Some perspectives for intergroup behavior. *Eur J Soc Psychol* 5:5-34.

Wallace SA, Miller KS, Forehand R. 2008. Perceived peer norms and sexual intentions among African

American preadolescents. *AIDS Educ Prev* 20 (4) (Aug.): 360-69.

Weitzman ER, Cole E, Kaci L, Mandl KD. 2011. Social but safe? Quality and safety of diabetes-related online social networks. *J Am Med Inform Assoc* 18 (3) (May 1): 292-97.

Wejnert B. 2002. Integrating models of diffusion of innovations: A conceptual framework. *Ann Rev Soc* 28:297-326.

Wylie JL, Jolly A. 2001. Patterns of chlamydia and gonorrhea infection in sexual networks in Manitoba, Canada. *Sex Transm Dis* 28 (1) (Jan.): 14-24.

Behavior Change at the Environmental Level

ANN KLASSEN, AMBER C. SUMMERS,
AND AMY R. CONFAIR

LEARNING OBJECTIVES

After completing the chapter, the reader will be able to

* Describe the benefits of intervening at the level of the environment to change individual-level health behaviors.
* Understand the characteristics and key elements of the geographic and nongeographic social environment as they pertain to health behaviors.
* Describe the important types of interventions conducted to date at the environmental level to modify food-related health behaviors, physical-activity-related health behaviors, and microfinance interventions related to HIV/AIDS prevention.
* Evaluate the strength of the evidence to date for environmental interventions for behavior change in key health areas (tobacco, diet, drug use, and sexual risk-taking).

Introduction

This chapter focuses on the **levels of influence** on human **health behaviors** that are less tangible than those discussed in the previous chapters and are less often the deliberate target of behavioral medicine approaches to health behavior change—those that influence behavior at the level of the **social environment**. Despite the increasing sophistication and success of intrapersonal and interpersonal behavior change strategies, there is growing recognition that even the most individually targeted efforts to improve behavior must take into account the social environmental factors in which those individually directed **interventions** occur, in order to have the maximum impact.

Increasingly, public health professionals are recognizing that factors beyond the individual level influence the adoption of unhealthful behaviors. In fact, as Hall and colleagues (2008) observe, our increasingly Westernized global society has become "a world that largely pulls for unhealthy behaviors as the default" as we navigate environments offering more opportunities for unhealthful lifestyles and fewer options for healthful choices. Atwood and colleagues (1997) argued that earlier behavioral medicine research had neglected the environmental, social, and political factors that affect health and that these factors were now ripe for reconsideration.

The **ecological model** allows for an integrative approach, which considers how multiple factors at the environmental level affect health and, conversely, how specific environmental factors might apply to various conditions. The ecological model has been applied to numerous areas of public health, including injury, obesity, infectious disease, and pollution (Stokols 2000a). Despite the vast scope of the environmental factors influencing behavior, we have ample evidence that the physical and social environment is often amenable to intervention. When we gain a greater understanding of the contextual factors that influence health behaviors, we are often successful at intervening on these factors, to prevent the adoption of unhealthful behaviors, reduce the occurrence of unhealthful behaviors, and/or support and encourage healthful behaviors at the population level.

Environmental interventions often deliver considerable "bang for the buck," in that negative environments tend to drive multiple unhealthful behaviors. Thus, even modest interventions at the environmental level may address related problems. For example, the Prevention Institute (2010) reviewed the compelling rationale for the connection between community-level violence and crime and poor nutrition and physical activity patterns among community residents. Reducing the culture of violence and crime in communities clearly leads to less vic-

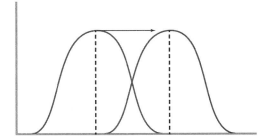

FIGURE 8.1. Structural-level interventions ("shift the curve"). *Source:* Reprinted from Cohen et al. 2000, 147. Used with permission from Elsevier.

timization and property loss, but, as a secondary level of benefit, it also improves the ability of residents to freely use their neighborhood for shopping, leisure activity, and socialization, giving individuals the potential to adopt more healthful lifestyles. An additional downstream benefit of such environmental change is that it may lead to uptake of community-level efforts to create resources such as community gardens or playgrounds as well as create the **social capital** needed to organize and collectively address other problems and **goals**.

Because intervening at the individual level is resource intensive, we often focus on the most problematic portions of the population and those who are at the greatest risk. For example, human immunodeficiency virus (HIV) prevention efforts are often targeted toward those at high risk of acquiring HIV, so that one tail of the distribution is lowered. The goal of interventions at the environmental level is to shift the entire curve (fig. 8.1) so that the population mean is lowered. Thus, populations can be impacted by interventions at the environmental level.

The Conceptualization of the Environment in Social and Behavioral Sciences

In the more biologically based areas of classical public health, such as epidemiology, the environment is often conceptualized as containing multiple discrete harmful **agents**, the health **consequences** of which may vary for different individuals because of differences in susceptibility. Environmental health considers both the degree of exposure and the toxicity of the harmful agent in assessing the level of risk to health. An individual's or a population's predisposing vulnerability to disease and health consequences may be conceptualized as the sum of all potentially harmful factors in their environment plus all biologically beneficial or protective factors.

In social and behavioral sciences, however, the conceptualization of the environment is more encompassing. As in classical environmental health, some of the most important elements of the social environment are spatially determined. The **geographic environment** not only comprises both the residential space of individuals and the location of their home within their neighborhood, city, and region, but also their so-called activity space (where they work, go to school, shop, and spend leisure time), as well as their travel routes to and from these nonresidential activity spaces. The geographically determined environment, including built and social characteristics and **influences**, is becoming increasingly important both conceptually and methodologically in behavior change **theory** and practice. Innovative new methodologies such as Geographic Information Systems (GIS) allow us to easily combine multiple types of spatially referenced data to clearly portray an individual's or a community's spatial influences on health-related behaviors (Cromley and McLafferty 2002).

The **social environment** extends beyond this geographic environment, as elaborated in chapter 7. Because of the ease with which we can measure and evaluate geographic environments, researchers may be tempted to place less emphasis on important nonspatial components of environmental influences on behavior. For example, culture and communication are some of the most constant environmental influences on behaviors. Included are mediated communication, which comes to individuals through formal mechanisms such as television, newspapers, popular culture, and the Internet, and interpersonal communication, from influences such as family, peers, and even public, cultural, or professional figures. Studies of influences on behaviors such as voting show that **networks** of influential discussions occur between individuals at work or at social gatherings, rather than solely in residential neighborhoods (Eagles et al. 2003). Religion; interest groups; and historical, racial, ethnic, and cultural identities can also link an individual or a community to a network of influences that exert very powerful influences on behavior, despite their distance in actual time or space. For example, the Spanish-language television network Univision reports on events taking place in Latin and South America to U.S. Hispanic viewers, creating opinions and shaping behaviors based on ethnic identity that are as influential as messages communicated in broadcasts from their "local" networks. In addition to culture and communication, nongeographic environmental influences can include laws or policies that are applied to groups or situations, rather than communities or geographic areas.

Environmental versus Individual Targets

Distinguishing whether an intervention is targeted toward achieving behavior change primarily through intervening with individuals or through changing the environment is often difficult. Indeed, the most successful and comprehensive interventions often target both the individual and his environment. For example, policies restricting smoking and increasing the costs of tobacco products, which are changing the tobacco use environment, have been shown to be most successful if accompanied by increased availability of quit-lines, cessation counseling, and other tools for individually focused behavior change.

Other interventions use social theory and identify influential individuals as **change agents**. Interventions with these initial individuals in a social group are often based on individually targeted interventions, but, given their influential roles in the **target population**, the rest of the group (as the theory goes) changes not through direct intervention effects but because of changes in the **norms** and **expectations** of the members of their social environment.

Finally, in market economies, changing the purchasing power and buying patterns of one group often causes changes in the pricing and availability of items in the stores where these individuals shop, which may impact the behavior of other shoppers. For example, **evaluations** of changes in the Women, Infants and Children's (WIC) food program found that as store owners began to stock more whole-grain bread products to comply with WIC recipients' needs, nonrecipients also began to purchase more of these products, and the overall food purchasing patterns in low resource communities improved for all residents (Altarum Institute 2011).

Cohen and colleagues (2000) makes the distinction that **individual-level interventions** must target factors that are within the control of the individual, whereas **structural interventions** are those that target factors external to the control of the individual. Others emphasize the unit of randomization or delivery of the intervention, as to whether an intervention should be thought of as primarily individual or community focused. For example, if researchers randomize entire communities to receive either the intervention or the control condition (because effects of individually targeted activities are thought to potentially influence others as well), then it is a community-level intervention, despite the mode of delivery (Jepson et al. 2006).

Still others have made the distinction between health behaviors and **health lifestyles** by pointing out that lifestyles are collectively shared behaviors that are developed in response to the social, cultural and economic environment and are collective, rather than individual, phenomena (Abel et al. 2000).

Compositional versus Contextual Environments

When describing environmental influences, social scientists conceptualize both **compositional** and contextual **environments** within communities (Macintyre et al. 2002). The *composition* of a neighborhood or group is simply the aggregate description of individual characteristics, such as the proportion of persons in a census tract having a college education. The *contextual* environment created by these individual-level characteristics might be a neighborhood that is regarded as well-educated and thought to have a certain collective culture. As described in more detail below, these distinctions have important consequences for behavioral interventions.

Communities have long been recognized as bringing enhanced health to their members through shaping behavior socially (Kawachi and Berkman 2003). Communities set norms, facilitating certain behaviors and restricting others; for example, communities modify smoking behaviors through both formal smoking bans and informal norms of where tobacco use is or is not acceptable. There is a well-developed sociologic literature demonstrating the added influence of social **context** on health. For example, the average income of a person's immediate neighbors affects individual health, over and above the effect of her own income, perhaps by creating shared resources that improve health, such as attracting high-quality health services. Similarly, individual wealth cannot protect someone completely from the reduced **quality of life** of a low-income neighborhood. Thus, individual and area-level social characteristics have complementary but separate health consequences (Cubbin et al. 2000; Cubbin et al. 2001; Diez-Roux et al. 2001; O'Campo et al. 1997).

Additionally, specific behaviors on the individual level likely combine to form contextual effects that become essentially social phenomena. **Social capital** is a concept based on individual actions, such as voting or community involvement, which, when combined in social groups or geographic areas, create an area-level contextual resource that offers benefits to all (Kawachi and Berkman 2003). Conceptually, social capital cannot be decomposed but draws its meaning as a characteristic of the entire larger unit. For example, knowing the aggregate charitable donations of a work group, a religious organization, or a neighborhood tells us something different from knowing each individual member's level of giving.

Similarly, we might speculate that a behavior such as reading a daily newspaper has both individual and contextual meaning. A news story about the connection between diet and cancer will have a different impact on each reader depending on whether everyone else or no one else in a person's immediate **social network** has also read the story. This area-level aggregate behavior, which we might term community-level story penetration, will modify the individual's interpretation of the story's message and perhaps may even determine how the person's knowledge, **attitudes**, and behaviors change as a result.

More subtly, the ratio of automobiles to residents in a neighborhood will provide insight into the contextual characteristics of the neighborhood itself (i.e., by describing levels of car use, an attribute that affects all residents through traffic patterns, norms for public transportation and walkway use, and pollution and noise levels). Individual-level behaviors such as diet, tobacco use, exercise, and medical utilization create norms in groups and communities and may influence the characteristics of the community for all its members. Dietary patterns shape the availability and quality of foods in a community's homes, restaurants, and stores; smoking preferences affect the number of places where smoking is allowed or discouraged; and the demand for goods and services, from screening tests to exercise venues, determines the local availability of such resources. These factors, in turn, can influence whether or not individual-level behaviors are taken up or sustained.

Environment Levels

Drawing on the classic work of Urie Bronfenbrenner (1992), health behavior change theorists have conceptualized multiple nested levels of influence on individual behavior, describing such models as *ecological* or *systems based*. The *macrolevel* of the social environment includes such influences as health care delivery systems, public policy and government, and large-scale social forces such as the media. An intermediate, or *mesolevel* of influence would include factors in the more local environment that influence behaviors of individuals and groups, such as the community, workplace, or school. In addition to these shared spheres of influence, each individual also functions within, and is influenced by, a *microenvironment,* which is made up of the person's social network, including family and peers.

Structural Interventions

In this section, we review three different health behavior areas and describe the evidence in each area for different types of structural interventions that improve health behaviors and outcomes. We look first at nutrition and food choices, focusing on interventions that change either the availability of food types or the information delivered to individuals at the point of food choice or purchase. Next, we focus on physical activity, and how the **built environment** influences energy expenditure and fitness in both residential and activity space, such as schools and workplaces. Third, we investigate the research evidence on the use of financial changes, including microfinance and conditional cash transfers (CCTs) to create empowerment and promote maternal and child health.

Nutrition and Food Choices

Much research has focused on downstream, or individual-level behavioral interventions, which show positive impact on dietary behaviors, such as reducing fat intake and increasing fruit and vegetable intake among populations with high disease risk, but not among healthy populations (Ammerman et al. 2002; Watters et al. 2007). Although we often emphasize the **individual-level factors** and behaviors that drive food choices and related effects on well-being or ill health, changing food-related behaviors depends not just on the individual, but also on the social environment in which the individual makes food choices. The social environment influences what, how, when, and how much we eat. For example, factors such food cost (Glanz et al. 1998), quality and availability of healthful food (Glanz and Yorach 2004), access to supermarkets and other food sources (Caldwell et al. 2008; French et al. 2001; Morland et. al. 2002; Morland et al. 2006; Zenk et al. 2005), prevalence of fast food restaurants (Reidpath et. al. 2002), culture (Gans et al. 2009), and social influence (Hargreaves et al. 2002) all contribute to our food-related behaviors. Structural interventions can be developed in a variety of settings, such as schools, work sites, and community retail food stores, to address these aspects of the social environment and improve food-related behaviors and health outcomes (Biener et al. 1999; Cullen et al. 2007; Lytle et al. 2006; Maston-Koffman et al. 2005; Song et al. 2009).

Structural interventions that address food availability or information in place at the point of food choice or purchase have shown success in influencing food choices. Food availability interventions increase the availability of healthful foods and may also involve decreasing the availability of less healthful foods. Information

delivered at the point of food choice or purchase, such as nutritional content, cost comparisons, and promotion of healthful selections, can help individuals choose the more healthful options. These interventions are sometimes implemented as individual strategies to influence food choices but are often used among a combination of strategies within a part of a larger socioecological intervention (Maston-Koffman et al. 2005; Seymour et al. 2004).

An example of a structural intervention that addressed food availability and incorporated point-of-purchase information comes out of Shape Up Somerville: Eat Smart, Play Hard (SUS) in Somerville, Massachusetts, a collaborative project involving Tufts University, the city of Somerville, and community agencies. SUS was originally kicked off as a three-year, controlled, community-based participatory research trial with the goal of creating small changes in the environments of children and families to help prevent and reduce obesity in children (Economos et al. 2007). Results from formative research completed at the school and community levels indicated that meals were frequently consumed outside the home by Somerville residents, underscoring the need to support a healthful environment by working with local restaurants within the community to both offer, and draw attention to, healthful options for children and families. Thus, as a component of SUS, a community-based restaurant initiative took place in 2003–4 with the **objective** to increase lower-fat choices, fruits, and vegetables in local community restaurants (Economos et al. 2009). Healthful menu criteria were established for a restaurant to qualify as an SUS restaurant, and restaurants that were able to meet the criteria with current menus or by modifying menu items were provided an SUS decal to place in their windows as one means of publicity. At completion of the **recruitment** phase, 21 restaurants were approved, which was 28% of those recruited. At the point of purchase, consumers were able to identify healthful menu options in SUS-approved restaurants by locating stickers strategically placed on menus. With commitment from key leaders in multiple sectors, other components of the SUS that addressed structural factors to improve food choices and physical activity included school food-service reform, an increase in the number of community gardens, park renovations, and improved public transit and **walkability**. Ownership among the community and cooperation from civic and cultural leaders strengthened the sustainability of the program. After the first year, school children in the intervention community were found to have a significant decrease in **body mass index** z-score compared to children in the control communities (Economos et al. 2007). At the end of the three-year grant, the initiative continued and, as of 2010, was led by the Shape Up Somerville Task Force (Economos and Curtatone 2010), with long-term evaluation results pending.

Structural interventions that address food availability can also be successful in more targeted settings (e.g., among employees in a worksite wellness program). In Howard County, Maryland, for example, the Wellness Works program is a comprehensive wellness program for Howard County government and allied agency employees. As a part of this program, a Healthy Vending policy was developed in collaboration with the Howard County Health Department to increase the availability of healthful options in on-site vending machines. This policy requires that at least 25% of food and beverages in vending machines must meet healthful nutrition criteria based on standards set by the Institute of Medicine.

The Black Churches United for Better Health Project is another structural intervention in a targeted setting. This National Cancer Institute–funded research project encouraged consumption of five or more daily servings of fruit and vegetables to promote cancer and chronic disease prevention and included 50 black churches from 10 rural counties in eastern North Caro-

lina. The primary objective was to increase daily servings of fruit and vegetables among participants by 0.5 servings per day. To achieve this goal, churches cultivated gardens to increase the availability of fruit and vegetables at church functions where food is commonly served. In addition to these strategies, other community-based intervention components took place at the individual, social network, and community levels and included educational sessions, recipe tastings, promotion of farmers' markets, encouragement of pastoral support, and involvement of lay health leaders and community **coalitions**. The project was successful in changing health behavior and resulted in an increase in servings of fruit and vegetables by 0.85 servings per day among participants (Campbell et al. 1999).

As these examples demonstrate, structural interventions not only have the potential to influence the availability of healthful food but can also be used as a method to engage community members and help prioritize healthful behavior. The Prevention Institute (2010) offers multiple strategies to engage communities to improve availability of healthful food through various institutions including restaurants, food retailers, churches, and other community settings by engagement of multiple **stakeholders**. The Prevention Institute suggests promoting community engagement in addition to utilizing federal resources, offering retailers **incentives** from the local government to provide healthful choices, and providing consumers with access to transportation to supermarkets, among other strategies.

Physical Activity

The **built environment** is the part of the physical environment that has been modified by humans. It includes transportation systems, land use, public resources (e.g., parks), zoning regulations, and buildings (i.e., schools, homes, workplaces). Inadequate access to exercise facilities such as safe recreational parks and side-walks is a structural factor leading to physical inactivity, whereas proximity to recreation sites such as parks, basketball courts, walking and running tracks, and public open space is associated with greater physical activity (Grow et al. 2008; Owen et al. 2004). Thus, the built environment—including those features that act as barriers to physical activity opportunities—influences health outcomes such as obesity (Northridge et al. 2003). Perceived neighbor-hood safety, **social support**, and social capital are aspects of the social environment that im-pact engagement in physical activity (McNeill et al. 2006).

The Community Preventive Services Task Force (2002) suggests methods to increase physical activity levels in communities. Among other strategies, such as informational ap-proaches (e.g., point-of-decision prompts to use stairs instead of elevators, community-wide campaigns) and behavioral and social ap-proaches (e.g., school-based physical education, social support interventions), the Task Force recommended improved access to physical ac-tivity opportunities by **targeting** physical and organizational structures based on evidence of **effectiveness**. Multiple initiatives have been set in action nationwide to address physical activ-ity and the built environment, such as the Rob-ert Wood Johnson Foundation's Active Living by Design and the Centers for Disease Control and Prevention's Active Community Environ-ments Initiative. These programs encourage interdisciplinary **partnerships** to enhance built environments.

The interventions highlighted below focus on walking programs, insofar as walking is a more acceptable and accessible form of exercise among previously sedentary adults (Siegel et al. 1995). The Walk with Us intervention (Riley-Jacome et al. 2010) is one example of how exist-ing community resources can be used to in-crease physical activity among previously sedentary individuals. Walk with Us began in

February 2005 in the Greenville School District in Greene County, a rural community in up-state New York. This pilot intervention, led by the University at Albany Prevention Research Center, was developed based on a community needs assessment to determine the social and environmental factors influencing diabetes self-care behaviors in two underserved communi-ties in upstate New York. During the needs assessment, community residents identified hav-ing a safe place to walk or exercise as a high priority and suggested indoor walking pro-grams among multiple solutions to alleviate barriers to physical activity. As a result, a nine-week indoor walking program using school buildings was developed as a pilot intervention. The program was evaluated through a mixed-method approach using surveys, daily logs, dia-ries, registration forms, interviews, and focus groups. Results indicated that social support is a primary benefit to program participation in addition to external or environmental benefits, such as safety, convenience of location, and lower cost. Although barriers were identified in both implementation and participation, includ-ing conflicts with other activities held at the school and distance between schools and resi-dences, the Walk with Us program helped to promote "community spirit," while increasing physical activity levels among participants.

Walking groups have also been incorporated into multicomponent interventions that sup-port physical activity. The High Point Walking for Health program was developed to increase physical activity levels among the diverse, low-income High Point Public Housing community in Seattle by making both the social *and* the physical environment supportive of walking (Krieger et al. 2009). Community mobilization and community-based participatory research were used to foster collaboration among resi-dents, community-based organizations, the Se-attle Housing Authority, researchers, practitio-ners, and other public agencies. Youth and adult residents participated in community action teams and worked to determine community conditions and concerns, which were used to develop relevant project activities. Community assessment employing qualitative interviews, focus groups, and surveys helped identify aspects within the community that discouraged walking, actions that were culturally appropriate, and existing assets and challenges. Modifications in the built environment included restoring staircases and advocating pedestrian safety through rallies and community forums, improving traffic signals, and dealing with street parking restrictions. Social environment components included the creation of walking groups and a walking information campaign. Participation among community stakeholders helped implement and sustain the project. For example, residents served as walk leaders and took on duties such as making calls to remind participants, checking in walkers, and timing walks. Changes in walking activity were evaluated among participants using pre- and post-program surveys, which indicated an increase in **self-reported** walking minutes per day from 64.6 minutes to 108.8 minutes at three-month follow-ups. Other benefits of the program included improvements in general health and social connectedness.

These examples demonstrate how existing community resources can be enhanced to support physical activity. The Ozark Heart Health Coalition in rural Missouri helped to enhance existing trails to encourage increased physical activity levels among community residents, but it also focused on developing new trails (Wiggs et al. 2008). The Ozark Heart Health Coalition focuses on multiple behavioral risk factors for heart disease, including physical activity, by delivering interventions at multiple levels of the ecological framework. For success, the coalition enlists early engagement on the part of key leaders and decision-makers in the construction of new trails, including local parks and recreation personnel, state departments of conservation and natural resources, and city and council members. They have helped with construction of more than 30 walking trails, varying in length from 0.13 miles to 2.38 miles, on land donated primarily by churches, schools, and local governments, which are incorporated as a new element of the community environment supporting physical activity. Evaluation findings to date show that 55.2% of users report increased activity since the trails were constructed, with women and those with less education showing the greater gains.

Microcredit, Microfinance, and Conditional Cash Transfers

In the final example for environmental influences on behavior, we consider the range of programs that offer economic incentives as a means of improving health-related behaviors among low-resource populations. In most societies, there are government and charity programs aimed solely at ameliorating the effects of poverty by offering material or financial aid, but programs relevant to behavior change are those that tie assistance to specific behaviors. In doing so, policymakers, whether representing government or **private sector** efforts, are using behavioral and social theory to incentivize behaviors that are believed to produce better outcomes for recipients, their families, or society as a whole.

Although these programs may appear to be at the individual level, they typically are designed to change economic dynamics at the group level, within families, collective groups of recipients, or social and economically dependent networks, such as villages. Furthermore, because these interventions tie economic resources to specific activities or behaviors, they serve to change behavioral norms among cultures and societies; therefore, they are intended to also change the behaviors of persons who are not direct funding recipients.

Microcredit interventions typically offer very small loans to impoverished individuals who would otherwise lack the collateral to borrow from banks or conventional loan sources. Loans are typically made to groups of persons who are all responsible for the entire sum borrowed; therefore, microcredit interventions use social control and group dynamics to maximize program success. In doing so, they create the capacity for group problem solving and empowerment in settings where borrowers, such as women, may not have previously had opportunity to work collectively with their own economic resources. For example, women may lack authority within their families to hold back sufficient earnings to repay their share of the loan, but if multiple households within a village will be affected, husbands may feel more pressure to support the initiative. Caldas and colleagues (2010) identify microcredit as a "minimalist" approach, compared to microfinance. Microfinance, described as "credit plus," is often coupled with other strategies to improve people's financial well-being, including insurance, savings programs, and business training. Additional interventions coupled with financial assistance often include literacy and education or targeted interventions for health or nutrition education.

Microfinance interventions have been used extensively to improve specific health outcomes and to change specific health-related behaviors. Microfinance is especially effective when the drivers of a disease or health-related risk are based in power imbalances and economic vulnerabilities. The Sonagachi Project in India, a sexually transmitted disease (STD)/HIV intervention for female sex workers, used four specific structural intervention strategies to empower women: community mobilization, rights-based framing, advocacy, and microfinance. Women in the **control groups** received standard STD care, condom promotion, and peer education (Swendeman et al. 2009). Significant effects of the intervention included increased disclosure of profession and reframing of sex work as valid work, while also expressing a more posi-

tive future orientation and desire for education. Other outcomes were increased social support and interpersonal networks, financial savings, and skills in both condom negotiation and refusing undesirable transactions.

Caldas and colleagues (2010) review multiple microfinance interventions designed to either prevent HIV risk behaviors among financially vulnerable groups or to intervene with persons living with HIV/AIDS (PLWHAs) to improve socioeconomic well-being and health outcomes. Although there is evidence that microfinance improves outcomes for some recipients, the authors note that many persons are not able to repay the loans owing to ill health or even death or because of overwhelming economic hardship and competing household demands. Additional issues are driven by changes to social dynamics introduced by financial independence for female PLWHAs, such as increases in interpersonal violence from male partners or boycotts of small business efforts by PLWHAs within communities. For such persons, the authors argue, conditional or even unconditional cash transfers may be more appropriate. The authors also note the **complexity** of rigorously evaluating the short- and long-term impact of such interventions, especially when the unit of intervention is a collective, such as a village. Additional criticisms of microfinance as a policy strategy focus on the relatively high interest rates charged to offset the risk for investors and the "bottom up" approach, which may not address other fundamental economic issues within these societies.

Conditional cash transfers (CCTs), as the name indicates, provide direct payments rather than loans; receipt of the payments is tied to behaviors or achievements. As with microfinance, transfers are made to break the cycle of poverty among the poorest members of communities. In a review of CCT programs in 13 Latin American countries, Lomeli (2008) notes the rapidity with which such programs were adopted during the 1990s and the first decade of the 2000s and the initial positive appraisal by policy experts that such programs were an efficient means to increase human capital and break the "inter-generational cycle of poverty." Lomeli explains that a key concept in CCT is that poverty persists owing to a lack of investment in the education, preventive health, and nutrition of children and that breaking this cycle is more important than addressing immediate financial needs. Therefore, CCT programs pay mothers for their children's school attendance, well-child medical visits, or nutrition-related behaviors. These efforts create "human capital" by ensuring that the child will become a healthy adult with maximum employment potential. Furthermore, the pressures on children to discontinue school are reduced, insofar as CCTs make it more financially advantageous for a family to allow a child to continue attending school rather to have the child work.

Despite the widespread enthusiasm of policymakers for CCTs, Lomeli reports mixed results across indicators of health, education, and nutrition in the countries and programs studied. For example, he reports the view of many policymakers that longer school attendance for very poor persons cannot be assumed to yield the same return on investment as it provides to persons in economically strong societies because of the lower quality of schooling and the failure of impoverished societies to accommodate an influx of well-educated job seekers.

As with microfinance, CCTs may improve, but also can often strain, social relationships within communities and within households. Although financial decision making may enhance the role of mothers within their families, Lomeli also notes that it may also increase their responsibilities and tasks, further burdening their lives and reinforcing the idea that women must serve as the vehicles for others' well-being.

In 2007 the City of New York, with private funding, began a CCT program called Opportunity NYC—Family Rewards. Cash incentives were tied to 22 specific activities and outcomes related to children's education but also to family preventive health care and parental employment. A randomized controlled trial awarded an average of $6,000 across 2 years to the intervention arm, which was made up of half of the participating 4,800 families and 11,000 children. Most payments went to parents, but high school students received payments directly for some achievements, such as taking an important school examination (Riccio et al. 2010). Financial improvements included increased savings and bank accounts and reduced reliance on check-cashing services. Health outcomes included increased preventive dental care by families and decreased reliance on emergency rooms visits for routine care. Children had improved school attendance, although improved achievement was seen only among certain well-prepared high school students.

Opportunity NYC—Family Rewards is reportedly the first use of municipally run CCTs in a developed country. As with programs outside the United States, Family Rewards resulted in unanticipated changes in social dynamics within families. For example, a greater number of relationship changes—both marriages and divorces—were observed in the intervention households than among controls. The evaluators hypothesize that greater financial stability may allow couples to make changes they would typically postpone during financially stressful times.

Stakeholder Roles

Planners of an intervention on the environment to impact behavior change must consider the role of **key stakeholders** (see chapter 4). Stakeholders in a behavior change intervention can include any person or institution who is influenced by that intervention or has influence over those involved. The input of stakeholders can have important impacts at every stage, from defining the problem and program design to the dissemination of results. For example, an intervention to increase physical activity in youth by encouraging them to walk to school could have stakeholders including residents (parents, children, and neighbors), schools (teachers and administrators), city authorities (government officials, police, and transportation), contractors and manufacturers (for sidewalks, streetlamps, and traffic signals), publicity specialists, health providers (school nurses and pediatricians), health plans or payers, neighborhood groups, and after-school programs. Especially with environmental behavior change interventions that aim to impact large groups of people, having a wide range of stakeholder groups means more perspectives from the whole group are considered in the design of the intervention. Including stakeholder perspectives can improve the cultural acceptability of an intervention because stakeholders provide insight into the pertinent circumstances of a community or environment that may otherwise go unnoticed. For example, outside evaluators of a neighborhood park may be unaware of the dynamic temporal nature of space use and they may design interventions that miss important evening or weekend users.

This **integration** of the intervention within the existing social and physical structure of the community creates more trust, buy-in, and active participation from community members during implementation and increases the sustainability of aspects of the intervention after its conclusion. In other words, an intervention is more likely to succeed if key stakeholders partner with the interventionists throughout (Israel, Parker, et al. 2005). The following examples further illustrate the role of stakeholders in environmental behavior change interventions.

Browne and colleagues (2009) describe partnership principles used and the lessons learned when forming a partnership with the goal of replicating a previously successful beauty-salon-based health education and promotion program with African American and Latino communities in Philadelphia. This partnership included an oversight committee of 6 key health care organizations and philanthropies in the area, 2 community-based organizations to help recruit salons as partners, 3 academic institutions (universities) for technical guidance and expertise, and 17 beauty salons for the intervention sites and to distribute and collect surveys. Local businesses such as barbershops and beauty salons have proved to be effective venues for community-based health promotion, both because of their social function as community gathering places and because of the common role of barbers and beauticians as lay health educators. In part owing to the involvement of many different kinds of stakeholders, the program was successful at increasing health knowledge about asthma and diabetes, decreasing negative health beliefs, and modifying the perception that such conditions were "not big risks." It also successfully created a meaningful partnership that continued beyond the original program to become a "consortium committed to health education of minority populations in Philadelphia," exemplifying how coalition building can result from stakeholder partnerships formed for environmental behavior change interventions.

Another example comes from the journal *Injury Prevention,* in which a commentary about how to bridge the gap between research and practice primarily recommended: "Researchers and practitioners should engage the community, including stakeholders, as equal partners in the initiation of community-based interventions. Scientific evidence and community knowledge should be integrated" (Mallonee et al. 2006). One example cited was work by Brussoni and colleagues in the field of injury prevention. These academic researchers completed systematic reviews of existing research evidence to capture information regarding effective practices and then brought together local stakeholders to plan practical strategies for incorporating those evidence-based effective practices into their community (Brussoni et al. 2006).

Conclusion

As we stated in the introduction to this chapter, interventions aiming to reach every person in a population on an individual level to encourage behavior change are both costly and complicated, and therefore individual-level interventions are usually aimed at changing only high-risk individuals' behavior. However, structural or environmental interventions can target and potentially affect everyone, whether or not they are individually at risk, thus having the potential to influence large numbers of people.

Thus, the choice of level of intervention may be guided by how prevalent a condition is, whether it is concentrated or diffuse in a population, and whether there are disparities in impact. If the goal is to influence a large number, structural interventions are appropriate. For example, to address obesity, a tax on sugary beverages could theoretically reduce consumption of the taxed beverages and improve health outcomes for everyone in a jurisdiction, regardless of body size. However, if the number of people at risk or affected is small, the individual level may be more appropriate (Cohen et al. 2000).

Jepson and colleagues (2006) undertook the task of conducting a "review of reviews," to consider the evidence for the effectiveness of interventions for changing health behaviors. They focused on six key health behaviors: cigarette smoking, alcohol use, physical activity, healthful diet, illicit drug use, and sexual risk-taking among young people. They focused on the best-established review procedures, including those in Cochrane reviews and the Database of Reviews of Effects reports, but also sought out high-quality reviews in the broader health literature. Among the 87 reviews discussed, they found 40 addressing tobacco use, 17 for physical activity, 12 for alcohol use, 8 for

food, 4 for illicit drug use, and 8 addressing sexual risk-taking among youth. Interestingly, the distribution of reviews focusing on individual-, community-, and population-level interventions differs substantially by behavior. For example, of the 40 reviews of tobacco interventions, 22 reviewed evidence for individual-level interventions, but of the 8 reviews of nutritional interventions, 6 focused on **community-level interventions** and only 2 on the individual level. The authors found evidence that community- and population-level interventions could be effective across a range of behaviors. For example, school-based approaches showed effectiveness across all behaviors, and workplace approaches were effective for diet, physical activity, and smoking cessation. Mass media approaches, if evaluated separately, showed modest but consistent effects on knowledge, attitudes, and behaviors in diet, tobacco, alcohol use and driving, and physical activity.

Ongoing work by the Centers for Disease Control and Prevention's Community Preventive Services Task Force (2011) similarly reviews evidence for prevention interventions on a range of health issues and compiles these into the Guide to Community Preventive Services (www.thecommunityguide.org). The 2011 *First Annual Report to Congress* reported a range of environmentally focused behavior change strategies as having enough evidence that the Task Force recommended them, including work site immunization availability; tobacco, alcohol, and motor vehicle policy approaches; and design-based approaches to physical activity, such as point-of-decision prompts for stair use.

Much of the evidence to date for the impact of the environment on behaviors is cross-sectional and observational. Even when causal time order is established, environmental changes often happen in the aggregate, leaving it difficult to tease apart the true drivers and mechanisms. Indeed, one methodological complexity arising from contextual and ecologically framed interventions is that their multilevel, community-based nature often makes it difficult to know which intervention elements, in which combinations, would deliver the same impact to other groups. Furthermore, controlling or even determining who has received an intervention, such as a mass media campaign, is often difficult, because of diffusion.

Reviews that attempt to synthesize the evidence across multiple studies often must choose whether to draw on only the most rigorous designs and results or incorporate a broader range of evidence. Randomized trials are often difficult to conduct for interventions that change large-scale aspects of the social or built environment; for example, a policy intervention affecting vending machine labeling or point-of-sale warnings for cigarettes for only one geographic area would be impractical both from a research and a policy standpoint. Reviews and other comprehensive appraisals of the evidence often reflect the inevitable lag time between intervention development and dissemination of findings and therefore may not fully inform our current choices of strategies. In addition, even the most thorough reviews may identify gaps in the evidence for specific topics or populations. For example, Jepson and colleagues (2006) found that the evidence was very sparse for interventions with older populations, revealing a need to review any existing studies but also to design rigorous trials of environmental interventions to improve health behaviors among older adults.

The role of the behavioral medicine specialist in this area is discussed in detail by Stokols (2000b). He argues that focusing only on personal health behaviors of individuals may be less effective than focusing on other-directed behaviors. For example, maximum impact at the population level might be possible if focus is put on changing the decisions and behaviors of key stakeholders, whose decisions influence the health of others. He also encourages the incorporation of ecologically based training programs in behavioral medicine and nursing, so that practitioners understand how to identify "high leverage" settings for patients and are able to make full use of the theory and tools at their disposal when they consider environmental influences on behavior change.

REFERENCES

Abel T, Cockerham W, Niemann S. 2000. A critical approach to lifestyle and health. In *Researching Health Promotion,* ed. J Watson, S Platt. London: Routledge.

Altarum Institute. 2011. WIC Food Package Evaluation Symposium proceeding report. Altarum Institute, Washington, DC.

Ammerman AS, Lindquist CH, Lohr KN, Hersey J. 2002. The efficacy of behavioral interventions to modify dietary fat and fruit and vegetable intake: A review of the evidence. *Prev Med* 35 (1): 25–41.

Atwood K, Colditz GA, Kawachi I. 1997. From public health science to prevention policy: Placing science in its social and political contexts. *Am J Public Health* 87:1603–6.

Biener L, Glanz K, McLerran D, et al. 1999. Impact of the Working Well Trial on the worksite smoking and nutrition environment. *Health Educ Behav* 26 (4): 478–94.

Bronfenbrenner U. 1992. Ecological systems theory. In *Six Theories of Child Development: Revised Formulations and Current Issues,* ed. R Vasta. London: Jessica Kingsley.

Browne N, Vaughn NA, Siddiqui N, et al. 2009. Community-academic partnerships: Lessons learned from replicating a salon-based health education and promotion program. *Prog Community Health Partnersh* 3 (3): 241–48.

Brussoni M, Towner EML, Hayes M. 2006. Evidence into practice: Combining the art and science of injury prevention. *Inj Prev* 12:373–77.

Caldas A, Arteaga F, Munoz M. 2010. Microfinance: A general overview and implications for impoverished individuals living with HIV/AIDS. *J Health Care Poor Underserved* 21 (3): 986–1005.

Caldwell EM, Kobayashi MM, DuBow WM, Wytinck SM. 2008. Perceived access to fruits and vegetables associated with increased consumption. *Pub Health Nutr* 12 (10): 1743–50.

Campbell MK, Demark-Wahnefried W, Symons M, et al. 1999. Fruit and vegetable consumption and prevention of cancer: The Black Churches United for Better Health project. *Am J Public Health* 89 (9): 1390–96.

Cohen DA, Scribner RA, Farley TA. 2000. A structural model of health behavior: A pragmatic approach to explain and influence health behaviors at the population level. *Prev Med* 30:146–54.

Community level HIV interventions in 5 cities: Final outcome data from the CDC AIDS Community Demonstration Projects. 1999. *Am J Public Health* 89:336-45, www.howardcountymd.gov/WW/WW _HealthVending.htm.

Community Preventive Services Task Force. 2002. Recommendations to increase physical activity in communities. *Am J Prev Med* 22 (suppl. 4): 67-72.

———. 2011. *First Annual Report to Congress and to Agencies Related to the Work of the Task Force.* Atlanta, GA: Centers for Disease Control and Prevention.

Cromley EK, McLafferty SL. 2002. *GIS and Public Health.* New York: Guilford Press.

Cubbin C, LeClere FB, Smith GS, et al. 2000. Socioeconomic status and injury mortality: Individual and neighborhood determinants. *J Epidemiol Commun Health* 54:517-24.

Cubbin C, Hadden WC, Winkleby MA, et al. 2001. Neighborhood context and cardiovascular disease risk factors: The contribution of material deprivation. *Ethn Dis* 11:687-700.

Cullen KW, Hartstein J, Reynolds KD, et al. 2007. Improving the school food environment: Results from a pilot study in middle schools. *J Am Diet Assoc* 107 (3): 484-89.

Diez-Roux AV, Kiefe CI, Jacobs DR, et al. 2001. Area characteristics and individual-level socioeconomic position indicators in three population-based epidemiological studies. *Ann Epidemiol* 11 (6): 395-405.

Eagles M, Belanger P, Calkins HW. 2003. The spatial structure of urban political discussion networks. In *Spatially Integrated Social Sciences,* ed. MF Goodchild, DG Janelle. New York: Oxford University Press.

Economos CD, Curtatone JA. 2010. Shape Up Somerville: A community initiative in Massachusetts. *Prev Med* 50 (suppl. 1): S97-S98.

Economos CD, Folta SC, Goldberg J, et al. 2009. A community-based restaurant initiative to increase availability of healthy menu options in Somerville, Massachusetts: Shape Up Somerville. *Prev Chronic Disease* 6 (3): A102.

Economos CD, Hyatt RR, Goldberg JP, et al. 2007. A community intervention reduces BMI z-score in children: Shape Up Somerville first year results. *Obesity* 15 (5): 1325-36.

French SA, Story M, Jeffery RW. 2001. Environmental influences on eating and physical activity. *Annu Rev Public Health* 22:309-35.

Gans KM, Risica PM, Kirtania U, et al. 2009. Dietary behaviors and portion sizes of black women enrolled in *SisterTalk* and variation by demographic characteristics. *J Nutr Educ Behav* 41 (1): 32-40.

Glanz K, Basil M, Maibach E, Goldberg J, Snyder D. 1998. Why Americans eat what they do: Taste, nutrition, cost, convenience, and weight control concerns as influences on food consumption. *J Am Diet Assoc* 98 (10): 1118-26.

Glanz K, Yaroch AL. 2004. Strategies for increasing fruit and vegetable intake in grocery stores and communities: Policy, pricing, and environmental change. *Prev Med* 39 (suppl. 2): S75-S80.

Grow HM, Saelens BE, Kerr J, Durant NH, Norman GJ, Sallis JF. 2008. Where are youth active? Roles of proximity, active transport, and built environment. *Med Sci Sports Exerc* 40 (12): 2071-79.

Hall PA, Elias LJ, Fong GT, Harrison AH, Borowsky R, Sarty GE. 2008. A social neuroscience perspective on physical activity. *J Sport Exerc Psychol* 30 (4): 432-49.

Hargreaves MK, Schlundt DG, Buchowski MS. 2002. Contextual factors influencing the eating behaviours of African American women: A focus group investigation. *Ethn Health* 7 (3): 133-47.

Israel BA, Parker EA, Rowe Z, et al. 2005. Community-based participatory research: Lessons learned from the Centers for Children's Environmental Health and Disease Prevention Research. *Environ Health Perspect* 113 (10): 1463-71.

Jepson R, Harris F, MacGillivray S, Kearney N, Rowa-Dewar N. 2006. *A Review of the Effectiveness of Interventions, Approaches, and Models at Individual, Community, and Population Level That Are Aimed at Changing Health Outcomes through Changing Knowledge, Attitudes, and Behaviour.* Stirling, UK: National Institute for Health and Clinical Excellence.

Kawachi I, Berkman LF, eds. 2003. *Neighborhoods and Health.* New York: Oxford University Press.

Krieger J, Rabkin J, Sharify D, Song L. 2009. High point walking for health: Creating built and social environments that support walking in a public housing community. *Am J Public Health* 99 (suppl. 3): S593-S599.

Lomeli EV. 2008. Conditional cash transfers as social policy in Latin America: An assessment of their contributions and limitations. *Ann Rev Soc* 34:475-99.

Lytle LA, Kubik MY, Perry C, Story M, Birnbaum AS, Murray DM. 2006. Influencing healthful food choices in school and home environments: Results from TEENS study. *Prev Med* 43 (1): 8-13.

Macintyre S, Ellaway A, Cummins S. 2002. Place effects on health: How can we conceptualise, operationalise, and measure them? *Soc Sci Med* 55 (1): 125-39.

Mallonee S, Fowler C, Istre GR. 2006. Building the gap between research and practice: A continuing challenge. *Inj Prev* 12:357-59.

Maston-Koffman DM, Brownstein JN, Neiner JA, Greaney ML. 2005. A site-specific literature review of policy and environmental interventions that promote physical activity and nutrition cardiovascular health: What works? *Am J Health Promot* 19 (3): 167-93.

McNeill LH, Kreuter MW, Subramanian SV. 2006. Social environment and physical activity: A review of concepts and evidence. *Soc Sci Med* 63 (4): 1011-22.

Morland K, Diez Roux AV, Wing S. 2006. Supermarkets, other food stores, and obesity: The atherosclerosis risk in communities study. *Am J Prev Med* 30 (4): 333-39.

Morland K, Wing S, Diex Roux A. 2002. The contextual effect of the local food environment on residents' diets: The Atherosclerosis Risk in Communities (ARIC) study. *Am J Public Health* 92 (11): 1761-68.

Northridge ME, Sclar ED, Biswas P. 2003. Sorting out the connections between the built environment and health: A conceptual framework for navigating pathways and planning healthy cities. *J Urban Health* 80 (4): 556-68.

O'Campo P, Xue X, Wang MC, Caughy M. 1997. Neighborhood risk factors for low birthweight in Baltimore: A multilevel analysis. *Am J Public Health* 87 (7): 1113-18.

Owen N, Humpel N, Leslie E, Bauman A, Sallis JF. 2004. Understanding environmental influences on walking: Review and research agenda. *Am J Prev Med* 27 (1): 67-76.

Prevention Institute. 2010. *Recipe for Change: Healthy Food in Every Community.* The Convergence Partnership Fund of the Tides Foundation, www.convergence partnership.org.

Reidpath DD, Burns C, Garrard J, Mahoney M, Townsend M. 2002. An ecological study of the relationship between social and environmental determinants of obesity. *Health Place* 8 (2): 141-45.

Riccio JA, Dechausay N, Greenberg DM, Miller C, Rucks Z, Verma N. 2010. *Towards Reduced Poverty across Generations: Early Findings from New York City's Conditional Cash Transfer Program.* New York: MDRC.

Riley-Jacome M, Gallant MP, Fisher BD, Gotcsik FS, Strogatz DS. 2010. Enhancing community capacity to support physical activity: The development of a community-based indoor-outdoor walking program. *J Primary Prev* 31 (1-2): 85-95.

Seymour JD, Yaroch AL, Serdula M, Blanck HM, Kahn LK. 2004. Impact of nutrition environmental interventions on point-of-purchase behavior in adults: A review. *Prev Med* 39 (suppl. 2): 108-36.

Siegel PZ, Brackbill RM, Heath GW. 1995. The epidemiology of walking for exercise: Implications for promoting activity among sedentary groups. *Am J Public Health* 85 (5): 706-10.

Song HJ, Gittelsohn J, Kim M, Suratkar S, Sharma S, Anliker J. 2009. A corner store intervention in a low-income urban community is associated with increased availability and sales of some healthy foods. *Pub Health Nutr* 12 (11): 2060-67.

Stokols D. 2000a. The social ecological paradigm of wellness promotion. In *Promoting Human Wellness: New Frontiers for Research, Practice, and Policy,* ed. MS Janner, D Stokols. Berkeley: University of California Press.

———. 2000b. Social ecology and behavioral medicine: Implications for training, practice, and policy. *Behav Med* 26:129-38.

Swendeman D, Basu I, Das S, Jana S, Rotheram-Borus MJ. 2009. Empowering sex workers in India to reduce vulnerability to HIV and sexually transmitted diseases. *Soc Sci Med* 69 (8): 1157-66.

Watters JL, Satia JA, Galanko JA. 2007. Associations of psychosocial factors with fruit and vegetable intake among African-Americans. *Pub Health Nutr* 10 (7): 701-11.

Wiggs I, Brownson RC, Baker EA. 2008. If you build it, they will come: Lessons from developing walking trails in rural Missouri. *Health Promot Practice* 9 (4): 387-94.

Zenk SN, Schulz AJ, Israel BA, James SA, Bao S, Wilson ML. 2005. Neighborhood racial composition, neighborhood poverty, and the spatial accessibility of supermarkets in metropolitan Detroit. *Am J Public Health* 95 (4): 660-67.

CHAPTER 9

Evaluating Behavior Change Programs

JANE BERTRAND AND DANNY SCHIEFFLER JR.

LEARNING OBJECTIVES

After completing the chapter, the reader will be able to

* Appreciate the importance of program evaluation as a core component of health behavior change interventions.
* Describe the three types of program evaluation.
* Provide several examples of program evaluations, including evaluations of smoking prevention and hand-washing interventions described in the chapter.

Introduction

Most organizations responsible for implementing behavior change programs will want to evaluate whether their **interventions** make a difference—that is, did the intervention have the desired impact? Others may want to know if their programs are on the right track and what they might do to improve them. Such questions have spawned a field of study known as **program evaluation**. Many activities may be included within this study, depending on the range of methodologies used, the level of scientific rigor, and differing levels of analysis and **complexity**. In this chapter, we will first present an overview of program evaluation and clarify several questions to help readers understand and classify the wide range of program evaluations conducted or reported in the scientific literature. We will then present two examples of program evaluations to illustrate the concepts discussed in the chapter.

Types of Evaluation

Although many people equate **evaluation** with "measuring impact," program evaluation takes three forms, each with a separate purpose: formative, process, and summative evaluations (and some researchers suggest a fourth form: **cost-effectiveness evaluation**, which we describe below).

Formative Evaluation

Formative evaluation is used to obtain information that will be useful in designing the intervention to be as effective as possible. Ideally, formative evaluation begins prior to the initiation of an intervention and continues throughout its initial steps. Rarely will an organization or program set out to design and implement an intervention without some formative research to guide the decision making.

Formative evaluation involves **primary data** collection and/or secondary analysis about the **target population** to gather the following information:

- the epidemiology of the disease or health condition
- the persons most affected
- the drivers of unhealthful behaviors
- the barriers to change
- the persons considered to be most credible as sources of information on the topic
- channels through which the population receives information
- any related matters

Formative evaluation draws on a wide range of data collection methods, both quantitative (e.g., surveys, epidemiological **surveillance**, observation checklists) and qualitative (e.g., focus groups, in-depth interviews, participant observation). Well-funded, large-scale interventions are likely to conduct extensive formative research. However, small organizations on a limited budget can, and should, perform some type of data collection. Alternatively, they may tap into existing sources of information about their target population in an effort to tailor the intervention to their specific population.

Formative research is similar to needs assessment. However, the latter often involves determining the current results, articulating the desired results, and establishing the distance between the two as the actual need (Kaufman and English 1979). Formative evaluation does not necessarily quantify the need but rather seeks to understand the factors that may facilitate or hinder desired behavior change.

Process Evaluation

Process evaluation is used to assess how well the intervention is being implemented. This form of evaluation occurs after the launch of the intervention, often during the first one-third to half of the intervention period, so that the results can point to any necessary mid-course corrections. At a minimum, process evaluation monitors which aspects of the planned intervention actually take place, referred to as **fidelity to design**. Other possible pieces of program evaluation include the following components:

- **Dose delivered:** assessment of the volume of activity or intended units of the program delivered by the implementers.
- **Reach:** extent to which the intervention reaches the target population.
- **Level of exposure:** extent to which the target audience has been exposed to the intervention (e.g., number of channels on which they saw or heard a message on the intended topic, often labeled *dose*) and their reaction (positive or negative) to the intervention.
- **Recruitment:** procedures used to approach and attract participants at individual or organizational levels; sociodemographic characteristics of participants in program activities.
- **Context:** aspects of the environment that may influence the implementation or study

of the intervention, such as **spillover** from the treatment to the control area. (Saunders et al. 2005)

Process evaluation can be invaluable for understanding the dynamics of the intervention and how it might be replicated elsewhere. However, it stops short of measuring behavior change (i.e., whether the target population actually changed their behavior after the launch of the intervention).

Summative Evaluation

Summative evaluation measures whether change occurred as a result of the intervention. This type of evaluation answers the question "Did the intervention work?" At the most basic level, summative evaluation measures whether change occurred on the outcomes of interest, which may include the following factors:

- increases in knowledge, **risk-perception**, or **self-efficacy**
- changes in **attitudes** and stated intentions
- (most importantly) changes in behavior

Although a health behavior change professional would ideally like to assess an intervention in terms of its long-term effect on health status (i.e., **mortality** or **morbidity**), this is rarely possible for interventions that last only a few months or years. Instead, evaluators measure changes in psychocognitive factors, such as knowledge and attitudes, as **initial effects** and **self-reported**, or observed, behavior as an **intermediate effect**.

For example, evaluators do not assess the **effectiveness** of an antismoking campaign based on rates of new cases of lung cancer, but rather on the intermediate effects of smoking cessation such as self-report of cigarette consumption in the past week or month. Using behavioral measures of outcome is particularly defensible when strong epidemiological evi-

dence exists to link the behavior to the long-term health outcome.

Summative evaluation generally attempts either to establish **causality** or (with weaker designs) to tease out causal inferences. Confidence in the findings relates directly to the strength of the study design used to demonstrate causality. Note that summative evaluation is a term that includes both outcome and impact evaluation. **Outcome evaluation** refers to assessing changes in a given outcome (either a health behavior, such as smoking, or a health status, such as lung cancer among smokers) without necessarily attributing it to an intervention. **Impact evaluation** carries at least two different meanings. Some use the term for research with a rigorous study design capable of demonstrating cause and effect, not just plausible attribution (e.g., a clinical trial of a new product designed to help smokers quit). Others use the term in relation to tracking the ultimate **objective** of a given intervention, such as reducing mortality related to smoking.

Cost-Effectiveness Evaluation

Where data permit, evaluators may go one step further to assess the intervention's **cost-effectiveness**, which is a specialized form of impact assessment. This type of evaluation extends beyond measuring the extent to which change occurred and quantifies the cost per unit of change. It requires both careful tracking of the costs of the intervention and numerous assumptions on the part of the evaluator. Despite its complexities, cost-effectiveness evaluation answers the question that decision-makers most often want to know, "What is the 'bang for the buck'?"

Key Evaluation Questions

Several factors and key questions are involved in designing an evaluation for a behavior change program:

1. How is the intervention expected to achieve the desired outcome?
2. Who is the target population for the intervention?
3. Does the evaluation focus on those enrolled in a particular program, or all persons who fall within the definition of the target population?
4. What study design will be used to evaluate impact?
5. What are the measures of program success?
6. What are the available data for answering these questions?

Achieving Desired Outcomes

Strong programs tend to draw on one or more theories of change, either implicitly or explicitly. Most common in the field of health education and behavior change are the **Health Belief Model**, the **Social Learning Theory (modeling)**, the **Theory of Reasoned Action**, the **Diffusion of Innovations Theory**, and the **Extended Parallel Process Model** (*fear management*) (Glantz et al. 2002; Witte 1992). Fundamental to any

evaluation is an understanding of the sequence of pathways that link the intervention to the ultimate outcome. This sequence of pathways goes under a number of different titles: **conceptual framework**, **logic model**, **program theory**, and **program impact pathway** (**PIP**), among others.

Having a framework is extremely useful both for those designing the intervention and for those evaluating the intervention. For designers of the intervention, a framework helps to clarify their thinking on the sequence of steps necessary for a successful outcome and also to promote a common vision of the intervention among **stakeholders**. For the evaluators of the intervention, a framework helps to identify relevant indicators for measuring success, in terms of initial, intermediate, and long-term outcomes. An example of a conceptual framework illustrating how a smoking ban might reduce morbidity and mortality appears in figure 9.1.

Interventions may focus on different **levels of influence** of health behaviors. We describe throughout this textbook the **ecological**, or *social ecological*, **model**, which describes several

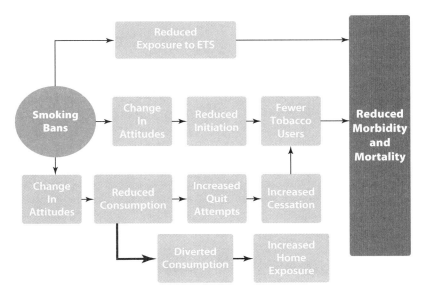

FIGURE 9.1. A conceptual framework: how smoking bans can result in reduced morbidity and mortality. ETS = environmental tobacco smoke.

levels of influence, including structural, environmental, organizational, interpersonal, and individual.

Structural intervention refers to implementation or changes in laws, policies, physical structures, social or organizational structures, or standard operating procedures to bring about environmental or societal change, independent of individual volition (e.g., seat belt laws decreasing mortality related to automobile accidents). **Environmental interventions** aim to change behavior by facilitating or inhibiting behaviors through changes in the surroundings (Sweat and Dennison 1995) (e.g., promoting breastfeeding by providing nursing mothers with a room in the workplace to nurse or pump, discouraging smoking by limiting it to certain designated areas). **Organizational intervention** relates to policies that facilitate the adoption of health behaviors, such as flextime to allow staff to exercise before or after work. **Interpersonal**, or *family-level,* **interventions** attempt to reach clusters of family members who can then reinforce specific behaviors (e.g., a nutrition intervention that targets all members of the family). Finally, **intrapersonal**, or *individual-level,* **interventions** generally involve health education and counseling provided to one individual at a time. These aim to change the behavior of individuals who collectively make up the population (e.g., getting a flu shot); however, even in this case, other **influences** (of family, workplace, society) tend to come into play.

Although an intervention can operate at a single level, the most effective behavioral interventions often work at multiple levels, for example, encouraging girls to become more physically fit by combining education or counseling along with implementing social and environmental interventions such as addressing the **built environment** (Elder et al. 2007). In this example, we see the power of the social ecological approach; individuals are far more likely to work toward fitness if their social and physical environment encourages and facilitates it.

The Target Population

Evaluating a given intervention should be done among the intended audience or **target population** for the intervention. Occasionally, this may be the general public (e.g., a mass media campaign to encourage people to get a seasonal flu shot), but even then, subpopulations might be of particular interest, such as adolescents, the immunocompromised, or older adults. Similarly, interventions may target a subgroup of the general population defined by age (e.g., ages 15-19 years) or by age and sex (e.g., females, ages 13-26 years, as is the case for the human papillomavirus vaccine). More often, the target population is more narrowly defined by additional criteria, such as income, race or ethnic group, geographical area, or workplace. Although we typically think of interventions as **targeting** the ultimate beneficiaries, in fact, they may target intermediaries who directly influence health outcomes of the ultimate beneficiaries. Examples include caretakers of young children (e.g., to encourage complete vaccination of the child) or clinicians (to encourage frequent hand-washing to avoid spreading infection).

Program-Based versus Population-Based Evaluation

Whether an evaluation should focus on those enrolled in a particular program or all persons who fall within the definition of the target population depends on the objective of the program. For example, a specific drug rehabilitation program evaluates its success based on those enrolled in the program, without consideration for others who might be eligible. By contrast, the Partnership for a Drug-free America campaign aimed to reduce drug use among youth in the United States and was consequently evaluated on a random sample of this group (Hornik et al. 2008). Evaluators refer to the former as **program-based evaluation** and the latter as **population-based evaluation** (Rossi et al. 2004).

Appropriate Study Design

The gold standard for measuring impact is the **experimental design**, used widely in clinical research to evaluate the effectiveness of a given drug or treatment regime. A randomized control trial is one type of experimental design. This design offers the strongest possible means of controlling potential **confounders** (such as **selection bias**, **testing effect bias**, **maturation bias**, and **history bias**, among other sources of bias), but it has been criticized for having a low **generalizability** to the larger population (Victora et al. 2004; West et al. 2008).

On the other end of the continuum are **nonexperimental designs** that control only some of the potential sources of bias but are nonetheless widely used (e.g., a pre-test–post-test design with no control group), under the philosophy that some evaluation is better than none. Many evaluators opt to use **quasi-experimental** designs, which tend to have greater generalizability and control for some but not all potential sources of bias. Quasi-experimental designs enjoy widespread use where it is not possible to randomize subjects into **treatment** and **control groups**. One such design is the time series, which is particularly useful for interventions that potentially reach all members of the target group—such as a mass media campaign—making it difficult, if not impossible, to have a control or comparison group. In recent years, evaluators have increasingly used observational studies (post-test only among the experimental population) and applied sophisticated analytic techniques (e.g., **propensity scoring**, **structural equations**) to tease out causal inferences (Babalola and Kincaid 2009).

The choice of study design will depend on multiple factors, including the importance of rigor to those sponsoring the research, the availability of human resources to conduct advanced statistical analysis, the budget available for evaluation, the time period available for the evaluation, the availability of existing data, and others.

Measures of Intervention Success

Behavior change programs often encourage members of the target population to perform a particular behavior that will result in decreased morbidity or mortality (e.g., encouraging youth to use condoms to avoid human immunodeficiency virus [HIV] transmission, encouraging clinicians to wash their hands between patients to reduce infection). Although the causal chain between the behavioral outcome (e.g., using the condom) and the ultimate outcome (HIV incidence) may be well known, program evaluation often focuses on the behavioral outcome (measured by self-report) rather than on the long-term outcome that is biological in nature (measured by some type of biomarker).

An alternative for measuring behavioral outcomes is observation, if the nature of the intervention lends itself to observation (e.g., does the clinician wash or sanitize his hands before each new patient?). Observation reduces the bias inherent in self-report but may introduce other biases (such as the **Hawthorne effect**, whereby participants perform better than under normal conditions precisely because they realize they are being observed).

Three reasons that many evaluators choose to use self-report data on behavioral outcomes rather than biomarkers are (1) self-report data are often less expensive, time-consuming, and intrusive to collect; (2) factors other than the intervention may influence the biological outcome; and (3) the effect of the intervention may not manifest itself within the evaluation period (e.g., HIV transmission).

However, self-reported data are subject to substantial reporting biases, especially on sensitive topics (e.g., sexual behaviors or topics subject to strong social disapproval). Certain techniques help to reduce this bias by giving respondents a greater sense of the confidentiality of their responses, such as audio computer-assisted self-interview (ACASI). Similarly, one can give the respondent a card with precoded response categories, so that she can simply read out a letter response rather than verbalizing the actual, potentially embarrassing response. In some evaluations, self-reported data can be confirmed with biomarker data. For example, Joffe and colleagues (2009) confirmed self-reported quit status with salivary nicotine levels in a study of adolescent smoking.

Data Collection

Ideally, evaluators will have the time and resources to obtain the most appropriate data for answering the key question(s) of their evaluation. However, it is often the case that funding for evaluation is limited; therefore, evaluators must either make do with existing data sources or at least tap into such sources in addition to collecting other data. In fact, where such data are well suited to answering the key questions, it is desirable to use them. For example, routinely collected service statistics in a clinical facility may provide the exact information needed to answer the key question of the evaluation, such as "Did the campaign to promote breast cancer screening result in a significant increase in mammograms in the main public and private facilities in the catchment area?"

Similarly, existing data can be useful for formative or process evaluation. In terms of formative evaluation, there is much to be gleaned from epidemiological reports for a given population, previous research conducted among the population, and clinical or program records that yield the sociodemographic profile of patients. With regard to process evaluation, it may be possible to tap into existing data systems within the organization (including the accounting system) to track the production of materials or to use radio or TV station logs to determine the frequency of broadcasts.

However, in the vast majority of cases, it will be necessary to design and conduct some type of primary data collection—for formative, process, or summative evaluation. Formative and process evaluations often include a combination of quantitative and qualitative methodologies. The most frequently used quantitative data come from surveys, routinely gathered statistics from clinical services, or program records, sales data, or performance checklists. Frequently used sources of qualitative data include focus groups, in-depth interviews, and ethnographic observation.

Examples of Evaluating Behavior Change Interventions

To illustrate how formative, process, and summative evaluation apply to behavior change interventions, we have selected two health behavior change campaigns in different institutional settings, reflecting the social ecological perspective that change at the individual level is strongly influenced by the individual's environment: friends and family, community, and society. The topic areas are

- reducing smoking among adolescents through a school-based program and
- increasing hand hygiene among clinicians to prevent infection in a hospital setting.

In the case of adolescent smoking, we present the three types of evaluation in relation to a single program. For hand-washing in a hospital setting, we were unable to identify a program that had published results for all three types of evaluation; so we draw on different studies to underscore the value of each type.

Case Example: Reducing Smoking among Adolescents through a School-Based Program

Interventions to prevent or reduce adolescent smoking abound, but the Acadiana Coalition of Teens against Tobacco (ACTT) program in Louisiana provides one of the best examples of a program with published results from all three types of evaluation. In response to the increase in adolescent smoking rates in the 1990s, numerous programs were implemented across the United States to prevent or reduce smoking among teens. The ACTT program was a clinical trial designed to reduce adolescent smoking in 10 schools in an area of south central Louisiana known locally as "Cajun country," where early initiation of both smoking and drinking is common. A unique feature of this intervention was to follow a cohort of incoming high school freshmen through their high school years.

FORMATIVE RESEARCH AND EVALUATION

Although national-level statistics existed on adolescent smoking behavior, adolescents from Louisiana were underrepresented in national surveys. Therefore, before launching a program to target the problem of smoking, the program planners wanted to learn more about this problem. To this end, Johnson and colleagues (2004) conducted a baseline survey to examine the prevalence of tobacco use among ninth grade students in the Acadiana region of south central Louisiana and to develop profiles of adolescent tobacco use. Formative research can include both **qualitative research** (which is particularly useful in understanding the mind-set of the target population, including their values, attitudes, beliefs, aspirations, and fears that strongly affect behavior) and **quantitative research**, especially where quantifying baseline levels is important. The type of quantitative study conducted by Johnson and colleagues (2004) served a dual purpose: (1) to guide the design of the intervention by identifying the characteristics of those at risk and learning more about their **social environment** and (2) to establish baseline levels of smoking prevalence, against which to evaluate the effectiveness of the program.

The baseline survey consisted of a cross-sectional sample survey among 4,808 ninth graders, almost evenly distributed by gender, which included Caucasian (61%), African American (33%), and other races (6%). The study pro-

vided useful baseline data: 59% reported some type of tobacco use, most of which was cigarette smoking; 25% had smoked in the past 30 days. In addition, it provided important insights for program design. White adolescents were much more likely to have ever smoked (62%) than black adolescents (46%), but within these groups there was no gender difference. For both groups, smokers had more spending money and lower academic performance or more lacked college aspirations than nonsmokers. Moreover, the influence of social relationships was a strong correlate of smoking in both groups: having friends who smoke, having friends who use smokeless tobacco, having friends who drink alcohol, having friends who get drunk at least once a week, being around people who used alcohol for "kicks," and the presence of parents or siblings who used tobacco.

These results formed the evidence base for the design of the ACTT intervention, which had two components. The first was a school-based media campaign that targeted adolescent smoking, which ran from 2001 to 2004 (Johnson et al. 2009). Because of higher levels of current smoking among whites than blacks, messages with encouragement to quit were directed primarily toward whites, whereas prevention messages were directed to both ethnic groups. The lack of gender differences signaled the need to target females and males with equal intensity. Here we can notice that formative research may not deliver up all the answers, as was the case in this study with respect to the strong influence of friends and family on smoking. The formative research identified the problem but did not yield any insights for an easy solution.

The second component was an activities program that targeted youth as they progressed through high school. It operated in 10 schools and worked on the premise that prevention programs couched within the school environment can change the broader social environment, which can influence youth behavior (Flay 2000). The main activities for the school-based intervention included a media campaign (posters hung on school walls that were changed every two months and a weekly public service announcement [PSA] broadcast read by a non-smoker student over the school public-address system) and interactive educational activities in the hallways and during recess that required students to actively initiate participation. Some activities included models of diseased mouths and lung tar infusion, roulette-style question and answer games with prizes, and interaction with pig lung tissue that had been exposed to the equivalent of 10 years of tobacco use (Johnson et al. 2009). The posters included several types: high quality stock posters obtained from the Centers for Disease Control and Prevention (CDC) and the American Cancer Society and two categories (high-budget and low-budget) of customized posters that depicted high-school-aged kids of different races. **Social Cognitive Theory** and **social marketing** principles guided the campaign. The main themes changed over the three years of the intervention: "Don't be a sucker" (year 1), "Say no to Big Tobacco" (year 2), and "The future is yours" (year 3, coinciding with the students' graduation). The ACTT logo—"ACTT Smart, Don't Start"—branded all material.

PROCESS EVALUATION

Hong and colleagues (2008) reported the results of the process evaluation of the ACTT intervention. Their evaluation addressed three of the variables commonly included in process evaluation: dose delivered, message reach, and student satisfaction with the messages. It also measured judged impact of the materials on smoking behavior (which has been used as a proxy for **behavioral intention** but should not be interpreted as a measure of behavior change). The main method for collecting data for the process evaluation was a survey conducted annually among students in the 10 schools (n = 1,823, 1,552, and 1,390 in years 1, 2, and 3, respectively).

Dose delivered. The ACTT program staff used observational journals to monitor the number and content of posters displayed, and they tracked the actual broadcast of the PSAs (confirming 97% compliance).

Reach. An annual survey of students in the selected schools measured recalled exposure to PSAs and posters and recognition of the campaign theme for that year. Students reported higher levels of exposure to the posters (approximately 80% a year over the three years) than to the PSAs (ranging from 51% to 68% over the years). The highest media exposure—for both the posters and the PSAs—occurred in year 2.

Reaction or Satisfaction. In addition, the survey measured judged impact of the antismoking poster advertisements and affective reactions to the poster advertisements. In terms of affective response to the posters, the percent reporting them to be "interesting" was highest in year 1 (59%), then dropped to 45% and 44% respectively in years 2 and 3, which may reflect campaign fatigue or "advertising wearout," especially by year 3. Students preferred the stock media posters (produced by CDC and the American Cancer Society) to the custom low- and high-budget posters made specifically for this campaign. This finding suggests that well-designed stock media campaign materials may be both cost-efficient and cost-effective in eliciting desirable emotional responses among adolescents (Hong et al. 2008).

SUMMATIVE EVALUATION

Johnson and colleagues (2009) reported on the results from this three-year intervention to prevent or reduce smoking among teens, using a randomized, controlled cohort study that involved 22 high schools in six Louisiana parishes (counties). Twenty of the schools were research schools and two were used for pilot-testing instruments and activities. The 20 schools were stratified by parish and randomized within parish to intervention or control conditions after baseline measurement, resulting in 10 intervention and 10 control schools. The baseline measurement, using the Health Habits Survey, occurred when the adolescents were in the 9th grade, two interim measurements occurred in the 10th and 11th grades, and a follow-up measurement took place in the 12th grade.

At baseline (9th grade), the 30-day smoking prevalence was 23.0% for the intervention schools and 26.1% for the control schools (a nonsignificant difference). By 12th grade, the difference in prevalence was 7 percentage points: 27.3% for the intervention schools and 34.3% for the control schools. Smoking prevalence had increased in both groups, but less in the intervention than in the control group. However, no **statistically significant** interaction between treatment condition and time was observed, resulting in a nonsignificant intervention effect. Researchers also found that the higher the percentage of white students in the school, the higher the prevalence rates of smoking, regardless of intervention or control status. Boys' and girls' smoking rates were similar. In the discussion section of the journal, the researchers (Johnson et al. 2009) commented that perhaps the intervention effect size was not strong enough to achieve statistical significance.

Of particular interest for this chapter, the researchers used the results from their process evaluation to explain why this might be the case: "Variables such as low reach or participation, inconsistent exposure to media, weak program dose, and contextual factors beyond the control of the program staff influenced program implementation." They concluded that a stronger focus on presentation of media through the use of social marketing principles would contribute significantly to any environmental tobacco control program (Johnson et al. 2009, 1313).

In reflecting on this experience, the researchers believed that the design was strong and the measurement appropriate. For example, they adopted the conventional practice of randomizing schools to a treatment and a con-

trol group, using the school as the unit of analysis. However, in hindsight, they recognized certain limitations related to the intervention. When they designed the study, they initially believed that the classroom activities would be the focal point of the intervention and the media a support arm. After they realized that classroom time was not an option, it was decided to conduct the antismoking and prevention activities in the school hallways at lunchtime. It is possible that this approach resulted in "preaching to the choir." (In other words, students who were smoking and did not want to quit would be unlikely to actively pursue involvement in these activities, whereas those who did get involved were probably already planning to quit or were nonsmokers.) Also, the intervention period did not allow the researchers the time to reach all or even most of the students, especially in large schools. That is one of the reasons why, in hindsight, they thought a more coordinated and stronger media campaign might have served to better focus the intervention/prevention. Also, results from exit focus groups conducted at the end of the program (which were presented at conferences but not published) showed that those students who did not smoke and had no intention of smoking were very critical of the program. They felt that it had nothing to do with them and therefore was a waste of their time when measurements were administered in the class periods or physical education periods. Similarly, 75% of students measured in the baseline survey had not had a cigarette in the past 30 days (the primary outcome), although the percentages of nonsmokers decreased as students progressed through their high school years. Still, an intervention that would engage *all* students would be far more likely to achieve success. One possible approach would have been to focus on passive smoking and to recruit students themselves to be champions of a smoke-free environment. In that way, their own pressure could have been brought to bear on smoking students as well as smokers within the family (CC Johnson, personal communication, 2010).

Case Example: Increasing Hand-Washing to Reduce Infections in Hospital Settings

Health-care-associated infections (HAIs) are the leading cause of complications in critically ill patients (NNISS 2004). Hand hygiene—including both traditional hand cleaning with a soap-and-water wash and hand decontamination using an alcohol-based hand rub—is the single most effective method of preventing the spread of HAIs. Unfortunately, despite the established benefits, health care workers tend to have suboptimal hand-hygiene practices, with reported **compliance** estimates from 1999 ranging between 30% and 50% (Boyce 1999). A sizable literature exists on interventions to increase hand-washing among physicians, nurses, and other clinical personnel in hospital settings and the implications of noncompliance (Aragon et al. 2005; Larson et al. 2009; Lederer et al. 2009; Zerr et al. 2005). Yet the large majority of these studies focus on the effectiveness of the intervention, without describing what formative or process evaluation—if any—was conducted. In the description that follows, our focus is on the types of evaluation and examples of each from the literature, rather than on the results themselves.

FORMATIVE EVALUATION

Important sources of formative research on this topic are literature reviews that synthesize other interventions and provide lessons learned that are relevant to the testing of (new) interventions in other facilities. For example, the review by Maskerine and Loeb (2006, 248) pointed to the difficulty of obtaining behavior change among clinicians. They report: "As a whole, the success of interventions to improve adherence to hand hygiene among health care professionals has been limited. Recent data suggest that a multifaceted intervention, including the use of feedback, education, the introduction of alcohol-based hand wash, and visual reminders, may increase adherence to hand-hygiene recommendations. Although the 'active ingredient' of such an intervention is unknown, there is evidence that the use of feedback may be key to increasing adherence."

PROCESS EVALUATION

For other health topics, we found articles titled "Process Evaluation of [health topic] Programs," but we were unable to identify any such articles for the promotion of hand-washing among clinicians. Rather, the large majority of articles involved summative evaluation (asking, Was the intervention effective?), with elements of process evaluation mentioned only in passing. For example, McKinley and colleagues (2005) describe an intervention that used a stepwise design by which information collected in one phase was used to enhance the next stage.

Specifically, a series of four posters, each 11×17 inches were developed over a 12-month period. Each poster (except the first) was designed using ideas, comments, and suggestions from focus group discussions conducted among health care professionals after the original poster had been displayed in a highly visible location for three months. Participants were asked to give their opinions on the effectiveness of each poster on compliance and to suggest ideas on intervention methods they believed would be effective to increase desired behaviors. The data from the focus groups were incorporated in the production of subsequent posters. This process was carried out three times in an effort to fine-tune these visual **cues**. Although the primary purpose of McKinley and colleagues' article was to report on the effectiveness of this intervention on compliance (measured through direct observation of hand-washing behaviors), their approach of "assess then revise, assess then revise" is one example of process evaluation used to improve the ultimate effectiveness of the intervention.

SUMMATIVE EVALUATION

Many of the studies on this topic represent attempts to test different approaches to increasing compliance with hand hygiene. For example, Thomas and colleagues (2009) tested whether (1) placement of hand-hygiene foam dispensers in more conspicuous positions and in closer proximity to patients and (2) increasing the number of dispensers would increase the use of infection control agents, as measured by the volume of the product that was used (the first did; the second did not).

The gold standard for testing an intervention is the experimental design, which would be the most rigorous type of summative evaluation. For example, Harbarth and colleagues (2002) used an interventional, randomized cohort study with four study phases to assess the introduction of an alcohol-based hand gel and multifaceted quality improvement interventions on hand-hygiene compliance. Other studies simply compare behaviors and test for significant differences before and after the intervention, such as a study by Assanasen and colleagues (2008), which tested two different levels of performance feedback on compliance with hand-hygiene compliance.

Although the purpose of promoting hand hygiene is to reduce the number of nosocomial infections, summative evaluation usually focuses on the desired change in behavior (hand hygiene) and not on the ultimate outcome (reducing infection). One exception is a three-year study from a teaching hospital in Switzerland that used nosocomial infection rates and methicillin-resistant *Staphylococcus aureus* transmission as outcome measures (Pittet et al. 2000).

Because the hand-hygiene case study examines the experience of multiple interventions rather than presenting the three types of evaluation for a single program, it is difficult to summarize the findings into "what would have worked better." However, the dearth of published information on formative evaluation of hand-hygiene interventions underscores the need for those designing such interventions to develop a clearer understanding of why hand-hygiene behavior is not more prevalent in medical care delivery settings. Similarly, tracking these interventions once they are in place to assess how well they are implemented and how members of the target group react to them (i.e., process evaluation) is important. Table 9.1 summarizes these three types of evaluation, including questions addressed, commonly used data collection methods, and study designs.

Conclusion

The three types of evaluation are conceptually clear. *Formative evaluation* serves to inform the design of the intervention (and thus must occur before it is implemented). *Process evaluation* focuses on how well the intervention is implemented; thus, by definition, it occurs while the intervention is ongoing. *Summative evaluation* seeks to determine whether the intervention results in the desired change and thus takes place after the period of implementation. As mentioned above, the results of a meta-analysis of intervention effectiveness (which is summative) can be used to inform the design of new programs—and the meta-analysis, in turn, may be thought of as formative. Similarly, summative evaluation often includes information on what elements of the program performed well and which did not, which might be considered the domain of process evaluation. Summative evaluation may also provide data on the reaction of participants to the intervention, which falls into the domain of process evaluation. In addition, a summative evaluation may identify barriers to behavior change, which become the basis for the design of a new intervention (and is thus formative). Despite this seeming blur, the distinctions between the three types of evaluation remain useful in designing and revising interventions and, finally, in assessing the impact of an intervention.

TABLE 9.1. Evaluation of behavior change interventions

Type of evaluation	Questions addressed	Data collection methods	Study designs
Formative (includes needs assessment) (Rossi et al. 2004)	What are the epidemiological patterns of this problem? What subgroups are most affected? What are the social determinants of this problem? What are barriers to change among the affected population? What would be the best channels/times to reach the affected population?	Use of existing data: epidemiological, service statistics, national-level surveys, market surveys Primary data collection: qualitative (focus groups, key-informant/ in-depth interviews, ethnographic observation) and quantitative (surveys)	One-time cross-sectional surveys (most common) or other forms of data collection
Process (Saunders et al. 2005)	Fidelity to design: Was the program operating as planned?	Desk review combined with field observations	Post-only assessment
	Reach: What percent of the intended audience did it reach?	Survey	Post-only survey among intended audience
	Dose delivered: How many units of each activity/ product were delivered (no. of trainings, no. of brochures distributed)	Program records	Desk review of program activities and records
	Dose received: How much exposure did members of the intended audience report having to the program?	Survey	Post-only survey among intended audience
	Reaction/satisfaction: What was the level of satisfaction among the intended audience with elements of the program?	Survey, focus group, or individual in-depth interviews with members of the intended audience	Post-test only among those exposed to the program
	Recruitment: Were those recruited similar in sociodemographic profile to those targeted by the program?	Desk review to compare program plan and data from program records on client/user profiles	Post-test only
	Context: What factors external to the program facilitated or hindered implementation?	Multiple sources of data	Continuous data collection over life of program
Summative Service utilization	Did service utilization increase (consistent with program objectives)?	Collection of routine service statistics or activity logs	Time-series designs; trend analysis

TABLE 9.1. (*continued*)

Type of evaluation	Questions addressed	Data collection methods	Study designs
Outcomes	Did the desired health behavior or health status change (consistent with program objectives)?	Surveys	Pre-post designs; or post-test only in an experimental and comparison population
Impact	To what extent can the change in behavior or health status be attributed to the intervention/program?	Surveys	Experimental or quasi-experimental designs; post-only with propensity score matching
Cost-effectiveness analysis	What is the cost per unit of change?	Surveys, collection of cost data	Experimental or quasi-experimental designs; post-only with propensity score matching; combined with costing exercise on the program

Practitioners of public health are coming to expect and demand **evidence-based programming** (refer to chapter 5). This chapter describes the specific types of evaluation—formative, process, and summative—that yield evidence with which to design interventions and evaluate their effectiveness. Not all programs will have sufficient funding to conduct comprehensive research that includes all three types of evaluation.

Historically, many have questioned the effectiveness of behavior change programs, given that undesirable health behaviors persist in society despite communication campaigns and other interventions to change behavior. However, we have now entered an era in which practitioners and evaluators work together in an effort to design, implement, and evaluate programming that will make a measurable difference in health behaviors and health status. This chapter shines additional light on what we mean by *evidence-based programming.*

REFERENCES

Aragon D, Sole ML, Brown S. 2005. Outcomes of an infection prevention project focusing on hand hygiene and isolation practices. *AACN Clin Issues* 16:121-32.

Assanasen S, Edmond M, Bearman G. 2008. Impact of 2 different levels of performance feedback on compliance with infection control process measures in 2 intensive care units. *Am J Infect Control* 36:407-13.

Babalola S, Kincaid DL. 2009. New methods for estimating the impact of health communication programs. *Commun Meth Meas* 3 (1): 61-83.

Boyce JM. 1999. It is time for action: Improving hand hygiene in hospitals. *Ann Intern Med* 130:153-55.

Elder JP, Lytle L, Sallis JF, et al. 2007. A description of the social-ecological framework used in the Trial of Activity for Adolescent Girls (TAAG). *Health Educ Res* 22 (2): 155-65.

Flay BR. 2000. Approaches to substance use prevention utilizing school curriculum plus social environment change. *Addict Behav* 25:861-85.

Glanz K, Rimer BK, Lewis FM, eds. 2002. *Health Behavior and Health Education: Theory, Research, and Practice.* 3rd ed. San Francisco: Wiley.

Harbarth S, Pittet D, Grady L, et al. 2002. Interventional study to evaluate the impact of an alcohol-based hand gel in improving hand hygiene compliance. *Pediatr Infect Dis J* 21:489-95.

Hong T, Johnson CC, Myers L, Boris N, Brewer D, Webber LS. 2008. Process evaluation of an in-school anti-tobacco media campaign in Louisiana. *Pub Health Rep* 123:781-89.

Hornik R, Jacobsohn L, Orwin R, Piesse A, Kalton G. 2008. Effects of the national youth anti-drug media campaign on youths. *Am J Public Health* 98 (12): 2229-36.

Joffe A, McNeely C, Colantuoni E, An MW, Wang W, Scharfstein D. 2009. Evaluation of school-based smoking-cessation interventions for self-described adolescent smokers. *Pediatrics* 124:e187-94.

Johnson CC, Myers L, Webber LS, Boris NW. 2004. Profiles of the adolescent smoker: Models of tobacco use among 9th grade high school students. Acadiana Coalition of Teens against Tobacco (ACTT). *Prev Med* 39:551-58.

Johnson CC, Myers L, Webber LS, Boris NW, He H, Brewer D. 2009. A school-based environmental intervention to reduce smoking among high school students: The Acadiana Coalition of Teens against Tobacco (ACTT). *Int J Environ Res Public Health* 6:1298-1316.

Kaufman R, English FW. 1979. *Needs Assessment: Concept and Application.* Englewood Cliffs, NJ: Educational Technology.

Larson EL, Quiros D, Giblin T, Lin S. 2007. Relationship of antimicrobial control policies and hospital and infection control characteristics to antimicrobial resistance rates. *Am J Crit Care* 16:110-20.

Lederer JW, Best D, Hendrix V. 2009. A comprehensive hand hygiene approach to reducing MRSA health care-associated infections. *Jt Comm J Qual Patient Saf* 35:180-85.

Maskerine C, Loeb M. 2006. Improving adherence to hand hygiene among health care workers. *J Contin Educ Health Prof* 26:244-51.

McKinley T, Gillespie W, Krauss J, et al. 2005. Focus group data as a tool in assessing effectiveness of a

hand hygiene campaign. *Am J Infect Control* 33:368-73.

National Nosocomial Infections Surveillance System (NNISS). 2004. National Nosocomial Infections Surveillance (NNIS) Systems Report, data summary from January 1992 through June 2004, issued October 2004. *Am J Infect Control* 32:470-85.

Pittet D, Hugonnet S, Harbarth S, et al. 2000. Effectiveness of a hospital-wide programme to improve compliance with hand hygiene: Infection control program. *Lancet* 356:1307-12.

Rossi PH, Lipsey MW, Freeman HE. 2004. *Evaluation: A Systematic Approach.* 7th ed. Thousand Oaks, CA: Sage.

Saunders RP, Evans MH, Joshi P. 2005. Developing a process-evaluation plan for assessing health promotion program implementation: A how-to guide. *Health Promot Practice* 6:134-47.

Sweat MD, Dennison JA. 1995. Reducing HIV incidence in developing countries with structural and environmental interventions. *AIDS* (suppl. A): S251-S257.

Thomas BW, Berg-Copas GM, Vasquez DG, Jackson BL, Wetta-Hall R. 2009. Conspicuous vs. customary location of hand hygiene agent dispensers on alcohol-based hand hygiene product usage in an intensive care unit. *J Am Osteo Assoc* 109:263-67.

Victora CG, Habicht JP, Bryce J. 2004. Evidence-based public health: Moving beyond randomized trials. *Am J Public Health* 94 (3): 400-405.

West SG, Duan N, Pequegnat W, et al. 2008. Alternatives to the randomized controlled trial. *Am J Pub Health* 98:1359-66.

Witte, K. 1992. Putting the fear back into fear appeals: The extended parallel process model. *Commun Monographs* 59:329-49.

Zerr DM, Allpress AL, Heath J, Bornemann R, Bennett E. 2005. Decreasing hospital-associated rotavirus infection: A multidisciplinary hand hygiene campaign in a children's hospital. *Pediatr Infect Dis J* 24:397-403.

Part II

STATE OF THE SCIENCE AND ROLES FOR KEY STAKEHOLDERS

CHAPTER 10

Tobacco and Behavior Change

ARNAB MUKHERJEA AND LAWRENCE W. GREEN

LEARNING OBJECTIVES

After completing the chapter, the reader will be able to

* Describe the magnitude, economic burden, demographic correlates, and trends of tobacco use in the United States.
* Detail determinants of tobacco use and classify them within levels in the social ecological model.
* Understand disparities in tobacco use patterns by diverse population segments in national and local populations.
* Characterize evidence-based interventions and their impact on reducing or preventing tobacco use.
* Describe CDC "Best Practices" and recommendations for comprehensive tobacco control interventions.
* Detail the successes of California's Tobacco Control Program as a model for other states and countries.
* Identify roles for key stakeholders in a comprehensive tobacco control program in countries such as the United States.

Introduction

The remarkable increase in adult use of tobacco to epidemic proportions in the first two-thirds of the 20th century and its remarkable reduction by half in the last third of the century make it, as illustrated in chapter 3, one of the great American public health success stories of the century. Similar reductions were achieved in other countries that undertook similarly aggressive tobacco control efforts. This chapter will take that history forward to the 21st century to examine how the reduction in tobacco use accounts for improvements in **morbidity** and **mortality** and reduction in the economic costs for several leading chronic disease causes of death and hospitalization. The centrality of behavior in the causes and solutions of the health problems associated with tobacco also make it a hallmark of the public health approach to behaviorally induced health problems. In this chapter we will assess the demographic and other **determinants** of tobacco use at individual, interpersonal, organizational, and policy levels. The combination of **individual-level interventions** in clinical and educational settings for smoking prevention and cessation, with organizational and policy-level restraints on industry promotions of an unhealthful product, make tobacco use a quintessential model for this book's central themes.

Widespread recognition of tobacco use as a health hazard is considered one of the 10 greatest public health achievements in the 20th century, based on its contribution to improving the health and life expectancy of persons living in the United States (CDC 1999b) and numerous other developed countries (Eriksen et al. 2007). These successes were largely initiated in the United States by the landmark 1964 surgeon general's report (USDHEW 1964), which concluded from authoritative and systematic reviews of the evidence that "cigarette smoking is a health hazard of sufficient importance in the United States to warrant appropriate remedial action" (Housman 2001; USDHEW 1964). The report followed decades of equivocation about the certainty of the evidence, fueled in part by tobacco industry strategies of casting doubt ("debunking," as they called it and as their public relations firms are now advising the petroleum energy industries to do with climate change science) on epidemiological and biological evidence. Such evidence was necessarily the limit of proof that could be brought to bear, insofar as trials of human beings randomized to smoking and nonsmoking groups could not be conducted ethically. The surgeon general's report was the impetus for more aggressive public health education and **counter-advertising** to offset the misinformation contained in the tobacco industry's communications and, eventually, for a wide array of comprehensive approaches to protect the public from environmental tobacco smoke, promote cessation, and prevent initiation of the smoking **habit** (Eriksen et al. 2007). Despite the widespread successes of these cumulative and comprehensive approaches, tobacco use remains a key **health behavior** contributing to major causes of mortality in the United States and globally.

Finally, this chapter will examine the major sources of evidence recommending **interventions** for the new challenges in tobacco control going forward. These sources of evidence have been submitted to systematic reviews by the Task Force on Community Preventive Services (CSPSTF 2013) and published with periodic updates on the Centers for Disease Control and Prevention's (CDC's) website.[1] The roles played by **key stakeholders** are also reviewed, including providers of health care; legislative and regulatory bodies; and public health agencies at federal, state and local levels (including government, voluntary, and philanthropic funding organizations). The tobacco industry itself as a key stakeholder presents major impediments to the larger successes of the tobacco control movement. The industry's infamous activities in deceiving the American public and suppressing research evidence led to a guilty finding of racketeering and fraud in U.S. Federal Court.[2] Some have likened the tobacco industry to a disease **vector** because of the manner in which it markets and promotes its products, much as a mosquito spreads malaria. Its sponsorship of youth programs and sports events, for example, gives it advertising venues, space, and the appearance of legitimacy and acceptability for its products; its placement of cigarettes in film scenes is known to influence youth perceptions and adoption of smoking as a result of role modeling "cool" behavior (Hendlin et al. 2010).

The Magnitude of the Tobacco Epidemic

Not only does tobacco produce enormous burdens on individual and public health; in addition it has significant social and economic **consequences**. Tobacco use is the leading cause of preventable death, disease, and disability in the United States, killing twice as many Americans as alcohol use, homicide, illicit substance abuse, and suicide *combined* (Mokdad et al. 2004). In addition to the deaths of smokers themselves—the estimated 443,000 Americans who die prematurely each year from smoking—some 50,000 nonsmokers die each year from exposure to environmental tobacco smoke (ETS). These latter deaths are disproportionately children who are exposed to ETS. An additional 8.6 million Americans have a serious illness caused by smoking. In total, more than 5 million years of life are lost yearly because of tobacco use. An additional growing body of evidence implicates tobacco residuals in carpeting, furniture, and other indoor objects as a long-lasting source of illness from third-hand smoke (Burton 2011).

The situation is even more dismal globally. The more than 5 million deaths attributable to tobacco use yearly account for approximately 10% of all global deaths (WHO 2008). It is estimated that by 2030, the death toll from tobacco will be more than 8 million a year. At the current pace, more than 1 billion people worldwide could be killed by tobacco by the end of the 21st century (WHO 2008). More than 80% of tobacco-related mortality will occur in low- and middle-income countries (Mathers and Loncar 2006). Although tobacco is predominantly consumed in the form of cigarettes, other smoked products (i.e., bidis, kreteks, and hookahs or shishas) and smokeless items (for example, *snus, gutka,* and chewing tobacco) are commonly used and gaining popularity (WHO 2008). Electronic cigarettes are the latest rapidly spreading arrival on the marketplace of tobacco products (Caponnetto et al. 2012), advertised as having no secondhand smoke. However, in truth, a nicotine vapor from the battery powered e-cigarette could be having a similar and possibly worse environmental effect on those exposed to it.

Tobacco use affects all major organ systems, with the most adverse consequences occurring in the pulmonary and cardiovascular systems. In the United States, smoking is responsible for an average of 150,000 deaths from cancer—including almost 130,000 lung cancer deaths—as well as more than 125,000 deaths from heart disease and almost 100,000 from chronic lung disease (CDC 2008). Besides cigarettes, pipe and cigar smoking increases risks of lip, oral, and lung cancers, whereas the use of smokeless tobacco is a major cause of oral cancers (e.g., cheek, gums, and lips).

The Economic Burden

In addition to severe health consequences, tobacco use places an economic burden on health care systems and more broadly on national economies. In the United States, it is responsible annually for $96 billion in medical expenditures and an additional $97 billion in lost economic opportunities such as loss of productivity in the workforce. The economic impact of ETS includes $5 billion in direct medical costs and another $5 billion in indirect losses, such as those for disability and lost wages (CDC 2002). Although global estimates of economic impact are incomplete, the net effect disproportionately burdens the poor, especially in impoverished countries.

Trends in Tobacco Use

Understanding temporal patterns in tobacco use across populations is important for **planning**, implementing, and evaluating tobacco control interventions and policies. The National Health Interview Survey, the Youth Behavioral Risk Factor Surveillance System, and for adults, the Behavioral Risk Factor Surveillance System (all administered by the CDC) and the National Survey on Drug Use and Health (SAMHSA 2012) collect ongoing national and regional data to estimate smoking prevalence in the United States, and they have their counterpart in the Global Youth Tobacco Survey (Warren et al. 2000) and others (McQueen and Puska 2003; WHO 1998). Other sources provide local, state, and national estimates and international comparison data. One of the features of the tobacco movement nationally and internationally has been the widespread adoption of consistent and uniform definitions and measures of current and lifetime smoking, smoking prevalence, and related measures (Warren et al. 2000). In 2011, 19.0% of Americans age 18 and older were current smokers, numbering approximately 43.8 million residents (CDC 2013). This is in sharp contrast to the peak rate of U.S. smoking prevalence, which was approximately 40% in 1965 (Rahilly and Farwell 2007), showing a reduction of almost 50%. The earlier rates were much higher for men. Their decline in prevalence has been greater than that for women, whose smoking rates continued to rise for some time after 1965. These trends contributed to significant differences between statistics for men and women regarding decreases over time in cases of, and deaths from, heart disease and cancers. Women's later declines in smoking rates are now beginning to show the time-lagged reductions in related cancers (OSH 2001). Smoking cessation rates combined with smoke-free ordinances that reduce exposure to secondhand smoke have been shown to produce much more immediate effects on reductions in heart attack rates (Barnoya and Glantz 2005).

Despite the sharp decline in smoking rates, the rate of decrease in the United States has stalled since 2005. In addition, there are substantial variations in use of tobacco among various subgroups in the United States. Approximately 20% of American adults smoke. According to a 2007 report, smoking levels were lowest for individuals age 65 and older and did not vary significantly in the same year across ages 18 to 24, 25 to 44, and 45 to 64 (CDC 2007). Nearly 90% of smokers start during adolescence, making youth (individuals younger than age 18) a primary target group for industry promotion and for public health intervention (Thomson et al. 2007). In the same time frame, the National Youth Tobacco Survey found that almost 24% of high school students and more than 8% of middle school students reported current use of tobacco. Despite overall declines from 2000 to 2009, neither of these groups demonstrated significant reductions between 2006 and 2009.

Demographic Correlates of Tobacco Use

In addition to differences by gender and age, there are differences in smoking rates for regions and ethnic groups. Western states have the lowest prevalence, and the South has the highest. Like national trends, rates of smoking did not decline in any of the four major regions—Northeast, Midwest, South, or West—from 2005 to 2009. Figure 10.1 provides a state-by-state comparison of smoking prevalence in the United States.

Differences in smoking prevalence in the United States follow socioeconomic gradients, usually measured by educational attainment and level of income (CDC 2010). For instance, smoking prevalence is inversely correlated with education; those holding a General Education Development (GED) certificate have a rate almost ten times as high as adults with a graduate degree. Although the income disparity is not as dramatic as that for educational gradations, almost one-third of individuals living below the federal poverty level smoked in 2011 (Agaku et al. 2012), while approximately one in five living at or above this threshold was a current smoker.

Considerable variations occur between racial and ethnic minority populations in the United States. Native Americans and Alaskan Natives had the highest prevalence rate (23.3%) of adults reporting a single race or ethnicity, whereas Asian Americans had the lowest (12.0%). However, individuals reporting multiple races had the overall highest prevalence rate at almost 30%. Table 10.1 details the percentage of current adult smokers, by race or ethnicity.

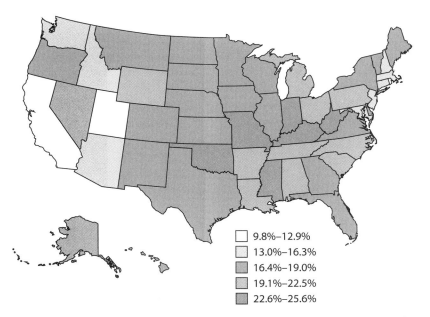

9.8%–12.9%
13.0%–16.3%
16.4%–19.0%
19.1%–22.5%
22.6%–25.6%

FIGURE 10.1. The percentage of persons age 18 or older who were current cigarette smokers in 2009 (persons who reported smoking at least 100 cigarettes during their lifetime and who, at the time of the survey, reported smoking every day or on some days), by state, according to the Behavioral Risk Factor Surveillance System, United States, 2009. *Source:* Agaku et al. 2011.

Regardless of racial and ethnic classification, individuals born in the United States are more likely to smoke than foreign-born people; the only exception is for Asian males born in the United States; their rates are slightly lower than their foreign-born counterparts (Baluja et al. 2003). Overall low smoking prevalence by Asians notwithstanding, when Asian and Pacific Islander immigrants are disaggregated into distinct subgroups, smoking rates for certain populations were significantly higher than non-immigrant ones, with estimated rates as high as 33% (Koreans). Asian female immigrants have much lower use rates of all tobacco products than do Asian male immigrants.

Alternative Forms of Tobacco

Tobacco users consume a range of products in addition to cigarettes, such as cigars, smokeless tobacco (e.g., "snuff"), and pipe tobacco. In 2011, the National Survey on Drug Use and Health found that between 18 and 23 million individuals used noncigarette forms of tobacco (SAMHSA 2012). Among youth, smokeless tobacco use prevalence is high among males, with some states reaching male rates of more than 20% of youth. These statistics do not take into account culturally specific tobacco products commonly used by various minority groups, such as South Asians, Pacific Islanders, and Native Americans, including *gutka, iqmik,* and betel quid (Kim et al. 2007; Mukherjea et al. 2012).

Global Trends

Globally, more than 1 billion males and 250 million females smoke (Eriksen et al. 2012). The number of female smokers is expected to double by 2025 if current trends continue. The majority of women smokers live in high-income countries, whereas most male smokers are in the developing world. More than two-thirds of the world's smokers are from 10 countries, and

TABLE 10.1. Percentage of persons age 18 and older who were
cigarette smokers in 2009, by race/ethnicity

Race/Ethnicity	Total		Men		Women	
White, non-Hispanic	22.1	(21.2–23.1)	24.5	(23.2–25.9)	19.8	(18.8–20.8)
Black, non-Hispanic	21.3	(19.6–22.9)	23.9	(21.5–26.2)	19.2	(17.1–21.3)
Hispanic	14.5	(13.2–15.8)	19.0	(16.9–21.1)	9.8	(8.5–11.0)
American Indian/Alaska Native	23.2	(12.9–33.5)	29.7	(15.4–44.0)	—[a]	—[a]
Asian, non-Hispanic[b]	12.0	(10.0–14.0)	16.9	(14.0–19.9)	7.5	(4.8–10.3)
Multiple race, non-Hispanic	29.5	(22.9–36.1)	33.7	(24.4–43.0)	24.8	(16.6–33.0)

Source: CDC 2010.
[a]Data not available.
[b]Does not include Native Hawaiians or Other Pacific Islanders.

300 million of them live in China (WHO 2008). This does not take into account countries (e.g., India, Taiwan, Papua New Guinea) where the bulk of users consume tobacco in the smokeless form (NCI and CDC 2002).

The World Health Organization (WHO) estimates that tobacco use causes 5.4 million deaths annually and will cumulatively kill 175 million persons between 2010 and 2030 if current trends continue (Eriksen et al. 2012). Of these deaths, 80% will occur in low- and middle-income countries.

In summary, despite tremendous success over the past decade in the United States and in Western Europe, Australia, Canada, New Zealand, Singapore, and some other countries, tobacco control continues to face formidable challenges—and even greater challenges in the emerging economies and the poorest countries. The significant disparities in tobacco use and related disease among subpopulations, coupled with slowing rates of decline in tobacco use, result in enormous health and economic burdens in the United States and globally, which will persist for at least 30 years after each cohort of the former smokers of each country quit. With rates continuing to climb in developing countries, and the tobacco industry turning its promotions increasingly toward those countries as it loses smokers in the United States and other developed countries, the epidemic of tobacco-related diseases and deaths will continue for decades to come, regardless of successes that some countries can claim. To ensure that current and future intervention strategies are effective and coordinated, increased understanding of the social, economic, and contextual milieu in which tobacco use is promoted by the industry in specific countries and adopted by people of those countries will be essential for continued progress in tobacco control.

Key Determinants

The **ecological model** posits a multilevel framework to understand **complex** and dynamic factors that influence smoking and other health behaviors. Tobacco use is determined by myriad factors, including individual, interpersonal, community, organizational, and structural components. In addition, these determinants often occur in a multidimensional sociocultural **context**, influenced by **social norms** and **expectations**, cultural values, and economic considerations (Unger et al. 2003). This section describes several of the central determinants of tobacco use.

Individual Determinants

At the biological level, the key mechanism sustaining tobacco use is the presence of nicotine in cigarettes and other tobacco products. Nicotine binds to specific receptors in the brain, which, in turn, initiate release of neurotransmitters (Benowitz 2010). Release of these chemical messengers—including dopamine and serotonin—signals a pleasurable sensation and reinforces continued use. In addition, nicotine contributes to mood modulation by reducing stress and anxiety and improving concentration and performance. As more nicotine is consumed, the brain adapts with repeated exposure, requiring sustained or increased levels to achieve the same outcomes. The withdrawal effects of nicotine—irritability, anxiety, restlessness, depression—contribute to its repeated use and addictive potential. Even after withdrawal symptoms subside, the urge to resaturate nicotinic receptors continues for long periods of time.

These processes are influenced by an individual's genetic profile. Of the variability in smoking initiation, 50% is associated with genetic factors, and genetic factors are also associated with 60% of the variance in smoking rates and up to 75% of differences in nicotine dependence (Schnoll et al. 2007). For instance, twin studies have demonstrated that biological siblings raised in separate environments have a three-to-five-times-higher likelihood of smoking if the other smokes. Gene coding for nicotine metabolism, dopamine biosynthesis, and serotonin transport play important roles in the heritability of smoking behavior.

Other significant individual determinants include various combinations of personality traits (e.g., extroversion, **self-efficacy**, locus of control, sensation seeking, global outlook), behavioral problems (e.g., school or work performance), presence of mental illness, and addiction to or abuse of other substances (van Loon et al. 2005). These factors become increasingly pertinent when tobacco use occurs at an earlier age, because younger people are more vulnerable to addiction and have both a larger propensity for neural **adaptation** and a greater likelihood of permanent biological and behavioral conditioning (Benowitz 2010).

Individual demographic characteristics are highly correlated with tobacco use. As indicated earlier, the age of initiation plays a significant role in maintaining tobacco use; 89% of current smokers began by age 18 (Lynch and Bonnie 1994). The level of individual education may have strong **influences** on accurate health knowledge, perceptions of risk regarding disease and disability, and immediacy of health and social consequences associated with tobacco use. Among smokers, education level is also negatively associated with frequency and intensity of smoking, and positively with quit attempts and likelihood of cessation (Eriksen et al. 2012). Similarly, an individual's lack of knowledge about or underestimation of lesser-known tobacco risks plays a significant role in whether the person continues smoking (Oncken et al. 2005).

Individual smoking behavior is also influenced by cues. **Cues** are sensations, moods, and situations that users associate with their use of tobacco. For regular tobacco users, behaviors and feelings associated with nicotine—rewards and withdrawal—become conditioned as cues for smoking behavior (Olausson et al. 2004). Such smoking-related cues include finishing a meal, drinking coffee or alcoholic beverages, experiencing heightened emotional states (stress, depression, excitement), and certain routine tasks (e.g., talking on the phone, driving).

Another set of individual determinants revolves around situational factors in the individual's immediate environment. These factors, such as job strain, professional or personal expectations, and reactions to physical or mental abuse, are largely responses to external stimuli (Anda et al. 1999; van Loon et al. 2005). They are considered to be **individual-level determinants** because they are factors over which the individual has a considerable degree of influence, if not control. Some of these interactions of the individual with his social and physical environments involve the ecological principle of **reciprocal determinism**, in which ecology recognizes (as does **systems thinking**) that every system is a subsystem of larger systems and that the larger systems are influenced by their subsystems (Green, Richard, and Potvin 1996; Richard et al. 1996). Individuals are not merely the victims of their environments; they also have agency to act upon their environments. They do so all the more effectively when they join forces with other individuals, as in collective action, advocacy, and policy influence. These interactions are explored further in the next section.

Interpersonal Determinants

Interpersonal determinants include influences from **social networks**, such as family members, friends or peers, and co-workers (Umberson 1987). For tobacco use, research has consistently shown that **norms**, behaviors, and the strength of ties with various social networks often influence smoking behavior (Christakis and Fowler 2008). For instance, the smoking status of parents or siblings, parent-child conflict, parental monitoring, the level of familial concern or involvement, and family rules all have associations with tobacco use (Kim et al. 2009). Similarly, smoking status among spouses has a high rate of concordance (Macken et al. 2000). Adolescents and adults with high exposure to peer groups who smoke are significantly more likely to smoke themselves (Bricker et al. 2006; Buttross and Kastner 2003; Green et al. 2008; Hoffman et al. 2007). For instance, actions of individuals in a given workplace, such as discouragement of quitting smoking and offering cigarettes to co-workers, have been strong predictors of smoking behavior in these social groups (Sorensen et al. 1986). (Ironically, the

recent **denormalization** of smoking, which accounts for much of the reduction of smoking at large, has actually pushed some smokers to the fringes of mainstream **social environments**; among these marginalized groups, the **density** and strength of ties actually reinforce smoking among these individuals.) As with individual tobacco-related cues, family settings or social environments normally involving tobacco use may be a conditional determinant of smoking, even when use of tobacco is not present (Benowitz 2010).

In addition to *actual* smoking behavior of various peer groups, the *perception* of tobacco use in a social group influences smoking intention and smoking initiation, especially among youth, and such perceptions tend to be higher than the actual smoking rates (Brown and Moodie 2009; Farrelly et al. 2009). The perception of peer smoking prevalence has also been shown to be inversely associated with perceptions of harm and disapproval of smoking (Lipperman-Kreda and Grube 2009). In sum, the perceived and actual behaviors of intimate peer and social groups have strong and varied influences on smoking initiation and maintenance.

Community and Neighborhood Determinants

Many **community-level determinants** are extensions of **interpersonal factors**. For instance, smoke-free homes—defined as households with voluntary restrictions on smoking by occupants—have been shown to influence smoking cessation among adults and prevent initiation among youth (Hyland et al. 2009; Trosclair et al. 2007). Somewhat counterintuitively, the increase in the number of smoke-free homes is largely associated with the adoption of local smoke-free public places, such as neighborhood restaurants and bars and local workplaces. Although it may be assumed that prohibitions in public venues may lead to a higher likelihood of smoking in private homes, this association may demonstrate the strong impact of the denor-malization of tobacco use (Borland et al. 2006; Farkas et al. 1999).

In addition to prohibitions and restrictions on tobacco use, concentrated exposure to to-bacco advertisements, such as at the neighbor-hood level, is linked to smoking among youth. Similarly, close proximity to tobacco outlets in a given community expands residents' access to tobacco, thereby increasing the likelihood of smoking behavior (Asumda and Jordan 2009; Gilpin et al. 2007). These determinants of smok-ing behavior are amplified in neighborhoods with more working-class or socioeconomically disadvantaged residents (Barbeau et al. 2004; Stead et al. 2001).

Communities not bound by geographic limi-tations are also subject to specific influences on tobacco use. For instance, specific groups with shared interests, affiliations, memberships, and identities (such as gender, age, race/ethnicity, religion, sexual orientation, and generational status) may be homogeneous with respect to tobacco behavior (Acevedo-Garcia et al. 2005; Fagan et al. 2004; Gillum et al. 2009; Lee et al. 2013; Pizacani et al. 2009; Simons-Morton and Farhat 2010). These commonalities in smoking behavior have been attributed to processes of **socialization** or **selection**, or both (Simons-Morton and Farhat 2010). As an indication of the social normative aspect of smoking, identities revolve around abstinence (e.g., "nonsmoker"), frequency (e.g., "light smoker"), purpose (e.g., "social smoker"), cosmetic effects (e.g., "smoker's breath"), and past behaviors (e.g., "ex-smoker"), rather than levels of addiction.

Certain racial and ethnic minority popula-tions may use tobacco as an expression of iden-tity and symbolizing specific meaning (Nichter 2003; Unger et al. 2003). Specific tobacco prod-ucts (such as pipes, hookahs, cigarillos, and chewable combinations of betel nut and to-bacco) may be used for certain purposes, mean-ings, and contexts (USDHHS 1994). For instance, the use of tobacco, often smoked in pipes, among

Native Americans serves ceremonial or medici-nal purposes, or both (Linton 1924; Spangler et al. 1997). For African Americans, tobacco has historical significance for entry into the em-ployment and civic sectors of American society (Foner 1981; Kaufman 1986). The sharing of cigarettes among Latinos demonstrates a high strength of friendship or filial respect within social relationships, especially among men (Un-ger et al. 2001; Marin et al. 1990). Similarly, shar-ing of cigarettes among certain Asian American subgroups signifies hospitality and respect (Tamir and Cachola 1994). Moreover, the use of specific tobacco products has symbolic value. For instance, many Pacific Islander communi-ties, as well as South Asians, use combined tobacco and betel nut concoctions to welcome guests, to observe religious and cultural events, and to avail themselves of perceived health ben-efits attributed to use (Mukherjea et al. 2012; Nelson and Heischober 1999; Sullivan et al. 2000). Especially in societies where certain eth-nic groups are minorities in the general popula-tion, use of these "indigenous" tobacco prod-ucts helps preserve and express native cultural attributes.

Organizational and Institutional Determinants

Much has been published about institutional and organizational influences on tobacco use in the United States and beyond. Many of these factors can be traced to the activities of the to-bacco industry. While other institutional and **organizational factors** and settings, such as schools and workplaces, are also important de-terminants of tobacco use, we concentrate our discussion here on the role of the tobacco indus-try, insofar as its activities have been so nefari-ous (as documented in court cases) and its **reach** so extensive.

The epidemiological analogy of a host-vector-agent relationship, often used to describe the role of the tobacco industry in spreading the epidemic of tobacco-related disease and death (WHO 2008; Yach and Wipfli 2006), positions the smoker as the **host**, with cigarettes and other tobacco products serving as the **agents** of disease and death and the tobacco industry as the **vector**. The **goal** of the tobacco industry is not simply to survive, but to maximize profit, influence the market, and promote its products. The industry has acknowledged that the cigarette was designed as a vector for efficient delivery of nicotine. The success of this business objective comes at the expense of disability and disease of the industry's customers. It is beyond the scope of this chapter to detail the numerous and complex activities employed by the tobacco industry to achieve its goals. The following history merely illustrates the tobacco industry's structural influence on tobacco use.

Despite concealing it from the public, the tobacco industry was acutely aware of the science behind the risk imparted by its products (Bero 2003). Specifically, the tobacco industry knew that nicotine was an addictive drug and that delivery via a smoked cigarette had unique psychological and biological advantages to initiate and maintain use (Hurt and Robertson 1998; Slade et al. 1995). Research conducted on adverse health effects by the tobacco industry confirmed the relationship between smoking and cancer (Hanauer et al. 1995). As the public absorbed the understanding that cigarettes were harmful, beginning with a *Reader's Digest* article in 1954, the tobacco industry engaged in substantial research to determine optimal nicotine absorption rates, while also portraying and marketing the image of creating "safer" cigarettes, despite internal research findings to the contrary (Kozlowski and O'Connor 2002; Pollay and Dewhirst 2002).

In light of its own findings, the tobacco industry knew that public acceptance of the harms associated with tobacco use would cause irreversible harm to its profits by reducing the number of current and future smokers. To counteract this possibility, the tobacco industry was keen to emphasize that the science sur-rounding adverse effects of smoking was "controversial" (Francey and Chapman 2000). By keeping the debate alive—usually by sponsoring credible third parties whose research findings and sources of funding were edited or omitted—the tobacco industry influenced legislation, defended itself from litigation, and influenced standards for regulation of tobacco products (Bero 2003).

The tobacco industry employed its advertising and marketing as another major strategy for countering the growing scientific and legal forces against its products. Despite assertions to the contrary, the industry strategically implemented a targeted promotion by segmenting the market and appealing to specific population groups, including youth and racial/ethnic populations (Ling and Glantz 2002; Pollay 2000). Understanding that users of its products were likely to die, and that older adults would quit as they endured symptoms of tobacco harms, the tobacco industry targeted youth and young adults as "replacement smokers" to assure sustainability of profit margins and expansion of the market (Cummings et al. 2002). The tobacco industry designed advertising campaigns, promotion schemes, and product characteristics aimed at women (USDHHS 2001; Haglund 2010), younger smokers (Katz and Lavack 2002; Wayne and Connolly 2002), racial and ethnic minorities, and low-income populations (Apollonio and Malone 2005; Balbach et al. 2003; Muggli et al. 2002). With the passage of the Master Settlement Agreement between the attorneys general of the states and the tobacco companies, which restricted marketing and required financial compensation in exchange for immunity from tort liability, the tobacco industry has implemented more covert strategies, including introduction of smoked and smokeless products with claims of reduced harm (e.g., *Snus*, e-cigarettes), marketing and promotion of its products via the Internet and movies, and increased point-of-sale advertising in disadvantaged communities (Freeman and Chapman 2009; John et al. 2009; Mejia and Ling 2010). These efforts facilitate tobacco use by impeding dissemination of accurate information, influencing legislation by manipulating research, and **targeting** population groups with a high propensity to become addicted users.

Structural and Policy-Level Determinants

Besides tobacco industry involvement, public policy (or lack thereof) is a key **structural determinant** of tobacco use. Public policies not only influence tobacco use through modification or maintenance of physical environments in which tobacco use may occur; they also shape and normalize smoking behavior. For instance, the lower the excise taxes are on cigarettes, the higher the number of cigarettes smoked (Chaloupka and Warner 2000). A lack of indoor smoking bans (e.g., for workplaces, airplanes, cars) influences tobacco use by increasing opportunities to smoke, portraying smoking as a socially acceptable or "normal" behavior, facilitating **modeling** of youth habits by subjecting them to adult smokers, and facilitating exchange of tobacco products among regular and infrequent users (Eriksen and Cerak 2008). Accessibility of tobacco, particularly to young persons, is a strong determinant of use and initiation of use. Unenforced age restrictions or allowance of tobacco vending machines facilitates ease of access to tobacco among youth (Powell and Chaloupka 2003). A lack of restrictions on the industry in such matters as commercial outlets, product packaging, addition of appealing flavoring and other additives to tobacco products, free samples and discounted products, and event sponsorship also enables initiation and maintenance of tobacco use.

Tobacco-Related Health Disparities

As indicated earlier, the determinants of tobacco use interact with each other in complex fashions. Their dynamic interplay results in numerous groups being disproportionately affected. Despite dramatic disparities within and between U.S. minority groups encompassing race and ethnicity, sexual orientation, **socioeconomic status**, and others, there is incomplete understanding of the causes of population differences in exposure and susceptibility to and consequences of tobacco use and related diseases (Fagan et al. 2004). Notwithstanding the multilevel influences discussed earlier, the *context* of tobacco use among diverse populations remains complicated by the variety and **complexity** of interactions among settings, cultures, tastes, politics, and language. Cultures shape many social and behavioral norms. In addition to methods and patterns of use, such as consumption of certain products and their use in specific environments, the values, meanings, and beliefs ascribed to tobacco play important (and understudied) roles in the existence of **health disparities** (Nichter 2003; Unger et al. 2003). The difficulty of operationalizing culture and testing associations between ambiguous variables and tobacco-related outcomes has often led health researchers to neglect investigating such complex relationships. Health professionals and advocates have increasingly urged collaborative approaches to better understand the social context of tobacco use in order to strengthen tobacco control and practice (Poland et al. 2006).

Exacerbating the consequences of the limited data examining tobacco-related health disparities are the tobacco industry's sophisticated demographic and psychographic marketing campaigns and products targeting cultural values and social norms of specific minority communities. This technique of population **segmentation** has helped the tobacco industry create niche products and normalize tobacco use among distinct social and cultural groups. For instance, billboards advertising cigarettes appear with significantly greater density in minority communities, often depicting models ethnically and socially concordant with the neighborhood in which they are placed. The industry has similarly segmented and targeted these populations in print media (Muggli et al. 2002; Washington 2002). Even within defined demographic categories, the tobacco industry identifies psychographic qualities of segments (e.g., sensation seekers, social "rebels") more amenable to adopting tobacco behavior (John et al. 2009; Ling et al. 2007).

Tobacco control stands to lose much of the momentum that has been gained if it fails to examine the role and context of tobacco use among diverse populations, particularly among the most vulnerable and disadvantaged. In recent years, health institutions have been created to address such disparities. For instance, California's Department of Health Services funded ethnically specific tobacco education **networks** to address distinct issues among the state's diverse populations; the National Cancer Institute and the American Legacy Foundation partnered to create the Tobacco Related Network on Disparities; the CDC has implemented the National Networks for Tobacco Control and Prevention, which sustains leading policy, advocacy, and community-based organizations to address tobacco use among population groups that experience significant tobacco-related disparities. Despite these promising initial efforts, the existence of disparities related to tobacco use remains one of the most pressing public health concerns and should be emphasized as a means to counteract the tobacco industry's established influence and pursue health equity in *all* affected communities.

Evidence-Based Interventions

In its relatively short history, the tobacco control movement has achieved notable success. This realization has been manifested in reductions in smoking rates and smoking-related diseases, largely through strategic, comprehensive, **multilevel interventions** that work in concert

across organizations and communities to reinforce prevention and change of tobacco-use norms.

Interventional components aim to reduce both the supply of and the demand for tobacco products, although researchers surmise that reducing demand is more effective (Jha and Chaloupka 2000). This section focuses on three major milestones in tobacco control: the Surgeon General's Report on Reducing Tobacco Use in 2000, the CDC's report on Best Practices for Comprehensive Tobacco Control Programs, and the California Tobacco Control Program (CTCP). The Surgeon General's Report in 2000 identified and categorized all the components necessary for tobacco control by reviewing the evidence for programmatic work and evaluating economic and regulatory approaches to reducing use (Eriksen and Green 2002; Mercer et al. 2003). To accelerate these efforts nationwide, the CDC generated a repository of **evidence-based practices** to enable states to create, implement, and evaluate comprehensive tobacco control programs (CDC 1999a, 2014). This publication provided the research, **program evaluation**, and econometric evidence supporting interventional components that had achieved demonstrable success in the reduction of tobacco use in California, Massachusetts, and a few other states relative to the other states. At the state level, the CTCP has been acclaimed as one of the most successful programs in comprehensiveness, **innovation, effectiveness**, and impact (Rogers 2010). The CTCP's demonstrable accomplishments have been attributed to its underpinning **theory**, which emphasizes an ecological and social-normative approach to addressing the multilevel influences on tobacco use and to denormalizing its use. In light of these approaches, which encompass a broad scope of intervention strategies, this section focuses on these three major milestones in tobacco control to frame the discussion of evidence-based strategies and practice-based evidence.

Case Example: Surgeon General's Report

In 2000, the congressionally mandated Surgeon General's Report on Tobacco and Health presented an extensive articulation of historical, social, economic, clinical, educational, and regulatory efforts designed to reduce tobacco use, especially among youth and racial/ethnic minority populations (USDHHS 2000). The report identified five key elements necessary for achieving successful tobacco control: clinical, educational, regulatory, and economic approaches, all coordinated in comprehensive programs.

CLINICAL INTERVENTION AND MANAGEMENT

Helping tobacco users quit produces a public health benefit that occurs sooner and in greater numbers of tobacco users reduced than approaches attempting to prevent the uptake of tobacco (USDHHS 1990). Among clinical prevention strategies, physician counseling and treatment of smokers has been deemed one of the most medically effective and cost-effective means of all disease prevention interventions (Mercer et al. 2003), even though the rate of successful quitting (between 20% and 30%) at best seems weak to physicians accustomed to higher rates of effectiveness with pharmaceutical and surgical interventions. Successes of *clinical interventions* are amplified with higher intensity as well as greater frequency and duration (USDHHS 2000). In addition to the effort's clinical efficacy, patients whose physicians discussed quitting tobacco use were more satisfied with the medical encounter (Solberg et al. 2001). As such, the primary care setting serves as a valuable venue for personalized clinical interventions. In addition to clinical practice **guidelines**, recommendations have been made regarding structural changes to facilitate a physician's ability to undertake cessation-related tasks, including ensuring reimbursement for cessation counseling sessions, implementing tobacco-user

identification systems, and expanding vital signs to include tobacco use (Fiore 2000; Hollis et al. 2000). Self-help programs have shown a lesser benefit in enabling users to quit, although **tailoring** materials to specific individuals may increase this effect (Niaura 2008).

EDUCATIONAL AND MASS MEDIA INTERVENTIONS

Most educational strategies have focused on intervention in elementary school settings and counter-advertising of tobacco products. Those in schools have been most effective when combined with school policies banning smoking on the premises, both by students and by faculty. Because most smokers start before age 18, school-based programs are pivotal components of a comprehensive tobacco control program. In conjunction with community- and media-oriented approaches, *educational interventions* can postpone or prevent initiation of smoking in up to 40% of adolescents (USDHHS 2000); many of these programs sustain their effect long after the intervention has ended (Mercer et al. 2003). Linking school-based programs with public **coalitions** and countermarketing programs—often utilizing mass media—has been shown to the bolster the strength of these strategies. Children and adults are more likely to consume tobacco when exposed to tobacco promotion and advertising, so strategies countering these influences hold promise for reducing tobacco use. For instance, the Legacy Foundation's Truth Campaign, a mass-media program with messaging that counters tobacco advertising and exposes the industry, accounted for 22% of the decline in youth smoking between 1999 and 2002, paralleling the successes of other countermarketing strategies (Farrelly et al. 2005; Wakefield et al. 2003).

REGULATORY INTERVENTIONS

Regulation and enforcement are key components of any comprehensive tobacco control program. The control of tobacco products, curtailing access by minors, and implementing clean indoor air policies are considered to be pivotal elements of tobacco control efforts (Farrelly et al. 2013; Mercer et al. 2003). Part of the argument for comprehensiveness is that the components of education, regulation, and economics are synergistic. If policies, for example, do not align with the message that children receive in schools, the inconsistency undercuts the credibility of the educational message. And if education does not build an informed electorate about tobacco and its regulation, policies are harder to pass and more difficult to enforce.

ECONOMIC INTERVENTIONS

As a manifestation of supply-demand theory, evidence demonstrates that the price of tobacco inversely correlates with overall tobacco consumption. For instance, a 10% increase in the price of cigarettes tends to produce a 3%-5% decrease in overall consumption in high-income countries and up to a 10% decrease in low-income nations (USDHHS 2000). Adolescents are especially sensitive to this price plasticity because they have less disposable income (Green 1997; Chaloupka et al. 1999). Therefore, a key focal point of *economic intervention* highlighted and supported by the 2000 Surgeon General's Report is to decrease the affordability of cigarettes in the form of higher tobacco excise taxes (Mercer et al. 2003; Grossman 1997).

COMPREHENSIVE PROGRAMS

The 2000 Surgeon General's Report, like the CDC's 1998 and 2007 guidelines for statewide programs, emphasized the importance of integrating the approaches outlined above in a comprehensive approach, using multiple channels of implementation and diffusion. **Multilevel interventions** address many of the factors influencing both individual- and population-level tobacco use in a simultaneous and mutually reinforcing fashion (NCI 2000). Evidence demonstrates that the success of comprehensive to-

bacco programs depends on the synergistic and dynamic interplay of the intervention strategies outlined above (Mercer et al. 2003). The importance of intersectoral collaboration, including the engagement of educational institutions, affected workplaces, the hospitality industry, and others, is essential to this notion of comprehensiveness (Green et al. 2006). Moreover, the success of these programs depends largely on the ability to adapt to changing contexts and new research evidence. They therefore require strong leadership, good administration, monitoring, and oversight to sustain optimal impact.

Case Example: CDC Best Practices for Comprehensive Tobacco Control Programs

Initially predating the 2000 Surgeon General's Report, the CDC created an integrated programmatic structure to reduce tobacco use across the United States (CDC 1999a, 2014). The initial recommendations (in 1999) and an updated set of recommendations (in 2014) critically examined the characteristics of the most effective programs (particularly the California and Massachusetts state programs). The CDC defined the most effective population-based approaches within nine core, overarching components (in the first edition) and later consolidated them into five components. These programmatic domains include statewide and community interventions, **health communication interventions**, cessation interventions, **surveillance** and **evaluation**, and administration and management. The CDC report also stipulated a recommended level of investment for each state to reach the specific goals outlined in the document, based on the per capita expenditures for the various components in the most successful state programs.

STATEWIDE AND COMMUNITY INTERVENTIONS

Statewide and **community-level interventions** work in parallel to address each state's unique sociodemographic and historical milieu. By providing skills, resources, and information, statewide programs facilitate the coordinated and strategic execution of effective community programs. This allows the community programs to counter aggressive pro-tobacco forces, influence affected populations in their homes and frequented venues, and change the context of tobacco use within various institutions, structures, and cultural groups. Because many communities cannot afford the more expensive elements of comprehensive programs (such as the development and air time for mass media messages and exposure), states can provide for the development and airing of such mass media, and communities can build upon them locally. Examples of appropriate state and community programs include California's Smoker Helpline, which provides linguistically and culturally appropriate cessation services for diverse audiences, and the Vermont Tobacco Disparities Program, which targets disproportionate smoking rates among the mentally ill, substance abusers, and persons in extreme poverty (Anderson and Zhu 2000; CDHS 2006; VDH 2007). Other states, such as Colorado, have integrated tobacco control into a larger chronic disease prevention program, allowing targeting of specific tobacco-related outcomes that afflict different populations (CDPHE 2007).

HEALTH COMMUNICATION
INTERVENTIONS

Health communication interventions facilitate targeted messages, using diverse vehicles of dissemination, to reduce tobacco use and create a supportive climate for intervention efforts. In addition to the aforementioned Truth campaign, statewide programs have demonstrated large successes in various aspects of tobacco control. For instance, Minnesota implemented a continuous youth prevention program featuring a high-profile media campaign from 2000 to 2003, reducing the smoking initiation rate among youth (Sly et al. 2004). Other multi-

method health communication programs have had success in reducing tobacco use among adults, slowing initiation among youth, and protecting the public from environmental tobacco (secondhand) smoke (CDC 2014).

CESSATION INTERVENTIONS

Cessation interventions include clinical advisement, pharmacotherapy, and intensive counseling, which are often provided through state quit lines. The combination of counseling and medication has been shown to be most effective for tobacco cessation. For instance, the Ohio Tobacco Quit Line received more than 100,000 calls between 2004 and 2007, attributed to an intensive media campaign, dissemination through organizational **partnerships**, and the offer of free nicotine replacement therapy (CDC 2014).

SURVEILLANCE AND EVALUATION

To ensure the implementation, progress, and ultimate effectiveness and reach of public funding for tobacco control, states and communities must provide ongoing monitoring, surveillance, and evaluation. These assess the short- and long-term quality of practices and outcomes of comprehensive tobacco programs, provide accountability of public officials, and inform programmatic and policy-level adjustments. Both process and outcome measures evaluate the allocation and deployment of services and resources in the context of the program's implementation standards, interim **objectives**, and ultimate goals. The CDC consistently publishes results of its Adult Tobacco Survey and Youth Tobacco Survey and, together with WHO, which disseminates global counterparts of these surveys, highlights population trends, elucidates potential influences on tobacco use, and identifies emerging disparities in tobacco use and outcomes among diverse communities for realignment of program resources and emphases. With estimates at the local, state, and national level and by demographic groups, data can be compared to determine whether certain geographic vicinities and populations are not equally benefiting from a comprehensive tobacco control program.

ADMINISTRATION AND MANAGEMENT

Because comprehensive tobacco control programs require substantial coordination of financial and human resources, maximizing administration and management capacity is imperative. As reducing tobacco use requires participation from multiple entities, the states of California, New York, Oklahoma, and Indiana each created an umbrella administrative and management unit, ensuring that oversight for all tobacco control programs was continuous and coordinated (e.g., Mueller et al. 2006; TEROC 2012). The National Cancer Institute's ASSIST evaluation also highlighted the significance of organizational infrastructure, experienced personnel, and strong collaborations in implementing a comprehensive tobacco control program (NCI 2005).

THE COMMUNITY GUIDE

In addition to the Best Practice recommendations, CDC's Office on Smoking and Health funded a systematic review of the scientific and program evaluation literature to lay out the range of evidence for effective community- and environmental-level prevention strategies. This review was included in the CDC's *Guide to Community Preventive Services* ("*The Community Guide*") (Zaza et al. 2005). The Community Preventive Services Task Force (2013), an independent body authorized by Congress, provides oversight on the conduct and quality of the reviews. The *Community Guide* resource summarizes the evidence for effective tobacco control strategies, by identifying all relevant studies and assessing their quality. *The Community Guide* addresses the following four overarching goals of comprehensive tobacco control:

1. To prevent initiation among youth and young adults;

2. To promote quitting among adults and youth;
3. To eliminate exposure to secondhand smoke; and
4. To identify and eliminate tobacco-related disparities among population groups.

Prevent Initiation among Youth and Young Adults. Evidence has supported two major intervention strategies to reduce the initiation of tobacco use. Increasing the unit price for tobacco products—through municipal, state, or federal legislation—is effective in reducing tobacco use among youth and adults. Mass media education campaigns using brief and recurring messages motivating individuals to remain tobacco free, combined with other interventions (e.g., price increases, school-based education and policies, community education), demonstrate success in reducing initiation among adolescents (Tworek et al. 2010).

Promote Quitting among Adults and Youth. Various strategies have been shown to be effective in promoting quitting. In addition to price increases and mass media education, health care provider reminder systems—either alone or as part of a multicomponent intervention—increase cessation rates by allowing providers to identify patients who use tobacco and reminding providers to advise those users to quit through direct communication and/or provision of patient education materials. Another element of a successful multicomponent intervention is telephone support for tobacco users, including cessation counseling and assistance with initiating and maintaining abstinence. By using trained counselors, health care providers, or standardized taped messages, this strategy, in conjunction with client education materials, in-person counseling, and/or nicotine-replacement therapies, has been shown to be effective in increasing individual tobacco cessation in both clinical and community settings.

Eliminate Exposure to Secondhand Smoke. Smoking bans and restrictions (defined as policies, regulations, and laws prohibiting or limiting the use of smoked tobacco products in designated public areas) are the only interventional strategies identified by *The Community Guide* as having been conclusively proven to reduce exposure to environmental tobacco smoke. In fact, analyses of smoke-free laws have demonstrably concluded that municipalities adopting such measures show significant, and early, drops in heart attacks, and these benefits grow over time (Lightwood and Glantz 2009). This is commensurate with international studies showing other decreases in tobacco-related diseases, such as asthma, that are associated with implementation of smoke-free legislation (Mackay et al. 2010).

Evidence has since accumulated showing the effectiveness of mass media in promoting smoke-free homes, resulting in increased percentages of households that have made family rules against smoking indoors and in automobiles. Some jurisdictions have now passed state or local ordinances against smoking in automobiles in which a passenger under a certain age is present. Local ordinances and **incentives** have begun to create smoke-free apartment complexes by prohibiting smoking in apartments that share walls with other apartments. Related evidence has also accumulated showing the hazards of "third-hand smoke"—that which accumulates in carpeting, covered furniture, and other housing material. These findings will likely produce an intensification of policies against smoking in public places not just when others are present, but where others may be exposed after the secondhand smoke has settled.

Identify and Eliminate Tobacco-Related Disparities among Population Groups. Although this goal of a comprehensive tobacco control strategy targets population groups, few strategies targeting minors and workers were identified as being effective. Specifically, community mobilization with additional interventions (such as strengthened laws targeting retailers, active enforcement of existing regulations, and retailer education with **reinforcement**) has dem-

onstrated effectiveness in reducing youth tobacco use and access to tobacco products from commercial sources. For worker protection, smoke-free policies, including **private sector** rules and public policies prohibiting smoking in indoor workplaces and designated public areas, decrease tobacco use in work sites when the policies are implemented by communities through ordinances and regulations, adopted by companies and organizations with multiple work sites, and implemented at individual work sites. Despite many federally funded reports demonstrating disparities, no studies were cited by the Task Force on Community Preventive Services report as targeting diversity of gender, race/ethnicity, sexual orientation, or specific occupation.[3] This problem of **generalizability** of the research literature beyond the settings and populations in which they were conducted is of growing concern in linking research to practice and policy recommendations (Green 2006). The problem applies also in translating clinical research from academic settings to practice in community clinical settings (Green 2008).

Case Example: California Tobacco Control Program

The California Tobacco Control Program (CTCP) is arguably the most successful state-level tobacco use prevention and control program both in the United States and worldwide. Though Utah has lower smoking prevalence and per capita consumption rates, these are largely attributed to the demographic and religious composition of that state. The state of Victoria in Australia had early success, similar to that of California, in lowering its rate of smoking (Green et al. 2001). The effectiveness and impact of the CTCP and Victoria state's program serve as models for other state, federal, and international efforts. These programs maintained an emphasis on implementing an integrated, comprehensive approach, as outlined in the previous subsections. (Victoria added the tactic of buying out sports and arts sponsorships where the tobacco industry had obtained advertising at sporting events.) This section will discuss the underlying theories that diffused through the CTCP's multilevel strategies and effective interventional components of the CTCP.

DENORMALIZATION

The theoretical basis of the CTCP is the concept of **social norm change** (Roeseler and Burns 2010). This concept aims to change the broader normative value of tobacco use and influence current and future users by creating a social and institutional environment in which tobacco use is less acceptable and desirable and where the promotion of and access to tobacco products are curtailed. Often termed *denormalization,* the approach aims to change the social norms of the community, which, in turn, influence the behavior of individuals. As the composition of social groups changes with demographic shifts and the passage of time, the population inherits, adopts, and conforms to norms that reflect a less tolerant threshold for social acceptability of tobacco use. The specific activities stemming from this core programmatic premise include reducing secondhand smoke; countering pro-tobacco influences by discrediting tobacco industry advertising methods and claims; reducing the availability of tobacco, including tobacco vending machines in youth-accessible places; and providing cessation services (Siegel 2007).

COUNTER-ADVERTISING

A key component of the CTCP's success revolves around exposing and countering the tobacco industry's practices. Counter-advertising campaigns were created to foster negative **attitudes** toward tobacco use and the tobacco industry (CDC 2003). As a result, as compared to those elsewhere, smokers in California were approximately 70% more likely to have made a quit attempt within the last 12 months and 60% more likely to have an intention to quit in the

following six months, and also held more negative attitudes toward the tobacco industry (Zhang et al. 2010). Even though the CTCP did not have a direct cessation component, it is considered to have had a profound impact on tobacco cessation outcomes through social norm change and mass media education, *despite* declining cigarette prices.

LOCAL EMPHASIS

From a policy standpoint, the effectiveness of the CTCP's programming was largely attributed to a focus on local efforts. At various junctures during its inception, the state bureaucracy was often a hostile environment for tobacco control efforts, resulting in the failure of initial statewide measures espousing smoke-free workplaces (Glantz and Balbach 2000). The tobacco industry could mount effective lobbying against state-level legislative efforts but could not simultaneously counter the many local smoke-free ordinances and other initiatives that could be undertaken. The CTCP involved local communities in statewide agenda-setting by engaging **stakeholders**, providing training and technical assistance, building local coalitions, supporting statewide media campaigns, and educating elected officials to facilitate informed decision making (CDHS 2006). Among these, the statewide media campaigns were producing growing public outrage and an informed electorate in support of local policy initiatives (Green and Kreuter 2010). Evidence also demonstrated that sustained effort on the part of county health departments predicted an increasing number of local tobacco control policies, such as retail licensing and secondhand smoke policies (Modayil et al. 2010). As a result, momentum built up at the local level, enabling passage of municipal and countywide smoke-free ordinances for public settings (Francis et al. 2010).

PRICE INCREASE

The groundswell of local policy activity, in turn, fueled and enabled the passage of California's Proposition 99, which imposed a 25-cent excise tax per pack of cigarettes, restrictions on cigarette vending machines in public settings, and a prohibition on the sale of individual cigarettes (Hu et al. 1994).

SMOKE-FREE WORKPLACES
AND RESTAURANTS

This was followed by Assembly Bill 13, which successfully enacted 100% smoke-free workplaces and restaurants, with a lagging moratorium for bars and card rooms. The strong emphasis on building capacity to influence local policies has been shown to have tremendous impact on support for and implementation of strong state-level tobacco control policies. Because tobacco control regulations are only as strong as the manner in which they are enforced, the CTCP enlisted the assistance and authority of the California attorney general's office, resulting in more than $24 million of payments, penalties, and fees levied against the tobacco industry since 2000; almost $2 million of this sum was earmarked for tobacco control activities (Roeseler et al. 2010).

ADDRESSING DISPARITIES

The CTCP also espoused another belief, that it must reflect the diverse and multicultural composition of California's population (this view was still relatively innovative in the implementation of statewide tobacco control programs in the early 1990s). In addition to providing culturally and linguistically appropriate messaging and services, the CTCP also recognized that the tobacco industry targeted racial and ethnic minority through promotion and advertising. Therefore, four statewide ethnic networks were established in 1990, and in 2004 a parallel movement was created for populations grouped by nonracial characteristics, who were also disproportionately affected by tobacco (Francis et al. 2010). In parallel, surveillance efforts incorporated an appreciation for this diversity; the state's Tobacco Control Section funded independent adult tobacco surveys for three of California's major ethnic groups as well as the Lesbian-Gay-Bisexual-Transgender and military populations (Bye et al. 2005; Carr et al. 2005a, 2005b; McCarthy et al. 2005).

SURVEILLANCE AND EVALUATION

In addition to these surveys, the CTCP used innovative methods to evaluate its progress and drive continuous change. By applying technology to improve the management of programmatic data, evaluate its media campaign and data collection efforts, and test culturally specific strategies, the CTCP was able to identify shortcomings and improve its programming with respect to its short-, intermediate-, and long-term outcomes. Another element of the CTCP's novel framework is its dissemination strategy, which has been shown to redefine and reshape social and institutional practices (Francis et al. 2010). Given its focus on social norm change and innovative programming, and thanks to its surveillance and evaluation efforts, the CTCP served as a model for other states' tobacco control programs, public health practices outside of tobacco control (such as obesity), and the establishment of standard cessation and prevention mechanisms federally and internationally (CDC 1999a, 2014; Francis et al. 2010; USDHHS 2000; Wingo et al. 2001).

The implementation of this novel, integrated, and comprehensive approach contributed to impressive objective impacts on population-based measures of tobacco use behavior in California. Even though per capita consumption of cigarettes at the time of Proposition 99's passing was already 20% lower than the average of the remaining states, by 2007 it had fallen by more than two-thirds. In 2009 California's per capita cigarette consumption was measured to be less than half that of the other states in the nation (TEROC 2009). California's smoking prevalence declined from 22.7% in 1988 to 13.8% in 2007 and 11.9% in 2010 (TEROC 2012). Among smokers, there was also a shift from heavy daily smoking to occasional smoking.

Among racial and ethnic minorities in California between 1990 and 2005, the reduction in smoking prevalence was relatively uniform at approximately 25%, with the exception of Hispanic males (almost 42% reduction) and Asian or Pacific Islander females (only an 11% reduction) (Al-Delaimy et al. 2008). Nevertheless, these declines were larger than those of the nation as a whole during the same time period. California's decline in tobacco consumption was twice the average rate of the other states during the first two years of its program, and it tripled the average state rate in the next few years.

A commensurate decline in tobacco-related disease followed these reductions in consumption and prevalence. Lung cancer rates declined in California at a rate four times as high as in the rest of the country between 1998 and 2004 (Cowling and Yang 2010); more rapid reductions were seen for heart disease (Fichtenberg and Glantz 2000). Researchers and California's Tobacco Education and Research Oversight Committee (2012) surmise that many of these reductions are associated with the CTCP's efforts, especially those targeting the denormalization of tobacco use (Lightwood et al. 2008; Roesler and Burns 2010). Population surveys of attitudes and experiences regarding smoking in public places, adoption of smoke-free homes, and exposure to secondhand smoke demonstrated that the CTCP did indeed have a profound impact on attitudes, which changed both population and individual behaviors (TEROC 2009). With respect to tobacco promotion, between 2000 and 2008, the number of public events with tobacco sponsorship and stores with cigarette advertisements in locations appealing to youth declined significantly (Roeseler et al. 2010).

ECONOMIC IMPACT

The economic benefits of the CTCP are also substantial. An evaluation of the CTCP's effects among males estimated that the program re-sulted in more than 700,000 **person-years** of life saved and averted more than 150,000 person-years of treatment (Miller et al. 2010). By 2012, cumulative savings over the first 15 years of the program totaled $86 billion, which was a 50-fold return on the $1.8 billion investment. And those costs were exceeded 10-fold by the tobacco industry's promotion and lobbying expenditures (TEROC 2009, 2012).

Other Evidence-Based Interventions

Several additional evidence-based interventions merit mentioning, based on the systematic reviews of evidence conducted by the Community Preventive Services Task Force, the U.S. Preventive Services Task Force, the Surgeon General Reports on Tobacco and Health, and others.

PHARMACEUTICALS

At the individual core of the ecological model, some pharmacological therapies have been shown to have significant impact on tobacco cessation. The 2008 update of the Public Health Service's Clinical Practice Guideline *Treating Tobacco Use and Dependence* articulates that the use of certain medications reliably increases long-term smoking abstinence rates (Fiore et al. 2008). For singular medications, the odds ratio of quitting ranged from 1.5-3.3 with use; combined pharmaceutical therapies demonstrated greater benefit. These medications include various forms of nicotine-replacement therapy, neurotransmitter-blocking agents, and partial nicotinic receptor agonists or antagonists.

INCENTIVES AND OUT-OF-POCKET COST COVERAGE

Monetary incentives for smoking cessation, with or without adjunctive treatment programs or pharmacological therapies, have been shown to be effective. Given the high costs of treating smoking-related disease, offering small financial incentives to promote quit attempts and maintenance has become a more common consideration in many populations such as employee groups. A recent randomized trial showed that small direct payments for attending tobacco cessation classes ($20 for each of up to five classes) and having a biochemically confirmed (via a urine test) quit attempt ($100 for being tobacco free after 30 days) led to significantly improved quit rates at 30 days (the effect declined in the difference between the intervention and **control groups** after six months) (Volpp et al. 2006). A larger follow-up study that included nearly 1,000 subjects in 85 separate work sites showed that slightly larger incentives ($100 for completing a smoking cessation program, $250 for biochemically confirmed cessation, and $400 for biochemically confirmed cessation for an additional six months) could effectively impact smoking rates for 18 months following enrollment in the study.

MASS MEDIA

On the community, state, and national levels, heightened frequency of exposure to smoking incidents in the media, namely, movies, has been shown to be associated with an increase in tobacco initiation and use among adolescents (Charlesworth and Glantz 2005). Conversely, when depictions of smoking in movies fell between 2005 and 2009, the national prevalence of ever having tried a cigarette declined significantly among high school students from 54.3% to 46.3% over the same time period. The CDC has therefore recently called for potential implementation of certain restrictions on smoking in movies, including an "R" rating for any movie with depictions of tobacco use and certification by producers that no payment was accepted to depict smoking behavior.

COMMUNITY SYNERGY

The recent experience led by the New York City Department of Health illustrates another example of leveraging a number of synergistic interventions at multiple **levels of influence** to promote health behavior change on a population level. Launched shortly after Mayor Michael Bloomberg took office in 2001, and based on the CDC's Best Practices recommendations, New York City (NYC) implemented a five-point plan to address tobacco control: taxation, legal action, cessation treatment, education, and evaluation.

Taxation to increase the cost of cigarettes, combined with indoor smoking bans, made it harder to smoke in NYC. Increases in state and city excise taxes increased the price of cigarettes to more than seven dollars per pack. Comprehensive indoor-air laws (the NYC Smoke-Free Air Act of 2002 and the New York State Indoor Air Act of 2003) prohibited smoking in almost all workplaces, including restaurants and bars. Concurrently, increased access to cessation treatments, services, and medications made it easier to quit for many residents. The Department of Health distributed more than 100,000 free, six-week courses of nicotine patches to heavy smokers; the department provided medications, technical assistance, and support to clinic- and community-based organizations to provide cessation services; the public health detailing program promoted systematic screening for tobacco use and delivery of cessation services by providers; and the tax revenue helped to increase enrollment and use of medications at cessation programs at public hospitals. Evaluation of the nicotine patch giveaways showed substantial benefits. After 34,000 courses of patches were distributed, more than 11,000 heavy smokers (33%) quit smoking after six months, which *doubled* expectations. Quit rates were found to be six times higher than for those not receiving nicotine replacement (Miller et al. 2005). As part of a robust public education campaign to counter tobacco industry marketing, NYC also set in motion a series of hard-hitting media campaigns. In January 2006, NYC launched the largest city campaign ever: "Every Cigarette Is Doing Damage." The ads were video testimonials of sick and dying smokers, followed by the tag "Quit Smoking To-day. Call 311." During this campaign, calls to 311 quit lines *quadrupled* to 30,000, compared with just 7,500 calls during the same time period the prior year.

Evaluation of the NYC programs revealed striking decreases in adult and teen smoking rates. From 1992 to 2002, adult smoking prevalence hovered at around 21.5%. From 2002 to 2011, the rate declined to 14.8% (Steier and Coady 2012). An estimated reduction of more than 200,000 smokers in New York by 2006, and more than 50,000 premature deaths, could be attributed to the combined effects of the several interventions. From 1999 to 2005, the prevalence of smoking in New York public high school students declined by 52%; by 2005, the rate stood at less than half that of the national average (NYC DHMH 2011). As part of the shift in social norms initiated by these programs, 90% of New Yorkers, and 70% of smokers, made their homes smoke-free, resulting in 125,000 fewer residents being exposed to environmental tobacco smoke at home (Perl et al. 2007).

Roles for Key Stakeholders

The previous sections describe how a comprehensive approach to tobacco control can have profound influences in reducing population-level tobacco use and tobacco-related disease at statewide and community levels. To sustain and improve upon these efforts, however, reducing the high burden attributable to tobacco use will require multidimensional, multilevel, and multisectoral efforts. The multiple *dimensions* of tobacco control call for strategic use of communications; advocacy and framing of policy initiatives; program planning, administration, monitoring, and evaluation; and countering tobacco promotion initiatives. In the context of an ecological model, the multiple *levels* apply to each of these dimensions: global, national, state or region, local-community, organizational, family, and individual. The *sectors* relevant to

tobacco control include commitments from within and outside the health sector, such as law enforcement to restrain sales to minors and to interdict smuggling of cigarettes, the educational sector for school policies, the media sector for mass communications, and so forth.

The diverse stakeholders within each of these dimensions, sectors, and levels require compelling reasons or justifications for actions. Such justifications usually must be framed for the nonhealth sectors within their mandates and missions, most of which are outside the realm of health reasons. One way to engage these other sectors is to offer reciprocal contributions between sectors, such as health sector support to schools in return for educational sector support for school anti-tobacco policies. A growing movement has developed in Canada, and now increasingly among states and communities in the United States, to require health impact assessments when any nonhealth sector proposes a new policy or initiative. Such assessments can have the effect of due diligence in examining the impact on health before passage of such policies or implementation of initiatives in other sectors.

Described below are some of the particular stakeholder groups that hold great promise for reducing and eliminating morbidity and mortality associated with tobacco use.

Providers and Health Care Systems

Health care providers, such as physicians and nurses, can have significant influence on smoking cessation. Meta-analysis of behavioral counseling treatment reveals that minimal counseling (less than three minutes) improves the likelihood of quitting by 30%, and higher-intensity counseling (10 minutes or longer) more than doubles the likelihood of quitting (Fiore 2000). Clinicians should routinely screen for tobacco use and offer brief, simple advice to users as a routine practice (Lancaster and Stead 2004). Clinical advice should follow established, evidence-based counseling guidelines, which usually include **Stages-of-Change** assessment (see chapter 7), motivational counseling and follow-up, and adjunctive aids such as self-help manuals; these integrated efforts increase the likelihood of quitting and of sustained cessation after 12 months.

Since interpersonal communication may be burdensome for both patient and provider, health care systems should adopt innovative methods to counsel and motivate smokers to quit. For instance, computer-generated letters, tailored to patients who use tobacco, have been demonstrated to have at least as much effect as interventions involving brief advice from providers (Meyer et al. 2008). As this and other approaches (e.g., those taking advantage of electronic communication systems) may be most cost- and time-effective, they should be implemented within health care provider settings after demonstrating effectiveness.

With or without physician advice, nicotine replacement therapy (NRT) in the form of gum, transdermal patch, inhaler, nasal spray, and oral tablet is an effective component of a clinical intervention strategy; this is true largely without regard to the specific type of NRT used (Silagy and Stead 2004). Thus, clinicians should be prepared to provide singular or combined forms of NRT to patients who use tobacco, based on the specific needs of the patient (such as tolerance) and considerations of cost and dosage. Physicians should also be prepared to dispel false claims or interpretations of any NRT product as a "magic cure" for tobacco use and take into account both benefits and adverse effects of any given pharmacotherapy for treatment of smoking. Moreover, physicians should be prepared to dispel false beliefs about nicotine and NRT that may limit its use as an adjunctive clinical tool; for example, in one survey, 53% of smokers believed that nicotine causes cancer and 11% believed that NRT was more likely than smoking to cause heart attacks (Cummings et al. 2006). In addition to relating health consequences to the individual smoker, clinicians should highlight the negative effects on family members, friends, and other peers caused by the patient's use of tobacco.

These endeavors require the institutions in which these clinicians practice to accommodate and support them. Because the consequences of tobacco use are burdensome to individual providers and care delivery systems, the health care infrastructure would benefit itself and its consumers by training personnel and providing supplementary resources to enable smokers to quit as rapidly as possible. Similarly, *health care plans* and *insurance companies* should provide benefits for clinical counseling, pharmacological aids, and individual- or group-level therapies to give the insured full access to clinical resources that facilitate cessation. In addition, insurers might provide incentives for quitting tobacco use by offering lower premiums or compensation to people who complete a comprehensive cessation program. Medicaid programs have already employed such strategies in some states (Greene 2007; Marteau et al. 2009). The consequences in terms of cost to the health care system attributable to tobacco use are well documented; much of this large expenditure can be mitigated by timely and well-focused clinical intervention, in conjunction with other components.

A recent entry within the health care sector to be mobilized in support of tobacco control is the pharmacy marketplace. Drugstores and their pharmacists are perceived to be dedicated to health. Selling tobacco in such places sends an inconsistent message to the tobacco-consuming public. San Francisco was the first municipality to ban tobacco sales in its local drugstores.

Researchers

The tobacco control movement has been bolstered by research that focuses on prevalence and predictors of tobacco use as well as studies of interventional effectiveness. Research has also elucidated organizational, social, environmental, and community factors that facilitate or encourage consumption. Researchers should continue to monitor the prevalence and trends of use to evaluate the effectiveness of interventional components, settings, and circumstances, as well as to identify populations who have disproportionate rates of use or disparities in tobacco-related disease. More emphasis should be placed on the role of newer research orientations, such as community-based participatory research, to identify novel or understudied determinants and contexts of use, to enhance surveillance systems to include alternative and culturally specific forms of tobacco, and to generate community-oriented intervention strategies that originate from and are most relevant to the populations locally affected by use. Engaging community members in the research enterprise will maximize the relevance and meaningfulness of the data generated for future study; it will also enhance the implementation and evaluation of targeted and multifaceted approaches to reduce tobacco use and related disease (Minkler and Wallerstein 2008). Such approaches are especially critical to identifying and addressing tobacco-related disparities in social and cultural contexts of use among multicultural populations (Green, O'Neill et al. 1996). These efforts will bolster ongoing research that examines the effectiveness of existing public health programs and multilevel prevention and cessation strategies.

Another major domain of research that has already demonstrated great impact is the exposure of tactics used by the tobacco industry to market and promote its products. These maneuvers were brought to public attention by the uncovering of previously secret industry documents mandated by the Master Settlement Agreement between the four largest tobacco companies and attorneys general of 46 states. Analyses of these papers have revealed the tobacco industry's knowledge about the harms of tobacco, contrary to its public statements, and a form of deception and racketeering (Brandt 2007; Glantz et al. 1997). Since these internal documents contain much information about the future goals and potential strategies of the industry, research should continue to focus on examining these materials to elucidate future directions of marketing and promotion as well as to develop countermarketing strategies that directly undermine the effectiveness of any such approach. Researchers should be especially critical of industry intentions to target developing countries, minority populations, and disadvantaged groups who may be disproportionately affected by a large-scale adoption of tobacco in these communities. Studies should also monitor the ongoing efforts of the tobacco industry—such as marketing efforts and influencing of public or regulatory agencies—to generate data that is relevant for multilevel intervention efforts.

Legislative and Regulatory Bodies

During the period when the rates of smoking were declining most rapidly, between the downturn in tobacco consumption in the mid-1960s and the end of the century, the legislative initiatives that were passing with the highest percentage of success were local initiatives, not state or federal efforts. As noted earlier, the tobacco industry could counter legislation in Congress and in state legislatures because it could exert powerful lobbying and financial influence at those levels. It could not, however, put out the hundreds of "brush fires" ignited in local communities with smoke-free initiatives for workplaces, restaurants, and other public places. The major resistance to these local initiatives came from restaurants and other commercial stakeholders who feared that their businesses would be disadvantaged by nonsmoking laws. Research demonstrated that this was not true when the local policies applied equally to all competitors, effectively "leveling the playing field" of competition for customers. When it was further demonstrated that many customers who had been avoiding the previously smoke-laden restaurants and bars began to come back as patrons, the resistance of the commercial stakeholders further declined (CDC 2005).

One of the national initiatives designed by stakeholders and intended to engage a wider range of federal regulatory stakeholders, particularly the Food and Drug Administration (FDA), was a legislative bill that had strong congressional support but eventually collapsed in the face of divisions within the anti-tobacco movement organizations and between their leaders (Pertschuk 2001). A later bill did pass to give enlarged responsibility to the FDA in regulating tobacco and to put strong, compelling images of the dangers of tobacco consumption on cigarette packages, similar to what has been implemented in Canada, Australia, and most European countries. This, however, was successfully challenged in the courts by the tobacco industry, leading to a watered-down role for the FDA in package labeling.

Public Health Agencies and Organizations

Public health agencies play a significant role in protecting and promoting health at the international, federal, regional, and local levels. Given their influence and authority, these entities bear a large responsibility to safeguard their constituencies from tobacco-related harm. To achieve this goal, public health agencies need to focus their efforts, ensuring that tobacco control remains a top public health priority insofar as it remains the leading preventable cause of death. Obesity is elbowing its way into that position of policy priority, but tobacco consumption rates remain unacceptably high and have stalled since 2004 in the downward trajectory they had since the mid-1960s.

Internationally, WHO has taken a substantial step in organizing member countries in negotiating the Framework Convention on Tobacco Control (FCTC) as a response to the globalization of the tobacco epidemic and to reaffirm the right of all people to attain the highest standard of health. The FCTC provides a legal cooperative framework that enables international standards for tobacco control by way of a treaty that had 168 signatory nations in 2014. To build from this momentum, WHO continues to add member nation signatories, provide technical support for implementation of the FCTC in diverse settings, and ensure that the objectives of this treaty are fulfilled through enforcement of its various provisions. A working group of signatory nations met in 2013 to draft the guidelines for price and tax measures to reduce demand for tobacco products.

At the federal level in the United States, entities such as the CDC have created independent infrastructures (such as the aforementioned Office on Smoking and Health) to facilitate comprehensive public protection from the harmful effects of tobacco. In 2010 the U.S. Department of Health and Human Services adopted a department-wide strategic plan to help the nation reach the objectives laid out in *Healthy People 2020* and support the FDA's role to regulate the manufacture, marketing, and distribution of tobacco products (USDHHS 2010). Such agencies need to ensure that tobacco control remains a key concern at the federal level, fund and generate research that supports local efforts, enhance surveillance for key indicators of tobacco use, and disseminate information to both the research and the lay community. Federal agencies need also to exert their authority to counteract the considerable influence of the tobacco industry by generating and advocating for evidence-based strategies that mitigate industry efforts. In addition, these entities need to provide technical assistance and resources, such as CDC's *Community Guide*, to serve as models of programmatic and policy-level implementation and evaluation to local groups.

As much of the innovation for the success of tobacco control has originated at the state and local levels, public health agencies and voluntary health organizations representing these regional constituencies play a significant role in tobacco control. In the United States, these entities have included most prominently the American Cancer Society, the American Heart Association, and the American Lung Association. Advocacy organizations such as Americans for Nonsmokers Rights have added a further dimension to the efforts of the voluntary health organizations. Together they identify issues unique to their constituent populations and create policies and programs that address these factors. Especially key is the protection of individuals and communities that do not consume tobacco but are affected by the lack of measures protecting them from secondhand smoke and other tobacco by-products. Taking the lead from international and federal recommendations as well as successes in other states and municipalities, regional public health agencies need not only to adopt evidence-based solutions, but also to ensure through monitoring and evaluation that those solutions are adapted to local circumstances and are implemented. Much of the discourse in public health has turned to the notion of health equity (through elimination of disparities) and place-based health (by creating social and physical conditions that allow for optimal community health), so local and state health agencies need to ensure that tobacco control remains one of the many foci in these more contemporary approaches (Carter-Porkas and Baquet 2002; Kawachi and Berkman 2003; Koh et al. 2011). The relative success of the tobacco control movement has invited more attention to newer public health threats; nonetheless, regional entities need to ensure that the gains are not reversed by diminishing the efforts needed to sustain and improve upon these milestones.

Funding Agencies

The base of tobacco research and the empirical evidence of effective prevention and cessation strategies is largely attributable to the commitment of both public and private funding agencies to examine the prevalence and determinants of tobacco use at the population level and approaches to combating it. The success of the tobacco control movement has, at times, obscured the necessity for research and programs, including provision of adequate resources, and has often shifted attention to other pressing public health priorities (NCI 2007).

Because tobacco control research traverses multiple academic and professional disciplines, funding agencies tend to specialize in parts of the multidimensional intervention strategies that aim to prevent or reduce use. The surveillance and program evaluation functions fall most clearly on the CDC as the federal agency funding state programs and, through them, many of the local initiatives within states. The CDC also funds Prevention Research Centers to assist with the practical application of research to the benefit of local and state jurisdictions. The Health Resources and Services Administration has the responsibility similarly for monitoring the enforcement of restrictions on sales of tobacco to minors in states and has the teeth of enforcement in the federal withholding of state highway funds when states are in violation of enforcement mandates. But more support is needed from other agencies in the form of research that balances scientific and theoretical interests with the practical and policy interests of federal, state, and local efforts. For instance, many of the National Institutes of Health focus on outcomes directly related to tobacco use, such as the National Cancer Institute; the National Heart, Lung, and Blood Institute; and the National Institute for Drug Abuse. As agencies charged with research on protecting the public's health, these entities might be well served to expand their portfolios to include more tobacco-related research and to focus more of their research on policy and program issues.

Similarly, *voluntary* health agencies and private foundations, such as the American Cancer Society, the American Heart Association, and the Robert Wood Johnson Foundation, have provided research and program support, but they are faced with constant trade-offs with competing priorities and the desire of their boards of directors to remain innovative in areas where the government has not yet been able to mount similar momentum. They could sustain and even increase the resources committed to assessing and evaluating the impact tobacco use has on their respective target conditions and populations (Bornemeier 2005; Eyre et al. 2004), but this requires continued advocacy from their constituencies as well as the resolve of their boards of directors to give priority to tobacco control over other pressing health issues. These resources are needed not only for tobacco research, but to build capacity in community-based organizations, schools, and other venues charged with protecting the health and well-being of large segments of the population. In the context of health disparities, agencies that fund academic and career development programs might focus on training a diverse generation of tobacco control researchers, enabling the elucidation of issues specific to tobacco behavior among minority and understudied communities. A sustained and enhanced infrastructure for research and practice is paramount to make sure that past successes continue, the investments of the past are not wasted, and the momentum toward a smoke-free society is not lost.

Workplaces and Employers

The tobacco control movement has had many of its successes through indoor clean air regulations and prohibitions on tobacco use in public settings, largely to protect the health of nonsmoking employees and patrons. Despite claims to the contrary by the tobacco industry, restaurants and the hospitality industry are not nega-tively affected financially and, in some cases, gain profit when subjected to smoke-free ordinances (Alamar and Glantz 2004; Huang et al. 2004; Scollo et al. 2003). A simulation model conducted by the surgeon general concluded that if all U.S. workplaces went smoke-free, we would see an initial benefit (in the first year) of 1.3 million fewer smokers, 950 million fewer cigarette packs smoked, 1,540 heart attacks and 360 strokes averted, and $49 million in direct medical cost savings, with the benefits increasing over time (USDHHS 2006). Even with this abundance of evidence, many states do not have 100% smoke-free laws and, as a consequence, many employees and patrons are not protected from the effects of second-hand smoke. Moreover, existing laws are often ignored or circumvented by claims of exemption by establishments that offer alternative forms of tobacco, such as *hookah* smoking (Noonan 2010).

In the absence of state or local ordinances, pressure should be placed on employers and entrepreneurs to adopt smoke-free policies voluntarily as a means to protect the health of workers and patrons. Moreover, other establishments currently not protected, such as casinos, should be encouraged to implement similar policies; research has indicated that adoption of such prohibitions does not negatively affect gaming revenue (Mandel et al. 2005). Since the levels of certain carcinogenic particles generated by tobacco smoke are up to six times higher inside casinos than outdoors, owners should be encouraged—if not required—to assume a 100% smoke-free policy in these high risk venues (Repace 2009). Many private entities with large publicly accessible outdoor facilities, such as universities, have implemented prohibitions on smoking; other similar venues might be well served by adopting similar measures (Halperin and Rigotti 2003). All in all, protecting the health of individuals who frequent any workplace should be a high priority for employers, both ethically and financially.

Conclusion

The tobacco epidemic has been characterized as proceeding through four stages over the course of about a century: First, male smoking begins and grows rapidly, but few women smoke, and tobacco-related health problems have not yet developed. Second, within a few decades, men continue to smoke at high rates, women are increasingly smoking, and health problems and premature deaths begin to accumulate among men. Third, male smoking begins to diminish, female smoking plateaus, and men and women both experience significant and rising rates of tobacco-related disease and premature death. Fourth, male smoking continues to decline and male mortality begins to fall, female smoking declines to about the same rate as that of males, but female mortality rates continue to rise (Lopez et al. 1994). This sequence reflects the lag time between smoking and most of the mortality impact, except for heart attacks.

In the United States, Canada, Australia, the United Kingdom, and Western Europe, we appear to be in stage four of this process. Continued political, social, environmental, and clinical progress must be nurtured to support further health behavior change and health protection in these developed nations. Though we have made much progress, a recent modeling study looking at the effect of combinations of policies and cessation interventions on future adult smoking rates concluded that a national, multi-level tobacco policy approach could decrease U.S. smoking rates significantly further. Leveraging a basket of policies, including tax increases, clean indoor air laws, media campaigns, access to evidence-based cessation medications and quit lines, and brief tobacco counseling in health care settings, could lower national smoking rates to 13% by 2020 (Levy et al. 2010). Still, much disparity exists among many subpopulations of U.S. residents, and care must be taken to extend policies and treatments to underserved and poorly represented groups and areas.

Most of the developing world, however, falls into earlier stages of tobacco epidemics and will likely accumulate significant disease, premature loss of life, and economic burden as the epidemics progress. With perhaps 1 billion or more lives hanging in the balance, tolerating what could be a century-long process through these four stages is unimaginable. Extension and application of the strategies outline in this chapter is a critical and urgent international public health and human rights mandate.

NOTES

1. See The Community Guide, www.thecommunity guide.org/tobacco/index.html.

2. *United States v. Philip Morris USA, Inc., et al.* (449 F.Supp. 2d 1 (U.S. D.D.C. 2006)).

3. See note 1.

REFERENCES

Acevedo-Garcia D, Pan J, Jun HJ, Osypuk TL, Emmons KM. 2005. The effect of immigrant generation on smoking. *Soc Sci Med* 61 (6): 1223–42.

Agaku I, King B, Dube SR. 2012. Current cigarette smoking among adults—United States, 2011. *MMWR* 61 (44): 889–94.

Alamar BC, Glantz SA. 2004. Smoke-free ordinances increase restaurant profit and value. *Contemp Econ Policy* 22 (4): 520–25.

Al-Delaimy W, White M, Gilmer T, Zhu SH, Pierce J. 2008. The California Tobacco Survey Control Program: Can we maintain the progress? Results from the California Tobacco Survey, 1990–2005. University of California–San Diego, La Jolla.

Anda RF, Croft JB, Felitti VJ, et al. 1999. Adverse childhood experiences and smoking during adolescence and adulthood. *JAMA* 282 (17): 1652–58.

Anderson CM, Zhu SH. 2000. The California smokers' helpline: A case study. California Department of Health Services, Sacramento.

Apollonio DE, Malone RE. 2005. Marketing to the marginalised: Tobacco industry targeting of the homeless and mentally ill. *Tobacco Control* 14 (6): 409–15.

Asumda F, Jordan L. 2009. Minority youth access to tobacco: A neighborhood analysis of underage tobacco sales. *Health Place* 15 (1): 140–47.

Balbach ED, Gasior RJ, Barbeau EM. 2003. RJ Reynolds' targeting of African Americans: 1988–2000. *Am J Public Health* 93 (5): 822–27.

Baluja KF, Park J, Myers D. 2003. Inclusion of immigrant status in smoking prevalence statistics. *Am J Public Health* 93 (4): 642-46.

Barbeau EM, Leavy-Sperounis A, Balbach ED. 2004. Smoking, social class, and gender: What can public health learn from the tobacco industry about disparities in smoking? *Tobacco Control* 13 (2): 115-20.

Barnoya J, Glantz SA. 2005. Cardiovascular effects of secondhand smoke: Nearly as large as smoking. *Circulation* 111 (20) (May 24): 2684-98.

Benowitz NL. 2010. Nicotine addiction. *N Engl J Med* 362 (24): 2295.

Bero L. 2003. Implications of the tobacco industry documents for public health and policy. *Annu Rev Public Health* 24 (1): 267-88.

Borland R, Yong HH, Cummings KM, Hyland A, Anderson S, Fong GT. 2006. Determinants and consequences of smoke-free homes: Findings from the International Tobacco Control (ITC) Four Country Survey. *Tobacco Control* 15 (suppl. 3): iii42-iii50.

Bornemeier J. 2005. Taking on tobacco: The Robert Wood Johnson Foundation's assault on smoking. In *To Improve Health and Healthcare,* ed. SL Isaacs, JR Knickman. San Francisco: Jossey-Bass.

Brandt AM. 2007. *The Cigarette Century: The Rise, Fall, and Deadly Persistence of the Product That Defined America.* New York: Basic Books.

Bricker JB, Peterson AV, Andersen MR, Leroux BG, Rajan KB, Sarason IG. 2006. Close friends', parents', and older siblings' smoking: Reevaluating their influence on children's smoking. *Nicotine Tob Res* 8 (2): 217-26.

Brown A, Moodie C. 2009. The influence of tobacco marketing on adolescent smoking intentions via normative beliefs. *Health Educ Res* 24 (4): 721-33.

Burton A. 2011. Does the smoke ever really clear? Third-hand smoke exposure raises new concerns. *Env Health Perspec* 119 (2): A70-A74.

Buttross LS, Kastner JW. 2003. A brief review of adolescents and tobacco: What we know and don't know. *Am J Med Sci* 326 (4): 235-37.

Bye L, Gruskin E, Greenwood G, Albright V, Krotki K. 2005. California lesbians, gays, bisexuals, and transgender (LGBT) tobacco use survey—2004. California Department of Health Services, Sacramento.

California Department of Health Services (CDHS). 2006. California releases new data and anti-smoking ads targeting diverse populations. News Release No. 06-82, October 2, www.dhs.ca.gov/tobacco/documents/press /PR-October-2006.pdf.

Caponnetto P, Campagna D, Papale G, Russo C, Polosa R. 2012. The emerging phenomenon of electronic cigarettes. *Expert Rev Respir Med* 6:63-74, doi: 10.1586 /ers.11.92.

Carr K, Beers M, Kassebaum T, Chen MS. 2005a. California Chinese American tobacco use survey—2004. California Department of Health Services, Sacramento.

———. 2005b. California Korean American tobacco use survey—2004. California Department of Health Services, Sacramento.

Carter-Porkas O, Baquet C. 2002. What is "health disparity"? *Public Health Rep* 117 (5): 421-34.

Centers for Disease Control and Prevention (CDC). 1995. Assessment of the impact of a 100% smoke-free ordinance on restaurant sales—West Lake Hills, Texas, 1992-1994. *MMWR* 44 (19) (May 19): 370-72.

———. 1999a. *Best Practices for Comprehensive Tobacco Control Programs.* National Center for Chronic Disease Prevention and Health Promotion, Office on Smoking and Health. Atlanta, GA: CDC.

———. 1999b. *Reducing Tobacco Use: A Report of the Surgeon General—Executive Summary.* Atlanta, GA: US Department of Health and Human Services, Centers for Disease Control and Prevention, National Center for Chronic Disease Prevention and Health Promotion, Office on Smoking and Health.

———. 2002. Smoking-attributable mortality, years of potential life lost, and economic costs: United States, 1995-1999. *MMWR* 51:300-303.

———. 2003. *Designing and Implementing an Effective Tobacco Counter-Marketing Campaign.* Atlanta, GA: U.S. Department of Health and Human Services.

———. 2004. Effect of ending an anti-tobacco youth campaign on adolescent susceptibility to cigarette smoking—Minnesota, 2002-2003. *MMWR* 53:301-4.

———. 2007. Cigarette smoking among adults—United States, 2006. *MMWR* 56 (44): 1157-61.

———. 2008. Smoking-attributable mortality, years of potential life lost, and productivity losses—United States, 2000-2004. *MMWR* 57 (45): 1226-28.

———. 2010. Vital signs: Current cigarette smoking among adults aged ≥ 18 Years—United States, 2009. *MMWR* 59 (35) 1135-40.

———. 2013. Cigarette smoking—United States, 2006- 2008 and 2009-2010. *MMWR* 62 (3) (supplements, Nov. 22).

———. 2014. *Best Practices for Comprehensive Tobacco Control Programs.* 3rd ed. National Center for Chronic Disease Prevention and Health Promotion, Office on Smoking and Health. Atlanta, GA: Center for Chronic Disease Prevention and Health Promotion, Office on Smoking and Health.

Chaloupka FJ, Tauras J, Grossman M. 1999. Economic models of addiction and applications to cigarette smoking and other substance abuse, 1-27. University of Illinois-Chicago.

Chaloupka FJ, Warner KE. 2000. The economics of smoking. *Handbk Health Econ* 1:1539-1627.

Charlesworth A, Glantz SA. 2005. Smoking in the movies increases adolescent smoking: A review. *Pediatrics* 116 (6): 1516-28.

Christakis NA, Fowler JH. 2008. The collective dynamics of smoking in a large social network. *N Engl J Med* 358 (21): 2249-58.

Colorado Department of Public Health and Environment (CDPHE). 2007. *Making a Difference in Colorado's Health: A Report on the Colorado Department of Public Health and Environment Programs Funded by Amendment 35.* Denver: Colorado Department of Public Health and Environment.

Community Preventive Services Task Force (CPSTF). 2013. *Annual Report to Congress and to Agencies Related to the Work of the Task Force.* Atlanta: Centers for Disease Control and Prevention.

Cowling DW, Yang J. 2010. Smoking-attributable cancer mortality in California, 1979-2005. *Tobacco Control* 19 (suppl. 1): i62-i67.

Crawford R, Olsen C, Thompson B, Barbour G. 2005. *California Active Duty Tobacco Use Survey—2004.* Sacramento: California Department of Health Services.

Cummings KM, Fix B, Celestino P, Carlin-Menter S, O'Connor R, Hyland A. 2006. Reach, efficacy, and cost-effectiveness of free nicotine medication giveaway programs. *J Public Health Man Pract* 12 (1): 37-43.

Cummings KM, Morley CP, Horan JK, Steger C, Leavell NR. 2002. Marketing to America's youth: Evidence from corporate documents. *Tobacco Control* 11 (suppl. 1): i5-i17.

Eriksen MP, Cerak RL. 2008. The diffusion and impact of clean indoor air laws. *Annu Rev Public Health* 29:171-85.

Eriksen MP, Green L. 2002. Progress and next steps in reducing tobacco use in the United States. In *Principles of Public Health Practice,* ed. FD Scutchfield, CW Keck. 2nd ed. New York: Thomson Delmar Learning.

Eriksen MP, Green LW, Husten CG, Pederson LL, Pechacek TF. 2007. Thank you for not smoking: The public health response to tobacco-related mortality in the United States. In *Silent Victories: The History and Practice of Public Health in Twentieth-Century America,* ed. JW Ward, CS Warren, 423-36. Oxford: Oxford University Press, 2007.

Eriksen M, Mackay JL, Ross H. 2012. *The Tobacco Atlas.* Atlanta, GA: American Cancer Society.

Escoffery C, Bundy L, Carvalho M, Yembra D, Haardörfer R, Berg C, Kegler MC. 2013. Third-hand smoke as a potential intervention message for promoting smoke-free homes in low-income communities. *Health Educ Res* 28 (5): 923-30.

Eyre H, Kahn R, Robertson RM, et al. 2004. Preventing cancer, cardiovascular disease, and diabetes: A common agenda for the American Cancer Society, the American Diabetes Association, and the American Heart Association. *CA* 54 (4): 190-207.

Fagan P, King G, Lawrence D, et al. 2004. Eliminating tobacco-related health disparities: Directions for future research. *Am J Public Health* 94 (2): 211-17.

Farkas AJ, Gilpin EA, Distefan JM, Pierce JP. 1999. The effects of household and workplace smoking restrictions on quitting behaviours. *Tobacco Control* 8 (3): 261-65.

Farrelly MC, Davis KC, Duke J, Messeri P. 2009. Sustaining "truth": Changes in youth tobacco attitudes and smoking intentions after 3 years of a national antismoking campaign. *Health Educ Res* 24 (1): 42-48.

Farrelly MC, Davis KC, Haviland ML, Messeri P, Healton CG. 2005. Evidence of a dose-response relationship between "truth" antismoking ads and youth smoking prevalence. *Am J Public Health* 95 (3): 425-31.

Farrelly MC, Loomis BR, Kuiper N, et al. 2013. Are tobacco control policies effective in reducing young adult smoking? *J Adolesc Health.* Epub ahead of print.

Farrelly MC, Pechacek TF, Thomas KY, Nelson D. 2008. The impact of tobacco control programs on adult smoking. *Am J Public Health* 98:304-9.

Fichtenberg CM, Glantz SA. 2000. Association of the California Tobacco Control Program with declines in cigarette consumption and mortality from heart disease. *N Engl J Med* 343 (24): 1772-77.

Fiore MC. 2000. US public health service clinical practice guideline: Treating tobacco use and dependence. *Respir Care* 45 (10): 1200-1262.

Fiore MC, Bailey WC, Cohen SJ, et al. 2008. *Treating Tobacco Use and Dependence. A Clinical Practice Guideline.* Rockville, MD: U.S. Department of Health and Human Services.

Foner P. 1981. *Organized Labor and the Black Worker, 1619-1981.* New York: International.

Francey N, Chapman S. 2000. "Operation Berkshire": The international tobacco companies' conspiracy. *Br Med J* 321 (7257): 371.

Francis JA, Abramsohn EM, Park HY. 2010. Policy-driven tobacco control. *Tobacco Control* 19 (suppl. 1): i16-i20.

Freeman B, Chapman S. 2009. Open source marketing: Camel cigarette brand marketing in the "Web 2.0" world. *Tobacco Control* 18 (3): 212-17.

Gillum F, Obisesan TO, Jarrett NC. 2009. Smokeless tobacco use and religiousness. *Int J Environ Res Public Health* 6 (1): 225-31.

Gilpin EA, White MM, Messer K, Pierce JP. 2007. Receptivity to tobacco advertising and promotions among young adolescents as a predictor of established smoking in young adulthood. *Am J Public Health* 97 (8) (Aug.): 1489-95.

Glantz SA, Balbach ED. 2000. *Tobacco War: Inside the California Battles.* Berkeley: University of California Press.

Glantz SA, Fox BJ, Lightwood JM. 1997. Tobacco litigation. *JAMA* 277 (9): 751-53.

Green KJ, Hunter CM, Bray RM, Pemberton M, Williams J. 2008. Peer and role model influences for cigarette smoking in a young adult military population. *Nicotine Tob Res* 10 (10): 1533-41.

Green LW. 1997. Taxes and the tobacco wars. *Can Med Assoc J* 156 (2): 205-6.

———. 2006. Public health asks of systems science: To advance our evidence-based practice, can you help us get more practice-based evidence? *Am J Public Health* 96 (3): 406-9.

———. 2008. Making research relevant: If it's an evidence-based practice, where's the practice-based evidence? *J Family Med* 25 (suppl. 1): 20-24. Full text online at http://fampra.oxfordjournals.org/cgi/reprint/25/suppl_1/i20.

Green LW, Kreuter MW. 2010. Evidence hierarchies versus synergistic interventions. *Am J Public Health* 100 (10) (Oct.): 1824-25.

Green LW, Nathan R, Mercer SL. 2001. The health of health promotion in public policy: Drawing inspiration from the tobacco control movement. *Health Prom J Aus* 12 (2): 12-18.

Green LW, O'Neill M, Westphal M, Morisky D. 1996. Editorial: The challenges of participatory action research for health promotion. *Promot Educ* 3 (4): 3-5.

Green LW, Orleans CT, Ottoson JM, Cameron R, Pierce JP, Bettinghaus EP. 2006. Inferring strategies for disseminating physical activity policies, programs, and practices from the successes of tobacco control. *Am J Prev Med* 31 (suppl. 4): S66-S81.

Green LW, Richard L, Potvin L. 1996. Ecological foundations of health promotion. *Am J Health Promot* 10 (4): 270-81.

Greene J. 2007. *Medicaid Efforts to Incentivize Healthy Behaviors.* Hamilton, NJ: Center for Health Care Strategies.

Grossman M, Chaloupka FJ. 1997. Cigarette taxes: The straw to break the camel's back. *Public Health Rep* 112 (4) (July-Aug.): 290-97.

Haglund M. 2010. Women and tobacco: A fatal attraction. *Bull World Health Org* 88 (8) (Aug. 1): 563.

Halperin AC, Rigotti NA. 2003. US public universities' compliance with recommended tobacco-control policies. *J Am Coll Health* 51 (5): 181-88.

Hanauer P, Slade J, Barnes DE, Bero L, Glantz SA. 1995. Lawyer control of internal scientific research to protect against products liability lawsuits. *JAMA* 274 (3): 234-40.

Hendlin Y, Anderson SJ, Glantz SA. 2010. "Acceptable rebellion": Marketing hipster aesthetics to sell Camel cigarettes in the US. *Tobacco Control* 19 (3) (June): 213-22.

Hoffman BR, Monge PR, Chou CP, Valente TW. 2007. Perceived peer influence and peer selection on adolescent smoking. *Addictive Behav* 32 (8): 1546-54.

Hollis JF, Bills R, Whitlock E, Stevens VJ, Mullooly J, Lichtenstein E. 2000. Implementing tobacco interventions in the real world of managed care. *Tobacco Control* 9 (suppl. 1): i18-i24.

Housman M. 2001. Smoking and health: The 1964 US Surgeon General's Report as a turning point in the anti-smoking movement. *Harvard Health Policy Rev* 2 (1): 119-27.

Hu TW, Bai J, Keeler TE, Barnett PG, Sung HY. 1994. The impact of California Proposition 99, a major anti-smoking law, on cigarette consumption. *J Public Health Policy* 15 (1): 26-36.

Huang P, De AK, McCusker ME. 2004. Impact of a smoking ban on restaurant and bar revenues—El Paso, Texas, 2002. *MMWR* 53 (7) (Feb.): 150-52.

Hurt RD, Robertson CR. 1998. Prying open the door to the tobacco industry's secrets about nicotine. *JAMA* 280 (13): 1173-81.

Hyland A, Higbee C, Borland R, et al. 2009. Attitudes and beliefs about secondhand smoke and smoke-free policies in four countries: Findings from the International Tobacco Control Four Country Survey. *Nicotine Tob Res* 11 (6): 642-49.

Jha P, Chaloupka FJ. 2000. The economics of global tobacco control. *Br Med J* 321 (7257): 358.

John R, Cheney MK, Azad MR. 2009. Point-of-sale marketing of tobacco products: Taking advantage of the socially disadvantaged? *J Health Care Poor Underserved* 20 (2): 489-506.

Katz SK, Lavack AM. 2002. Tobacco related bar promotions: Insights from tobacco industry documents. *Tobacco Control* 11 (suppl. 1): i92-i101.

Kaufman RL. 1986. The impact of industrial and occupational structure on black-white employment allocation. *Am Sociol Rev,* 310-23.

Kawachi I, Berkman LF, eds. 2003. *Neighborhoods and Health.* New York: Oxford University Press.

Kim MJ, Fleming CB, Catalano RF. 2009. Individual and social influences on progression to daily smoking during adolescence. *Pediatrics* 124 (3): 895-902.

Kim SS, Ziedonis D, Chen KW. 2007. Tobacco use and dependence in Asian Americans: A review of the literature. *Nicotine Tob Res* 9 (2): 169-84.

Koh HK, Piotrowski JJ, Kumanyika S, Fielding JE. 2011. Healthy people: A 2020 vision for the social determinants approach. *Health Educ Behav* 38 (6) (Dec.): 551-57.

Kozlowski LT, O'Connor RJ. 2002. Cigarette filter ventilation is a defective design because of misleading taste, bigger puffs, and blocked vents. *Tobacco Control* 11 (suppl. 1): i40-i50.

Lancaster T, Stead LF. 2004. Physician advice for smoking cessation (Cochrane Review). *Cochrane Database Syst Rev* 4:CD000165 4.

Lee YO, Jordan JW, Djakaria M, Ling PM. 2013. Using peer crowds to segment black youth for smoking intervention. *Health Promot Practice.* Epub ahead of print, April 29.

Levy DT, Mabry PL, Graham AL, Orleans CT, Abrams DB. 2010. Exploring scenarios to dramatically reduce smoking prevalence: A simulation model of the three-part cessation process. *Am J Public Health* 100 (7): 1253-59.

Lightwood JM, Dinno A, Glantz SA. 2008. Effect of the California tobacco control program on personal health care expenditures. *PLoS Med* 5 (8): e178.

Lightwood JM, Glantz SA. 2009. Declines in acute myocardial infarction after smoke-free laws and individual risk attributable to secondhand smoke. *Circulation* 120 (14): 1373-79.

Ling PM, Glantz SA. 2002. Why and how the tobacco industry sells cigarettes to young adults: Evidence from industry documents. *Am J Public Health* 92 (6): 908-16.

Ling PM, Neilands TB, Nguyen TT, Kaplan CP. 2007. Psychographic segments based on attitudes about smoking and lifestyle among Vietnamese-American adolescents. *J Adolesc Health* 41 (1): 51-60.

Linton R. 1924. *Use of Tobacco among North American Indians.* Anthropology Leaflet 15. Chicago: Field Museum of Natural History.

Lipperman-Kreda S, Grube JW. 2009. Students' perception of community disapproval, perceived enforcement of school antismoking policies, personal beliefs, and their cigarette smoking behaviors: Results from a structural equation modeling analysis. *Nicotine Tob Res* 11 (5): 531-39.

Lopez AD, Collishaw NE, Piha T. 1994. A descriptive model of the cigarette epidemic in developed countries. *Tobacco Control* 3:242, doi:10.1136/tc.3.3.242.

Lynch BS, Bonnie RJ, eds. 1994. *Growing Up Tobacco Free: Preventing Nicotine Addiction in Children and Youths.* Washington, DC: National Academy Press.

Mackay D, Haw S, Ayres JG, Fischbacher C, Pell JP. 2010. Smoke-free legislation and hospitalizations for childhood asthma. *N Engl J Med* 363 (12): 1139-45.

Macken LC, Yates B, Blancher S. 2000. Concordance of risk factors in female spouses of male patients with coronary heart disease. *J Cardiopulm Rehabil Prev* 20 (6): 361-68.

Mandel L, Alamar B, Glantz S. 2005. Smoke-free law did not affect revenue from gaming in Delaware. *Tobacco Control* 14 (1): 10.

Marin BV, Perez-Stable EJ, Marin G, Sabogal F, Otero-Sabogal R. 1990. Attitudes and behaviors of Hispanic smokers: Implications for cessation interventions. *Health Educ Behav* 17 (3): 287-97.

Marteau TM, Ashcroft RE, Oliver A. 2009. Using financial incentives to achieve healthy behaviour. *Br Med J* 338:b1415.

Mathers CD, Loncar D. 2006. Projections of global mortality and burden of disease from 2002 to 2030. *PLoS Med* 3 (11): e442.

McCarthy WJ, Divan H, Shah D, Maxwell A, Freed B, Bastani R. 2005. California Asian Indian Tobacco Use Survey: 2004. California Department of Health Services, Sacramento.

McQueen D, Puska P, eds. 2003. *Global Behavioral Risk Factor Surveillance.* New York: Kluwer Academic / Plenum.

Mejia AB, Ling PM. 2010. Tobacco industry consumer research on smokeless tobacco users and product development. *Am J Public Health* 100 (1): 78-87.

Mercer SL, Green LW, Rosenthal AC, Husten CG, Khan KL, Dietz WH. 2003. Possible lessons from the tobacco experience for obesity control. *Am J Clin Nutr* 77 (4): 1073S-1082S.

Meyer C, Ulbricht S, Baumeister SE, et al. 2008. Proactive interventions for smoking cessation in general medical practice: A quasi-randomized controlled trial to examine the efficacy of computer-tailored letters and physician-delivered brief advice. *Addiction* 103 (2): 294-304.

Miller LS, Max W, Sung HY, Rice D, Zaretsky M. 2010. Evaluation of the economic impact of California's Tobacco Control Program: A dynamic model approach. *Tobacco Control* 19 (suppl. 1): i68-i76.

Miller N, Frieden TR, Liu SY, et al. 2005. Effectiveness of a large-scale distribution programme of free nicotine patches: A prospective evaluation. *Lancet* 365 (9474): 1849-54.

Minkler M, Wallerstein N, eds. 2008. *Community Based Participatory Research.* 2nd ed. San Francisco: Jossey-Bass.

Modayil MV, Cowling DW, Tang H, Roeseler A. 2010. An evaluation of the California community intervention. *Tobacco Control* 19 (suppl. 1): i30-i36.

Mokdad AH, Marks JS, Stroup DF, Gerberding JL. 2004. Actual causes of death in the United States. *JAMA* 291 (10): 1238-45.

Mueller NB, Luke DA, Herbers SH, Montgomery TP. 2006. The best practices: Use of the guidelines by ten state tobacco control programs. *Am J Prev Med* 31 (4): 300-306.

Muggli ME, Pollay RW, Lew R, Joseph AM. 2002. Targeting of Asian Americans and Pacific Islanders by the tobacco industry: Results from the Minnesota Tobacco Document Depository. *Tobacco Control* 11 (3): 201-9.

Mukherjea A, Morgan PA, Snowden LR, Ling PM, Ivey SL. 2012. Social and cultural influences on tobacco-related health disparities among South Asians in the USA. *Tobacco Control* 21 (4): 422-28.

National Cancer Institute (NCI). 2000. *Population Based Smoking Cessation: Proceedings of a Conference on What Works to Influence Cessation in the General Population.* Smoking and Tobacco Control Monograph No. 12, NIH Publication. No. 00-4892, November 2000. Bethesda, MD: U.S. Department of Health and Human Services, National Cancer Institute.

———. 2005. *ASSIST: Shaping the Future of Tobacco Prevention and Control.* Tobacco Control Monograph No. 16, NIH Pub. No. 05-5645. Bethesda, MD: U.S. Department of Health and Human Services, National Institutes of Health, National Cancer Institute.

———. 2007. *Greater than the Sum: Systems Thinking in Tobacco Control.* Tobacco Control Monograph No. 18. Bethesda, MD: US Department of Health and Human Services, National Institutes of Health, National Cancer Institute.

National Cancer Institute, Centers for Disease Control and Prevention (NCI and CDC). 2002. Smokeless tobacco fact sheets. Stockholm Centre of Public Health. Third International Conference on Smokeless Tobacco, Stockholm, Sept. 22-25.

Nelson BS, Heischober B. 1999. Betel nut: A common drug used by naturalized citizens from India, Far East Asia, and the South Pacific Islands. *Ann Emergency Med* 34 (2): 238-43.

New York City Department of Health and Mental Hygiene (NYC DHMH). 2011. Epi data brief: Trends in cigarette use among adults in New York City, 2002-2010. New York City Department of Health and Mental Hygiene, New York.

Niaura R. 2008. Nonpharmacologic therapy for smoking cessation: Characteristics and efficacy of current approaches. *Am J Med* 121 (4): S11-S19.

Nichter M. 2003. Smoking: What does culture have to do with it? *Addiction* 98 (suppl. 1): 139-45.

Noonan D. 2010. Exemptions for hookah bars in clean indoor air legislation: A public health concern. *Pub Health Nurs* 27 (1): 49-53.

Office on Smoking and Health (OSH). 2001. *Women and smoking: A report of the surgeon general.* Centers for Disease Control and Prevention, Atlanta, GA.

Olausson P, Jentsch JD, Taylor JR. 2004. Repeated nicotine exposure enhances responding with conditioned reinforcement. *Psychopharmacology* 173 (1-2): 98-104.

Oncken C, McKee S, Krishnan-Sarin S, O'Malley S, Mazure CM. 2005. Knowledge and perceived risk of smoking-related conditions: A survey of cigarette smokers. *Prev Med* 40 (6): 779-84.

Perl SB, Ellis JA, Vichinsky LE, et al. 2007. Smoking cessation strategies in New York City: 2002-2006. In *Progress in Smoking and Health Research,* ed. TC Jeffries, 89-115. New York: Nova Biomedical Books.

Pertschuk M. 2001. *Smoke in Their Eyes: Lessons in Movement Leadership from the Tobacco Wars.* Nashville, TN: Vanderbilt University Press.

Pizacani BA, Rohde K, Bushore C, et al. 2009. Smoking-related knowledge, attitudes, and behaviors in the lesbian, gay, and bisexual community: A population-based study from the US Pacific Northwest. *Prev Med* 48 (6): 555-61.

Poland B, Frohlich K, Haines RJ, Mykhalovskiy E, Rock M, Sparks R. 2006. The social context of smoking: The next frontier in tobacco control? *Tobacco Control* 15 (1): 59.

Pollay RW. 2000. Targeting youth and concerned smokers: Evidence from Canadian tobacco industry documents. *Tobacco Control* 9 (2): 136-47.

Pollay RW, Dewhirst T. 2002. The dark side of marketing seemingly "light" cigarettes: Successful images and failed fact. *Tobacco Control* 11 (suppl. 1): i18-i31.

Powell LM, Chaloupka FJ. 2003. *Parental Influences, Public Policy, and Youth Smoking Behavior.* Chicago: ImpacTeen.

Rahilly CR, Farwell WR. 2007. Prevalence of smoking in the United States: A focus on age, sex, ethnicity, and geographic patterns. *Curr Cardiovasc Risk Rep* 1 (5): 379-83.

Repace JL. 2009. Secondhand smoke in Pennsylvania casinos: A study of nonsmokers' exposure, dose, and risk. *Am J Public Health* 99 (8): 1478-85.

Richard L, Potvin L, Kishchuck N, Prlic H, Green LW. 1996. Assessment of the integration of the ecological approach in health promotion programs. *Am J Health Promot* 10:318-28.

Roeseler A, Burns D. 2010. The quarter that changed the world. *Tobacco Control* 19 (suppl. 1): i3-i15.

Roeseler A, Feighery EC, Cruz TB. 2010. Tobacco marketing in California and implications for the future. *Tobacco Control* 19 (suppl. 1): i21-i29.

Rogers T. 2010. The California Tobacco Control Program: Introduction to the 20-year retrospective. *Tobacco Control* 19 (suppl. 1): i1-i2.

Schnoll RA, Johnson TA, Lerman C. 2007. Genetics and smoking behavior. *Curr Psychiatry Rep* 9 (5): 349-57.

Scollo M, Lal A, Hyland A, Glantz S. 2003. Review of the quality of studies on the economic effects of smoke-free policies on the hospitality industry. *Tobacco Control* 12 (1): 13-20.

Siegel MB, Biener L, Rigotti NA. 2007. Effect of local youth-access regulations on progression to established smoking among youths in Massachusetts. *Tobacco Control* 16 (2): 119-26.

Silagy C, Stead LF. 2004. Physician advice for smoking cessation. *Cochrane Library* 3:CD000165.

Simons-Morton BG, Farhat T. 2010. Recent findings on peer group influences on adolescent smoking. *J Primary Prev* 31 (4): 191-208.

Slade J, Bero LA, Hanauer P, Barnes DE, Glantz SA. 1995. Nicotine and addiction. *JAMA* 274 (3): 225-33.

Sly D et al. 2004. Effect of ending an antitobacco youth campaign on adolescent susceptibility to cigarette smoking—Minnesota, 2002-2003. *MMWR* 53 (14): 301-4.

Solberg LI, Boyle RG, Davidson G, Magnan S, Link Carlson C, Alesci NL. 2001. Aids to quitting tobacco use: How important are they outside controlled trials? *Prev Med* 33 (1): 53-58.

Sorensen G, Pechacek T, Pallonen U. 1986. Occupational and worksite norms and attitudes about smoking cessation. *Am J Public Health* 76 (5): 544-49.

Spangler JG, Dignan MB, Michielutte R. 1997. Correlates of tobacco use among Native American women in western North Carolina. *Am J Public Health* 87 (1): 108-11.

Stead M, MacAskill S, MacKintosh AM, Reece J, Eadie D. 2001. "It's as if you're locked in": Qualitative explanations for area effects on smoking in disadvantaged communities. *Health & Place* 7 (4): 333-43.

Steier JB, Coady M. 2012. Qualitative data on young adult, non-daily smokers in New York City. Epi Data Brief, May, No. 17. New York City Department of Health and Mental Hygiene, New York.

Substance Abuse and Mental Health Services Administration (SAMHSA). 2012. *Results from the 2011 National Survey on Drug Use and Health: Summary of National Findings*. NSDUH Series H-44, HHS Publication No. (SMA) 12-4713. Rockville, MD: Substance Abuse and Mental Health Services Administration.

Sullivan RJ, Allen JS, Otto C, Tiobech J, Nero K. 2000. Effects of chewing betel nut (Areca catechu) on the symptoms of people with schizophrenia in Palau, Micronesia. *Br J Psychiatry* 177 (2): 174-78.

Tamir A, Cachola S. 1994. Hypertension and other cardiovascular risk factors. In *Confronting Critical Health Issues of Asian and Pacific Islander Americans*, ed. NWS Zane, DT Takeuchi, KNJ Young. Thousand Oaks, CA: Sage.

Thomson CC, Hamilton WL, Siegel MB, Biener L, Rigotti NA. 2007. Effect of local youth-access regulations on progression to established smoking among youths in Massachusetts. *Tobacco Control* 16 (2): 119-26.

Tobacco Education and Research Oversight Committee (TEROC). 2009. *Endangered Investment: Toward a Tobacco-Free California, 2009-2011: Master Plan of the Tobacco Education Research Oversight Committee*. Sacramento: California Department of Public Health.

———. 2012. *Saving Lives, Saving Money: Toward a Tobacco-Free California, 2012-2014: Master Plan of the Tobacco Education and Research Oversight Committee*. Sacramento: California Department of Public Health.

Trosclair A, Babb S, Murphy-Hoefer R, et al. 2007. State-specific prevalence of smoke-free home rules—United States, 1992-2003. *MMWR* 56:501-4.

Tworek C, Yamaguchi R, Kloska DD, et al. 2010. State-level tobacco control policies and youth smoking cessation measures. *Health Policy* 97 (2): 136-44.

Umberson D. 1987. Family status and health behaviors: Social control as a dimension of social integration. *J Health Soc Behav* 28 (3): 306-19.

Unger JB, Cruz T, Baezconde-Garbanati L, et al. 2003. Exploring the cultural context of tobacco use: A transdisciplinary framework. *Nicotine Tob Res* 5 (suppl. 1): S101-S117.

Unger JB, Rohrbach LA, Cruz TB, et al. 2001. Ethnic variation in peer influences on adolescent smoking. *Nicotine Tob Res* 3 (2): 167-76.

U.S. Department of Health and Human Services (USDHHS). 1990. *The Health Benefits of Smoking Cessation: A Report of the Surgeon General*. DHHS Publication No. CDC 90-8416. Washington, DC: U.S. Government Printing Office.

———. 1994. *Preventing Tobacco Use among Young People: A Report of the US Surgeon General*. Executive Summary. Washington, DC: Government Printing Office.

———. 2000. *Reducing Tobacco Use: A Report of the Surgeon General*. Atlanta, GA: US Department of Health and Human Services, Centers for Disease Control and Prevention, National Center for Chronic Disease

Prevention and Health Promotion, Office on Smoking and Health.

———. 2001. Women and smoking: A report of the surgeon general. Washington, DC: HHS, Public Health Service, Office of the Surgeon General.

———. 2006. *The Health Consequences of Involuntary Exposure to Tobacco Smoke: A Report of the Surgeon General.* Washington, DC: U.S. Department of Health and Human Services, Centers for Disease Control and Prevention, National Center for Chronic Disease Prevention and Health Promotion, Office on Smoking and Health.

———. 2010. *Healthy People 2020.* Washington, DC: Office of Disease Prevention and Health Promotion.

U.S. Department of Health, Education, and Welfare (USDHEW). 1964. *Smoking and health: Report of the Advisory Committee to the Surgeon General of the Public Health Service.* Public Health Service Publication No. 1103. Washington, DC: Public Health Service, Centers for Disease Control and Prevention.

U.S. District Court for the District of Columbia. 2006. United States v. Philip Morris USA, Inc., et al. 449 F. Supp. 2d 1 (U.S. D.D.C. 2006).

Van Loon AJM, Tijhuis M, Surtees PG, Ormel J. 2005. Determinants of smoking status: Cross-sectional data on smoking initiation and cessation. *Eur J Public Health* 15 (3): 256-61.

Vermont Department of Health (VDH). 2007. Bridging the gap: Partnering to address tobacco disparities in Vermont, www.ttac.org/tcn/peers/pdfs/09.07.11/VT_Addressing_Tobacco_Disparities_July_2007.pdf.

Volpp KG, Gurmankin AD, Gomez A, et al. 2006. A randomized controlled trial of financial incentives for smoking cessation. *Cancer Epidem Biomarkers Prev* 15 (1): 12-18.

Wakefield M, McLeod K, Smith KC. 2003. Individual versus corporate responsibility for smoking-related illness: Australian press coverage of the Rolah McCabe trial. *Health Promot Int* (4) :297-305.

Warren, CW, Riley LA, Asma S, Eriksen MP, Green LW, Yach D. 2000. Tobacco use by youth: A surveillance report from the Global Youth Tobacco Survey Project. *Bull World Health Org* 78:868-76.

Washington HA. 2002. Burning love: Big tobacco takes aim at LGBT youths. *Am J Public Health* 92 (7): 1086-95.

Wayne GF, Connolly GN. 2002. How cigarette design can affect youth initiation into smoking: Camel cigarettes, 1983-93. *Tobacco Control* 11 (suppl. 1): i32-i39.

Wingo C, Kiser D, Boschert T, Hunting P, Buffington T, Wellman-Bensen J. 2001. Eliminating smoking in bars, restaurants, and gaming cubs in California: The California Smoke-Free Workplace Act. California Department of Health Services, Tobacco Control Section, Sacramento.

World Health Organization (WHO). 1998. *Guidelines for Controlling and Monitoring the Tobacco Epidemic.* Geneva: World Health Organization.

———. 2008. *WHO report on the global tobacco epidemic, 2008: The MPOWER package.* Geneva: World Health Organization.

Yach D, Wipfli H. 2006. A century of smoke. *Ann Trop Med Parasitol* 100 (5-6): 5-6.

Zaza S, Briss PA, Harris KW, eds. 2005. *The Guide to Community Preventive Services: What Works to Promote Health? What Works to Promote Health?* New York: Oxford University Press.

Zhang X, Cowling DW, Tang H. 2010. The impact of social norm change strategies on smokers' quitting behaviours. *Tobacco Control* 19 (suppl. 1): i51-i155.

Alcohol and Behavior Change

HAROLD HOLDER

LEARNING OBJECTIVES

After completing the chapter, the reader will be able to

* Understand the differences in utilization and relevance between individual-directed approaches and environmental or public policy approaches to the reduction of alcohol problems.
* Define limitations in utilizing educational strategies alone to reduce alcohol problems and understand how such approaches can be utilized within environmental or policy approaches to prevention of alcohol problems.
* Recognize which policy approaches have shown the strongest evidence of potential effectiveness in reducing alcohol problems at the population level.
* Identify the major stakeholders in any public health approach to prevention of alcohol problems and identify the natural conflicts of interest as well as the possible points of collaboration existing among and between these stakeholders.
* Define the "prevention paradox" and understand why this concept is important in understanding policy efforts to reduce alcohol problems at the population level.

Introduction

Although alcohol is used to provide considerable pleasure and satisfaction to millions of consumers worldwide, it is also a psychoactive substance that can diminish clarity of thought and inhibitions, personal judgment, and eye and hand coordination to perform skilled (or dangerous) tasks. While these features are a part of the attraction of alcohol in many social settings, excessive drinking can also have both acute and long-term negative effects. Long-term effects result from regular heavy drinking, which affects the health of the drinker and often leads to early death.

Alcohol can also exert life-threatening effects on others. For example, heavy drinking during pregnancy increases the risk of fetal alcohol syndrome for the infant. Further, acute effects that result from impairment in thinking, judgment, and physical skills increase the risk for intoxicated-driving crashes, falls, drowning, and other accidental deaths as well as violence. Such harmful possibilities create a challenge for public health.

Alcohol is identified as the cause of more than 100,000 deaths annually in the United States. For adolescents, it is the most commonly abused drug. Alcohol-related motor vehicle crashes are the leading cause of death in teenagers. More than half of the high school seniors in the United States have reported on recent national surveys that they drink alcohol, which increases the risk of involvement in violence, traffic crashes, crime, high-risk sexual behavior, and injuries for this age group. According to a 2011 publication, people who consume at least four drinks per occasion cost the U.S. economy $223.5 billion a year, and governments pay more than 60% of their health care costs (Bouchery et al. 2011).

Key Determinants and Conceptual Framework

An **ecological approach** to alcohol abuse, as to the other **health behaviors** discussed in this textbook, is an effective means to reduce health and social problems at the population level. Alcohol might be thought of as a form of legal drug that, when used inappropriately or without care, can increase problems for the individual drinker as well as for others. Thus, a drinking driver increases her risk of injury or death as well as risking death and injury for others on the roadway, railway, boat or airplane. From a public health perspective, the major important variable is reducing alcohol availability or easy access to it. The cost of the product reflects economic availability and is related to the final price for the consumer as well as the consumer's ability to pay. Physical availability reflects how convenient it is for the consumer to acquire alcohol, so the days and hours of alcohol sale, the minimum age to purchase alcohol, and the location of alcohol outlets are important public health considerations.

Evidence-Based Interventions

In this chapter, we will address both **environmental** and **individual interventions**. *Environmental-based approaches* seek to alter the physical, social, economic, and geographical or physical environment to reduce alcohol-involved social and health problems, whereas *individual approaches* focus on the individual's drinking pattern, including addiction or dependency, with the specific **goal** to alter harmful patterns. These, of course, are not mutually exclusive approaches, and they are often pursued jointly.

Individual Interventions

Individual strategies are central to screening for alcohol misuse and for the treatment of alcoholism and consumption that is seen as a threat to the health or social well-being of individuals, families, and the community.

Treatment of alcoholism as an effort to support recovery represents a substantial societal investment to reduce dependency upon alcohol. Following detoxification, a variety of therapeutic modalities have been incorporated to treat drinking problems, promote abstinence from alcohol, and prevent relapse. Alcohol treatment is typically provided in outpatient and inpatient hospital settings, but it can also be delivered in psychiatric clinics, social service agencies, and other health care settings (Finney et al. 1996). Various methods are used within the **context** of outpatient and residential treatment services. The approaches with the strongest supporting evidence are behavior therapy, group therapy, family treatment, and motivational enhancement. Research suggests that Alcoholics Anonymous (AA) or Twelve Step Facilitation is as effective as more **theory**-based therapies (Ouimette et al. 1999), even including those that combine behavior change with medication (Kranzler and Van Kirk 2001).

Providing treatment services has been shown to reduce alcohol-related deaths from liver cirrhosis (Holder and Parker 1992) and medical costs for alcoholics (Holder 1998; Holder and Blose 1992). However, there is as yet little evidence that individual treatment reduces population-level acute problems, such as traffic crashes, injuries, or violence (Holder 1997).

One individual approach that has been encouraged internationally is brief **intervention** with problem drinkers, typically within health care settings, as a means to encourage them to seek further services or to cut down voluntarily on drinking levels and frequency. Strong evidence demonstrates that brief interventions can contribute to reductions in drinking and associated alcohol-related problems (Whitlock et al. 2004). However, one major limitation of this approach is the consistent complacency or resistance of medical personnel when it comes to carrying out such interventions.

The U.S. Preventive Services Task Force (USPSTF) has reviewed the available evidence on individual-level clinical interventions to reduce alcohol misuse. These reviews conclude that there is only fair evidence that primary care screening and behavioral counseling helps to reduce alcohol misuse in adults, including pregnant women. In children, the USPSTF concluded, the evidence is insufficient to recommend for or against primary care screening and behavioral counseling interventions for adolescents.

These very conservative findings may be attributed to the limitations of the research and to the reality that interventions in the clinical setting are inevitably limited by the brevity and the relative infrequency of medical encounters

in which to counsel patients on such a **complex** problem. When considered within the web of lifestyle, human biology, **social environment**, cultural history, family codependency, employment and housing conditions, and other social and environmental circumstances not largely under the control of the individual, it is perhaps no wonder that brief clinical interventions are of limited value on their own.

Recently, interest has grown in conducting brief individual interventions as a component of comprehensive community prevention efforts, which also emphasize policy or environmental strategies. In one example, Hingson and colleagues (2005) found that five communities that received a comprehensive mix of prevention and intervention experienced an approximately 20% decline in alcohol-related fatal crashes, compared with comparison (control) communities.

Mass media campaigns have been used to inform the population about the dangers of heavy drinking. They have specifically been used to reduce drinking and driving. In a review of eight studies, Elder and colleagues (2004) concluded that well-designed and well-executed mass media campaigns implemented in conjunction with other ongoing prevention activities can contribute to overall **effectiveness** in reducing alcohol-related harms. In contrast, mass media campaigns implemented without more comprehensive prevention activities are not likely to be effective. Ditter and colleagues (2005) reviewed nine campaigns that either encouraged designated driver use or provided **incentives** for people to act as designated drivers and found insufficient evidence of effectiveness of such programs. In short, no existing evidence shows that mass media campaigns *alone* can reduce alcohol-related problems.

One version of public education has been the mandated alcoholic beverage container warning labels, which began in the United States in 1989 to warn of the risk of birth defects when alcohol is consumed during pregnancy, of driving or operating machinery after drinking, and of general health risks. Some states require posted warnings of alcohol risks in establishments that serve or sell alcohol. Greenfield and Kaskutas (1998) and Greenfield and co-workers (1999) have found that warning labels can increase knowledge regarding the risks of drinking and driving and drinking during pregnancy among some subgroups (e.g., light drinkers). Argo and Main (2004), in a meta-analysis of 48 studies of warning labels, which included some studies of alcohol, found that warning labels had some impact on consumers' attention, reading, comprehension, and recall but resulted in only moderate **self-reported** behavior changes. This is consistent with other reviews (Agostinelli and Grube 2002; Grube and Nygaard 2005), all of which conclude that alcohol warning labels have little or no measurable effects on drinking behavior. Further, no direct effects of warning labels on population-level alcohol-related problems have been reported.

Counter-advertising involves disseminating information about a product, its effects, and the industry that promotes it, in order to decrease its appeal and use. It is distinct from other types of informational campaigns in that it directly addresses the fact that the particular commodity is promoted through advertising (Agostinelli and Grube 2002). State legislative initiatives to place warnings directly on alcohol advertisements, particularly electronic messages, have not succeeded in the United States (Giesbrecht 2002; Greenfield et al. 1999). While counter-advertising has the potential to increase advertising awareness in the general population, there is insufficient evidence that such awareness alone reduces alcohol-related problems.

Environmental Interventions

In contrast to the limited data on individual interventions, the evidence for population-level improvements in alcohol abuse and alcohol-related problems is extensive (Babor et al. 2010).

The remainder of this chapter will focus on policy and environmental approaches to reducing alcohol-involved health and safety problems (i.e., those acute problems associated with "in the moment" drinking and harm such as traffic crashes, violence, and unintended injuries). Policies can be effective to reduce alcohol-involved problems by producing changes in the environment or reducing the opportunities for drinking.

The rationale for **targeting** communities, as opposed to individuals, is compelling. First, alcohol problems often occur largely within community or neighborhood contexts, and the prevention strategies available to communities are extensive. For example, in the case of underage drinking, communities exert some control (e.g., zoning and business licensing of alcohol establishments) over the means through which alcohol is typically obtained, including restrictions on sales to underage persons. Second, many of the social and health effects associated with alcohol are born collectively at the community level, producing victims other than just the person or persons abusing alcohol, for example in motor vehicle crashes and acts of violence. Like other health problems, alcohol-related harms also impose shared medical care costs and burdens on the capacity of health care systems to serve the community. Third, to the extent that individuals cannot, or will not, restrict their alcohol intake within safe boundaries, community-level restraints, controls, and penalties to deter or buffer the individual's potential to do harm to others is a justified community undertaking.

The Task Force on Community Preventive Services, based on its systematic reviews, has recommended "the use of multicomponent interventions with community mobilization on the basis of strong evidence of their effectiveness in reducing alcohol-impaired driving. Effective programs included most or all of the following: sobriety checkpoints; responsible beverage service training; efforts to limit access to alcohol, particularly among youth; public education campaigns; and **media advocacy** efforts to gain the support of policymakers and the public" (Shults et al. 2009, 71).

THE ECONOMIC AVAILABILITY OF ALCOHOL

As a legal product, demand for alcohol is inversely related to its retail price (i.e., as price increases, demand declines, and vice versa). Economists call this relationship **elasticity**, or the sensitivity of demand for a product to retail price. A number of estimates of the elasticity of various alcoholic beverages exist across the world (see the international summary of elasticities in Babor et al. 2010). A recent meta-analysis of research papers on price elasticity of alcohol concluded that averages across reported elasticities are −0.46 for beer, −0.69 for wine, and −0.80 for spirits. The price sensitivity of heavy drinking (which typically has the greatest risk of producing harm) has an average elasticity of −0.28 (Wagenaar, Salois, et al. 2009). Although taxation and price increases can be effective prevention strategies, price elasticities are moderated by social, environmental, and economic factors. As a result, the price sensitivity of alcohol may vary considerably across time, states, and countries, depending on drinking patterns and **attitudes** and on the presence of other alcohol policies.

Alcohol is a specially taxed product at both the federal and the state level, such that the retail price of alcohol can be changed through excise tax changes (Chaloupka et al. 2002; TF-CPS 2010). Historically the real prices of alcoholic beverages (i.e., the prices after accounting for the effects of inflation) have declined significantly. Between 1975 and 1990, the real price of distilled spirits fell by 32%, wine by 28%, and beer by 20%. Coate and Grossman (1988) found in early research that as the price of beer went up, the frequency of beer consumption went down. A recent study of Alaska (Wagenaar, Maldonado-Molina, et al. 2009) found that intentional public health policy increases in alcohol

excise in 1983 and 2002 were each significantly associated with reductions in alcohol-related **mortality** of between 11% and 29%. Ohsfeldt and Morrisey (1997) focused on workplace accidents in the United States between 1975 and 1985, concluding that an increase of $0.25 in beer taxes would have resulted in 4,587 fewer workdays lost through injuries.

A substantial body of literature has examined the links between alcohol taxes (and prices) and road traffic accidents, predominantly in the United States, beginning with Cook (1981), who found that states that had increased their alcohol taxes between 1960 and 1975 experienced lower-than-average increases in road traffic fatalities. Econometric advances produced cross-sectional time-series analyses, which found significant relationships between taxes and fatality rates for the general population (Ruhm 1996; Saffer and Grossman 1987).

Studies that look at drinking by youth generally find even larger effects of taxes and prices than for the overall population, suggesting that increases in prices are particularly effective in reducing youth drinking and its **consequences**. McCarthy (2003), using 18 years of data from California, finds that crashes involving younger drivers are more related to alcohol prices, although the effect of price is still significant for drivers age 60 and older. Similarly, Eisenberg (2003) finds that beer taxes are most strongly related to crashes involving young people (age 21 or younger) and to crashes that occur on weekend nights (a proxy for alcohol involvement). Ponicki and colleagues (2007) examined data from 48 U.S. states between 1975 and 2001 and state that alcohol price has been significantly related to youth traffic fatalities, although its effect has diminished somewhat since the introduction of the minimum legal drinking age of 21.

Several studies have examined the impact of the price of alcoholic beverages on homicides and other crimes, including rape, robbery, assaults, motor vehicle thefts, domestic violence, and child abuse (Chaloupka et al. 2002; Cook 2007; Markowitz and Grossman 2000; Sen 2006; Sivarajasingam et al. 2006). These studies suggest that raising the price of alcohol is likely to result in a reduction in violence. Finally, a growing literature links alcohol regulation and sexually transmitted diseases, with a number of studies in the United States finding significant relationships between alcohol taxation rates and rates of gonorrhea (Chesson et al. 2000; Grossman et al. 2004; Markowitz et al. 2005).

THE PHYSICAL (RETAIL) AVAILABILITY OF ALCOHOL

In addition to economic accessibility for those with less disposable income, the physical or retail availability of alcohol has been an essential aspect of public policy. Retail availability includes on-premise outlets, such as bars or restaurants, as well as off-premise outlets, such as grocery stores, liquor stores, and other retail outlets licensed to sell alcohol within their community. In general, when retail alcohol is cheap, convenient, and easily accessible, people drink more, and the rates of alcohol problems are higher. Aspects of retail availability such as privatization, hours and days of alcohol sales, and outlet density have been associated with changes in alcohol sales to underage youth, shifts in beverage choice to more readily accessible alcoholic beverage types, and drinking behavior (Campbell et al. 2009; TFCPS 2009).

Underage Drinking Laws. Underage drinking and minor in possession (MIP) laws are the formal rules, regulations, and laws concerning purchase, possession, and use of alcohol by persons under a specific age, uniformly age 21 in the United States. States differ on the specific provisions of their statutes. Wagenaar and Toomey (2002) analyzed 57 published studies that assessed the effects of changes in the minimum legal drinking age (MLDA) on indicators of consumption and harm related to drinking from 1960 to 1999. They concluded that increasing the legal age appears to have been more ef-

fective than any other prevention strategy for reducing drinking and drinking problems among high school students, college students, and other youth. An analysis of state-level data in the United States found that raising the MLDA to age 21 reduced alcohol-related crashes among youth by as much as 19% (Voas et al. 2003). Similarly, the MLDA of 21 in the United States has been associated with a 47% decrease in fatal crashes involving young drivers with high blood alcohol concentrations (BACs) (0.08% and higher) and a 40% decrease in such crashes involving young drivers with positive BACs (BAC > 0.0) (Dang 2008). Conversely, a review of research indicated that the trend to decrease the MLDA in the United States from 21 to 18 years during the 1970s was associated with a 7% *increase* in traffic fatalities for the affected age groups (Cook 2007). Other studies have provided similar findings (Carpenter and Dobkin 2007; Carpenter et al. 2007; Voas et al. 2003). The U.S. National Highway Traffic Safety Administration (NHTSA) estimated that a MLDA of 21 reduced traffic fatalities by 846 deaths in 1997 and had prevented a total of 17,359 deaths since 1975 (NHTSA 1998).

Despite higher minimum age drinking laws, young people can and do purchase alcohol (e.g., Grube 1997; Paschall et al., "Alcohol outlet characteristics," 2007). Studies show that anywhere from 30% to 90% of outlets will sell to a minor, depending on geographical location. Even moderate increases in enforcement can reduce sales of alcohol to minors by as much as 35% to 40%, especially when combined with media and other community and policy activities (Grube 1997; Wagenaar et al. 2000). Additional evidence comes from recent studies showing that **compliance** and enforcement at the community level are inversely associated with youth consumption, problem consumption, and use of commercial sources for alcohol (Dent et al. 2005; Paschall et al., "Alcohol availability," 2007). According to a study in New Orleans, enforcement of underage sales laws increased compliance with the laws from 11% to 39% (Scribner and Cohen 2001). The greatest gains in compliance occurred among those retailers who had been cited (51%), but substantial gains were also seen for those not cited (35%).

One example of enforcement is compliance checks (checking by law enforcement whether a licensed establishment actually sells or serves alcohol to underage persons or "underage looking persons"). Studies of enforcement effects show that enforcement has reduced sales to youth (Scribner and Cohen 2001). Some evidence suggests that enforcement primarily affects the specific establishments targeted in compliance checks, with limited diffusion, and that any effects on sales may decay relatively quickly (Wagenaar, Toomey, and Erickson 2005a, 2005b). Dent, Grube, and Biglan (2005) found that stronger enforcement of MIP laws, as indexed by the student's average perceived level of enforcement in the community, was significantly related to lower levels in the communities' general frequency of use and binge drinking.

Concentration of Outlets Licensed to Sell or Serve Alcohol. Restricting the number of places where alcohol can be sold or served has been widely used as a policy to reduce consumption and, therefore, alcohol-related problems. In general, this has been accomplished using the state licensing apparatus, with limitations either formally legislated or emerging through individual licensing decisions. Studies find significant relationships over time between outlet density and violence rates, drinking and driving, and child abuse (see Gruenewald 2007; Gruenewald and Remer 2006; Livingston 2008; Stockwell and Gruenewald 2001 for reviews). Outlet density in close proximity to college campuses is related to heavy drinking and frequent drinking but also to drinking-related problems for the college-age resident students (Weitzman et al. 2003). Studies also find evidence that frequency of underage drinking and driving and riding with drinking drivers increased with outlet density (Dent et al. 2005; Treno et al. 2003).

Based upon reviews of the scientific evidence, the Task Force on Community Preventive Services (2009) and Campbell and colleagues (2009) confirm the potential of limiting alcohol outlet density as a means to reduce excessive consumption and alcohol-related harms.

Legal Hours and Days of Week for Selling or Serving. Restricting the days and times of alcohol sale reduces opportunities for purchasing alcohol (and thus its availability). A recent review of studies on the effects of changes in hours of sale included 48 relevant studies from eight countries across four decades with a wide variety of research designs (Stockwell and Chikritzhs 2009). The authors concluded that, based upon controlled studies, the evidence supports the **expectation** that changes in hours of sale will be associated with changes in harms involving alcohol. Recent studies in Western Australia (Chikritzhs and Stockwell 2002, 2006) and Canada (Vingilis et al. 2005; Vingilis et al. 2007) find that late-night trading hours can contribute to increases in alcohol-related motor vehicle injuries and increases in other injuries (such as assault and fall-related injuries).

Kelly-Baker and co-workers (2000) found that temporary bans on the sale of alcohol from midnight Friday through 10 a.m. Monday (because of federal elections in Mexico) reduced cross-border drinking by young Americans of ages 14–25; early closings on Friday night produced a 34% net reduction in the number of persons with high BACs, and earlier bar closing hours in Juarez, Mexico, reduced the number of young adult American pedestrians with high BAC levels by 89%. In short, increased hours and days of sale increase the ease of purchasing alcohol and thereby increase drinking, whereas reductions in such availability have the potential to reduce alcohol-related harms.

State Retail Monopolies for Off-Premise Alcohol Sales. Retail alcohol monopolies are a public policy means to reduce drinking; this tactic goes back in U.S. history to the end of Prohibition in December 1933. The rationale supporting the policy is that eliminating a private profit reduces physical access and convenience of access to alcohol and facilitates the enforcement of rules against selling to minors or to individuals who are already intoxicated (Her et al. 1999). For example, Miller and colleagues (2006) found that underage drinking rates, including heavy drinking as well as youth-involved traffic crashes, were lower in states that had retail sale monopolies, controlling for other factors.

The formal powers and resources of state alcohol beverage control agencies place them in a position to regulate access to alcoholic beverages through restrictions on retail distribution and sales. For example, monopoly states restrict access to spirits, and sometimes wine, by allowing retail sales only through state stores. Both license and monopoly states restrict sales through the use of price posting and fixing provisions. States or provinces that eliminate government retail monopolies typically have increased consumption and/or substantial increases in alcohol outlets (see Holder and Wagenaar 1990; Trolldall 2005).

Service Regulation and Training in Bars, Restaurants, Pubs, and Clubs. The primary policy approach to preventing overserving alcohol in on-premise licensed establishments has been a combination of policies on training and establishment serving practices and local regulatory enforcement of them.

Responsible Beverage Service (RBS) describes a policy to prevent serving alcohol to minors and intoxicated patrons and to intervene so that intoxicated patrons do not drive. RBS programs have been shown to be effective in some circumstances, reducing the numbers of intoxicated patrons leaving a bar, car crashes, sales to intoxicated patrons, sales to minors, and incidents of violence surrounding outlets (e.g., Wallin et al. 2003). Establishments with firm and clear policies (e.g., checking IDs for all patrons who appear younger than age 30) and a system for monitoring staff compliance are less likely to sell alcohol to minors (Wolfson, Toomey,

Forster, et al. 1996; Wolfson, Toomey, Murray, et al. 1996). Evidence shows that state-mandated training for alcohol servers can produce lower alcohol-involved traffic crash rates (Holder and Wagenaar 1994).

The Minimum Age to Sell Alcohol. The minimum age of alcohol sellers, which is set in some countries, could affect the extent to which underage sales occur; that is, younger persons may find themselves less able to detect underage buyers and may be more willing to sell to underage buyers (Treno et al. 2000).

UNDERAGE SOCIAL ACCESS TO ALCOHOL

A substantial portion of the alcohol obtained by underage persons is from social sources (friends, parties, homes, etc.) and other persons who purchase alcohol and provide it to them (both persons who are themselves under the legal purchase age and persons who are of legal age). See reviews that confirm that social alcohol sources are more strongly related to underage drinking than are commercial alcohol sources and the perceived ease of obtaining alcohol (Harrison et al. 2007; Paschall et al., "Alcohol availability," 2007). This illustrates a combined effect of social context (e.g., a party) and low cost per drink of alcohol. Given that young people use multiple sources for alcohol, **social availability** is a significant means for underage youth to obtain alcohol. The social availability may be through friends, at parties, or from strangers.

Policy approaches such as shoulder-tap laws, party patrols, and keg registration can restrict social availability. Such strategies share a similar theoretical basis (association with alcohol availability and alcohol harms) and thus have the potential to be effective insofar as other strategies with a similar theoretical basis have been shown to be effective. However, they need more extensive **evaluation**.

Youth Curfews. Curfews establish a time when children and young people below certain ages must be home. Although this policy was not initially considered an alcohol problem prevention strategy, research has shown positive effects. The strategy reduces both the availability of alcohol to youth through social sources and the convenience of obtaining alcohol at gatherings of youth; it also reduces the amount of evening time they have to consume alcohol at those gatherings. Therefore, they are less likely to be involved in a crash. In states that have established such curfews, alcohol-involved traffic crashes for young people below the curfew age have declined (Preusser et al. 1984; Williams et al. 1984).

Social Host Liability. Under social host liability, adults who provide alcohol to a minor or serve intoxicated adults in social settings can be sued through civil action for damages or injury caused by that minor or intoxicated adult (Grube and Nygaard 2005). There is very little research on the effectiveness of social host liability laws, and what evidence exists is conflicting. In one study in the United States, social host liability laws were associated with decreases in alcohol-related traffic fatalities among adults but not among minors (Whetten-Goldstein et al. 2000). Social host statutes were not related to single-vehicle nighttime crashes for either group. In a second study, social host liability laws were associated with decreases in reported heavy drinking and in decreases in drinking and driving by lighter drinkers (Stout et al. 2000). Although social host liability may send a powerful message, that message must be effectively disseminated before it can have a deterrent effect.

Third-Party Provision of Alcohol to Youth. A person of legal age can purchase alcohol on behalf of an underage person. Often, the underage person approaches a legal-age stranger outside an alcohol-selling establishment and asks the stranger to purchase alcohol for him. Toomey, Fabian, Erickson, and Lenk (2007) found that 19% of young males older than age 21 were willing to purchase alcohol for youth who appeared to be underage when they were "shoulder-tapped" outside a convenience or liquor store. Shoulder-tap enforcement interventions occur when an underage person, or a person who appears to be underage, stands outside a licensed alcohol outlet and approaches an older person to ask the older person to purchase alcohol for her. If the older person actually makes the alcohol purchase and gives it to the youth, that older person can be arrested or cited by the police. Strategies addressing shoulder taps are promising ways to reduce third-party sources of alcohol for minors, but such strategies have not been seriously tested in replicated controlled studies.

Party Patrols. Another place where underage drinkers commonly gain access to alcohol is at parties (e.g., Wagenaar et al. 1993). Party patrols use law enforcement officers to (1) enforce laws prohibiting adult provision of alcohol to minors and prohibiting underage drinking at private parties and (2) disrupt one of the highest-risk settings for alcohol availability and misuse (i.e., private drinking parties) by conducting weekend patrols of areas known to be regular drinking locations. Party patrols increase law enforcement's responsiveness to reports of teenage drinking parties by community members. Party patrols are a local enforcement strategy in which police arrive at a social event in which alcohol is being served and check the IDs of party participants. Evidence of effectiveness is limited. For example, Oregon implemented a weekend drunk-driving and party-patrol program that has law enforcement officers working with schools to identify in advance the anticipated location of teen parties, which the officers then patrol. An unpublished evaluation of this program revealed that arrests of youth for possession of alcohol increased from 60 to 1,000 individuals in one year (with a corresponding decrease of 35% in underage drunk-driving accidents) (Little and Bishop 1998; Radecki 1993).

Keg Registration. The consumption of beer, the primary beverage of choice for underage drinkers, was found to be a potential factor in underage alcohol-related harm, especially traffic fatalities. Beer kegs are often a main source of alcohol at teenage parties. Without keg tagging, there is no way to trace who purchased the keg, so that that person can be held accountable for breaking the law. Wagenaar, O'Malley, and LaFond (2001) examined existing beer keg registration policies in all states and found no controlled studies of the effects of keg registration laws, which might include measurement of the rates of keg sales, bottled beer sales, beer consumption, or intoxication among teens and teen parties; or the frequency of disturbance calls to police could be studied; a study could also more directly measure teen consumption of keg beer. It has been found that most state alcohol control agency survey respondents noted very low levels of enforcement of extant keg registration laws and high levels of leniency in imposing penalties (Wagenaar, Toomey, and Erickson 2005a). However, keg registration laws are associated with a significant decrease in traffic fatalities. Cohen and colleagues (2001) found that the presence of a local keg registration law was associated with lower alcohol fatality rates as a part of a composite score for level of alcohol regulation. No controlled longitudinal studies of the passage of a beer keg registration exist, and its specific effects on alcohol-involved traffic crashes by underage persons or other alcohol problems are also as yet unknown.

PREVENTING ALCOHOL-INVOLVED MOTOR VEHICLE CRASHES

While regular enforcement and punishment of drinking and driving have substantially reduced the prevalence and level of alcohol-involved traffic crashes in the United States, alcohol remains a major contributor to injuries and death on the roadway. The major prevention strategies have involved enforcement, including stopping drivers to check their blood alcohol level (BAC) based upon individual driver behavior or in routine enforcement checks.

Random Breath Testing. Random breath testing (RBT) involves extensive and continuous random stops of drivers, who are required to take a breath test to establish their BAC. Tests of RBT in Australia (Homel 1990), Canada (Mercer 1985) and Great Britain (Ross 1988a, 1988b) indicate that RBT reduces car crashes. For example, in Australia, RBT resulted in a 24% reduction in nighttime crashes, especially in metropolitan areas and especially when accompanied by publicity to give public salience to enforcement (e.g., Cameron et al. 1997; Drummond et al. 1992). Increased public expectations of arrest must be reinforced with actual increased enforcement to have a sustained effect (Hingson et al. 1988; Vingilis and Coultes 1990). A limited version of RBT, sobriety checkpoints, is commonly implemented in individual U.S. states under prescribed circumstances, often involving prenotification about when and where they will be implemented. Even under these restricted circumstances, evidence shows that they reduce drinking and driving and related traffic crashes. See a review by Shults and coworkers (2001).

Zero Tolerance Laws. Zero-tolerance laws set lower BAC limits for underage drivers and/or create the risk that an underage youth who has been found to be drinking will lose his driver's license, even if he was not driving. Usually this limit is set at the minimum that can be reliably detected by breath-testing equipment (i.e., .01-.02 BAC). Zero-tolerance laws also commonly invoke penalties such as license revocation, which can be handled administratively by the officer. This punishment can be a major deterrent to youthful drinkers who drive (Ross and Gilliland 1991) insofar as a driving permit confers high status and is a valuable possession for young people. A study of all 50 U.S. states and the District of Columbia found a net decrease of 24% in the number of young drivers with positive BACs as a result of the implementation of zero-tolerance laws (Voas et al. 1998). Similarly, a 19% reduction in self-reported driving after any drinking and a 24% reduction in driving after five or more drinks was found using Monitoring the Future survey data from 30 states (Wagenaar et al. 2001). While it is a potentially effective policy, differences in the level of zero-tolerance law enforcement, as with other policy options, have been identified as a key issue in understanding why some programs are less successful than others (Voas et al. 2003).

Administrative License Revocation. Laws permitting the withdrawal of driving privileges without court action have been adopted by a majority of states to prevent traffic crashes caused by unsafe driving practices, including driving with a BAC over the legal limit, and have been associated with declines in nighttime fatal crashes in some studies (Hingson 1993; Zador et al. 1989). Administrative license revocation is one type of punishment that has been shown to be effective in reducing repeated incidents of drinking and driving. In practice, if the state has a provision for the zero-tolerance enforcement with regard to underage drivers or alcohol possession, then an officer can confiscate drivers' licenses.

Automobile Ignition Interlock Devices. Automobile ignition interlocks are devices that prevent drivers from starting their cars if their BAC is above a preset limit. This device has been discussed as a potential means to reduce all drinking and driving but has been used in the United States primarily as a means to prevent a multiple drinking and driving offender from starting her auto after drinking (Voas and DeYoung 2002; Elder et al. 2011). As the price of these devices comes down, requiring them in cars that adolescents drive as well as for multiple-offense drinking drivers could become feasible.

RESTRICTIONS ON ALCOHOL ADVERTISING AND PROMOTIONS

Each year, the alcohol industry in the United States spends more than $1 billion on "measured media" advertising (i.e., television, radio, print, and outdoor ads), according to the Federal Trade Commission.[1] Snyder and co-workers (2006) found that exposure to alcohol advertisements affects youth alcohol consumption and that the youth in markets with greater alcohol advertising expenditures drank more (each additional dollar spent per capita raised the number of drinks consumed by 3%). Policies that restrict advertising of alcohol to young people could conceivably reduce consumption; studies consistently find small but significant relationships between awareness of and appreciation of alcohol advertising, on one hand, and adolescents' drinking beliefs and behaviors, on the other. Saffer (2002), in a review of published research literature on the potential effects of alcohol advertising on consumption (in particular, the effects on youth drinking), concluded that alcohol advertising does increase consumption, but that an alcohol advertising ban alone is insufficient to limit all forms of promotion. A comprehensive ban on advertising (a ban in which all alcohol advertising was prohibited) would receive substantial public support, however, according to his review. Saffer and Dhaval (2002), following an analysis of national alcohol consumption related to total advertising expenditures, concluded that alcohol advertising bans decrease alcohol consumption. But Nelson (2003) concluded that "bans of advertising alone do not reduce total alcohol consumption, which partly reflects substitution effects." In short, the research evidence is mixed concerning the potential effects on consumption of policies to restrict advertising and promotion of alcohol, perhaps in part because these studies have been conducted at the country level and because of the lack of precision in measurement.

Roles for Key Stakeholders

Key stakeholders relevant to alcohol policies include the alcohol industry, the public health and safety community, and government policymakers.

The Alcohol Industry

The alcohol industry is a major participant in the process of establishing public policy concerning alcohol. The challenge faced by the industry is that more than half of the alcohol produced and sold is consumed by approximately 10% of drinkers, who consume alcohol frequently and in large amounts, though many of these heavy drinkers are not dependent or alcoholics. Thus, this small population of consumers make major contributions to the sales levels of alcohol as well as to the profits of the alcohol industry. The alcohol industry in the United States operates at three levels, according to the rules established at the end of American Prohibition (1933): producers, wholesalers and distributors, and retailers. All of these levels do not necessarily share the same goals and approaches. For example, all retailers exist within communities and are in direct interaction with local residents and local values, which can shape their potential for profit. They obtain a retail license to sell and/or serve alcohol as well as a local business license. Wholesalers do not typically engage local residents but may be active in influencing the actions of elected officials who establish regulations, which affect the distribution and wholesale or retail sale of alcohol. Producers of alcohol products are also diverse; they may produce wine, beer, or spirits and do not necessarily share the same strategies or goals in the sale of their products. The producers, especially those who are national in scope, politically oppose state and national legislation that can affect the sales of alcohol. This is especially true when increases to excise taxes are being discussed at the national or state level. Although wine is popularly associated with moderate consumption and food, low-quality wine distributed by the larger producers is often mixed with juices and sweeteners to increase sales, especially among youth. Beer, historically, has been the beverage of choice (and abuse) by youth and young adults and has increased in popularity in recent years as sales of spirits have declined.

The alcohol industry has been historically opposed to any public policy restrictions on alcohol advertising, especially in mass media. Nevertheless, for a number of years, the liquor industry upheld a voluntary ban on the advertising of spirits. This ban has ended in recent years as spirits sales have diminished.

The options for the alcohol industry as participants in public policy discussions are somewhat handicapped by the large consumption of alcohol by a relatively few customers *and* by the fact that almost any policy designed to reduce alcohol problems is likely to result in lower potential sales and profits. The segment of the alcohol industry that appears to have the greatest potential for positive participation in public policy (at the local level) is local alcohol retailers. Overselling and overserving by retail outlets can lower their acceptance in the community but also (and especially importantly) reduce the sales and profits of more responsible outlets. Thus, even though local regulations and enforcement can potentially reduce sales, some owners and managers of licensed establishments are (and have been) willing to participate in local policy prevention efforts, including those described previously.

The Public Health and Safety Community

Many organizations and agencies have an interest in the health and safety aspects of alcohol problems. The use of local public health policy approaches to reduce alcohol-related harms is not naturally limited to a specific target group or service group and, as such, loses some of the public advocacy that can be associated with special concerns (e.g., Children of Alcoholics or AA). There is a large treatment and recovery segment concerned with individual dependent drinkers that provides recovery opportunities for these persons in most communities.

Organizations and support groups such as AA concerned with recovery have historically stayed out of public policy discussions and, in some instances, have dismissed such efforts because their perspective is that alcoholism and dependency are like a disease and there is little that prevention can do. However, over the past 30 years, numerous organizations and agencies have been established with the goal to reduce alcohol-related problems in states and communities. One key example of such an organization is Mothers Against Drunk Driving (MADD), which began as a victims' advocacy group of people who had lost a family member to a drunk-driving crash. Over time, this unique focus has been expanded, and MADD has become an active participant in national and state legislation that establishes public policy directed at reducing alcohol problems. Examples of such legislation include creating incentives for each state to raise its minimum drinking or alcohol purchase age to 21 for all beverages, lowering the legal BAC for drinking and driving, and establishing a very low BAC limit for drivers younger than age 21.

Over the past 20 years, in response to federal and state funding and other incentives and the support of nongovernmental agencies such as Community Anti-Drug Coalitions of America (CADCA), a significant percentage of communities have established working groups or **coalitions** of people interested in reducing alcohol and other drug problems. Such groups can become an essential foundation for future public policy approaches, but they face the challenge of selecting and supporting the approaches with the best research evidence of potential effects.

At the local level, however, policy or environmental strategies have at least two major difficulties. First, they are often controversial and thus politically difficult to implement. Political will and public support are required for such strategies. Second, policy strategies often do not provide the level of immediate public attention or evidence of success or even satisfaction

and personal reward to program staff that educational or service strategies provide. This can mean that environmentally focused policy strategies may not be as attractive to everyone, especially volunteers.

Community-action projects that make specific use of public policy are intended to address the total community system and require local leadership in designing, implementing, and supporting effective policies. Although local alcohol policy strategies have the greatest potential to be effective when they draw on scientific evidence, many community prevention projects involve interventions that research has indicated are unlikely to reduce the population level of local alcohol problems. Public education efforts designed to increase community knowledge and change attitudes are focused on information alone and carry the assumption that an informed community will necessarily experience a reduction in alcohol problems. No research supports the effectiveness of public education strategies alone, but public education could be used to increase support for policy strategies.

Public Policymakers

Public policymakers have a major role in establishing and supporting alcohol policies. Local visibility of enforcement and maintenance of policies are essential to effectiveness and are key aspects of effective local policies. Many strategies that involve restricting retail or social access to substances have little or only modest effects without deterrence or a public sense of potential for detection and consequences. Federal as well as state laws (e.g., governing the legal alcohol purchase or drinking age, licensing of alcohol outlets, the legal BAC for drinking and driving) often serve as the foundations for local policies. Local governments, in turn, are responsible for implementing and enforcing these laws. The relative emphasis that local police departments give to different enforcement is an example of the kind of administrative policy decision that is made locally, often in the face of competing demands for limited police resources.

As a legal product, alcohol often enjoys unique status among potentially abusable substances. Since tobacco has in recent years achieved a negative status even as a legal drug, alcohol and its retail sale are sometimes viewed with less concern than tobacco by elected officials. For example, the alcohol industry at all levels is a major employer and contributes to local, state, and federal tax income, and elected officials often view it politically from such perspectives. Thus, in discussions of public policy, policymakers are confronted with supporting potential regulations or restrictions on alcohol that are opposed by the alcohol industry but supported by the public health and safety community. The challenge for policymakers is to become more informed about the actual cost to government and the community of alcohol abuse and to evaluate the potential cost savings of reducing alcohol problems, cost savings that can result from effective public policy. The difficulty with this cost approach is that such cost savings are not easily experienced or measured by public agencies and that reduced alcohol sales result in reduced state and federal excise tax income and sales taxes from alcohol retail sales.

One of the challenges faced by policymakers and policy approaches that are effective in restricting access to alcohol is the potential substitution of another abusable substance. As access to one substance is limited (e.g., tobacco or alcohol), other substances may be substituted. The most important downside to raising alcohol taxes is the possibility of alternatives to taxed alcoholic beverages, particularly through illegal smuggling or illegal in-country alcohol production. An important empirical question is, What are the effects of higher prices for alcohol on other substances of abuse (e.g., tobacco or marijuana)? Several studies have found that alcohol and tobacco, or marijuana and tobacco, are complements, not necessarily substitutes— that is, use of one may result in greater use of the other (Alter et al. 2006; Chaloupka et al. 1999; Farrelly et al. 2001).

Conclusion

Alcohol and its associated abuse and misuse have been a major part of public discussion and debate for well over 100 years. Efforts to reduce alcohol harm have included public policies to ban the product (e.g., Prohibition) as well as efforts to restrict the product in the interest of public safety and health. The producers, distributors, and retailers of alcohol represent a major economic and political force in most countries in the world. As a result, efforts to restrict the availability of alcohol are often met with political resistance, and elected officials find themselves facing conflicting and competing demands for supporting and implementing efforts to reduce the harm associated with drinking.

The evidence of policy effects, based upon the research cited, has a reasonable level of **generalizability** (what has been shown to be effective in one state or community has a strong potential to have a similar effect elsewhere). One of the attributes of public health policy concerning alcohol is that it is enacted and developed by state and local governments and is not based upon researcher-designed studies. Although alcohol regulation in the United States is largely in the hands of the state government (e.g., the state issues and controls licenses for alcohol sales and sets excise tax levels), communities are able to complement the state policies. This is especially true if the basic elements of minimum enforcement and compliance are maintained. For example, the minimum purchase age by itself has saved many lives. Yet local enforcement of alcohol sales to underage persons clearly affects the total impact of the policy both at the state and the local level.

There are some natural limits and counter-forces that must be addressed or accounted for in implementing public health alcohol policy. With considerable public concern about alcohol problems, especially for youth, comes public support for prevention. However, this public support rests upon existing values in communities and neighborhoods, a fact that is illustrated by differences across states in the existing policies and approaches to adolescent drinking-related problems. Effective implementation of a public policy can be limited by the willingness of community leaders to support effective policies.

In summary, any public health approach to alcohol-involved problems faces the "**prevention paradox**": although alcohol-dependent or alcoholic individuals have the greatest individual risk for alcohol problems, the greatest contribution to total acute alcohol problems in the population arises from persons who are heavy drinkers (but not necessarily dependent drinkers) as well as moderate and light drinkers. This occurs because nondependent drinkers are a much larger part of the population than alcoholics, even if their individual risk is lower. Their risk drinking can be reduced by effective public policy. A much wider public health perspective is essential in approaching alcohol problems on a population level, and policy priorities cannot be based upon treatment or health screening or public education alone.

NOTES

1. See the Federal Trade Commission website, www.ftc.gov/reports/alcohol/appendixb.htm.

REFERENCES

Agostinelli G, Grube J. 2002. Alcohol counter-advertising and the media: A review of recent research. *Alcohol Res Health* 26:15-21.

Alter RJ, Lohrmann DK, Greene R. 2006. Substitution of marijuana for alcohol: The role of perceived access and harm. *J Drug Educ* 36 (4): 335-55.

Argo JJ, Main KJ. 2004. Meta-analyses of the effectiveness of warning labels. *J Public Policy Marketing* 23 (2): 193-209.

Babor T, Caetano R, Casswell S, et al. 2010. *Alcohol: No Ordinary Commodity: Research and Public Policy.* New York: Oxford University Press.

Bouchery EE, Harwood HJ, Sacks JJ, et al. 2011. Economic costs of excessive alcohol consumption in the U.S., 2006. *Am J Prev Med* 41 (5): 516-24.

Cameron M, Diamantopoulou K, Mullan N, Dyte D, Gantzer S. 1997. Evaluation of the country random breath testing and publicity program in Victoria, 1993-1994. Monash University Accident Research Centre, Report 126, Victoria, Australia.

Campbell CA, Hahn RA, Elder R, et al. 2009. The effectiveness of limiting alcohol outlet density as a means of reducing excessive alcohol consumption and alcohol-related harms. *Am J Prev Med* 37 (6) (Dec.): 556-69.

Carpenter CS, Dobkin C. 2007. The effect of alcohol consumption on mortality: Regression discontinuity evidence from the minimum drinking age. NBER Working Paper 13374. National Bureau of Economic Research, Cambridge, MA.

Carpenter CS, Kloska DD, O'Malley P, Johnston L. 2007. Alcohol control policies and youth alcohol consumption: Evidence from 28 years of monitoring the future. *BE J Econ Anal Policy* 7 (1): 1-21.

Chaloupka FJ, Grossman M, Bickel WK, Saffer H. 1999. *The Economic Analysis of Substance Use and Abuse: An Integration of Econometric and Behavioral Economic Research.* Chicago: University of Chicago Press.

Chaloupka FJ, Grossman M, Saffer H. 2002. The effects of price on alcohol consumption and alcohol-related problems. *Alcohol Res Health* 26 (1): 22-34.

Chesson H, Harrison P, Kassler WJ. 2000. Sex under the influence: The effect of alcohol policy on sexually transmitted disease rates in the United States. *J Law Econ* 43 (1): 215-38.

Chikritzhs T, Stockwell T. 2002. The impact of later trading hours for Australian public houses (hotels) on levels of violence. *J Stud Alcohol* 63 (5): 591-99.

———. 2006. The impact of later trading hours for hotels on levels of impaired driver road crashes and driver breath alcohol levels. *Addiction* 101 (9): 1254-64.

Coate D, Grossman M. 1988. Effects of alcoholic beverage prices and legal drinking ages on youth alcohol use. *J Law Econ* 31 (1): 145-71.

Cohen D, Mason K, Scribner R. 2001. The population consumption model, alcohol control practices, and alcohol-related traffic fatalities. *Prev Med* 34:187-97.

Cook PJ. 1981. The effect of liquor taxes on drinking, cirrhosis, and auto accidents. In *Alcohol and Public Policy: Beyond the Shadow of Prohibition,* ed. MH Moore, DR Gerstein, 255-85. Washington, DC: National Academy Press.

———. 2007. *Paying the Tab: The Costs and Benefits of Alcohol Control.* Princeton, NJ: Princeton University Press.

Dang JN. 2008. Statistical analysis of alcohol-related driving trends, 1982-2005. National Highway Traffic Safety Administration, Washington, DC.

Dent CW, Grube JW, Biglan A. 2005. Community level alcohol availability and enforcement of possession laws as predictors of youth drinking. *Prev Med* 40:355-62.

Ditter SM, Elder RW, Shults RA, et al. 2005. Effectiveness of designated driver programs for reducing alcohol-impaired driving: A systematic review. *Am J Prev Med* 28 (suppl. 5): 280-87.

Drummond AE, Sullivan G, Cavallo A. 1992. *An Evaluation of the Random Breath Testing Initiative in Victoria, 1989-1990.* Quasi-experimental time series approach (37). Melbourne, Australia: Monash University Accident Research Centre.

Eisenberg D. 2003. Evaluating the effectiveness of policies related to drunk driving. *J Policy Anal Man* 22 (2): 249-74.

Elder RW, Shults RA, Sleet DA, et al. 2004. Effectiveness of mass media campaigns for reducing drinking and driving and alcohol-involved crashes: A systematic review. *Am J Prev Med* 27 (1): 57-65.

Elder RW, Voas R, Beirness D, et al. 2011. Effectiveness of ignition interlocks for preventing alcohol-impaired driving and alcohol-related crashes: A community guide systematic review. *Am J Prev Med* 40 (3): 362-76.

Farrelly MC, Bray JW, Zarkin GA, Wendling BW. 2001. The joint demand for cigarettes and marijuana: Evidence from the National Household Surveys on Drug Abuse. *Health Econ* 20:51-68.

Finney JW, Hahn AC, Moos RH. 1996 The effectiveness of inpatient and outpatient treatment for alcohol abuse: The need to focus on mediators and moderators of setting effects. *Addiction* 91:1773-96.

Giesbrecht N. 2002 Roles of commercial interests in alcohol policies: Recent developments in North America. *Addiction* 95 (12s4): 581-95.

Greenfield TK, Kaskutas LA. 1998 Five years' exposure to alcohol warning label messages and their impacts: Evidence from diffusion analysis. *Appl Behav Sci Rev* 6:39-68.

Greenfield TK, Giesbrecht N, Johnson SP, et al. 1999 *US Federal Alcohol Control Policy Development: A Manual.* Berkeley, CA: Alcohol Research Group.

Grossman M, Kaestner R, Markowitz S. 2004. An investigation of the effects of alcohol policies on youth STDs. NBER Working Paper, New York.

Grube JW. 1997. Preventing sales of alcohol to minors: Results from a community trial. *Addiction* (suppl. 2), S251-S260.

Grube JW, Nygaard P. 2005. Alcohol policy and youth drinking: Overview of effective interventions for young people. In *Preventing Harmful Substance Use: The Evidence Base for Policy and Practice,* ed. T Stockwell, PJ Gruenewald, JW Toumborou, W. Loxley, 113-127. West Sussex, England: Wiley.

Gruenewald P. 2007. The spatial ecology of alcohol problems: Niche theory and assortative drinking. *Addiction* 102 (6): 870-78.

Gruenewald PJ, Remer L. 2006. Changes in outlet densities affect violence rates. *Alcoholism* 30 (7): 1184-93.

Harrison PA, Fulkerson JA, Maldonado-Molina MM, et al. 2007. Who needs liquor stores when parents will do? The importance of social sources of alcohol among young urban teens. *Prev Med* 44 (6): 471-76.

Her M, Giesbrecht N, Room R, et al. 1999. Privatizing alcohol sales and alcohol consumption: Evidence and implications. *Addiction* 94:1125-39.

Hingson R. 1993. Prevention of alcohol-impaired driving. *Alcohol Health Res World* 17 (1): 28-34.

Hingson RW, Howland J, Levenson S. 1988. Effects of legislature reform to reduce drunken driving and alcohol-related traffic fatalities. *Public Health Rep* 103 (6): 659-67.

Hingson RW, Zakocs RC, Heeren T, Winter MR, Rosenbloom D, DeJong W. 2005. Effects on alcohol related fatal crashes of a community based initiative to increase substance abuse treatment and reduce alcohol availability. *Inj Prev* 11 (2): 84-90.

Holder HD. 1997. Can individually directed interventions reduce population-level alcohol-involved problems? *Addiction* 92 (1) (Jan.): 5-7.

———. 1998. Cost benefits of substance abuse treatment: An overview of results from alcohol and drug abuse. *J Ment Health Policy Econ* 1 (1): 23-29.

Holder HD, Blose JO. 1992. The reduction of health care costs associated with alcoholism treatment: A 14-year longitudinal study. *J Stud Alcohol* 53 (4) (July): 293-302.

Holder HD, Parker RN. 1992. Effect of alcoholism treatment on cirrhosis mortality: A 20-year multivariate time series analysis. *Br J Addict* 87 (9) (Sept.): 1263-74.

Holder HD, Wagenaar AC. 1990. Effects of the elimination of a state monopoly on distilled spirits' retail sales: A time-series analysis of Iowa. *Br J Addict* 85 (12) (Dec.): 1615-25.

———. 1994. Mandated server training and reduced alcohol-involved traffic crashes: A time series analysis of the Oregon experience. *Accident Anal Prev* 26 (1): 89-97.

Homel R. 1990. Random breath testing and random stopping programs in Australia. In *Drinking and*

Driving: Advances in Research and Prevention, ed. RJ Wilson, RE Mann, 159-202. New York: Guilford Press.

Kelly-Baker T, Johnson MB, Voas R, et al. 2000. To reduce youthful binge drinking: Call an election in Mexico. *J Safety Res* 31 (2): 61-69.

Kranzler HR, Van Kirk J. 2001 Naltrexone and acamprosate in the treatment of alcoholism: A meta-analysis. *Alcoholism* 25:1335-41.

Little B, Bishop M. 1998. Minor drinkers/ major consequences: Enforcement strategies for underage alcoholic beverage violators. *Impaired Driv Update* 2 (6):88.

Livingston M. 2008. A longitudinal analysis of alcohol outlet density and assault. *Alcoholism* 32 (6): 1074-79.

Markowitz S, Grossman M. 2000. The effects of beer taxes on physical child abuse. *J Health Econ* 19 (2): 271-82.

Markowitz S, Kaestner R, Grossman M. 2005. An investigation of the effects of alcohol consumption and alcohol policies on youth risky sexual behaviors. *Am Econ Rev* 95 (2) (May): 263-66.

McCarthy PS. 2003. Effects of alcohol and highway speed policies on motor vehicle crashes involving older drivers. *J Transport Statist* 6 (2-3): 51-65.

Mercer G. 1985. The relationship among driving while impaired charges, police drinking-driving checkpoint activity, media coverage, and alcohol-related casualty traffic accidents. *Accident Anal Prev* 17 (6): 467-74.

Miller T, Snowden C, Birckmayer J. et al. 2006. Retail alcohol monopolies, underage drinking, and youth impaired driving deaths. *Accident Anal Prev* 38 (6): 1162-67.

National Highway Traffic Safety Administration (NHTSA). 1998. *Traffic Safety Facts, 1997.* Washington, DC: U.S. Government Printing Office.

Nelson J. 2003. Advertising bans, monopoly, and alcohol demand: Testing for substitution effects using state panel data. *Rev Industr Org* 22:1-25.

Ohsfeldt RL, Morrisey MA. 1997. Beer taxes, workers' compensation, and industrial injury. *Rev Econ Statist* 79 (1): 155-60.

Ouimette PC, Finney JW, Gima K, Moos RH. 1999 A comparative evaluation of substance abuse treatment: Examining mechanisms underlying patient-treatment matching hypotheses for 12-step and cognitive-behavioral treatments for substance abuse. *Alcoholism* 23:545-51.

Paschall MJ, Grube JW, Black C, Flewelling RL, Ringwalt CL, Biglan A. 2007. Alcohol outlet characteristics and alcohol sales to youth: Results of alcohol purchase surveys in 45 Oregon communities. *Prev Science* 8:153-59.

Paschall MJ, Grube JW, Black C, Ringwalt CL. 2007. Is commercial alcohol availability related to adolescent alcohol sources and alcohol use? Findings from a multi-level study. *J Adolesc Health* 41:168-74.

Ponicki WR, Gruenewald PJ, LaScala EA. 2007. Joint impacts of minimum legal drinking age and beer taxes on US youth traffic fatalities, 1975 to 2001. *Alcoholism* 31 (5): 804-13.

Preusser DF, Williams AF, Zador RD, Blomberg PL. 1984. The effect of curfew laws on motor vehicle crashes. *Law Policy* 6:115-28.

Radecki T. 1993. *Compliance Checks and Other Enforcement Methods to Deter Underage Drinking.* Rockville, MD: U.S. Department of Health and Human Services, Center for Substance Abuse Prevention.

Ross HL. 1988a. Deterrence-based policies in Britain, Canada, and Australia. In *The Social Control of the Drinking Driver*, ed. M Laurence, JR Snortum, FE Zimring, 64-78. Chicago: University of Chicago Press.

———. 1988b. Editorial: British drink-driving policy. *Br J Addict* 83:863-65.

Ross HL, Gilliland EM. 1991. *Administrative License Revocation for Drunk Drivers: Options and Choices in Three States.* Washington, DC: AAA Foundation for Traffic Safety.

Ruhm CJ. 1996. Alcohol policies and highway vehicle fatalities. *J Health Econ* 15 (4): 435-54.

Saffer H, Dhaval D. 2002. Alcohol consumption and alcohol advertising bans. *Appl Econ* 5:1325-34.

Saffer H, Grossman M. 1987. Beer taxes, the legal drinking age, and youth motor vehicle fatalities. *J Legal Stud* 16 (2): 351-74.

Scribner RA, Cohen DA. 2001. The effect of enforcement on merchant compliance with the minimum legal drinking age law. *J Drug Issues* 31:857-66.

Sen B. 2006. The relationship between beer taxes, other alcohol policies, and child homicide deaths. *Topics Econ Anal Policy* 6 (1): 1-17.

Shults RA, Elder RW, Nichols JL, et al. 2009. Effectiveness of multicomponent programs with community mobilization for reducing alcohol-impaired driving. *Am J Prev Med* 37 (4): 360-71.

Shults RA, Elder RW, Sleet DA, et al. 2001. Reviews of evidence regarding interventions to reduce alcohol-impaired driving. *Am J Prev Med* 21 (4S): 66-88.

Sivarajasingam V, Matthews K, Shepherd J. 2006. Price of beer and violence-related injury in England and Wales. *Injury* 37 (5): 388-94.

Snyder LB, Milici FF, Slater M, Sun H, Strizhakova Y. 2006. Effects of alcohol advertising exposure on drinking among youth. *Arch Pediatr Adolesc Med* 160:18-24.

Stockwell T, Chikritzhs T. 2009 Do relaxed trading hours for bars and clubs mean more relaxed drinking? A review of international research on the impacts of changes to permitted hours of drinking. *Crime Prev Commun Safety* 11 (3): 153-70.

Stockwell T, Gruenewald P. 2001 Controls on the physical availability of alcohol. In *International Handbook of Alcohol Dependence and Problems,* ed. N Heather, TJ Peters, T Stockwell, 699-720. New York: Wiley.

Stout EM, Sloan FA, Liang L, Davies HH. 2000. Reducing harmful alcohol-related behaviors: Effective regulatory methods. *J Stud Alcohol* 61 (3): 402-12.

Task Force on Community Preventive Services (TFCPS). 2009. Recommendations for reducing excessive alcohol-related harms by limiting alcohol outlet density. *Am J Prev Med* 37 (6) (Dec.): 570-71.

———. 2010. Increasing alcoholic beverage taxes is recommended to reduce excessive alcohol consumption and related harms. *Am J Prev Med* 38 (2) (Feb.): 230-32.

Toomey TL, Fabian LEA, Erickson DJ, Lenk KM. 2007. Propensity for obtaining alcohol through shoulder tapping. *Alcoholism* 31 (7): 1218-23.

Treno A, Grube J, Martin SE. 2003. Alcohol availability as a predictor of youth drinking and driving: A hierarchical analysis of survey and archival data. *Alcoholism* 27 (5): 835-40.

Treno AJ, Gruenewald PJ, Johnson FW, et al. 2000. The geographic distribution of the service of alcoholic beverages to intoxicated and underage patrons: Implications for policy at the local level. Paper presented at the Annual Meetings of the Research Society on Addiction, Denver, CO, June 24-29.

Trolldal B. 2005. An investigation of the effects of privatization of retail sales of alcohol on consumption and traffic accidents in Alberta, Canada. *Addiction* 100:662-71.

Vingilis E, Coultes B. 1990. Mass communications and drinking-driving: Theories, practices, and results. *Alcohol, Drugs, Driving* 6 (2): 61-81.

Vingilis E, McLeod AI, Seeley J, Mann R, Beirness D, Compton C. 2005. Road safety impact of extended drinking hours in Ontario. *Accident Anal Prev* 37 (3): 549-56.

Vingilis E, McLeod AI, Stoduto G, Seeley J, Mann RE. 2007. Impact of extended drinking hours in Ontario on motor-vehicle collision and non-motor-vehicle collision injuries. *J Stud Alcohol Drugs* 68 (6): 905-11.

Voas RB, DeYoung DJ. 2002. Vehicle action: Effective policy for controlling drunk and other high-risk drivers? *Accident Anal Prev* 34:263-70.

Voas RB, Lange JE, Tippetts SA. 1998. Enforcement of the zero tolerance law in California: A missed opportunity? In *42nd Annual Proceedings of the Association for the Advancement of Automotive Medicine,*

369-383. Charlottesville, VA: Association for the Advancement of Automotive Medicine.

Voas RB, Tippetts AS, Fell JC. 2003. Assessing the effectiveness of minimum legal drinking age and zero tolerance laws in the United States. *Accident Anal Prev* 35 (4): 579-87.

Wagenaar AC, Finnegan JR, Wolfson M, Anstine PS, Williams CL, Perry CL. 1993. Where and how adolescents obtain alcoholic beverages. *Public Health Rep* 108 (4): 45964.

Wagenaar AC, Maldonado-Molina MM, Wagenaar BH. 2009. Effects of alcohol tax increases on alcohol-related disease mortality in Alaska: Time-series analyses from 1976 to 2004. *Am J Public Health* 99 (1): 1-8.

Wagenaar AC, Murray DM, Toomey, TL 2000. Communities mobilizing for change on alcohol: Outcomes from a randomized community trial. *J Stud Alcohol* 51 (1): 85-94. Wagenaar AC, O'Malley PM, LaFond C. 2001. Lowered legal blood alcohol limits for young drivers: Effects on drinking, driving, and driving-after-drinking behaviors in 30 states. *Am J Public Health* 91 (5): 801-4.

Wagenaar A, Salois M, Komro K. 2009. Effects of beverage alcohol price and tax levels on drinking: A meta-analysis of 1003 estimates from 112 studies. *Addiction* 104:179-90.

Wagenaar AC, Toomey TL. 2002. Effects of minimum drinking age laws: Review and analyses of the literature from 1960 to 2000. *J Stud Alcohol* (suppl. 14): 206-25.

Wagenaar AC, Toomey TL, Erickson DJ. 2005a. Complying with the minimum drinking age: Effects of enforcement and training interventions. *Alcohol* 29 (3): 255-62.

———. 2005b. Preventing youth access to alcohol: Outcomes from a multi-community time-series trial. *Addiction* 100 (3): 335-45.

Wallin E, Norstrom T, Andreasson S. 2003. Alcohol prevention targeting licensed premises: A study of effects on violence. *J Stud Alcohol* 64 (2): 270-77.

Weitzman ER, Folkman A, Folkman KL, Wechsler H. 2003. The relationship of alcohol outlet density to heavy and frequent drinking and drinking-related problems among college students at eight universities. *Health Place* 9 (1): 1-6.

Whetten-Goldstein K, Sloan FA, Stout EM, Liang L. 2000. Civil liability, criminal law, and other policies and alcohol-related motor vehicle fatalities in the United States, 1984-1995. *Accident Anal Prev* 32 (6): 723-33.

Whitlock EP, Polen MR, Green CA, Orleans T, Klein J, U.S. Preventive Services Task Force. 2004. Behavioral counseling interventions in primary care to reduce risky/harmful alcohol use by adults: A summary of the evidence for the U.S. Preventive Services Task Force. *Ann Intern Med* 140 (7): 557-68.

Williams A, Lund A, Preusser D. 1984. Night driving curfews in New York and Louisiana: Results of a questionnaire survey. Insurance Institute for Highway Safety, Washington, DC.

Wolfson M, Toomey TL, Forster JL, Wagenaar AC, McGovern PG, Perry CL. 1996. Characteristics, policies, and practices of alcohol outlets and sales to underage persons. *J Stud Alcohol* 57 (6): 670-74.

Wolfson M, Toomey TL, Murray DM, Forster JL, Short BJ, Wagenaar AC. 1996. Alcohol outlet policies and practices concerning sales to underage people. *Addiction* 91 (4): 589-602.

Zador P, Lund A, Fields M, Weinberg K. 1989. Fatal crash involvement and laws against alcohol-impaired driving. *J Public Health Policy* 10:467-85.

Substance Abuse
and Behavior Change

ERIC C. STRAIN AND D. ANDREW TOMPKINS

LEARNING OBJECTIVES

After completing the chapter, the reader will be able to

* Describe for the United States the prevalence of illicit substance use by individuals age 12 and older.
* Characterize the economic cost of illicit drug use for the United States.
* Identify at least one individual-level, one interpersonal-level, and one community-level factor that affects the risk for using or not using an illicit drug.
* Identify at least three different medications that can be used to treat a substance use disorder.
* Identify an environmental-level intervention that can decrease the risk of people engaging in substance abuse.

Introduction

The misuse of psychoactive substances and the **consequences** of that misuse are not new phenomena. They are noted in the Old Testament of the Bible:

> Who has woe? Who has sorrow? Who has strife? Who has complaints? Who has needless bruises? Who has bloodshot eyes? Those who linger over wine, who go to sample bowls of mixed wine. Do not gaze at wine when it is red, when it sparkles in the cup, when it goes down smoothly! In the end it bites like a snake and poisons like a viper. Your eyes will see strange sights, and your mind imagine confusing things. You will be like one sleeping on the high seas, lying on top of the rigging. "They hit me," you will say, "but I'm not hurt! They beat me, but I don't feel it! When will I wake up so I can find another drink?" (Proverbs 23:29-35, New International Version)

Despite the long history of substance misuse, social perceptions of the nature of drug use have remained an area of controversy even in the past 100 years. At various times various proponents have seen it as a moral weakness, a medical disease (such as diabetes), a legal problem, a need for self-medication (for painful affects or to address earlier life experiences), and a character flaw, among other perspectives. In some instances, advocates have sought to understand *why* a person uses a substance, as a necessary step toward stopping the use, while in other instances advocates have cared little about why a person uses and have focused primarily on the *consequences* of the use. In still other cases, some have viewed substance use as a social judgment that would be alleviated simply by removing restrictions on access and use.

In keeping with the overall theme of this book, this chapter looks at substance use from the perspective of behavior in its ecological **context**. While there are valuable reasons for doing so, it is also important to note that some see substance misuse as a disease (most notably, individuals who have found benefit from attending self-help programs, such as Alcoholics Anonymous or related groups). The view of drug misuse as a disease has clearly benefited hundreds of thousands who have suffered from these disorders, and the goal of this chapter is not to argue that this approach is wrong. Rather, the term *disease* in this case is being used in a broad sense—that is, similar to the term *illness*. While medical professionals consider *disease* to have a specific meaning and use it in this precise way, *disease* can also have a more general lay use that serves the needs of many people who suffer from addictive disorders.

Description and Definitions of Problem Behavior

Various approaches have been used to define problematic substance use and to identify typologies of misuse (most commonly for alco-

holics). Perhaps one of the earliest and most commonly identified among such approaches is the one proposed by E. M. Jellinek in his book *The Disease Concept of Alcoholism* (1960), although this was neither the first (nor the last) effort to define problematic drinking. Jellinek's work created five different typologies of alcoholism (alpha, beta, gamma, delta, and epsilon), although these categories have generally not been sustained in research or clinical practice and have primarily historical interest today. However, the concept of alcoholism as a medical condition that could be identified and characterized was perpetuated, and a classic paper by Edwards and Gross, titled "Alcohol Dependence: Provisional Description of a Clinical Syndrome," provided a set of seven elements that were thought to cluster as a syndrome in those who had alcoholism: (1) a narrowing in the repertoire of drinking behavior, (2) salience of drink-seeking behavior, (3) increased tolerance to alcohol, (4) repeated withdrawal symptoms, (5) repeated relief or avoidance of withdrawal symptoms by further drinking, (6) subjective awareness of a compulsion to drink, and (7) reinstatement of the syndrome after abstinence (Edwards and Gross 1976). An attractive feature of these elements for clinicians is that they are not culturally or socially based; there is not, for example, an element that is based upon having legal problems associated with alcohol use (which could vary over time as definitions of intoxicated blood levels varied, or could vary from one geographical region to another, or could depend upon the particular local laws). However, several elements are dimensional in nature (i.e., they can vary along a continuum), and the problem with dimensional elements is defining where along a dimension the individual has achieved an element (e.g., when does the repertoire become narrowed?). This can become a subjective decision; there may not be agreement across settings or clinicians.

The Edwards and Gross paper clearly influenced the subsequent editions of the American

Psychiatric Association's Diagnostic and Statistical Manual (*DSM-III, IIIR, IV, IV-TR,* and *5*) in its sections on substance use disorders. The current *DSM-5* definition of substance use disorder (SUD) has a set of criteria that represent a combining of the abuse and dependence diagnoses used in *DSM-IV-TR* (along with an item regarding craving). It also specifically states that at least two of the 11 are needed to qualify for a diagnosis of SUD, and it varies the severity depending upon the number of criteria fulfilled (i.e., mild, moderate, severe).

In part, the shift in *DSM-5* away from the term *dependence* as a diagnosis in *DSM* reflects the potential for confusion between physical dependence and syndromic dependence. The former is generally viewed as a state of physiological adaptation that occurs with repeated exposure to a substance and is generally indicated by tolerance and/or withdrawal; for example, the person who takes opioid analgesics each day for cancer pain. While such a person could manifest opioid withdrawal signs and symptoms with abrupt cessation of use (e.g., forgetting pain medicine when going out shopping), generally such patients are not thought to have problematic or pathological use of the substance. On the other hand, *syndromic* dependence is problematic use. Confusion can arise because physical dependence (tolerance, withdrawal) is a feature of syndromic dependence. However, physical dependence is neither necessary nor sufficient for a diagnosis of syndromic dependence. The dropping of the diagnosis of dependence in *DSM-5* has helped to rectify this confusion.

However, the ambiguous use of terms in the field of substance abuse is a recurring problem. Indeed, references to "substance abuse" have caused difficulties in recent years, given the definition of an abuse diagnosis in *DSM-IV-TR* versus the lay sense of abuse as a catchall term to indicate some form of problematic use. Other phrases, such as *methadone detoxification* (implying that methadone is a toxin), and *recreational use* (often linked to cannabis use, which is then

seen as analogous to activities such as after-school sports or clubs), are also problematic.

Thus, defining abnormal use of a substance is difficult. Most people exposed to a substance do not develop some form of problematic use. But some do, and efforts to identify those individuals in a unique and defining way continue. Clearly, physical dependence upon a substance does not mean that the person has pathologic use—as illustrated by the patient with cancer who is on opioid pain medications and develops physical dependence but otherwise has no evidence of problematic use. Culturally based definitions of problematic use are no more effective. Diagnosing as an alcoholic the person who is caught driving while intoxicated (or under the influence of alcohol) is hardly effective for a community where few people drive or for a wealthy athlete who simply has an assistant to drive him home from the party. Quantity or frequency of use certainly can be helpful when screening patients for problematic use, but the person who limits drinking to the weekend may still have significant problems associated with use despite infrequent rates of use, as does the person who uses cocaine only on the weekends but spends excessive amounts of money on the drug for a time limited period.

Craving has been proposed as a defining feature of problematic use. Although craving has an intuitive attraction—the idea that a person develops an overwhelming hunger for a substance—a problem with craving is that studies with simple approaches to measuring it (e.g., visual analog scales) have generally not found craving particularly useful. More complicated assessments of craving have been developed and can have value in the study of craving and its psychological features and components. Such assessments have limited use in clinical settings, although this is an area that may still prove fruitful in the future.

Finally, another potential approach to defining problematic use is to say the person demonstrating pathological use of a substance has lost control of choice, what can be called **dysregulation of choice**. The idea that substance use disorders are *disorders of choice* has attractive features. It moves the definition away from an internal state (i.e., craving) and focuses upon the action of interest, which is the behavior of consumption. The act of using a substance is a choice for the person. Adults who drink alcohol can choose to drink, but the person who does not have problematic use may choose to not drink (e.g., she is the designated driver for the evening). In contrast, the person who has pathologic use of a substance feels he has lost the ability to choose whether to use the substance. Choice also highlights that these disorders ultimately have some volitional component, and it places them within their settings, the surrounding physical and **social environments**.

Magnitude: The Public Health Burden of Substance Use Disorders

Estimates of the extent of substance abuse vary by geographical regions of the world, and some countries and regions have more sophisticated assessment methods than do other regions. In addition, some national assessments of substance use are probably better understood in terms of changes over time, rather than valid snapshots of use for a particular year.

The United States has conducted essentially annual national assessments of drug use for more than 30 years. For many years, these were called the National Household Survey on Drug Abuse, but in 2002 the title of the reports was changed to the National Survey on Drug Use and Health (NSDUH). The most recent survey results as the time of this writing are from 2011, and they report that 22.5 million adolescents and adults (age 12 and older, 8.7%) had used an illicit drug in the previous month, 15.9 million (6.2% of the population age 12 and older) had engaged in heavy drinking (defined as binge drinking on at least five days out of the past 30, with a binge defined as five or more drinks on

an occasion of drinking), and 68.2 million were tobacco users (26.5% of the population age 12 and older) (SAMHSA 2012). While cannabis continued to be the most common illicit drug used in the past month, the second most commonly used illicit drug was psychotherapeutics (e.g., misuse of prescription opioids)—something that has clearly become a substantial problem in the United States. Interestingly, the NSDUH provides evidence of increasing rates of drug use by older individuals (ages 55–59), suggesting that the aging baby boomer population could influence substance abuse treatment services (Lofwall et al. 2008).

The European Union also conducts assessments of drug use in its member countries through the European Monitoring Centre for Drugs and Drug Addiction (EMCDDA). For 2009, the EMCDDA reported that 12 million people had used cannabis in the past month (3.6% of individuals age 15 and older), 1.5 million had used cocaine (0.4% of the population age 15 and older), and about the same number were users of opioids (approximately 1.4 million) (EMCDDA 2009). The prevalence of smoking tobacco in the EU varies widely between countries, but overall it is approximately 28% for individuals age 15 and older.[1] The prevalence of alcohol use disorders also varies considerably across countries of the EU, although less variability occurs among countries in the average volumes consumed. Nevertheless, prevalence rates in the past 12 months for an alcohol use disorder among men have been estimated to be 6.1%, and for women 1.1%, for EU countries (Rehm et al. 2005).

Australia also conducts periodic national assessments of drug use (AIHW 2008). Interestingly, different ages are used in the reports by the United States, the EU, and Australia: age 12 and older in the United States, age 15 and older in the EU, and age 14 and older in Australia. Also, Australia differs by primarily reporting past-year use, rather than past-month use. For 2007 in Australia, past-year tobacco use occurred in 19.4% of individuals, alcohol use in 82.9%, and cannabis use in 9.1%. Past-year cocaine use was reported by 1.6%, methamphetamine use by 2.3%, and heroin use by 0.2%. Of the Australia population, 13.4% used any illicit drug in the past year.

Although rates of drug use vary across countries, some general themes arise. For example, *licit* drugs (alcohol, tobacco) have much higher rates of use than do *illicit* drugs. Among illicit drugs, cannabis has a high rate of use, and heroin tends to have a low rate of use. And there is evidence (especially in the United States, but in other developed countries as well) of a growing problem with prescription drug misuse—especially misuse of opioids (Birnbaum et al. 2006; SAMHSA 2012; Strassels 2009). However, rates of use of drugs provide only one perspective on the magnitude of substance abuse. The costs and burdens of drug use also should be considered when assessing the impact of drug abuse.

The magnitude of the public health burden of substance abuse disorders can be considered several different ways, including the impact on crime, lost employment, secondary acute and chronic physical effects, and social disruption. Various assessments are periodically conducted to measure the extent of substance use and its impact, and the recurring conclusion is that substance use disorders produce an immense effect on public health.

For example, the Global Burden of Disease study found that worldwide, two of the top five leading causes of disease were related to substance abuse: tobacco (fourth) and alcohol use (fifth) (Ezzati et al. 2002; Rehm et al. 2006). In developed regions of the world, tobacco use was the top cause of disease, alcohol use was the third-most-common cause, and illicit drug use was the eighth leading cause. (In developing regions of the world, alcohol was the top cause and tobacco was the third cause.)

In the United States, the federal Office of National Drug Control Policy (ONDCP) estimated that in 2002 the cost associated with drug abuse (not including alcohol and tobacco use) was $180.9 billion, an increase from $107.6 billion in 1992. The majority of this cost was related to lost productivity (71.2%), followed by health care (8.7%) and other costs (20.1%). The rate of increase for substance-abuse-related health care costs generally was lower than that for overall health care cost increases between 1992 and 2002 (but it totaled nearly $16 billion in 2002). Finally, other costs included dollars devoted to the criminal justice system and crime victim and social welfare system costs. As noted by the ONDCP in this report, the costs for drug abuse are comparable to those reported for other major disease entities, such as heart disease ($183.1 billion in 1999) and cancer ($96.1 billion in 1990) (ONDCP 2004).

While rates of use and the economic impact of such use can be quantified in various reports, surveys, and studies, we should note that substance abuse affects the individual, the family, and the community in ways that may not be fully captured by various dollar amounts. These are disorders that disrupt lives—they lead to problems in the person's emotional, physical, social, and spiritual life. Persons struggling with substance abuse run a high risk of losing relationships with family and friends, they often lose their ability to work, and they become a burden to our communities. We must recognize that these effects are real, they are highly disruptive, and they create problems that extend beyond the struggles of the person who uses a drug. At the level of the individual, the magnitude of drug use can be immense, and not uncommonly, a person's drug use becomes the organizing feature of her life.

Key Determinants

The initiation of use of a substance can be governed by factors inside the individual as well as external factors, such as the social and physical environment. Likewise, continued use is a function of both internal and external factors, although the profile of such factors may vary as a function of initiation versus maintenance of use (e.g., physical dependence on a substance may maintain use but does not contribute to initiation of use).

No single factor explains why a person uses a substance or why a person who tries a substance develops problematic use. As with other **complex** lifestyle health problems, attempts to arrive at a single explanation for substance abuse are inherently simplistic and, more importantly, ineffective in helping to prevent the start of use or to halt ongoing use. Indeed, even more textured efforts to prevent use may overlook important **determinants** of use. For example, an effort that comprehensively and longitudinally addresses alcohol use through a school-based program may be ineffective if a strong genetic vulnerability to alcohol dependence exists, and if a child's parents encourage alcohol use in the home. However, a growing body of evidence suggests what can be effective in mitigating substance use, and data from alcohol and tobacco studies can be informative when considering approaches for illicit drug use.

Individual-Level Factors

Not all people who try a drug go on to develop problematic use of it. For example, findings from the NSDUH have shown that for most drug classes, less than half of the individuals who used a drug in the past year have a *DSM-IV* substance use disorder for that drug (SAMHSA 2005). (The exception is heroin, for which approximately two-thirds have a *DSM-IV* abuse or dependence diagnosis for opioids.) **Individual-level factors** that may contribute to problematic use of a substance include genetics, demographic characteristics, the affective reaction, physical dependence, associated disorders, and behavioral factors.

GENETICS

Studies have shown that genetic vulnerabilities influence substance use (Agrawal and Lynskey

2008). Alcohol use disorders tend to run in families. Sons of male alcoholics show a particular propensity to be at increased risk for developing alcoholism. There is also evidence of genetic vulnerabilities for use of other types of drugs, such as nicotine and even caffeine (Bierut 2010; Pedersen 1981; Swan et al. 1997), both of which are more likely to be used by twins. Genetic vulnerability to alcohol misuse is generally estimated to be about 50% (Schuckit 2009), and evidence links genetic variations in the serotonin transporter to alcohol dependence (McHugh et al. 2010) and also variations in the mu opioid receptor, which might predict an alcoholic's treatment response to the opioid antagonist naltrexone (Anton et al. 2008). However, genetics do not dictate drug use (i.e., not all sons of alcoholics are destined to be alcoholics), and environmental factors can certainly influence use (Kendler et al. 2008).

DEMOGRAPHICS

Demographic features can also be associated with *illicit* drug use, although such associations should certainly not be interpreted as **causations**. In general, males are more likely than females to use illicit drugs : 11.1% versus 6.5% for current illicit drug use, according to the 2011 NSDUH, although, over the past several years, the gap between males and females seems to be growing smaller. Current illicit drug use also varies among races, with the lowest rate for Asians (3.8%), then Hispanics (8.4%), then whites (8.7%), then African Americans (10.0%); individuals with two or more races have the highest rate (13.5%). Current illicit drug use by individuals age 18 and older also varies as a function of educational experience, with the lowest rates for college graduates (5.4%), followed by high school graduates (8.9%), people who have some college (10.4%), and those who are not high school graduates (11.1%). Finally, there are higher rates of current illicit drug use in individuals who are unemployed (17.2%), than in those employed part time (11.6%) or full time (8.0%) (SAMHSA 2012).

The pattern of demographic features associated with illicit drug use is not the same as that seen for alcohol use. For example, although overall rates of any alcohol use are generally higher in males versus females, in some groups (e.g., 12-17-year-olds), rates of use by males and females are now identical (13.3%), which is a change from historically higher rates in young males. Whites tend to have the highest rates of alcohol use and the highest (or nearly the highest) rates of binge and heavy alcohol use. And higher rates of use tend to be associated with more education and being employed (SAMHSA 2012).

AFFECTIVE REACTION

Another important individual-level factor that can contribute to drug use is the affective (or emotional) reaction the person has to that substance. An individual tends to use substances that produce subjectively good feelings for him. Numerous human laboratory studies have shown that the acute effects of opioids produce subjectively good effects in those with opioid use disorders (e.g., Comer et al. 2005; Stoops et al. 2010; Strain et al. 2000), as is the case with other drugs of abuse, such as cocaine. However, studies also show that individuals without a history of abuse of a substance (e.g., opioids) generally do not report positive effects associated with that drug (e.g., Azorlosa et al. 1994; Zacny and Gutierrez 2009), although there can be considerable variability between individuals in their response to an opioid (Zacny 2003).

Caffeine is a good model for this point regarding the relationship between the use of a substance and the effect it produces. Although most people experience the acute effects of caffeine as positive and mildly stimulating, individuals with anxiety disorders tend to experience caffeine as anxiety-provoking and aversive (Boulenger et al. 1984; Bruce et al. 1992), and evidence shows that anxiety-prone groups tend to avoid caffeine use (Boulenger and Uhde 1982; Boulenger et al. 1984; Lee et al. 1988). Users of a substance tend to develop a desire for that particular substance; commonly, they avoid other drugs in favor of their preferred one.

PHYSICAL DEPENDENCE

In addition to the effects produced by the substance, continued use of a substance can be driven by physical dependence upon the substance. For some substances, withdrawal from the substance can be extremely uncomfortable (e.g., opioids) or even life threatening (e.g., alcohol, benzodiazepines). However, as noted earlier in this chapter, physical dependence upon a substance is neither necessary nor sufficient to consider a person addicted to it. Conversely, medically supervised withdrawal from a substance, such as alcohol or an opioid (e.g., heroin), is less successful as a stand-alone treatment for the addicted person than are more comprehensive and enduring forms of treatment.

ASSOCIATED DISORDERS

Non-substance-use psychiatric disorders can also be associated with use of a drug. Although some patients will report to a clinician that they use a drug such as heroin or alcohol to help with an underlying depression (hence, what such a person thinks is needed is an antidepressant, not necessarily to stop the drug use), depressive symptoms commonly improve with abstinence from a drug (Brown and Schuckit 1988; Strain et al. 1991). However, other psychiatric disorders may be associated with drug use, and among these, antisocial personality disorder (APD) is particularly likely to be found at higher than expected rates among individuals with illicit drug use disorders (Brooner et al. 1997).

Although APD is associated with substance use, not all individuals with APD have a substance use disorder; likewise, many individuals with substance use do not have APD. Indeed, efforts to find a particular personality typology that would explain substance use (either licit or illicit) have been fruitless, and the idea of an "addictive personality," while attractive to lay audiences and talk show hosts, is not supported by research studies. Similarly, efforts to identify other particular psychological characteristics that explain why certain people use a substance (e.g., measures of intelligence, having a "dependent" personality, demonstrating "unmet developmental needs") have not been fruitful.

THE BEHAVIORAL FACTOR

In part, such efforts to find individual-level explanatory factors for substance use are efforts that distract from the fundamental behavioral aspect of substance use. Finding something else that explains why people use substances would suggest that addressing that underlying feature would stop the use. Stopping substance use is both simple and complicated—it depends upon stopping the behavior of ingestion of the substance (simply not using, which is easy to say and complicated to do). Stopping use is easy; maintaining that stopping is difficult. (An old joke among smokers is, "Quitting smoking is easy—I do it a dozen times a day.") People resume use of a substance (and engage in any other behavior that they wish to stop, such as overeating, gambling, reading pornography, etc.) for a variety of reason related to factors inside themselves (e.g., changes in reward mechanisms in subcortical systems, physical dependence, how the substance makes them feel) and factors outside themselves (**cues** in the environment, availability, lack of alternate activities). However, the use of a substance is ultimately a *choice* to engage in the behavior of ingesting that substance.

Interpersonal Factors

In general, **interpersonal factors** play a more prominent role in the initiation (or the prevention of initiation) of drug use, which typically occurs during adolescence or young adulthood. However, the role of interpersonal relationships, including peer and family relationships, in ongoing use becomes less prominent than that seen for initiation and early use. Once a person has developed some degree of regular use—and especially for the person who has become addicted—that use is less dependent upon use by peers and less influenced by interpersonal relationships. However, if the peer group has become distilled to those who use that substance, the group may exert some continued social pressure to use it, especially if the person has achieved some initial period of abstinence.

PEER FACTORS

Interactions that make drug use seem normal (the "everyone else is doing it" phenomenon) are associated with an increased likelihood of use by the person. Conversely, the impression that use of a substance is not the **social norm** is likely to lead to a lower likelihood of use. Thus, peer factors can play an important role in substance use; peers who use a substance can influence a person (typically an adolescent) to use that substance (Cleveland et al. 2008; Ellickson et al. 2001; Ellickson et al. 2008; Guxens et al. 2007; Scal et al. 2003; Shortt et al. 2007).

Evidence also shows that exposure to violence can increase the risk of subsequent substance use (Kilpatrick et al. 2000; Martin et al. 2003; Roberts et al. 2003; Sartor et al. 2008; Smith et al. 2010), although the magnitude of this effect and the particular associations (e.g., if more likely in females than in males, if limited to subsequent alcohol use or both alcohol and other drug use) vary from study to study. Conversely, positive **social support** can be an important factor in maintaining drug abstinence (Booth et al. 1992; Havassy et al. 1991), although simple support alone may be insufficient—the support may need to be directly related to the **goal** of abstinence (Gordon and Zrull 1991; Wasserman et al. 2001). Engagement in religious activities is also associated with less risk of substance use according to some studies (Kendler et al. 1997; Kliewer and Murrelle 2007; Miller et al. 2000). This is consistent with the idea that being around others who are not using is likely to influence individuals to likewise forgo use.

FAMILY FACTORS

Family-related factors also can either increase or decrease the likelihood of drug use. For example, problematic relationships with parents are associated with an increase in the likelihood of drug use (Barnow et al. 2002; Castro et al. 2006; Guxens et al. 2007). In a study that looked at the number of adverse childhood experiences (up to 10, grouped into categories of abuse, neglect, and household dysfunction), it was found that higher numbers of adverse childhood experiences were associated with increased risk of illicit drug and alcohol use (Dube et al. 2003; Dube et al. 2006). Conversely, good relationships with parents can be protective in the development of substance use (Branstrom et al. 2008; Petrie et al. 2007; Sale et al. 2003; Sale et al. 2005; Stronski et al. 2000).

Organizational and Community Factors

Organizational factors such as school can also influence the likelihood of substance use. For example, the environment in a school setting can influence the likelihood of drug use by students (Bond et al. 2007; Fletcher et al. 2008; Shortt et al. 2007). Some factors increase the likelihood that there will be less drug use (e.g., a positive atmosphere in the school, increased student participation and school connectedness, parental involvement in education), and others may contribute to an increased likelihood of drug use (e.g., poor relationships between teachers and students, lack of involvement in the school), especially for boys.

Although this seems self-evident, a community-level aspect of substance use is access to the substance (or lack thereof). Thus, for example, restricting youth's access to cigarettes

(e.g., through requiring confirmation of age when someone tries to purchase cigarettes) reduces the use of cigarettes by youth (Richardson et al. 2009). Similarly, the number and density of outlets for alcohol may influence alcohol use and alcohol-related problems (Livingston et al. 2007).

Another community-level aspect that can affect substance use is media presentations of use. Most work in this area has focused upon tobacco and alcohol use, rather than illicit drug use. Positive media portrayals of tobacco use, either through films or in advertising, generally promote the use of tobacco, especially in children (Lovato et al. 2003; Wakefield et al. 2003b; Wellman et al. 2006). Similarly, advertising for alcohol is associated with an increased likelihood of alcohol use by adolescents and young adults (Anderson, de Bruijin, et al. 2009; Collins et al. 2007; Ellickson et al. 2005; Smith and Foxcroft 2009; Snyder et al. 2006). The fact that advertising is effective in promoting the use of a substance should be no surprise, given that the purpose of advertising is to encourage people to engage in a behavior (purchase a product, take some action). However, the impact of alcohol and tobacco advertising on youth is particularly worrisome. While most advertising seeks to encourage alcohol and tobacco use, antismoking media portrayals can also be effective (Bala et al. 2008; Wakefield et al. 2003a), and media campaigns targeting reductions in drinking also are associated with less alcohol-related driving (Elder et al. 2004).

Policy Factors

Policy factors in substance use overlap to some degree with other factors addressed above. Thus, for example, some policy **interventions** can play out in school settings, or they may attempt to address parental involvement. This reflects the **complexity** of the factors addressed here (individual, interpersonal, organizational, etc.), which contribute to initiation and continued use of a substance, and it reinforces the notion that a simple answer to the use of substances (e.g., a simple school-based intervention or raising the price of a drug through taxation) does not exist. However, some policy-level interventions can affect substance use, such as manipulating cost and access as well as using **surveillance**.

COST

Not surprisingly, the use of a substance varies as a function of the cost. Thus, for licit drugs (i.e., alcohol, nicotine), raising the cost (e.g., through taxing at higher rates) results in decreased consumption and experimentation by nonusers (Anderson, Chisholm, et al. 2009; Forster et al. 2007; Tauras 2005). Oddly enough, this relatively simple policy decision, which can both influence the use of substances that have adverse consequences (alcohol, tobacco) and generate increased government revenue, is not used very frequently (as noted below in the discussion of interventions).

ACCESS

Restricting *access* to illicit drugs should likewise decrease their use, but this effect has not been as clearly demonstrated as making them harder to obtain by raising their *cost*. It is beyond the scope of this chapter to consider all of the pros and cons of legalization of illicit drugs (and to even consider the nuances of legalization, such as through medical access versus **social availability**; the latter issue comes into play with current licit drugs). However, three points do seem worth noting. First, if illicit drugs were legalized in some way, government revenues (taxation) from those drugs would likely be a motivating factor, as has been the case with the trend to legalize gambling. (And the legalization of gambling has had tragic and demoralizing consequences, both in the increased numbers of individuals pathologically gambling and in conveying a cultural message that the way to achieve happiness is to get suddenly lucky and

have a lot of money.) Second, wider access to currently illicit drugs (and the message that they are now legal to use in some fashion) would seem likely to increase experimentation and use, with a consequent increase in the number of individuals developing problematic use. And finally (and ironically), we are living in an era in which efforts to control the use of licit drugs (e.g., nicotine and prescription opioids), are concurrent with calls to relax the availability of illicit drugs. However, the cost of current approaches to control illicit drug use is immense; perhaps a middle ground exists that can address this use without unduly expanding experimentation and problematic use.

Another way that access to a substance can be restricted relates to the availability of a place where use of that substance can occur. For example, banning tobacco smoking in certain areas, as a part of efforts to decrease exposure to secondhand smoke, not only decreases secondhand smoke exposure; it may also decrease overall smoking (Callinan et al. 2010). Similarly, restricting access by youth and young adults to tobacco products has beneficial effects on subsequent nicotine experimentation and regular use (Botello-Harbaum et al. 2009; DiFranza et al. 2009; Forster et al. 2007; Tauras et al. 2005).

SURVEILLANCE

Different types of surveillance interventions for substance use can be effective. For example, increasing the presence of police as a means to decrease alcohol-related driving impairment appears to be generally effective (Goss et al. 2008). A technologically sophisticated surveillance system to prevent drunk driving is the required use of ignition systems that will activate only after the driver provides a breath sample that is negative for alcohol. Although such systems have been shown to be effective (Willis et al. 2004), their effects are not clearly sustained once the devices are removed.

Evidence-Based Interventions

Interventions for substance abuse can be broadly conceptualized as those that seek to prevent the initiation of use and those that treat the person who has developed some level of problematic use. While this is somewhat of a generalization, proactive efforts to prevent the initiation of use tend to be targeted at groups of individuals (e.g., students in a particular grade), although it is certainly the case that parents might tailor prevention efforts directly to the particulars of their child (e.g., spending time with their child in weekend sports activities rather than allowing the child to be with peers that are suspected of using drugs). Conversely, treatments for a person who has developed problematic use of a substance generally need to be individualized for that specific individual (e.g., designed for the particular type of drug she uses, allowing for physical dependence if present, addressing the particular **triggers** that can precipitate use, and accounting for other **comorbidities** that may complicate treatment). Note that costs for prevention tend to be relatively low on a per-person basis (insofar as they are applied to larger groups and in a relatively standardized and homogeneous way), whereas costs for treatment are higher on a per-person basis (given the need for individualized **planning** and interventions).

A discussion of prevention efforts is provided elsewhere in this chapter, particularly in the section on organizational (school and work site) factors that influence substance use. This section will address treatments for substance use disorders, although it is beyond the scope of this chapter to address all aspects of these evidence-based interventions. A few general points can be made and examples of treatments provided. Evidence is also provided, below, that defined steps can be taken to address substance abuse (including raising taxes, decreasing advertising that encourages use, increasing advertising that discourages use, instituting effective programs in schools and possibly workplace settings). Such steps can have beneficial effects for the individual, his relationships with others, and the community.

Treatment

Substance abuse treatment is effective to decrease drug use (Agboola et al. 2010; Amato et al. 2008b; Gowing et al. 2009; Mattick et al. 2009; Stitzer and Vandrey 2008) and to deal with other areas indirectly related to drug use (e.g., improvements in employment, decreases in legal problems) (Ball and Ross 1991; Hubbard et al. 1989; Strain et al. 1993, 1994, 1996). However, not all treatments have clearly demonstrated efficacy, and certain treatments may be more effective than others. Although treatments are effective, scant data shows which specific treatments are particularly effective for certain groups of patients. Thus, despite the intuitive appeal of the idea that patient-treatment matching should improve outcomes, relatively little evidence supports it (Strain 2004).

The treatments for a person with a substance use disorder can be broadly characterized as pharmacological and nonpharmacological interventions.

PHARMACOLOGICAL TREATMENTS

In the United States and some other parts of the world, several approved medications treat individuals who have alcohol, nicotine, and opioid use disorders. There are no approved medications to treat disorders related to the use of amphetamine, cannabis, cocaine, or other substances (although considerable research has been conducted attempting to find a medication to treat cocaine use). In brief, in the United States, approved medications to treat alcohol dependence are acamprosate, disulfiram, and naltrexone (the latter available in both an oral and an injectable, extended-release form) (CSAT 2009). Medications approved for the treatment of nicotine dependence are bupropion, various nicotine products (e.g., gum, inhaler, nasal spray, and patch), and varenicline (Eisenberg et al. 2008). For opioid dependence treatment, approved medications are buprenorphine (with and without naloxone), LAAM, methadone, and naltrexone (Strain and Stitzer 2006). As indicated by their status as medications approved by the Food and Drug Administration (FDA), each of these pharmacotherapies has demonstrated efficacy with a tolerable safety profile. In addition to these approved medications, several other medications are approved for other uses but may also be used in the treatment of disorders related to the use of alcohol (e.g., topiramate, benzodiazepines), nicotine (e.g., nortriptyline), and opioids (e.g., clonidine).

Medications are broadly used for one of two purposes, either to withdraw a person who is physically dependent upon a substance (e.g., buprenorphine for opioids, benzodiazepines for alcohol, nicotine gum for nicotine dependence), or to maintain cessation of use of a substance (e.g., naltrexone for alcoholism or opioid dependence, methadone or buprenorphine for opioid dependence). Medically supervised withdrawal with medications can be effective (Amato et al. 2010; Gowing et al. 2009; Stead et al. 2008), although for opioid dependence, medically supervised withdrawal is often followed by relapse (Kakko et al. 2003; Sees et al. 2000). Maintenance treatment with medications, especially for opioid and alcohol dependence, can be highly effective for many patients (Johnson et al. 2000; Mattick et al. 2008; Mattick et al. 2009; Srisurapanont and Jarusuraisin 2005; Strain et al. 1999).

New medications to treat substance use disorders, and especially illicit drug use disorders, are developed rarely, and their development is heavily influenced by other factors beyond need, efficacy, or safety. Buprenorphine, an opioid that is effective and safe for the treatment of opioid dependence, can serve as an excellent example of this point. It illustrates lessons

learned based upon past successes and failures in the process of developing a medication to treat a substance use disorder. Buprenorphine was first identified as a potential medication for opioid dependence treatment in the late 1970s (Jasinski et al. 1978). However, despite a market that was primarily occupied by one approved medication (methadone), with little use of a second approved medication (naltrexone), work supporting buprenorphine's development moved at a slow pace through the 1980s. An Institute of Medicine report published in 1995 (Fulco et al. 1995) called for the development of new medications to treat substance use disorders and led to the creation of the Medications Development Division (MDD) at the National Institute on Drug Abuse (NIDA). The MDD focused upon the development of buprenorphine and also sought to bring LAAM (a mu agonist opioid similar to methadone, but with a longer duration of action that allowed dosing thrice weekly rather than daily as is the case with methadone) to FDA approval.

LAAM was approved by the FDA in 1993 for use in the treatment of opioid dependence. However, LAAM could be provided only through the methadone clinic system in the United States. Uptake of LAAM was extremely limited, in part because of the restrictive nature of the methadone clinic system, and its availability did not significantly affect treatment capacity. As buprenorphine approached approvable status in the United States (it was approved for the treatment of opioid dependence in France in 1996), policymakers realized that its success in expanding treatment capacity would depend on making it available through other means besides the methadone clinic system. This resulted in the passage of the Drug Addiction Treatment Act of 2000, which allowed certain opioids (e.g., buprenorphine) to be prescribed for the treatment of opioid dependence by physicians in office settings. The result was a substantial increase in treatment capacity for individuals with opioid dependence.

Buprenorphine (and LAAM) were both effective medications that, at the time of their approval, were considered safe. (Subsequent studies with LAAM questioned whether it produced cardiac toxicity, although it was not pulled from the U.S. market for this reason and could still be marketed in the U.S. today.) The availability and uptake of these medications was driven, in part, by factors beyond the science demonstrating their efficacy and safety. While controlled studies contributed to the ways in which buprenorphine was subsequently used (i.e., in office settings), a political and cultural decision was the key in how it became available. Unlike medications to treat other medical disorders (e.g., diabetes, hypertension), the use of medications for substance use disorders seems particularly influenced by broader cultural factors.

PSYCHOSOCIAL (NONPHARMACOLOGICAL) TREATMENT

Nonpharmacological treatments for substance use disorders can be very effective, and for some classes of drugs that have no approved pharmacotherapies (e.g., stimulants such as cocaine and amphetamines, cannabis, inhalants), these are the primary treatment options available. Considerable progress has been made in the standardization of different treatment approaches, the development of treatment manuals (Budney and Higgins 1998; Carroll 1998; Kadden et al. 1994; Mercer and Woody 2000; Miller et al. 1994; Nowinski et al. 1994), and studies testing the efficacy of different modalities.

In general, reviews and meta-analyses have shown that nonpharmacological (or **psychosocial**) treatments used for substance use disorders are effective (Dutra et al. 2008) and that common components across approaches can be identified (Moos 2007). For example, the addition of psychosocial therapies improves outcomes for both opioid dependence and opioid withdrawal treatments when combined with medications (Amato et al. 2008a, 2008b), although there is insufficient evidence to support the use of psychosocial treatments without concurrent medications for opioid dependence treatment (Mayet et al. 2005).

Given the evidence that psychosocial treatments work, two more specific questions arise: (1) Are there particular types of treatment that are more effective than others (i.e., is it a general effect that anything is good, or are there particular types of treatment that are better)? and (2) Is more treatment better than less (just because some treatment is good, does that mean that even more would be better)?

Regarding the first question, good evidence shows that behavioral therapies are particularly effective for the treatment of substance use disorders (Carroll and Onken 2005), and among the approaches used, **contingency management** has shown the most consistent and robust efficacy (Dutra et al. 2008; Prendergast et al. 2006). However, other treatments (cognitive-behavioral therapy, **motivational interviewing**, and family and couples counseling) have also demonstrated efficacy (Carroll and Onken 2005; Lundahl and Burke 2009; Powers et al. 2008). Important features of nonpharmacological treatment include the amount of treatment provided and the type of treatment (e.g., contingency management) that can be effective.

Dose of Treatment. In a classic study, McLellan and colleagues demonstrated that the efficacy of psychosocial services in opioid dependent patients treated with methadone was dose related; that is, that patients who received more psychosocial services had better outcomes, as measured by treatment retention and rates of opioid-positive urine samples (1993). The study tested three levels of services, and interestingly, follow-up **evaluation** from that study found that the most cost-effective level of service was the moderate amount of nonpharmacological treatment, rather than the highest amount (even though the best outcomes were associated with the highest amount of services) (Kraft et al. 1997). A variation on this dose effect for nonpharmacological services is the use of different levels of service intensity for patients in substance abuse treatment. For example, outpatient programs typically provide two or three levels of service (partial hospitalization programs [PHPs], which operate five to six days per week and provide services for 20 or more hours per week; intensive outpatient programs [IOPs], which operate three to five days per week and provide services for at least nine hours per week; and outpatient [OP] counseling, which may be an individual or a group service, which typically consists of services for one to two hours per week) (ASAM 2001). Patients usually move from more intensive levels of treatment early in the course of their care (e.g., PHP) to less intensive levels (IOP or OP) as they stabilize in their drug use. Although these different levels of service make sense, remarkably little well-controlled research has addressed whether these approaches are necessary and cost-effective—and if they are, whether they are such for all patients or only for certain ones.

Although findings from at least some research suggest that providing some nonpharmacological services (in the McLellan study, specifically in the case of methadone treatment) is effective, this conclusion should be balanced by other work that suggests providing medication (methadone) without psychosocial services may also be of significant benefit. For example, a study of interim methadone treatment (i.e., methadone medication with essentially no concurrent psychosocial services) found that this treatment of essentially medication alone was more effective than being placed on a waiting list (Schwartz et al. 2006).

Type of Treatment. The voucher **incentive** program is one form of contingency management that has been extensively tested and shown to be particularly useful in the treatment of individuals with substance use disorders (Higgins et al. 1994; Higgins et al. 2002; Lussier et al. 2006; Preston et al. 1999; Silverman et al. 1996; Stitzer and Petry 2006; Stitzer and Van-

drey 2008). In brief, this form of contingency management involves giving patients a voucher (typically in the form of a piece of paper) that has a monetary value and that is received for objective evidence of drug abstinence such as a negative urine sample. Vouchers are tracked by treatment staff and can be used to purchase items (e.g., movie passes, items for a hobby) that are consistent with the patient's treatment goals and prosocial activities. This approach, and variations on this theme (Lott and Jencius 2009; Peirce et al. 2006; Petry and Bickel 2000; Petry et al. 2002), is effective in initiating and sustaining abstinence in a variety of **target populations**, including individuals with cocaine dependence.

Other nonpharmacological treatments and services that should be noted include various forms of couples or family counseling (Fals-Stewart et al. 1996; O'Farrell and Fals-Stewart 2002); self-help groups such as AA, Narcotics Anonymous (NA), Smart Recovery (Moos and Moos 2006); therapeutic communities (De Leon 2000); and novel approaches that capitalize upon Internet or computer forms of service delivery (Carroll et al. 2008). In general, these approaches can be useful in targeted situations. For example, couples therapy can be useful when an appropriately trained therapist is available and the patient has a supportive and non-drug-using significant other.

Self-help groups such as AA and NA can be very useful for some individuals with substance use disorders, although these should be recognized as patient-driven forms of service, not treatment delivered by professionals. Although such self-help groups can result in good outcomes for some, others may not find them to be a good match for their needs and perspectives.

Other approaches, such as **therapeutic communities** (long-term residential settings with a strong emphasis on the use of community to enact long-term change), can also be useful for some patients, although the availability of this form of treatment has become much more limited in recent years. A detailed review of all these approaches is beyond the scope of this chapter, although books and chapters of textbooks on substance abuse treatment are typically devoted to these topics and can provide the interested reader with information about them.

Finally, despite evidence that nonpharmacological treatments are effective, and that particular behavioral treatments are effective and supported by a clear evidence base, the uptake of evidence-based approaches by substance abuse treatment providers in the community is not as extensive as we might hope (Benishek et al. 2010; Kirby et al. 2006). However, this problem is not limited to nonpharmacological treatments; similar difficulties have occurred with substance abuse pharmacotherapies, such as office-based buprenorphine for the treatment of opioid dependence and having physicians become qualified to prescribe this medication.

Environmental Interventions

As noted earlier in this chapter, interventions can occur in the environment (e.g., schools, the local community, or the more extended community) through entities that seek to act upon and mitigate determinants of drug use. These types of interventions are generally preventive in nature and are related to policy (usually through laws, rules, and regulations). Some examples of **environmental interventions** are provided here to illustrate how these can influence drug use.

SCHOOLS

School systems are a particularly prominent area in which environmental interventions have been used and studied. With respect to such interventions, efforts that focus upon simply educating students about the perils of drug use do not decrease the risk of subsequent use (Botvin and Griffin 2007). This is not to say that school-based interventions are uniformly ineffective, but rather that school-based interventions that are broader in their features, continue

over time, and have aspects that are appropriate for the target age group (e.g., differing for elementary versus middle school versus high school students) are more likely to be effective. These interventions include features such as skill and competence training, they utilize multiple components in such training, and they also provide information from surveys, for example, information showing that perceptions regarding the extent of substance use in a school are not valid (Botvin and Griffin 2007; Faggiano et al. 2005, 2008; Peters et al. 2009).

Although there is good evidence for school-based interventions directed at the prevention of substance use when they are broad-based, the same degree of research related to non-school-based settings for interventions **targeting** young people (Gates et al. 2006) does not exist, nor for work-based interventions (Webb et al. 2009), although there is some evidence that work-based programs can affect alcohol use (Bennett et al. 2004). It has also been found that non-school-based interventions that target parents can be effective in decreasing drug (at least alcohol) use (Smit et al. 2008).

School-based interventions can be effective, but they are not the only mechanism that can decrease drug use by youth. Thus, for example, restricting access to cigarettes (e.g., through requiring confirmation of age when someone tries to purchase cigarettes) reduces the use of cigarettes by youth (Richardson et al. 2009).

POLICY

Although school-based interventions are generally designed with the specific goal of preventing the use of both licit and illicit drug use, other interventions that affect drug use are not as specifically tailored to do so. For example, another environmental intervention that can be effective in decreasing drug use is to raise the cost of the drug (either the **direct cost** [the amount to purchase the drug], or the **indirect cost** [such as the effort that must be expended to obtain the drug]). This can be most easily accomplished with legal drugs and through taxation or through altering access to a drug. As noted previously, increasing the cost of a drug through taxes is associated with decreased use and experimentation, which in turn can affect both current use and the potential for new users to be exposed to the drug at an early age (Anderson, Chishold, et al. 2009; Forster et al. 2007; Tauras 2005).

While taxes are a relatively easy way to conceptualize altering cost (and one that seems to be attractive to politicians, given that it can be touted as being for the social good while providing more funds for the politicians to spend), another method is to change access to a substance—that is, to make it more costly (or difficult) in some way to get the substance. Two examples of the relationship between access alteration and use can be found in studies that have looked at alcohol. The first example comes from studies of changes in the age at which people can purchase alcohol. Such studies show that raising the minimum legal age for alcohol is clearly associated with beneficial outcomes related to the consequences of alcohol use, such as motor vehicle accidents (Birckmayer and Hemenway 1999; McCartt et al. 2010; Wagenaar and Toomey 2002). Thus, making access to a drug more difficult has beneficial effects. The second example comes from studies that have considered the density of establishments that sell alcohol. Having more availability to access alcohol (more establishments) is associated with violence of various forms and other alcohol-related consequences (Gruenewald et al. 2006; Lipton and Gruenewald 2002; Livingston 2008; Livingston et al. 2007; Treno et al. 2007). Both of these access issues (minimum drinking ages and density of outlets) suggest that environmental and policy manipulations (such as raising the legal drinking age and restricting the licenses issued for bars) can serve as effective interventions to decrease use of a drug. Although a similar research base for illicit drugs does not exist, the general principle that restricting access can lead to less use and use-related consequences would seem to be sound.

If restricting access and availability is an effective way to decrease early experimentation, use, and consequences of use, then steps that might make illicit drugs easier to obtain would seem to run counter to the lessons learned with alcohol and nicotine. A review of the pros and cons of drug decriminalization (and the related topics of depenalization and legalization) could easily encompass a whole book and is beyond the scope of this chapter.

Decriminalization refers to the elimination, reduction, or nonenforcement of penalties for the sale, purchase, or possession of illicit drugs (Joffe 2004). Laws related to decriminalization can vary widely when implemented. The primary intended effects of decriminalization are to reduce burdens on the criminal justice system, the negative consequences of drug convictions for individuals, the negative social consequence of use, and the risk of adverse consequences of use of a drug. When implemented, these policies can also reduce the **stigma** associated with use of a drug. For example, the perceived risk of regular use of cannabis has a strong inverse relationship with **self-reports** of adolescents who have used it (Johnston et al. 2011). A risk associated with reduced stigma is that the use of a drug becomes more acceptable, which in turn may increase rates of experimentation with it. An interesting peculiarity of the present era is that on one hand there has been a substantial social reaction against the use of one smoked legal product, nicotine (in effect, a drive to make smoking tobacco an illegal activity), while there is a concurrent interest in the legalization of another smoked product, cannabis. Environmental and some political policies would seem somewhat contradictory in these approaches (although the point here is not to advocate for smoking nicotine products).

Other policy interventions can be politically attractive to some groups but lack evidence for efficacy. An example is school-based drug testing, for which there was considerable federal support in the United States several years ago. However, no good evidence shows that such testing affects drug use by students, although, as is often the case, more definitive studies would be useful (Roche et al. 2009). Somewhat surprisingly, researchers found that workplace drug screening—either as part of a preemployment process or at random times during employment—is likewise not clearly effective and may even be ineffective, in deterring drug use (Kraus 2001; Levine and Rennie 2004), although studies of such interventions can be **confounded** (e.g., by inadequate testing procedures). Furthermore, some evidence shows that workplace drug testing can be effective when coupled with peer counseling regarding substance use (Miller et al. 2007; Spicer and Miller 2005).

In summary, some environmental interventions for substance use show evidence of efficacy, either in preventing use (e.g., multimodal school-based programs, minimum drinking ages) or in decreasing use (e.g., taxes on cigarettes). The evidence base is generally stronger for environmental interventions that relate to licit drugs rather than those for illicit drugs, but the conclusions drawn from studies of licit drugs provide direction for illicit-drug interventions.

INTERVENTIONS SUMMARY

Well-tested mechanisms can be effective in enhancing prevention of substance use and can help those who have developed problematic use to stop the use. Both pharmacological and nonpharmacological treatments can help people withdraw from substance use (although withdrawal does not necessarily mean the person will sustain abstinence). Given the ample evidence that at least some interventions for substance use disorders are effective, why are they not more commonly used? For example, despite well-controlled studies showing that methadone maintenance is effective for the treatment of opioid dependence, expansion of methadone treatment in the United States over the last 20 or

more years has been slow, and methadone treatment capacity historically has been much lower than the need (although the availability of office-based buprenorphine treatment appears to have relieved some of this demand for opioid-dependence treatment). Similarly, school-based prevention programs have been shown to be effective yet remain underutilized by schools.

Although cost is undoubtedly one driving factor, the lack of utilization also may be related to cultural ambivalence about the nature of substance use disorders—and especially the behavioral aspect of these disorders. Given the feature of choice and personal responsibility, perhaps we tend to think that the using person just needs to take charge in her life and accept responsibility to stop substance use (or not start its use). The volitional component to taking a substance exists, but once use has begun, the decision to stop becomes much more difficult for the individual—the drive to use the substance takes on a life of its own (especially as brain reward systems become hijacked by drug use).

Thus, addictive disorders evoke different reactions and perceptions. On one hand, some see these disorders as medical diseases (the "just like diabetes" argument). However, while curing diabetes—that is, curing the dysregulation of glucose control that is the defining feature of diabetes—seems possible, "curing" dysregulation of choice seems less likely. On the other hand, viewing addictive disorders as solely based on bad decisions fails to appreciate the overwhelming (and tragic, as clinicians can attest) loss of control that drives the person who uses a substance. Adaptive changes in the central nervous system become associated with the substance use, and these changes make the drive to use more compelling, salient, and organizing than similar actions of a non-substance-abusing person.

Ultimately, substance use disorders are medical disorders, and interventions can both help prevent their initiation and help those who have lost control in their use. The benefits of substance abuse treatments need to be weighed against their costs (as is the case with all medical treatments). For substance abuse treatments, much of the benefit in achieving and maintaining abstinence occurs in nonmedical areas, such as increased employment and decreased crime (Gerstein et al. 1994). These are important societal benefits, but medical insurers have little **motivation** to recognize and appreciate decreases in crime and increases in employment. Thus, while treatment is effective, its efficacy does not necessarily impact savings in the health care arena (unlike, for example, better glucose control in a diabetic, which may save money on subsequent medical complications and short-term inpatient hospitalizations for the diabetic).

Implementation Considerations

Addressing substance use is complicated, consistent with a behavioral perspective for these conditions. Designing and implementing effective strategies to address substance use can vary depending upon whether we are targeting initiation of use (prevention) or continued use (treatment) and also can depend upon the substance used (licit or illicit) and the characteristics of the particular user (physically dependent or not, comorbid conditions complicating the intervention, etc.).

When considering implementation issues, several topics should be considered: cultural **attitudes** toward substance abuse (addressed above), funding (also addressed above), workforce or treatment capacity, and research needs. Each of these is briefly considered here.

TREATMENT CAPACITY

As discussed in the intervention summary above, broad cultural acceptance that these are complicated medical disorders and funding that appreciates the benefits from treating them are necessary. Even with these requirements met, however, the United States currently has insuf-

ficient treatment capacity to address the needs of the substance-abusing population (and the same is true of many other countries). Hand in hand with this lack is the need for a trained and professional workforce. Substance abuse is unusual in the medical arena, because there is more emphasis on specialty care than on treatment by primary care providers (McLellan 2010). Expanding treatment capacity is essential, not just in the United States, but in other countries—for example, China is markedly expanding its methadone treatment system (Li et al. 2010). However, such expansion cannot occur overnight, especially if the goal is to provide quality treatment, and the expansion will require increases in treatment capacity and capability by the primary care system as well as a larger substance abuse treatment workforce.

RESEARCH NEEDS

Finally, despite the current extensive research base for addictive disorders, multiple questions are still in need of research. These vary from the basic science, to medications development and treatment, to epidemiology and broad policy implications. Implementation of changes should be driven by data. Studies are needed to continue to better understand the biological basis of reward, to develop medications for these disorders, to improve the nonpharmacological treatments used, and to optimize when and how they should be combined with medication, to both improve prevention services and assess the impact of policy and treatment interventions. Perhaps equally critical, the scientific community needs to effectively communicate to the broader culture the nature of these disorders—as medical conditions that can be addressed and treated by health care professionals.

Roles for Key Stakeholders

Substance abuse is a topic for which essentially everyone is a **key stakeholder**. Substance abuse disorders affect everyone, either directly (e.g., through self-use or use by a loved one), or indirectly (e.g., through crime, persons driving under the influence, loss of productivity by co-workers). No one is immune from the effects of substance use, and no one can view it as a problem that he has no stake in addressing.

First, among members of the research community, continued research is necessary on these disorders and the nature of substance abuse and all of its facets (e.g., biology, behavior, cognition, treatment outcome, epidemiology, policy). Equally importantly, the scientific community must help instruct the broader culture about the nature of these disorders and help people understand them as complicated and nuanced medical conditions. Oversimplifying messages can produce a loss of credibility. For example, periodically someone will proclaim, "We need to lose the stigma of substance abuse." Although at the surface level this may sound good (after all, isn't stigma bad?), in actuality, stigma can serve a useful social function in prevention efforts. We do not want to discourage people from seeking medical treatment, but concurrently we want to discourage children from thinking drug use is okay.

Second, the health care community needs to accept the treatment of these patients and expand the capacity to do so. This is no small matter. It requires both more providers in the specialty treatment system (which in turn require increases in funding for treatment) and more general medical providers who screen and provide interventions for individuals with substance use disorders. Ample evidence shows that the latter can be highly effective under the proper circumstances (Babor et al. 2007; Schaus et al. 2009; Whitlock et al. 2004). However, there is a need for ownership of substance abuse prevention and treatment on the part of the broader community of health care providers as an important step forward in expanding treatment capacity.

Third, policymakers have an opportunity to improve the funding for research, prevention, and treatment of substance abuse. These would be resources well spent, given the evidence for decreased social costs associated with lower rates of substance abuse.

Finally, we as a culture need to accept substance abuse as a medical condition and one that can be effectively treated by health care providers. In part, doing so requires an awareness of science by the broader population, an understanding of scientific principles, and an appreciation of how oversimplifications of medical illnesses run counter to helping people. The medical field is periodically accused of "making everything a disease," and the accusation is not an unfair one. Although the general population may not know what substance abuse is (in the more subtle features, as this chapter attempts to address), the general population seems to know what it is not. Researchers, including health care professionals, have an opportunity to teach the broader population about these disorders, and the broader population may well welcome such an opportunity to learn.

Conclusion

Substance use is complicated. Everyone seems to have an opinion about it, and not uncommonly, each person believes that she has some special expertise and understanding of how substance use disorders should be addressed. In part, this may reflect the pervasiveness of substance abuse—if an individual has not personally struggled with substance use, a family member, a neighbor, or a friend likely has. Peculiarly, a nonusing individual might show only limited support for expanding treatment and acknowledgment of substance use as a medical disorder, even though the same individual might well have personally experienced the struggles of loved ones with a substance use disorder.

A marked gap exists between the intuitive beliefs that many have about substance abuse and the nature of these disorders. Progress is being made, as evidenced by controlled studies of prevention and treatment interventions, by education in the political and policy arenas, and by our understanding of the biological and environmental determinants of substance use. However, as noted in the biblical passage at the beginning of this chapter, substance use is not a new struggle for humans. Nevertheless, misuse of substances can be prevented and can be treated, and we continue to improve in our abilities to do both.

NOTES

1. See EU Public Health Information & Knowledge System, www.euphix.org/object_document/o4754n 27423.html (accessed Aug. 4, 2010).

REFERENCES

Agboola S, McNeill A, Coleman T, Leonardi Bee J. 2010. A systematic review of the effectiveness of smoking relapse prevention interventions for abstinent smokers. *Addiction* 105:1362-80.

Agrawal A, Lynskey MT. 2008. Are there genetic influences on addiction? Evidence from family, adoption, and twin studies. *Addiction* 103:1069-81.

Amato L, Minozzi S, Davoli M, Vecchi S, Ferri MM, Mayet S. 2008a. Psychosocial and pharmacological treatments versus pharmacological treatments for opioid detoxification. *Cochrane Database Syst Rev,* CD005031.

———. 2008b. Psychosocial combined with agonist maintenance treatments versus agonist maintenance treatments alone for treatment of opioid dependence. *Cochrane Database Syst Rev,* CD004147.

Amato L, Minozzi S, Vecchi S, Davoli M. 2010. Benzodiazepines for alcohol withdrawal. *Cochrane Database Syst Rev* 3:CD005063.

American Society of Addiction Medicine (ASAM). 2001. *Patient Placement Criteria for the Treatment of Substance-Related Disorders.* ASAM PPC-2R. 2nd ed. rev. Chevy Case, MD: American Society of Addiction Medicine.

Anderson P, Chisholm D, Fuhr DC. 2009. Effectiveness and cost-effectiveness of policies and programmes to reduce the harm caused by alcohol. *Lancet* 373:2234-46.

Anderson P, de Bruijn A, Angus K, Gordon R, Hastings G. 2009. Impact of alcohol advertising and media exposure on adolescent alcohol use: A systematic review of longitudinal studies. *Alcohol Alcohol* 44:229-43.

Anton RF, Oroszi G, O'Malley S, et al. 2008. An evaluation of mu-opioid receptor (OPRM1) as a predictor of naltrexone response in the treatment of alcohol dependence: Results from the Combined Pharmacotherapies and Behavioral Interventions for Alcohol Dependence (COMBINE) study. *Arch Gen Psychiatry* 65:135-44.

Australian Institute of Health and Welfare (AIHW). 2008. *2007 National Drug Strategy Household Survey: Detailed Findings.* Drug statistics series. Canberra: Australian Institute of Health and Welfare.

Azorlosa JL, Stitzer ML, Greenwald MK. 1994. Opioid physical dependence development: Effects of single versus repeated morphine pretreatments and of subjects' opioid exposure history. *Psychopharmacol (Berl)* 114:71-80.

Babor TF, McRee BG, Kassebaum PA, Grimaldi PL, Ahmed K, Bray J. 2007. Screening, Brief Intervention, and Referral to Treatment (SBIRT): Toward a public health approach to the management of substance abuse. *Subst Abus* 28:7-30.

Bala M, Strzeszynski L, Cahill K. 2008. Mass media interventions for smoking cessation in adults. *Cochrane Database Syst Rev,* CD004704.

Ball JC, Ross A. 1991. *The Effectiveness of Methadone Maintenance Treatment.* New York: Springer-Verlag.

Barnow S, Schuckit MA, Lucht M, John U, Freyberger HJ. 2002. The importance of a positive family history of alcoholism, parental rejection and emotional warmth, behavioral problems and peer substance use for alcohol problems in teenagers: A path analysis. *J Stud Alcohol* 63:305-15.

Benishek LA, Kirby KC, Dugosh KL, Padovano A. 2010. Beliefs about the empirical support of drug abuse treatment interventions: A survey of outpatient treatment providers. *Drug Alcohol Depend* 107:202-8.

Bennett JB, Patterson CR, Reynolds GS, Wiitala WL, Lehman WE. 2004. Team awareness, problem drinking, and drinking climate: Workplace social health promotion in a policy context. *Am J Health Promot* 19:103-13.

Bierut LJ. 2010. Convergence of genetic findings for nicotine dependence and smoking related diseases with chromosome 15q24-25. *Trends Pharmacol Sci* 31:46-51.

Birckmayer J, Hemenway D. 1999. Minimum-age drinking laws and youth suicide, 1970-1990. *Am J Public Health* 89:1365-68.

Birnbaum HG, White AG, Reynolds JL, et al. 2006. Estimated costs of prescription opioid analgesic abuse in the United States in 2001: A societal perspective. *Clin J Pain* 22:667-76.

Bond L, Butler H, Thomas L, et al. 2007. Social and school connectedness in early secondary school as predictors of late teenage substance use, mental health, and academic outcomes. *J Adolesc Health* 40:357 e9-18.

Booth BM, Russell DW, Soucek S, Laughlin PR. 1992. Social support and outcome of alcoholism treatment: An exploratory analysis. *Am J Drug Alcohol Abuse* 18:87-101.

Botello-Harbaum MT, Haynie DL, Iannotti RJ, Wang J, Gase L, Simons-Morton B. 2009. Tobacco control policy and adolescent cigarette smoking status in the United States. *Nicotine Tob Res* 11:875-85.

Botvin GJ, Griffin KW. 2007. School-based programmes to prevent alcohol, tobacco, and other drug use. *Int Rev Psychiatry* 19:607-15.

Boulenger JP, Uhde TW. 1982. Caffeine consumption and anxiety: Preliminary results of a survey comparing patients with anxiety disorders and normal controls. *Psychopharmacol Bull* 18:53-57.

Boulenger JP, Uhde TW, Wolff EA 3rd, Post RM. 1984. Increased sensitivity to caffeine in patients with panic disorders: Preliminary evidence. *Arch Gen Psychiatry* 41:1067-71.

Branstrom R, Sjostrom E, Andreasson S. 2008. Individual, group, and community risk and protective factors for alcohol and drug use among Swedish adolescents. *Eur J Public Health* 18:12-18.

Brooner RK, King VL, Kidorf M, Schmidt CW Jr., Bigelow GE. 1997. Psychiatric and substance use comorbidity among treatment-seeking opioid abusers. *Arch Gen Psychiatry* 54:71-80.

Brown SA, Schuckit MA. 1988. Changes in depression among abstinent alcoholics. *J Stud Alcohol* 49:412-17.

Bruce M, Scott N, Shine P, Lader M. 1992. Anxiogenic effects of caffeine in patients with anxiety disorders. *Arch Gen Psychiatry* 49:867-69.

Budney AJ, Higgins ST. 1998. *A Community Reinforcement Plus Vouchers Approach: Treating Cocaine Addiction.* DHHS Publication No. 98-4309. Rockville, MD: Department of Health and Human Services.

Callinan JE, Clarke A, Doherty K, Kelleher C. 2010. Legislative smoking bans for reducing secondhand smoke exposure, smoking prevalence, and tobacco consumption. *Cochrane Database Syst Rev* 4:CD005992.

Carroll KM. 1998. *A Cognitive-Behavioral Approach: Treating Cocaine Addiction.* DHHS Publication No. 98-4308. Rockville, MD: Department of Health and Human Services.

Carroll KM, Ball SA, Martino S, et al. 2008. Computer-assisted delivery of cognitive-behavioral therapy for addiction: A randomized trial of CBT4CBT. *Am J Psychiatry* 165:881-88.

Carroll KM, Onken LS. 2005. Behavioral therapies for drug abuse. *Am J Psychiatry* 162:1452-60.

Castro FG, Brook JS, Brook DW, Rubenstone E. 2006. Paternal, perceived maternal, and youth risk factors as predictors of youth stage of substance use: A longitudinal study. *J Addict Dis* 25:65-75.

Center for Substance Abuse Treatment (CSAT). 2009. *Incorporating Alcohol Pharmacotherapies into Medical Practice.* Rockville, MD: U.S. Substance Abuse and Mental Health Services Administration, Center for Substance Abuse Treatment.

Cleveland MJ, Feinberg ME, Bontempo DE, Greenberg MT. 2008. The role of risk and protective factors in substance use across adolescence. *J Adolesc Health* 43:157-64.

Collins RL, Ellickson PL, McCaffrey D, Hambarsoomians K. 2007. Early adolescent exposure to alcohol advertising and its relationship to underage drinking. *J Adolesc Health* 40:527-34.

Comer SD, Sullivan MA, Walker EA. 2005. Comparison of intravenous buprenorphine and methadone self-administration by recently detoxified heroin-dependent individuals. *J Pharmacol Exp Ther* 315:1320-30.

De Leon G. 2000. *The Therapeutic Community: Theory, Model, and Method.* New York: Springer.

DiFranza JR, Savageau JA, Fletcher KE. 2009. Enforcement of underage sales laws as a predictor of daily smoking among adolescents: A national study. *BMC Public Health* 9:107.

Dube SR, Felitti VJ, Dong M, Chapman DP, Giles WH, Anda RF. 2003. Childhood abuse, neglect, and household dysfunction and the risk of illicit drug use: The adverse childhood experiences study. *Pediatrics* 111:564-72.

Dube SR, Miller JW, Brown DW, et al. 2006. Adverse childhood experiences and the association with ever using alcohol and initiating alcohol use during adolescence. *J Adolesc Health* 38:444 e1-10.

Dutra L, Stathopoulou G, Basden SL, Leyro TM, Powers MB, Otto MW. 2008. A meta-analytic review of psychosocial interventions for substance use disorders. *Am J Psychiatry* 165:179-87.

Edwards G, Gross MM. 1976. Alcohol dependence: Provisional description of a clinical syndrome. *Br Med J* 1:1058-61.

Eisenberg MJ, Filion KB, Yavin D, et al. 2008. Pharmacotherapies for smoking cessation: A meta-analysis of randomized controlled trials. *CMAJ* 179:135-44.

Elder RW, Shults RA, Sleet DA, Nichols JL, Thompson RS, Rajab W. 2004. Effectiveness of mass media campaigns for reducing drinking and driving and alcohol-involved crashes: A systematic review. *Am J Prev Med* 27:57-65.

Ellickson PL, Collins RL, Hambarsoomians K, McCaffrey DF. 2005. Does alcohol advertising promote adolescent drinking? Results from a longitudinal assessment. *Addiction* 100:235-46.

Ellickson PL, Tucker JS, Klein DJ. 2008. Reducing early smokers' risk for future smoking and other problem behavior: Insights from a five-year longitudinal study. *J Adolesc Health* 43:394-400.

Ellickson SL, Tucker JS, Klein DJ, McGuigan KA. 2001. Prospective risk factors for alcohol misuse in late adolescence. *J Stud Alcohol* 62:773-82.

European Monitoring Centre for Drugs and Drug Addiction (EMCDDA). 2009. 2009 annual report on the state of the drugs problem in Europe. European Monitoring Centre for Drugs and Drug Addiction, Lisbon.

Ezzati M, Lopez AD, Rodgers A, Vander Hoorn S, Murray CJ. 2002. Selected major risk factors and global and regional burden of disease. *Lancet* 360:1347-60.

Faggiano F, Vigna-Taglianti FD, Versino E, Zambon A, Borraccino A, Lemma P. 2005. School-based prevention for illicit drugs' use. *Cochrane Database Syst Rev,* CD003020.

———. 2008. School-based prevention for illicit drugs use: A systematic review. *Prev Med* 46:385-96.

Fals-Stewart W, Birchler GR, O'Farrell TJ. 1996. Behavioral couples therapy for male substance-abusing patients: Effects on relationship adjustment and drug-using behavior. *J Consult Clin Psychol* 64:959-72.

Fletcher A, Bonell C, Hargreaves J. 2008. School effects on young people's drug use: A systematic review of intervention and observational studies. *J Adolesc Health* 42:209-20.

Forster JL, Widome R, Bernat DH. 2007. Policy interventions and surveillance as strategies to prevent tobacco use in adolescents and young adults. *Am J Prev Med* 33: S335-S339.

Fulco CE, Liverman CT, Earley LE. 1995. *The Development of Medications for the Treatment of Opiate and Cocaine Addictions: Issues for the Government and Private Sector Institute of Medicine.* Washington, DC: National Academy Press.

Gates S, McCambridge J, Smith LA, Foxcroft DR. 2006. Interventions for prevention of drug use by young people delivered in non-school settings. *Cochrane Database Syst Rev,* CD005030.

Gerstein DR, Johnson RA, Harwood HJ, Fountain D, Suter N, Mallow K. 1994. *Evaluating Recovery Services: The California Drug and Alcohol Treatment Assessment (CALDATA) General Report.* Sacramento: California Department of Alcohol and Drug Progams.

Gordon AJ, Zrull M. 1991. Social networks and recovery: One year after inpatient treatment. *J Subst Abuse Treat* 8:143-52.

Goss CW, Van Bramer LD, Gliner JA, Porter TR, Roberts IG, Diguiseppi C. 2008. Increased police patrols for preventing alcohol-impaired driving. *Cochrane Database Syst Rev,* CD005242.

Gowing L, Ali R, White JM. 2009. Buprenorphine for the management of opioid withdrawal. *Cochrane Database Syst Rev,* CD002025.

Gruenewald PJ, Freisthler B, Remer L, Lascala EA, Treno A. 2006. Ecological models of alcohol outlets and violent assaults: Crime potentials and geospatial analysis. *Addiction* 101:666-77.

Guxens M, Nebot M, Ariza C, Ochoa D. 2007. Factors associated with the onset of cannabis use: A systematic review of cohort studies. *Gac Sanit* 21:252-60.

Havassy BE, Hall SM, Wasserman DA. 1991. Social support and relapse: Commonalities among alcoholics, opiate users, and cigarette smokers. *Addictive Behav* 16:235-46.

Higgins ST, Alessi SM, Dantona RL. 2002. Voucher-based incentives: A substance abuse treatment innovation. *Addictive Behav* 27:887-910.

Higgins ST, Budney AJ, Bickel WK, Foerg FE, Donham R, Badger GJ. 1994. Incentives improve outcome in outpatient behavioral treatment of cocaine dependence. *Arch Gen Psychiatry* 51:568-76.

Hubbard RL, Marsden ME, Rachal JV, Harwood HJ, Cavanaugh ER, Ginzburg HM. 1989. *Drug Abuse Treatment: A National Study of Effectiveness.* Chapel Hill: University of North Carolina Press.

Jasinski DR, Pevnick JS, Griffith JD. 1978. Human pharmacology and abuse potential of the analgesic buprenorphine: A potential agent for treating narcotic addiction. *Arch Gen Psychiatry* 35:501-16.

Jellinek EM. 1960. *The Disease Concept of Alcoholism.* New Haven, CT: College and University Press.

Joffe A. 2004. Legalization of marijuana: Potential impact on youth. *Pediatrics* 113:1825-26.

Johnson RE, Chutuape MA, Strain EC, Walsh SL, Stitzer ML, Bigelow GE. 2000. A comparison of levomethadyl acetate, buprenorphine, and methadone for opioid dependence. *N Engl J Med* 343:1290-97.

Johnston LD, O'Malley PM, Bachman JG, Schulenbert JE. 2011. *Monitoring the Future National Results on Adolescent Drug Use: Overview of Key Findings, 2010.* Ann Arbor: University of Michigan.

Kadden R, Carroll K, Donovan D, et al. 1994. *Cognitive-Behavioral Coping Skills Therapy Manual.* Rockville, MD: National Institute on Alcohol Abuse and Alcoholism.

Kakko J, Svanborg KD, Kreek MJ, Heilig M. 2003. 1-year retention and social function after buprenorphine-assisted relapse prevention treatment for heroin dependence in Sweden: A randomised, placebo-controlled trial. *Lancet* 361:662-68.

Kendler KS, Gardner CO, Prescott CA. 1997. Religion, psychopathology, and substance use and abuse: A multimeasure, genetic-epidemiological study. *Am J Psychiatry* 154:322-29.

Kendler KS, Schmitt E, Aggen SH, Prescott CA. 2008. Genetic and environmental influences on alcohol, caffeine, cannabis, and nicotine use from early adolescence to middle adulthood. *Arch Gen Psychiatry* 65:674-82.

Kilpatrick DG, Acierno R, Saunders B, Resnick HS, Best CL, Schnurr PP. 2000. Risk factors for adolescent substance abuse and dependence: Data from a national sample. *J Consult Clin Psychol* 68:19-30.

Kirby KC, Benishek LA, Dugosh KL, Kerwin ME. 2006. Substance abuse treatment providers' beliefs and objections regarding contingency management: Implications for dissemination. *Drug Alcohol Depend* 85:19-27.

Kliewer W, Murrelle L. 2007. Risk and protective factors for adolescent substance use: Findings from a study in selected Central American countries. *J Adolesc Health* 40:448-55.

Kraft MK, Rothbard AB, Hadley TR, McLellan AT, Asch DA. 1997. Are supplementary services provided during methadone maintenance really cost-effective? *Am J Psychiatry* 154:1214-19.

Kraus JF. 2001. The effects of certain drug-testing programs on injury reduction in the workplace: An evidence-based review. *Int J Occup Environ Health* 7 (2): 103-8.

Lee MA, Flegel P, Greden JF, Cameron OG. 1988. Anxiogenic effects of caffeine on panic and depressed patients. *Am J Psychiatry* 145:632-35.

Levine MR, Rennie WP. 2004. Pre-employment urine drug testing of hospital employees: Future questions and review of current literature. *Occup Environ Med* 61:318-24.

Li J, Ha TH, Zhang C, Liu H. 2010. The Chinese government's response to drug use and HIV/AIDS: A review of policies and programs. *Harm Reduct J* 7:4.

Lima MS, Reisser AA, Soares BG, Farrell M. 2001. Antidepressants for cocaine dependence (Cochrane Review). *Cochrane Database Syst Rev,* 4.

Lipton R, Gruenewald P. 2002. The spatial dynamics of violence and alcohol outlets. *J Stud Alcohol* 63:187-95.

Livingston M. 2008. Alcohol outlet density and assault: A spatial analysis. *Addiction* 103:619-28.

Livingston M, Chikritzhs T, Room R. 2007. Changing the density of alcohol outlets to reduce alcohol-related problems. *Drug Alcohol Rev* 26:557-66.

Lofwall MR, Schuster A, Strain EC. 2008. Changing profile of abused substances by older persons entering treatment. *J Nerv Ment Dis* 196:898-905.

Lott DC, Jencius S. 2009. Effectiveness of very low-cost contingency management in a community adolescent treatment program. *Drug Alcohol Depend* 102:162-65.

Lovato C, Linn G, Stead LF, Best A. 2003. Impact of tobacco advertising and promotion on increasing adolescent smoking behaviours. *Cochrane Database Syst Rev,* CD003439.

Lundahl B, Burke BL. 2009. The effectiveness and applicability of motivational interviewing: A practice-friendly review of four meta-analyses. *J Clin Psychol* 65:1232-45.

Lussier JP, Heil SH, Mongeon JA, Badger GJ, Higgins ST. 2006. A meta-analysis of voucher-based reinforcement therapy for substance use disorders. *Addiction* 101:192-203.

Martin SL, Beaumont JL, Kupper LL. 2003. Substance use before and during pregnancy: Links to intimate partner violence. *Am J Drug Alcohol Abuse* 29:599-617.

Mattick RP, Breen C, Kimber J, Davoli M. 2009. Methadone maintenance therapy versus no opioid replacement therapy for opioid dependence. *Cochrane Database Syst Rev,* CD002209.

Mattick RP, Kimber J, Breen C, Davoli M. 2008. Buprenorphine maintenance versus placebo or methadone maintenance for opioid dependence. *Cochrane Database Syst Rev,* CD002207.

Mayet S, Farrell M, Ferri M, Amato L, Davoli M. 2005. Psychosocial treatment for opiate abuse and dependence. *Cochrane Database Syst Rev,* CD004330.

McCartt AT, Hellinga LA, Kirley BB. 2010. The effects of minimum legal drinking age 21 laws on alcohol-related driving in the United States. *J Safety Res* 41:173-81.

McHugh RK, Hofmann SG, Asnaani A, Sawyer AT, Otto MW. 2010. The serotonin transporter gene and risk for alcohol dependence: A meta-analytic review. *Drug Alcohol Depend* 108:1-6.

McLellan AT. 2010. Treatment given high priority in new White House drug control policy: Interview by Bridget Kuehn. *JAMA* 303:821-22.

McLellan AT, Arndt IO, Metzger DS, Woody GE, O'Brien CP. 1993. The effects of psychosocial services in substance abuse treatment. *JAMA* 269:1953-59.

Mercer DE, Woody GE. 2000. *An Individual Drug Counseling Approach to Treat Cocaine Addiction: The Collaborative Cocaine Treatment Study Model.* USDHS Pub. No. 00-4380. NIDA Therapy Manuals for Addiction. Bethesda, MD: U.S. Department of Health and Human Services.

Miller L, Davies M, Greenwald S. 2000. Religiosity and substance use and abuse among adolescents in the

National Comorbidity Survey. *J Am Acad Child Adolesc Psychiatry* 39:1190-97.

Miller TR, Zaloshnja E, Spicer RS. 2007. Effectiveness and benefit-cost of peer-based workplace substance abuse prevention coupled with random testing. *Accident Anal Prev* 39:565-73.

Miller WR, Zweben A, DiClemente CC, Rychtarik RG. 1994. *Motivational Enhancement Therapy Manual.* National Institute on Alcohol Abuse and Alcoholism. Rockville, MD: U.S. Dept. of Health and Human Services.

Moos RH. 2007. Theory-based active ingredients of effective treatments for substance use disorders. *Drug Alcohol Depend* 88:109-21.

Moos RH, Moos BS. 2006. Participation in treatment and Alcoholics Anonymous: A 16-year follow-up of initially untreated individuals. *J Clin Psychol* 62:735-50.

Nowinski J, Baker S, Carroll K. 1994. *Twelve Step Facilitation Therapy Manual.* National Institute on Alcohol Abuse and Alcoholism. Rockville, MD: U.S. Dept. of Health and Human Services.

O'Farrell TJ, Fals-Stewart W. 2002. Behavioral couples and family therapy for substance abusers. *Curr Psychiatry Rep* 4:371-76.

Office of National Drug Control Policy (ONDCP). 2004. *The Economic Costs of Drug Abuse in the United States, 1992-2002.* Washington, DC: Office of National Drug Control Policy.

Pedersen N. 1981. Twin similarity for usage of common drugs. In *Twin Research 3, Part C: Epidemiological and Clinical Studies,* ed. L Gedda, P Parisi, W Nance, 53-59. New York: Alan R. Liss.

Peirce JM, Petry NM, Stitzer ML, et al. 2006. Effects of lower-cost incentives on stimulant abstinence in methadone maintenance treatment: A National Drug Abuse Treatment Clinical Trials Network study. *Arch Gen Psychiatry* 63:201-8.

Peters LW, Kok G, Ten Dam GT, Buijs GJ, Paulussen TG. 2009. Effective elements of school health promotion across behavioral domains: A systematic review of reviews. *BMC Public Health* 9:182.

Petrie J, Bunn F, Byrne G. 2007. Parenting programmes for preventing tobacco, alcohol or drugs misuse in children <18: A systematic review. *Health Educ Res* 22:177-91.

Petry NM, Bickel WK. 2000. Gender differences in hostility of opioid-dependent outpatients: Role in early treatment termination. *Drug Alcohol Depend* 58:27-33.

Petry NM, Kirby KN, Kranzler HR. 2002. Effects of gender and family history of alcohol dependence on a behavioral task of impulsivity in healthy subjects. *J Stud Alcohol* 63:83-90.

Powers MB, Vedel E, Emmelkamp PM. 2008. Behavioral couples therapy (BCT) for alcohol and drug use disorders: A meta-analysis. *Clin Psychol Rev* 28:952-62.

Prendergast M, Podus D, Finney J, Greenwell L, Roll J. 2006. Contingency management for treatment of substance use disorders: A meta-analysis. *Addiction* 101:1546-60.

Preston KL, Silverman K, Umbricht A, DeJesus A, Montoya ID, Schuster CR. 1999. Improvement in naltrexone treatment compliance with contingency management. *Drug Alcohol Depend* 54:127-35.

Rehm J, Room R, van den Brink W, Jacobi F. 2005. Alcohol use disorders in EU countries and Norway: An overview of the epidemiology. *Eur Neuropsychopharmacol* 15:377-88.

Rehm J, Taylor B, Room R. 2006. Global burden of disease from alcohol, illicit drugs, and tobacco. *Drug Alcohol Rev* 25:503-13.

Richardson L, Hemsing N, Greaves L, et al. 2009. Preventing smoking in young people: A systematic review of the impact of access interventions. *Int J Environ Res Public Health* 6:1485-1514.

Roberts TA, Klein JD, Fisher S. 2003. Longitudinal effect of intimate partner abuse on high-risk behavior among adolescents. *Arch Pediatr Adolesc Med* 157:875-81.

Roche AM, Bywood P, Pidd K, Freeman T, Steenson T. 2009. Drug testing in Australian schools: Policy implications and considerations of punitive, deterrence, and/or prevention measures. *Int J Drug Policy* 20:521-28.

Sale E, Sambrano S, Springer JF, Pena C, Pan W, Kasim R. 2005. Family protection and prevention of alcohol use among Hispanic youth at high risk. *Am J Commun Psych* 36:195-205.

Sale E, Sambrano S, Springer JF, Turner CW. 2003. Risk, protection, and substance use in adolescents: A multi-site model. *J Drug Educ* 33:91-105.

Sartor CE, Agrawal A, McCutcheon VV, Duncan AE, Lynskey MT. 2008. Disentangling the complex association between childhood sexual abuse and alcohol-related problems: A review of methodological issues and approaches. *J Stud Alcohol Drugs* 69:718-27.

Scal P, Ireland M, Borowsky IW. 2003. Smoking among American adolescents: A risk and protective factor analysis. *J Commun Health* 28:79-97.

Schaus JF, Sole ML, McCoy TP, Mullett N, O'Brien MC. 2009. Alcohol screening and brief intervention in a college student health center: A randomized controlled trial. *J Stud Alcohol Drugs,* suppl., 131-41.

Schuckit MA. 2009. An overview of genetic influences in alcoholism. *J Subst Abuse Treat* 36: S5-S14.

Schwartz RP, Highfield DA, Jaffe JH, et al. 2006. A randomized controlled trial of interim methadone maintenance. *Arch Gen Psychiatry* 63:102-9.

Sees KL, Delucchi KL, Masson C, et al. 2000. Methadone maintenance vs 180-day psychosocially enriched detoxification for treatment of opioid dependence: A randomized controlled trial. *JAMA* 283:1303-10.

Shortt AL, Hutchinson DM, Chapman R, Toumbourou JW. 2007. Family, school, peer, and individual influences on early adolescent alcohol use: First-year impact of the Resilient Families programme. *Drug Alcohol Rev* 26:625-34.

Silverman K, Wong CJ, Higgins ST, et al. 1996. Increasing opiate abstinence through voucher-based reinforcement therapy. *Drug Alcohol Depend* 41:157-65.

Smit E, Verdurmen J, Monshouwer K, Smit F. 2008. Family interventions and their effect on adolescent alcohol use in general populations: A meta-analysis of randomized controlled trials. *Drug Alcohol Depend* 97:195-206.

Smith CA, Elwyn LJ, Ireland TO, Thornberry TP. 2010. Impact of adolescent exposure to intimate partner violence on substance use in early adulthood. *J Stud Alcohol Drugs* 71:219-30.

Smith LA, Foxcroft DR. 2009. The effect of alcohol advertising, marketing, and portrayal on drinking behaviour in young people: Systematic review of prospective cohort studies. *BMC Public Health* 9:51.

Snyder LB, Milici FF, Slater M, Sun H, Strizhakova Y. 2006. Effects of alcohol advertising exposure on drinking among youth. *Arch Pediatr Adolesc Med* 160:18-24.

Spicer RS, Miller TR. 2005. Impact of a workplace peer-focused substance abuse prevention and early intervention program. *Alcohol Clin Exp Res* 29:609-11.

Srisurapanont M, Jarusuraisin N. 2005. Opioid antagonists for alcohol dependence. *Cochrane Database Syst Rev,* CD001867.

Stead LF, Perera R, Bullen C, Mant D, Lancaster T. 2008. Nicotine replacement therapy for smoking cessation. *Cochrane Database Syst Rev,* CD000146.

Stitzer M, Petry N. 2006. Contingency management for treatment of substance abuse. *Annu Rev Clin Psychol* 2:411-34.

Stitzer ML, Vandrey R. 2008. Contingency management: Utility in the treatment of drug abuse disorders. *Clin Pharmacol Ther* 83:644-47.

Stoops WW, Hatton KW, Lofwall MR, Nuzzo PA, Walsh SL. 2010. Intravenous oxycodone, hydrocodone, and morphine in recreational opioid users: Abuse potential and relative potencies. *Psychopharmacol (Berl)* 212:193-203.

Strain EC. 2004. Patient-treatment matching and opioid addicted patients: Past methods and future opportunities. *Heroin Addict Related Clin Problems* 6:5-16.

Strain EC, Bigelow GE, Liebson IA, Stitzer ML. 1999. Moderate- vs high-dose methadone in the treatment of opioid dependence: A randomized trial. *JAMA* 281:1000-1005.

Strain EC, Stitzer ML. 2006. *The Treatment of Opioid Dependence.* Baltimore: Johns Hopkins University Press.

Strain EC, Stitzer ML, Bigelow GE. 1991. Early treatment time course of depressive symptoms in opiate addicts. *J Nerv Ment Dis* 179:215-21.

Strain EC, Stitzer ML, Liebson IA, Bigelow GE. 1993. Methadone dose and treatment outcome. *Drug Alcohol Depend* 33:105-17.

———. 1994. Outcome after methadone treatment: Influence of prior treatment factors and current treatment status. *Drug Alcohol Depend* 35:223-30.

———. 1996. Buprenorphine versus methadone in the treatment of opioid dependence: Self-reports, urinalysis, and addiction severity index. *J Clin Psychopharmacol* 16:58-67.

Strain EC, Stoller K, Walsh SL, Bigelow GE. 2000. Effects of buprenorphine versus buprenorphine/naloxone tablets in non-dependent opioid abusers. *Psychopharmacol (Berl)* 148:374-83.

Strassels SA. 2009. Economic burden of prescription opioid misuse and abuse. *J Manag Care Pharm* 15:556-62.

Stronski SM, Ireland M, Michaud P, Narring F, Resnick MD. 2000. Protective correlates of stages in adolescent substance use: A Swiss National Study. *J Adolesc Health* 26:420-27.

Substance Abuse and Mental Health Services Administration (SAMHSA). 2005. *Results from the 2004 National Survey on Drug Use and Health: National Findings.* DHHS Publication No. SMA 05-4062. National Survey on Drug Use and Health. Substance Abuse and Mental Health Services Administration, Office of Applied Studies. Rockville, Maryland: U.S. Dept. of Health and Human Services.

———. 2012. *Results from the 2011 National Survey on Drug Use and Health: National Findings.* Substance Abuse and Mental Health Services Administration, Center for Behavioral Health Statistics and Quality. Rockville, MD: U.S. Dept. of Health and Human Services.

Swan GE, Carmelli D, Cardon LR. 1997. Heavy consumption of cigarettes, alcohol, and coffee in male twins. *J Stud Alcohol* 58:182-90.

Tauras JA. 2005. Can public policy deter smoking escalation among young adults? *J Policy Anal Man* 24:771-84.

Tauras JA, Markowitz S, Cawley J. 2005. Tobacco control policies and youth smoking: Evidence from a new era. *Adv Health Econ Health Serv Res* 16:277-91.

Treno AJ, Johnson FW, Remer LG, Gruenewald PJ. 2007. The impact of outlet densities on alcohol-related crashes: A spatial panel approach. *Accident Anal Prev* 39:894-901.

Wagenaar AC, Toomey TL. 2002. Effects of minimum drinking age laws: Review and analyses of the literature from 1960 to 2000. *J Stud Alcohol* (suppl. 14), 206-25.

Wakefield M, Flay B, Nichter M, Giovino G. 2003a. Effects of anti-smoking advertising on youth smoking: A review. *J Health Commun* 8:229-47.

———. 2003b. Role of the media in influencing trajectories of youth smoking. *Addiction* 98 (suppl. 1): 79-103.

Wasserman DA, Stewart AL, Delucchi KL. 2001. Social support and abstinence from opiates and cocaine during opioid maintenance treatment. *Drug Alcohol Depend* 65:65-75.

Webb G, Shakeshaft A, Sanson-Fisher R, Havard A. 2009. A systematic review of work-place interventions for alcohol-related problems. *Addiction* 104:365-77.

Wellman RJ, Sugarman DB, DiFranza JR, Winickoff JP. 2006. The extent to which tobacco marketing and tobacco use in films contribute to children's use of tobacco: A meta-analysis. *Arch Pediatr Adolesc Med* 160:1285-96.

Whitlock EP, Polen MR, Green CA, Orleans T, Klein J, U.S. Preventive Services Task Force. 2004. Behavioral counseling interventions in primary care to reduce risky/harmful alcohol use by adults: A summary of the evidence for the U.S. Preventive Services Task Force. *Ann Intern Med* 140 (7): 557-68.

Willis C, Lybrand S, Bellamy N. 2004. Alcohol ignition interlock programmes for reducing drink driving recidivism. *Cochrane Database Syst Rev,* CD004168.

Zacny JP. 2003. Characterizing the subjective, psycho-motor, and physiological effects of a hydrocodone combination product (Hycodan) in non-drug-abusing volunteers. *Psychopharmacol (Berl)* 165:146-56.

Zacny JP, Gutierrez S. 2009. Within-subject comparison of the psychopharmacological profiles of oral hydrocodone and oxycodone combination products in non-drug-abusing volunteers. *Drug Alcohol Depend* 101:107-14.

CHAPTER 13

Obesity and Eating Behaviors and Behavior Change

SCOTT KAHAN AND LAWRENCE J. CHESKIN

LEARNING OBJECTIVES

After completing the chapter, the reader will be able to

* Appreciate the complexity of obesity as a unique public health problem that goes beyond simplistic notions of "self-control."
* Define body mass index and describe the relevance for using this concept to measure obesity.
* Provide several determinants of obesity risk at multiple levels of influence.
* Describe several potential interventions that have evidence for effectiveness in addressing or preventing obesity.

Introduction

Since 1960, the entire distribution curve of weight has shifted for the U.S. population; the average American has gained approximately *25 pounds* (Flegal and Troiano 2000). One in three American adults is now classified as clinically *obese,* with an additional one in three classified as *overweight.* Indeed, nearly everyone is gaining weight; the majority of persons in the "normal" weight category are steadily gaining, such that studies suggest that by 2030 nearly every American will be overweight and more than 50% of Americans will be obese (Wang et al. 2008). Excess weight has become the **norm**.

At the core of many people's beliefs about obesity is personal responsibility (i.e., just *eat less and exercise more*). We assume that what we eat, how much we move, and ultimately our weight is purely a matter of personal choice—after all, we decide what we put on our forks, what we put in our mouths, and whether we spend our evenings in front of the television or at the gym, right?

Yet, a large and consistent body of knowledge, from nutrition science to social science to psychology to public health, shows that our behaviors are shaped, and often determined, by numerous factors that extend beyond individual control. "Willpower," or personal responsibility, though a piece of the puzzle, is too simplistic an explanation; pointing at willpower masks the intricacies of the problem, the multitude of **influences** on eating behaviors, physical activity, and weight. To dismiss weight gain and obesity as simply a matter of willpower or self-control implicates nearly all Americans, and much of the world's population, as essentially failures.

As discussed throughout this textbook, health behaviors—and **health behavior** change—are shaped by a multitude of influences. As shown in the fields of tobacco control (chapter 10), alcohol abuse (chapter 11), unintentional injuries (chapter 15), and other behavior-related public health problems, expecting individuals to change behavior without addressing the environment in which their behavior develops and occurs is rarely productive. Addressing the environment without simultaneously addressing individuals is similarly unproductive. This chapter will address the health behaviors related to weight gain and obesity following this principle, the **ecological model** of health behaviors.

Obesity is now firmly established as one of the most serious public health concerns throughout the Western world. Rates of obesity in developed countries approach epidemic levels, and even in most developing countries, rates are increasing dramatically. Few parts of the world are unaffected. Although obesity is an age-old problem that has been described in print and in art for millennia, much has changed in recent decades:

- Rates of weight gain, after increasing slowly for at least two centuries in the United States, have escalated since the last third of the 20th century at rates previously unheard of, resulting in the tripling in prevalence of adult and childhood overweight and obesity since the 1980s. Similar increases have occurred elsewhere.
- Rates of obesity-related chronic diseases—especially diabetes—have also ballooned, resulting in extensive **morbidity**, **mortality**, and economic cost to society.
- Many people now view weight gain and obesity as a medical problem, rather than simply an aesthetic one (in part as a result of the previous two points). Most public health authorities, scientific organizations, and physicians now regard obesity (beyond overweight) as a medical condition that requires aggressive and sustained **evaluation** and treatment. This has led to an increase in funding, research, and dissemination of education (to practitioners and the public), which has begun to address some of the drivers and **consequences** of weight gain.

Though the statistics of obesity rates in the United States and worldwide are sobering, significant progress has recently been made, suggesting the potential for future additional success. Indeed, perhaps for the first time in the course of the obesity epidemic, and even as obesity rates continue to grow in much of the world, hope for the future is emerging. Public health messages about obesity and a healthful diet have penetrated much of American society: the majority of Americans know that weight affects health; more Americans are now concerned about their weight and use weight as a key driver for dietary changes (there are, of course, unintended consequences of this awareness, such as potential increases in body image disorders, but that issue goes beyond the scope of this chapter) (IFIC 2010). Further, we are now in a climate of incredible pace of discovery and progress in the field of obesity prevention and treatment. With the discovery of leptin in 1995, we identified a key hormone produced by adipose (fat) cells that signals the brain and body of stored energy reserves and affects appetite and metabolic rate, among other physiological processes. We have entered an age of rapid biological, pharmaceutical, and genetic discoveries regarding weight and obesity. The Food and Drug Administration (FDA) has recently approved two new medications for the long-term treatment of obesity, and several others are being studied. Most importantly, focus has shifted to environmental and social **determinants** of weight gain, and political and social will now exists for addressing the underlying causes of weight gain in developed countries.

A chapter on obesity is included in this book because obesity is a key public health topic (as well as the primary area of expertise and passion of this book's editor-in-chief). However, it is paramount to recognize that *obesity is not a behavior*. Rather, weight gain and obesity are the outcome of numerous ongoing health behaviors. Because chapter 14 describes the determinants and **interventions** related to physical activity, this chapter will primarily concentrate on the issues of eating and caloric intake. Thus, we will discuss the individual, social, and societal factors that affect what we eat and what interventions have been shown to be effective in mitigating the risk for obesity or addressing and treating existing obesity. For the specific background, determinants, and interventions related to physical activity, we refer readers to chapter 14. Moreover, we primarily concentrate on adults and the U.S. obesity epidemic, although much of our discussion applies to childhood obesity and to other societies as well.

Magnitude

Numerous measures can be used to describe adiposity (amount of body fat) and obesity. Weight is the simplest, although it is **confounded** by several factors, including height, lean tissue (e.g., muscle, bone), and others. That is, two persons of the same weight might have very different levels of body fat and health risk. For example, someone who is six feet tall and weighs 200 pounds is leaner than someone who is five feet tall and weighs 200 pounds. Moreover, one who is frail will weigh less than a person of the same height who is muscular. Clearly, simply using weight to measure fat is problematic. Among the numerous more accurate measures to estimate body fat percentage are CT and MRI scans. But although these tests can be highly accurate for individuals, they are time-consuming and expensive. The primary indicator for measuring obesity on a population level is **body mass index** (**BMI**), which is a measure of weight related to height (calculated by dividing weight in kilograms by height in meters squared). This measure has been shown to correlate well with body fat on a population level (Gallagher et al. 2000). For adults, a normal BMI is considered to be 18.5-25 kg/m^2; overweight (i.e., elevated body weight that potentially indicates a "pre-obesity" state) is defined as a BMI of 25.0-29.9 kg/m^2; obesity is indicated by a BMI of 30 kg/m^2 or greater; and a BMI of 40 kg/m^2 or greater indicates severe obesity (NHLBI 1998; WHO Expert Committee 1995).

Rates of overweight and obesity in adults have increased dramatically since the 1980s. The most current estimates show that nearly 70% of Americans have a BMI greater than 25 kg/m^2 and 35.7% of American adults fit the classification for obesity (CDC 2009-10). Rates of obesity have more than doubled in most sectors of the population and have tripled in children and adolescents in just the past three decades. Rates of severe obesity have increased even more significantly (Sturm 2007). Similar trends are seen in other developed countries (Berg et al. 2005; Gutierrez-Fisac et al. 2000; Heitmann 2000; Kautiainen et al. 2002; Lindstrom et al. 2003). Additionally, developing countries, where malnutrition, hunger, and underweight continue to ravage, are paradoxically seeing more and more overweight and obesity.

Worldwide, at least 1 billion people are overweight and more than 300 million have a BMI greater than 30 (WHO 2008). Overweight and obesity rates are expected to double worldwide by 2015 (James 2008).

From 1971 to 2000, obesity rates increased from 5% to 10.4% in children 2–5 years old, from 4% to 15.3% in children 6–11 years old, and from 6.1% to 15.5% among adolescents 12–19 years old (Ogden et al. 2002). Overweight children are more likely to have obesity as adults.[1] In one study, 6–8-year-old children with obesity were 10 times as likely to be obese as adults than were lower-weight children (Freedman et al. 2005).

Distribution

Several ethnic disparities exist in rates of overweight and obesity. Rates of overweight in African American and Mexican American women are approximately 35% greater than age-adjusted rates for Caucasian women; rates of obesity in African American and Mexican American women are approximately 50% greater than the rates for age-adjusted Caucasian women. Childhood obesity rates are highest in non-Hispanic black girls and Hispanic boys. Rates of obesity in four-year-old children are two to three times more common in Native American children than in white or Asian children (Anderson and Whitaker 2009). Socioeconomic disparities are also common. Women with higher BMIs tend to have lower income (Chang and Lauderdale 2005). Nearly 40% of white women who qualify for nutrition assistance have obesity (Ogden et al. 2007). Nearly 35% of adults with less than a high school education have obesity, compared with 21% of those with a college degree (Pleis et al. 2008).

Consequences

Obesity affects disease risk in virtually every organ system, including certain cancers (NHLBI 1998). The risks for hypertension (high blood pressure), elevated cholesterol levels, heart disease, stroke, breathing difficulties and lung disease, infertility, and arthritis all increase precipitously with increasing weight, and more than 60 diseases are associated with obesity (Kopelman 2007). In particular, obesity is a strong risk factor for type 2 diabetes, and the increase in obesity rates appears to be driving an epidemic of diabetes, including the emergence of type 2 (previously called "adult-onset") diabetes in children (CDC 2003; Fagot-Campagna 2000; Harris et al. 1998). The vast majority of individuals with diabetes are overweight or have obesity, and a graded relationship exists between BMI and diabetes risk, with a BMI >35 resulting in more than a 10-fold increased risk for developing diabetes. One-third of all children born in the United States today (and as many as half of African American and Mexican American children) are expected to develop diabetes in their lifetime (Narayan et al. 2003). Largely because of obesity and unhealthful lifestyles, 70% of U.S. children have at least one risk factor for heart disease (Freedman et al. 2007).

Mortality and Economic Burden

Approximately 100,000 to 300,000 deaths per year in the United States alone are attributed to obesity (although precisely quantifying deaths caused by obesity is technically complicated, and different study approaches have yielded a wide range of estimates). If the high end of this estimate proves true, obesity will soon overtake tobacco use as the number one preventable cause of death in the United States. Yet, even in the "best-case" scenario of 112,000 deaths per year, obesity would be America's second most prevalent underlying cause of death (Mokdad et al. 2004).

Finally, the economic costs associated with obesity are immense. The **direct costs** (health care costs) and **indirect costs** (job absenteeism, decreased productivity, and others) of obesity are estimated to exceed $200 billion yearly in the United States (Cawley and Meyerhoefer 2012), accounting for 10% of all health-care-related costs and more than one-fourth of recent health care spending increases (Daviglus et al. 2004; Finkelstein et al. 2003; Thorpe et al. 2004).

Key Determinants

Weight gain and obesity are related to numerous physiological, psychological, environmental, and social factors. Each side of the energy balance equation (calorie intake and energy expenditure) is affected by **proximal determinants**, such as knowledge, behaviors, and genetics, as well as **distal determinants**, such as **sociocultural norms** and the food and **built environments**. Knowing what the **key determinants** are helps us understand how to address a public health problem, including what factors to intervene upon, where to invest resources, and what to address. Below we describe many of the determinants that influence food intake, body weight, and risk for obesity. An exhaustive list is beyond the scope of this chapter. We refer readers to chapter 14, on physical activity, for a description of the determinants of physical activity behaviors.

Some factors that affect the propensity to weight gain and obesity are more easily addressed (e.g., knowledge) and others less easily (e.g., environmental **cues**); still others are essentially not (or not yet) modifiable (e.g., genetics). We categorize the determinants here as individual, familial and interpersonal, community and environmental, and policy-societal. Each level of influence can affect health behavior. Moreover, influences among and between the levels are likely to be particularly salient. For example, having a parent with obesity increases the risk of childhood obesity by more than 10%, and the increased risk is likely due to a **complex** interaction between genetics, **epigenetics**, reinforced behavioral patterns, the home environment, and familial norms; societal **stereotypes** and **stigmas** toward people who have obesity are known to diminish **self-efficacy** and attempts at behavior change; unhealthful nutrition, obesity, and the development of gestational diabetes in a pregnant woman can affect the genetic expression (epigenetics) and lifelong risk of obesity and cardiovascular disease in her child; and increasing individuals' knowledge throughout the population, such as via **social marketing** or public awareness campaigns, helps to build an informed electorate, which in turn can initiate and support broad societal measures.

Individual-Level Factors

Individual characteristics that influence eating behaviors and weight, for the purposes of this chapter, are categorized as genetic and epigenetic factors, **psychosocial** and **lifestyle factors**, and dietary factors. Many of these observations make sense in an evolutionary **context**; that is, survival in the face of historical food scarcity is likely to have been enhanced by behaviors that maximized food consumption when food was plentiful (Brown and Konner 1987).

GENETICS AND EPIGENETICS

The impact of genetics on body weight and obesity risk has been shown repeatedly in twin adoption studies. In these studies, sets of biological twins who were adopted and reared apart were compared with their biological parents and their adoptive parents. Stronger weight relationships exist between the biological parents and the adoptees than between the adoptive parents' BMIs and the adoptees' weight class (Sunkard et al. 1986), suggesting that genetics is a key contributor to weight trajectory and the risk of obesity. Recent discoveries of genes (e.g., the FTO gene), hormones (e.g., leptin, ghrelin), neurotransmitters (e.g., neuropeptide Y), and numerous other biochemicals will continue to shed light on the mechanisms of genetic and biological influences on energy balance and body weight.

At the heart of weight and weight management is a homeostatic biological system that regulates energy balance. This regulatory system is primarily genetically determined and includes genes, neurochemicals, hormones, and complex metabolic factors that regulate metabolism, hunger, **satiety**, and physiological responses to food cues (e.g., specific smells, tastes, etc.) and eating. This system is generally fine-tuned. Consider that over the course of a year, an average person consumes approximately 1 million calories yet gains just one-half pound or so. Despite this enormity of calories consumed, eating opportunities, physical activity opportunities, and metabolic activities, the regulatory system is able to match almost identically the intake of calories with the expenditure or use of them—estimated to be within 0.17%.

Research indicates that some people with obesity have overly responsive appetite systems; this predisposition is largely genetically determined. Until recent decades, food scarcity masked it in most individuals; however, in the current environment of food abundance, such metabolic tendencies are exposed and lead to weight gain unless they are overridden by deliberate and consistent control (Butland et al. 2007, 44). Thin persons versus individuals with obesity often differ in the sensitivity of their neural, hormonal, and metabolic responses to external stimuli (such as tastes, sight, smell, and the availability of foods), in sensitivity of reward pathways in response to foods and other stimuli, and in appetite and satiety. Individual appetite and responsiveness to foods appears to be heritable (Wardle 2007). Evidence is mounting that certain individuals are predisposed to increased appetite and weight gain because they have more sensitive physiological responses to highly palatable foods, intense sweetness, and other food-related factors, which can overwhelm physiological control mechanisms and intentional counterbehaviors (e.g., dieting) (Lei-

bowitz 2002; Rolls 2007). In contrast, significant metabolic differences do not appear to exist between people with higher and lower weights. In fact, heavier persons generally have higher metabolisms, in part because more energy is needed to maintain a larger body size (Prentice 2007).

Epigenetics is the study of how gene function is affected by prenatal and early life experiences and exposures. Several periods and exposures during early life play critical roles in a person's risk for obesity as well as other health outcomes, such as heart disease (Barker et al. 2005). The intrauterine environment, determined by the mother's diet, circulating hormones, presence or absence of gestational diabetes, psychological and physical stress levels, and other factors, plays a central role in fetal development. Children born to women who smoked, gained excessive weight, or developed diabetes during pregnancy have increased risk of childhood obesity (Gilman 2008). Prenatal and early life exposures may affect metabolism, neurological and hormonal responses to food, fat storage, and other factors related to obesity (Barker 2007; Levin 2005).

A particularly salient early life exposure is breastfeeding. Infants who are breastfed tend to grow more slowly and have lower risks of childhood obesity and adult obesity, compared with formula-fed infants. Moreover, the longer breastfeeding lasts, the lower the risk of ensuing obesity; exclusive breastfeeding appears to confer a significantly lowered risk (Singhal and Lanigan 2007). One possible explanation for this phenomenon is that systematic exposure to the varied flavors of, and nutrients in, breast milk can promote healthier taste preferences (Menella et al. 2001). Other early life factors that may be related to later obesity risk include, among others, the child's birth weight, growth pattern during the initial weeks of life, early weight gain, and amount of sleep during the first year of life.

Psychosocial and lifestyle factors affecting the risk for obesity are numerous and include cognitive factors (e.g., knowledge, **attitudes**, beliefs, awareness), preferences, personality traits, perceived stress tendencies, outcome expectancies, health beliefs, types of **motivation**, self-efficacy, skills, **habits**, emotional regulation skills, perceived time, and many others.

Knowledge. Knowledge is essential for the intentional performance of healthful behaviors. Knowledge of target behaviors (e.g., eating fewer calories, decreasing sugar consumption) is a necessary prerequisite for behavior change, and knowledge has been shown to increase self-efficacy, or confidence, for healthful eating (Schnoll and Zimmerman 2001). In many areas of America, knowledge regarding eating and weight management remains poor, as indicated by a recent survey showing that just 12% of Americans accurately estimated the number of daily calories they should eat, on average, to maintain a healthful weight. Less than half knew how many calories they burned in a day or knew how to balance caloric consumption and caloric expenditure in order to manage their weight. Americans continue to be confused about macronutrients (carbohydrates, fats, and proteins), sweeteners (sugar, high-fructose corn syrup, artificial sweeteners), and other aspects of eating behaviors and weight management (IFIC 2010). However, studies do not *consistently* show that increasing one's knowledge influences one's eating behavior, weight gain, or behavior change in general, in part because of methodological limitations of such studies but also because of other factors that overwhelm intellectual food choice decisions, such as food palatability, availability, and advertising (Wardle et al. 2000). Thus, knowledge is necessary, but not sufficient, for healthful eating behaviors and weight management.

Behavioral Skills. Behavioral skills are an additional prerequisite for behavior change. Once an individual identifies a given target behavior to perform, he must have certain skills to accomplish the behavior. For example, once an individual knows that moderating calorie intake is essential for weight loss, she must be able to identify low-calorie foods, decipher the labeling that lists ingredients and nutrition facts, and shop for and prepare low-calorie foods that are enjoyable to eat; she may also have to prepare the foods in the context of a specific cuisine (e.g., Kosher) or limitation (e.g., gluten intolerance) (Taylor et al. 2005). Further, general process skills, such as problem-solving skills, **goal-setting skills**, self-monitoring skills, communication skills (e.g., how to ask questions of and negotiate with a dietitian) are also linked with behavior change (Hill-Briggs and Gemmell 2007; Povey et al. 1999).

Perceptions, Beliefs, and Perceived Control. A person's perceptions, beliefs, and perceived control over his eating behaviors and weight are associated with his actual eating behavior and successful behavior change (Furst et al. 1996; O'Dea 2003; Povey et al. 1999). Diet- and weight-related behavior change is also affected by a person's awareness and perception of her weight status (i.e., overweight versus normal weight) (Maximova et al. 2008), her beliefs about modifiable causes of obesity (Wang and Coups 2010), her perceptions of obesity as a health risk, her beliefs about the **expectations** (i.e., approval or disapproval) of others (family, physician, friends, etc.), and similar factors. If people think they lack the necessary time and money to eat healthfully, they are likely to eat poorer diets.

Stress. Stress has an effect as well. Studies suggest that in response to mild and moderate stress, both animals and humans overeat (extreme stress may cause undereating) and show preference for high-calorie and highly palatable foods, such as sweet and fatty foods (Wardle and Gibson 2002).

Self-Efficacy. **Self-efficacy**, or confidence in one's ability to achieve a target behavior in the face of barriers, is also associated with behavior and behavior change. Observing others who carry out healthful behaviors, especially those who are sociodemographically similar, has been shown to increase a person's self-efficacy.

Access. Another essential is access to the resources needed to enact the target behaviors, such as convenient sources of healthful foods and support options for gaining knowledge (i.e., "Who can teach me about nutrition? Does my insurance cover dietitian counseling?").

Motivation. Having the motivation to perform or change a given health behavior is an important, but limited, factor for engaging in healthful behaviors. In essence, motivation is essential for behavior change, but only after other prerequisites for behavior change have been achieved, including knowledge, skills, awareness, and access to resources (Miller and Rollnick 2002).

Food Preferences. Preference is most often shaped by taste and liking, especially in children and adolescents (Drewnowski 1997). Preference for a specific food strongly determines intake of that food, which may lead to an improved diet that protects against weight gain (e.g., fruits and vegetables) or a less healthful diet that predisposes to weight gain (e.g., processed sugar or fatty foods, fast foods, vending machine snacks) (Drewnowski et al. 1999; French et al. 1999; Resnicow et al. 1997; Shepherd et al. 2001). Food preferences developed in childhood will often persist into adulthood, and the quality of a person's diet often declines with age (CDC 1997; Johnson and Nicklas 1999). Taste and liking are related to several factors, including inherent properties of foods (e.g., palatability [see below]), physiology (e.g., neurophysiological responses to sweet or fatty foods), habit, social and cultural background, and environmental cues. Some individuals have an innate physiological tendency to prefer sweet, salty, or fatty foods, which may result in higher responsiveness to external food cues than to internal satiety cues. Several studies have associated such differences between lean individuals and persons with obesity (Schachter 1968). In particular, external factors, such as environmental cues and defaults, shape preferences. For example, having a McDonald's right next door to an individual's workplace increases not only intake of McDonald's food but also the individual's preference for it; the presence of a popular cartoon character on a food package influences children's preference for the food (Roberto et al. 2010). Further, experiences and habits tend to shape preferences; studies have shown that purposeful, repeated exposure to foods can increase acceptance and preference, such as for vegetables in those who previously disliked them (Myers and Sclafani 2006; Wardle et al. 2003).

Habits. **Habits** are learned, often automatic, behaviors that are commonly **triggered** by environmental and social cues and often have become decoupled from the original reason for the behavior (Wood et al. 2005). Habits are less guided by intent, knowledge, attitude, and motivation, making them often occur in contrast to conscious **goals** such as weight loss (Webb and Sheeran 2006). Ingrained habits often determine food preferences and intake. Moreover, habits lead to "tunnel vision," so that attempted changes in knowledge, attitudes, motivation, and other factors are less influential on behavior when habits are already formed (Maio et al. 2007). Meal structure appears to be a key habit in consumption and weight management. Having more structured and habitual meal plans, meal patterns and timing, and set grocery lists is associated with improved weight loss. Consistently eating breakfast and consuming a diet with little variety, both of which may be related to a more structured diet, are associated with improved weight-loss maintenance (Wing 2004).

Psychological and Emotional Factors. These influences, including self-esteem, body image, restrained eating (chronic on-and-off dieting), personality traits, mood, and the ability to regulate emotions, affect what and how much we eat—in part because what we eat can affect our mood and psychological well-being. Eating is an emotional and contextual event. Low self-esteem, low body image, and restrained eating have been shown to increase eating, unhealthful eating, binge eating, and emotional eating (eating in response to uncomfortable emotions, such as stress or anxiety). Food is commonly used to manage uncomfortable moods or emotional states, and skills for regulating one's emotions may be associated with eating and weight. Some studies have shown that, since food choices affect psychological well-being, healthful eating can negatively affect psychological health, even as it improves physical health (McFarlane et al. 1988; Polivy 1996; Polivy and Herman 2005; Stice et al. 2002).

Situational Factors and Life Events. Finally, situational factors and life events, including life changes and transitions (such as pregnancy and new parenthood, menopause, job changes, relationship changes, divorce), stressful events (such as physical or sexual abuse), smoking cessation, and others often contribute to weight difficulties.

DIETARY FACTORS

Distinct from the genetic, psychosocial, and lifestyle factors discussed above, numerous dietary factors affect eating behaviors, weight, and risk for obesity. In general, there are many limitations to studying the effect of diet on body weight. One such limitation is the difficulty of measuring dietary intake in real-world settings. In most cases, dietary intake is underreported, often by 25% or more (Livingstone and Black 2003). Nonetheless, several dietary factors are important to consider, including macronutrient composition, portion size, energy density, "liquid calories," and meal pattern.

Macronutrients. Macronutrient composition is an oft-discussed and argued aspect of obesity treatment and prevention, and yet it is still poorly understood. Many observational studies show that high-fat diets are associated with

weight gain and low-fat diets cause modest weight loss and improved maintenance of weight loss, but some randomized controlled studies show that macronutrient composition matters little in terms of weight loss (Howard et al. 2006; Wing 2004). In contrast, fiber consumption is consistently linked with body weight in an inverse relationship, and controlled studies show that increasing fiber intake can support weight loss (Howarth et al. 2001).

Portion Size. This is a particularly strong determinant of increased intake and weight gain. Portion sizes have increased precipitously as obesity rates have increased. People eat more when presented with larger portions (Ello-Martin et al. 2005), in part because increasing portions results in higher intake but not increased satiety—we tend to eat what is in front of us, regardless of hunger or fullness. Moreover, there is usually minimal compensation at later meals for the extra amounts eaten earlier (Rolls et al. 2005).

Energy Density. This is a measure of the caloric content of foods per unit of weight. Modern foods, particularly processed foods, tend to be more calorie-dense than traditional foods, such as vegetables and fruits; that is, they are (significantly) higher in calories for a given volume of food. Increased water and fiber content lower the energy density, since they contribute to the weight and volume of the food but do not contain calories. We tend to eat more when we consume energy-dense foods. For a given number of calories, foods that have low energy density take up more volume and take longer to eat than do foods of high energy density, resulting in increased satiety and less intake. Moreover, energy-dense foods may undermine biological appetite control mechanisms, resulting in passive overconsumption before satiety kicks in (Rolls et al. 2005; Stubbs et al. 2000). That is, when people eat energy-dense foods, the volume of food eaten is not decreased to match the greater number of calories being consumed. Studies show that ad libitum calorie intake is higher when more energy-dense foods are con-sumed (Stubbs et al. 2000).

High energy density may be the primary reason that fatty foods and restaurant and "fast" foods, both of which tend to be higher in fat and more energy dense compared with tradi-tional foods, cause weight gain (fat is more than twice as energy dense as carbohydrate or pro-tein) (Prentice and Jebb 2003). Consumption of restaurant foods and fast foods has increased significantly in recent decades, including a more than threefold increase in children's diets (Nielson et al. 2002). Consumption of liquid calories, especially sugar-sweetened beverages (SSBs, or "sodas") has also increased signifi-cantly in recent decades, including a more than tenfold increase in some portions of the popula-tion; SSBs now compose 7%-10% of daily intake, on average, for adults and children (McGinnis et al. 2006; Nielsen and Popkin 2004; Prynne et al. 1999). SSB consumption is associated with a poor diet and risk for obesity, diabetes, and heart disease (Vartanian et al. 2007). Moreover, the increased consumption of sweetened drinks has displaced the consumption of milk, which is an important source of numerous nutrients, is more satiating than sweetened drinks, and may prevent excess weight gain (Barba et al. 2005; Skinner et al. 2003). Liquid calories are likely not registered by the body as well as solid calories are—even if the composition of the calories is essentially identical (e.g., soda versus jelly beans); thus, consumption of liquid calo-ries is not significantly offset by lesser con-sumption of other foods, so it leads to increase caloric intake and propensity toward weight gain, compared with eating solid calories.

In contrast, fruit and vegetables are consis-tently associated with lowered weight gain, and nuts and dairy products may also be protective against weight gain and obesity (He et al. 2004; Sabate 2003). Certain dietary patterns may also be protective, such as increased protein intake (Simpson and Raubenheimer 2005) and adhering to a Mediterranean diet that emphasizes vegeta-

bles, fruits, nuts, unrefined carbohydrates, and olive oil (Sanchez-Villegas et al. 2006).

Environmental Cues. Environmental cues strongly shape behaviors and can overwhelm innate control mechanisms for regulation of food intake, energy balance, and weight. Food-related cues, such as the smell of a favorite food, the sight of someone eating, or the presence of highly palatable and preferred snack foods in the house, tend to increase the subjective feel-ing of hunger or the desire to eat, even when an individual's appetite is low. Nonfood cues, such as social situations (e.g., dinner party, business lunch) and environmental stimuli, and emo-tional and cognitive cues (e.g., "I had a tough day, so I deserve a treat.") also lead to food con-sumption, even in the absence of physiological hunger (Mattes 1997; Weingarten 1983).

Palatability. Particularly in the case of pro-cessed foods, palatability can overwhelm one's innate control mechanisms for food intake, espe-cially in susceptible individuals (Bobroff and Kis-sileff 1986). Studies have begun to unravel how certain foods, food combinations, tastes, and textures modulate and overwhelm reward and executive control systems in the brain; in some cases there is a similarity to the way addictive substances work (Volkow and O'Brien 2007). The overlap in addictive and reward pathways between certain foods and drugs of abuse con-tinues to be studied and shared among corporate and manufacturing entities, such as tobacco sci-entists and food scientists (Callahan et al. 2006).

In addition to those described in the sub-sections above, numerous other dietary factors, including eating rate, meal timing, snacking, meal skipping, food variety, and food availabil-ity, are also associated with weight control and obesity (Otsuka et al. 2006; Rolls 1985; Rolls 2007; Rolls et al. 1983).

Familial and Interpersonal Factors

Our social and familial environment influences our eating, especially since eating is often a social behavior. The opinions, thoughts, behavior, advice, criticisms, and support of those who surround us make a difference in our feelings and behavior. Family, friends, and peers provide social identity, support, and role definition. As we observe the people around us, we learn from them, imitate them, and emulate them, and we, in turn, affect their lives and choices. Social influences serve as a reference point for behavior and attitudes. In particular, social and **interpersonal factors** probably influence eating behavior through shaping our perceptions of eating and consumption norms (Polivy and Herman 2005).

Social networks, which include family members, friends, co-workers, and others, have a strong influence on behavior. This influence occurs via social processes that include information sharing, perceptions of others' behaviors and attitudes, observations of others' health behaviors, and positive or **negative reinforcement** of our own behaviors, **social norms**, and social monitoring. Numerous phenomena and behaviors, including those leading to obesity, have been shown to "spread" via social networks. Although this terminology is more often used for traditional infectious diseases, mounting evidence shows that attitudes, perceptions, tolerances, and adoption of behaviors can be similarly affected by social influence. A landmark study of more than 12,000 people who were followed for 32 years suggests that obesity spreads through social ties. Although neighbors and acquaintances who were close geographically did not affect the chance of weight gain (a finding that argues against a shared environmental exposure), closely socially related pairs, particularly mutual friends, had a strong effect on each other's weight gain (Christakis and Fowler 2007; Valente 2012).

Family and the *home environment* are the context for food choices, particularly for children, and the home environment is where dietary behaviors and patterns are learned and practiced. Family factors are particularly important

for children, since so much of how they live is dependent on their adult caretakers. A child born to obese parents has a 10% increased risk of obesity, which is likely mediated by a combination of genetic and familial contributions. Family can positively or negatively influence eating behaviors such as healthfulness of food selection, amounts of fruits and vegetables consumed, calories consumed, eating patterns, and disordered eating (Polivy and Herman 2005). Food availability and preparation, family dynamics, meal dynamics, parental nutrition knowledge, parental **modeling**, and parental interest in children's health behaviors affect dietary behaviors in children and adolescents. Children's perceptions of their parents' attitudes and behaviors are strongly related to their own behaviors (Baker et al. 2000; Baker et al. 2003).

The relationship between family and obesity is seen in the role of maternal employment in childhood weight gain. Children with working mothers engage in several behaviors that predispose them to weight gain. For example, they watch more television; spend less time cooking and eating with their mothers; and consume more prepared foods, including fast foods. They also spend more time in child care centers, and such children also are more likely to become obese than are children cared for by parents, nannies or nonparental relatives (Cawley and Liu 2007; Fertig et al. 2009). The increase in maternal weekly work hours between 1975 and 1994 is estimated to explain up to 35% of the rise in childhood obesity in families of high **socioeconomic status** (Anderson et al. 2003).

Social support is an important predictor of health behaviors. Having peer support strongly improves weight loss and maintenance of weight loss, as does having family support and support from a spouse (Black et al. 1990; Brownell et al. 1978; Renjilian et al. 2001). Obese children lose significantly more weight, and maintain the weight loss significantly longer, when their parents are actively involved in their treatment

(Epstein et al. 1998; Golan and Crow 2004). As children get older, peer and social encounters outside the home, or the lack thereof (such as social isolation), take precedence over familial influence as determinants of eating behaviors, weight, and obesity (Baranowski et al. 1999; Polivy and Herman 2005). Studies have shown that adolescents who perceive that their friends do not eat healthfully are less likely to have positive attitudes or intentions about healthful eating, and the weights of mutual friends were most highly correlated with an individual's weight gain over time (Christakis and Fowler 2007).

Structural and Community Factors

The social and cultural contexts in which we live also influence our eating and weight. Communities are central in developing and shaping opportunities, environments, and ultimately behaviors. Organizational and community settings that may be involved in the development or prevention of obesity include work sites, schools, child care settings, faith-based and social institutions, health care systems, recreational facilities, restaurants and food service establishments, and other community sites, as well as the community at large. Community factors also include norms, or standards, that exist among individuals, groups, and organizations.

Community organizations are composed of structures and cultures. *Structures* include regulations, rules, policies, mandates, commitments, and accountabilities that shape the physical and **social environment**. *Cultures* include patterns of interaction, norms, shared beliefs, and priorities that exist within the formal structures. These areas and settings are targets for intervention to shift the context of the organization or the community to become supportive of healthful behaviors and obesity prevention (Riley et al. 2007). For example, flexible work hours, healthful cafeteria choices, menu labeling with calories, vending machine options, op-

portunities for physical activity during the workday, wellness programs, and newsletters can promote healthful behaviors.

Community organizations and settings can serve as locations to reach individuals (e.g., through educational programs such as nutrition classes in schools, blood pressure screening drives in workplaces, vaccination programs in schools or hospitals), since they are key environments where we spend many of our waking hours and perform many health behaviors (e.g., eating, sitting, smoking), and they can also serve as opportunities to initiate or further obesity prevention programs in other systems or **levels of influence** (e.g., family physical activity challenge, healthful cooking classes for spouses, shared recreational facilities). These are therefore important areas for consideration regarding obesity prevention, both to address issues that may be contributing to the problem and to identify areas and implement interventions that may be part of the solution to the problem (Riley et al. 2007).

Health care settings, especially interactions with physicians and other health care providers, can have a central impact on patient behaviors. Studies show that most primary care physicians do not discuss weight with their patients, even very overweight patients (Galuska et al. 1999). While many studies show that physician screening and counseling for obesity can be highly effective (Moyer et al. 2012), other studies suggest that many clinical interactions between health care providers and overweight patients are counterproductive: providers may build less rapport or spend less time with obese patients than with other patients; they may show less respect or may even ridicule, label, or otherwise stigmatize these patients (Beach et al. 2006; Gudzune et al. 2013; Huizinga et al. 2009; Puhl and Brownell 2006). Of course, experiences like these can make patients unwilling to use health care services, further perpetuating declines in their health behaviors and health outcomes (Puhl and Heuer 2009).

Policy and Societal Factors

Laws, policies, and the social and physical environment dictate the health resources to which people have access. Policies can be powerful drivers of availability or can function as constraints. Policies can determine the affordability, appeal, and convenience of foods and food choices; access to health information; and access to facilities that support healthful eating and physical activity. They can make available the resources necessary to engage in healthful behaviors. In particular, availability, accessibility, and marketing of foods affect consumption by enabling or constraining food choices or affecting biological pathways that affect appetite and other determinants of eating behavior (Huang et al. 2009).

FOOD ACCESS AND AVAILABILITY

Food access and *availability* affects choices, intake, and weight gain. Where people live predicts their dietary patterns and obesity rates, even when adjusted for socioeconomic factors (White 2007). One reason for this is ease of access to unhealthful food options (Pereira et al. 2005; Thompson et al. 2004). The number and density of fast food restaurants has increased precipitously, and more fast food outlets reside in poorer areas (Block et al. 2004; Tillotson 2004). Fast food generally has higher energy density (which might make it seem a good buy for poorer people), more fat, sugar, and salt, and fewer nutrients than foods prepared at home. Similarly, the availability of healthful foods may be limited in many areas, especially poorer neighborhoods, in part because residents have limited access to large food supermarkets; obesity rates are higher in areas with fewer supermarkets and higher numbers of convenience stores; such areas are referred to as "food deserts" (Morland et al. 2006; White 2007), but they might also be called "food swamps" when the available food outlets are mostly for fast food.

PRICE

Price frames the context in which decisions are made and is an important determinant of eating behavior and obesity (Plassmann et al. 2008). The great decline in food prices in recent decades (adjusted for inflation) accounts for as much as 43% of the rise in young adults' BMIs between 1981 and 1994 (Lakdawalla and Philipson 2002). In general, foods that have higher calorie density are significantly cheaper than lower-calorie foods, and foods that are more healthful, as measured by nutrient density, cost much more than less healthful, high-fat and high-sugar foods. For example, fats and oils have many times more calories per unit of weight than raw vegetables, yet they are orders of magnitude cheaper per calorie and contain far fewer healthful nutrients (Drewnowski and Darmon 2005). Research shows that diets that meet nutrition **guidelines** are costlier than those that do not (Mooney 1990), which is attributable in part to distortions in our agricultural subsidy policies. Moreover, healthful foods are continuing to get more costly compared with unhealthful foods. From 1985 to 2000, the cost of fresh fruits and vegetables *increased* by nearly 40%, whereas prices *decreased* by 25% for soft drinks, 15% for fats and oils, and 10% for sugars and sweets.[2] Between 1990 and 2007, the inflation-adjusted price of Coca-Cola decreased by 35% and a McDonald's quarter-pounder by 5.4%, whereas the price of fruits and vegetables rose 17% between 1997 and 2003. Studies have linked these price fluctuations to higher BMIs in children and adolescents (Auld and Powell 2009; Christian and Rashad 2009; Powell and Bao 2009).

Put simply, more healthful diets cost more— and for many people this cost difference limits the opportunity to have healthful diets. Data suggests that food choices made by low-income consumers to manage a limited food budget result in consumption of fewer fruits, vegetables, meats, and dairy products and consumption of more cereals, sweets, and added fats (Darmon et al. 2002; Ellaway and Macintyre

2000). Families with easy access to affordable, high-quality fruits and vegetables are more likely to consume them (Sallis and Glanz 2006).

AGRICULTURAL POLICIES

Agriculture policies appear to be an important determinant of eating behavior and obesity by affecting access to and prices of foods. Nationwide, caloric supply has increased by approximately 25% since the 1970s, and it is believed that this is fueling the 10%–20% increase in average caloric intake over the same period (US-DAERS 2000; Wright et al. 2004). Increases in agricultural food production occurred following policies enacted in the mid-20th century that encouraged—and heavily subsidized—production of commodity crops, such as corn and soybeans. The U.S. government provides nearly $20 billion per year in agriculture subsidies and price supports, which primarily support the production and subsidize the cost of relatively unhealthful foods. For example, corn and soybeans are the most heavily subsidized foods. Corn and soybean crops are primarily used as substrates for processed foods. Soybeans are mostly converted to soybean oil for use in processed foods and packaged snacks, and corn is primarily used for sweeteners (corn syrup), carbohydrate flour for snack foods, and feed for livestock. These subsidies partly explain why fast food restaurants charge lower prices for "supersized" burger and fry meals, compared with salads or fruits. Despite government nutrition recommendations to consume more fruits and vegetables, scant agriculture subsidizing supports these. For example, apples, which are the most highly subsidized noncommodity fruit or vegetable, receive just 1/200th of the funding corn receives.[3] This distortion of funding may be a driver of weight gain and obesity and may be one of the reasons that Americans eat few fruits and vegetables. Although some surveys suggest that we eat about four servings daily, this number is greatly exaggerated because French fries and potato chips are counted as vegetables along with spinach, carrots, and broccoli. In fact, 25% of the vegetables consumed in the United States are fried potatoes, making the daily consumption of healthful fruits and vegetables closer to two servings—and likely lower in many at-risk populations, such as children and inner-city residents.

ADVERTISING

Advertising also strongly affects consumer choice and decisions (Finnegan and Viswanath 2002). Food marketing, in particular, has a strong influence on our food preferences, decisions, and consumption. Studies show that television viewing is associated with obesity, and recent data shows that this effect is primarily due to viewing television commercials, rather than television shows (Zimmerman and Bell 2010). Food marketing increased significantly during the second half of the 20th century and now occurs in numerous forms, such as Internet, video games, text messaging, sponsorships, billboards, and logos, in addition to television commercials (Linn and Novosat 2008). More than $11 billion is spent yearly on food marketing, and less than 1% of it supports fruits and vegetables (Nestle 2013). High-calorie foods and fast foods receive significantly more marketing and advertising than lower-calorie foods, fruits, and vegetables. (Advertising Age 2007).

Food marketing affects neuropsychology and physiological responses in the brain, increases purchases and consumption of the advertised foods, and promotes weight gain and obesity (McClure et al. 2004; McGinnis et al. 2006). Advertising aimed at young children is an especially powerful environmental cue for food consumption that molds children's preferences, food choices, purchases, and intake. It is particularly worrisome in young children, insofar as they cannot accurately distinguish advertising from entertainment or from truth (Mc-

Ginnis et al. 2006). On average, children view 15 food advertisements on television daily—or more than 5,000 per year. Of ads seen by children, 98% promote "junk" foods (i.e., foods high in fat, sugar, or salt) and snacking; children preferentially consume foods associated with popular commercials and cartoon characters; and studies show that kids eat more after viewing food commercials than after viewing nonfood commercials, regardless of their hunger (Halford et al. 2004; Harris et al. 2009; Powell et al. 2007; Roberto et al. 2010; USFTC 2007). Taken together, food advertising is an incredibly strong factor in children's eating behaviors. One study estimated that if children were to eat a diet consistent with the foods marketed to them during primetime and Saturday morning television, they would consume 25 times the recommended daily allowance of sugar, 20 times the recommended servings of fat, and less than half the recommended servings of fruits, vegetables, and most vitamins (Mink et al. 2010).

Evidence-Based Interventions

As discussed previously, attempts to address obesity by badgering or cajoling people to eat less and to exercise more are unproductive. Neither simplistic admonitions aimed at dieting and exercise nor "one-size-fits-all" approaches are suited to address the complex causes and contributors to weight gain and obesity. Success that has been achieved in addressing other public health epidemics, such as tobacco use (see chapter 3), indicates that multilevel, ecological combinations of individual approaches, such as health education and provision of clinical services, combined with environmental approaches, such as legislation and fiscal policies, can effectively stem the rise of obesity rates and ultimately reverse them. Below we describe several types of interventions that have been implemented with varying degrees of success and impact.

Individual-Level Interventions

Although **individual-level interventions** are limited in being cost- and effort-intensive (and often cannot take into account the many contextual factors at play when individuals make decisions), several individual interventions are effective for obesity, particularly when accompanied by other measures as part of a multicomponent intervention.

Nutrition and weight loss counseling can be effective for weight loss and weight maintenance. Good evidence also shows that intensive counseling by physicians for patients with obesity produces significant weight loss as well as improved blood sugar, blood pressure, and cholesterol levels (McTigue et al. 2003). Further, frequent support and **reinforcement** via in-person or telephone counseling enhances weight loss and maintenance attempts, and newer studies assessing the **effectiveness** of Internet or e-mail support are promising (Digenio et al. 2009; Wing et al. 2006). Technology-supported counseling (e.g., the use of computers, the Internet, e-mail, phone counseling, video conferencing) and group counseling and support may be as effective as individual counseling (Avenell et al. 2004). Education and support to improve weight-related behaviors is also effective, such as guidance for parents and children to decrease "screen time" (TV, videos, games, Internet), which leads not only to less screen time, but also to less sedentary behavior, improved nutrition intake, and improvements in weight and weight-related outcomes.

Behavioral interventions to modify eating and activity behaviors and improve weight management skills are a core set of principles and techniques for weight management. They aim at increasing awareness of target behaviors (e.g., decreasing calorie intake, decreasing high-calorie and energy-dense foods, increasing fruit and vegetable intake), modifying the situations and settings that predispose to unhealthful behaviors, and reinforcing positive behavior changes. Self-monitoring of behaviors and goals related to eating and physical activity—for example, via a food "diary," recording caloric intake or food "points," tracking activities or daily steps, or recording thoughts and moods that surround eating—has been shown to predict both short- and long-term weight loss and maintenance (Berkowitz et al. 2003). Self-monitoring feedback, for example via regular weighing, is also associated with improved long-term maintenance of weight loss (Wing and Hill 2001). Goal-setting and stimulus control strategies, such as adjusting food cues (e.g., putting a jar of cookies out of sight instead of on the countertop, avoiding stocking snack foods in the home), or restricting the location where eating takes place (e.g., eating only in the kitchen rather than in front of the television or while driving), are central behavioral interventions for weight control and other behavior changes (Wing 2004). The use of meal or snack replacement products, which are portion-controlled, prepackaged servings of low-calorie shakes, bars, or other foods, has been shown consistently to be safe and to improve weight loss and long-term maintenance. Studies that distribute premade meals to patients also show significant weight loss and maintenance beyond behavioral treatment alone (Jeffery et al. 1993). Probably the effectiveness of meal replacements derives primarily from the structure they provide. Studies assessing the differential effect of provided foods, meal plans, and grocery lists suggest that the provision of meals may not be the key element; rather, the structure provided (regular meal patterns, changing the availability of food in the home) is the most valuable feature.

Several medications can assist with weight loss and maintenance. Traditional medications are usually stimulants that decrease a person's appetite or food impulsivity, or both. These have been shown to decrease weight over the course of several weeks to months. Newer medications have additional targets of action, in-

cluding decreasing fat or calorie absorption, adjusting neurochemicals (e.g., serotonin, norepinephrine) involved in weight balance or appetite, or other mechanisms. In particular, when coupled with behavioral therapy and regular follow-up, medications can be particularly helpful, often achieving significant long-term weight losses and risk factor improvements that nearly approach the magnitude of some types of bariatric surgery interventions (Garvey et al. 2012).

Bariatric surgery, a group of surgical treatment options for obesity, on average, leads to greater sustained weight loss than any other intervention currently available; it can no longer be ignored as a valuable treatment for severe obesity. While surgery has significant up-front costs and potentially serious complications, numerous studies show that surgery in appropriate patients is safe and can lead to significant, sustained weight losses, health improvements, and cost savings (Sjostrom et al. 2007). Further study is necessary to better understand which patients are best suited for surgical intervention and why some patients fare poorly with surgery (i.e., regain lost weight, experience severe psychological or physical complications, etc.). Further study will also help us understand how surgery works and may lead to innovative approaches (such as medications) that mimic the effectiveness of surgery.

Combining effective strategies is a particularly useful way to maximize the likelihood of sustained weight loss and health improvement. For example, combining education and counseling with weight medication is more effective than either alone (Wadden et al. 2005). Several long-term, randomized controlled trials of such multicomponent interventions now exist, showing very positive results and ultimately disproving the old adages "nothing works for weight loss" and "everyone regains lost weight."

The "Look AHEAD" (Action for HEAlth in Diabetes) study tested a set of weight strategies in more than 5,000 individuals who had obesity and diabetes. A **control group** received basic diabetes education, and the lifestyle intervention group received intensive individual counseling for diet and weight loss, group counseling and support, regular follow-up (via phone, mail, or e-mail), education in weight loss and self-management strategies, meal replacement products, and, in some cases, weight medications when appropriate. Over the initial year, the intervention group lost an average of 8.6% of body weight, compared with 0.7% in the control group, and there were several concurrent health improvements, including lower blood sugar and cholesterol (Look AHEAD 2007). Many of the health improvements continued through the initial four years of the study, and even after more than *10 years,* the intervention group maintained more than 5% of their weight loss, which is considered a key benchmark for successful weight loss, and showed numerous sustained health improvements (Look AHEAD 2013).

The Diabetes Prevention Program was another important, multicomponent randomized trial that compared intensive lifestyle intervention with diabetes medication in patients with obesity and prediabetes. Compared with the control group, participants in the lifestyle intervention group reduced their risk of developing diabetes by 58% (participants taking the diabetes medication fared well but reduced their risk of developing diabetes by only 31%) (Knowler et al. 2002). These promising experimental trials left much to be investigated, and they are currently being translated from controlled clinical settings to public health community settings and studied further (Garfield et al. 2003; Green and Ottoson 2004).

The Louisiana Obese Subjects Study tested whether primary care practices could effectively implement a multicomponent weight loss program for adults with severe obesity. Compared with a control group that received basic weight loss guidance via an Internet program, the intervention group started with a brief medically monitored diet, which was followed by individual and group behavioral counseling, structured diet support, and use of weight medications as necessary. After two years, 31% of the intervention group achieved more than 5% weight loss, and 7% achieved more than 20% weight loss, along with many additional health improvements; in the control group, just 9% achieved more than 5% weight loss and only 1% lost more than 20% of their weight (Ryan et al. 2010). This study demonstrated the feasibility of primary care practices providing effective initial medical management for extreme obesity; ongoing weight loss maintenance remains to be studied using this approach, and further refinements and **adaptations** are necessary to be able to **scale up** and generalize such services to wide or disparate populations at reasonable financial and resource costs (Brownson et al. 2012; Green 2001).

Community-Based Interventions

Community-level interventions aimed at behavioral settings (i.e., the places where residents engage in—and which set the stage for—healthful (or unhealthful) behaviors) are important targets to address obesity. Behavioral settings include schools, work sites, health care settings, recreational settings, and other parts of communities. **Structural interventions**, which target conditions outside individual control, such as the availability of healthful food options in a given area or the prevalence of vending machines in schools, are an important component of community interventions. They can affect behavior directly by improving availability and accessibility or indirectly by altering the acceptability of healthful or unhealthful weight-related behaviors.

The school environment is one area that has received a lot of attention, and studies addressing the school environment show varying degrees of benefit. Some targets of school-based interventions include increasing access to healthful foods (e.g., fruits and vegetables), decreasing access to unhealthful foods (e.g., vending machine snacks or "competitive foods" such as candy bars, which compete with more healthful U.S. Department of Agriculture (USDA)–regulated school lunches), increasing physical activity in schools (via physical education classes, extracurricular or after-school activities such as sports or dance, or walking opportunities within and outside the school day), and increasing nutrition- or other weight-related education opportunities (e.g., classroom curricula intended to decrease television viewing or increase knowledge of healthful foods, parent-focused programs such as sending home newsletters to educate parents and families, or health fairs).

Many school-based interventions aim to change weight or related behavior outcomes, such as food consumption quality or physical activity levels. The USDA's Fruit and Vegetable Pilot Program led to increased interest in and consumption of fruits and vegetables among students in 107 elementary and secondary schools when they were given access to free fruits and vegetables (Buzby et al. 2003). The National Cancer Institute's 5 A Day for Better Health program, which encourages consumption of vegetables and fruit daily, and related elementary school behavioral and food service interventions, led to a significant increase in servings of fruits and vegetables consumed (Potter et al. 2006). Shape Up Somerville: Eat Smart, Play Hard, a three-year intervention designed to increase physical activity options and improve dietary choices in culturally diverse, high risk, first- to third-graders in Somerville, Massachusetts, led to an average one-pound reduction of weight gain over eight months— quite a large benefit for a sizable population (Economos et al. 2007). A public-school-based study in Chicago, Health-Kids, led to significantly reduced rates of overweight over the course of one year (Wang et al. 2006). A randomized trial of 1,349 urban fourth- to sixth-grade children, which involved nutrition education,

nutrition policy changes, free or reduced-price meals, social marketing, and parent **outreach**, resulted in a 50% reduction in the incidence of becoming overweight over two years (Foster et al. 2008). Another grade-school-based randomized trial including 4,603 high risk, primarily minority students in 42 schools resulted in lower rates of overweight and obesity, decreased BMI, and decreased waist circumference and fasting insulin levels (risk factors for diabetes) (HEALTHY Study Group et al. 2010). And a combined analysis of 19 school-based studies over 13 years showed convincing evidence of reducing childhood obesity (Gonzalez-Suarez et al. 2009).

Given the multiple and complex influences on body weight, it is not unreasonable to doubt that solely aiming at the school environment will be enough. Indeed, alongside these and other school-based studies with meaningful outcomes are many well-designed, intensive interventions that have failed to find significant changes in weight-related outcomes, and even when results have been positive, the benefits have been difficult to sustain beyond relatively short periods. For example, the Pathways Study, a four-year randomized controlled trial including 1,704 third- to fifth-grade students at 41 Native American schools tested a multicomponent intervention aimed at dietary intake, physical activity, curriculum changes focused on healthful eating and lifestyles, and a family involvement program (Caballero et al. 2003). Although the intervention led to decreased dietary fat intake and improved knowledge, attitudes, and some health behaviors, no significant changes in BMI, body fat percentage, or activity levels resulted. The researchers concluded that more intense or longer interventions might be needed to reduce weight outcomes significantly. As we have discussed throughout this textbook, even fairly broad and intensive interventions such as this are likely to be insufficient unless attention is simultaneously paid to other levels of influence.

A notable intervention that did address multiple levels of influence on food intake, activity, and weight-related behaviors was the "EPODE" projects conducted in two towns in France over the course of nearly two decades (Romon et al. 2009). Beginning in 1992, schools in the intervention towns began teaching children about nutrition and healthful eating. In the schools of intervention towns, students were taught to read food labels, attended healthful-cooking classes, visited supermarkets, and were given healthful breakfasts. Soon thereafter, community initiatives outside the schools began, including nutrition classes for adults, new sporting facilities, family fitness and healthful living activities, walking school bus programs, and others; several dietitians and physical education specialists were hired to support these and other programs. Home-based preventive care checkups incorporating family-oriented health and nutrition advice were also offered, and intensive media coverage supported the school, home, and community programs. After 12 years, childhood obesity rates in the intervention towns fell to 8.8%, compared with 17.8% in the control towns that did not receive this multicomponent intervention (and childhood and adult obesity in France overall rose significantly during the same time period).

Just as schools are an important area for intervention—in part because children spend most of their waking hours in school—work sites are optimal places for intervention because they are where adults spend much of their time. Work site interventions have included strategies aimed at increasing healthful nutrition options, increasing opportunities for physical activity, and providing health and nutrition education, **incentives** for weight loss or healthful behavior choices, preventive care services, and the like. Such programs require further study and **innovation**, but many studies show modestly improved weight outcomes, reduced absenteeism, improved productivity, and lower health care costs (IOM 2012, 2013).

Policy-Based Interventions

Policy and societal interventions are undoubtedly essential to address the obesity epidemic. Yet, they are challenging to develop, implement, and evaluate (IOM 2010, 2013). It has been difficult to achieve political will and consensus for policy changes to address society's obesogenic environments. Determining the optimal focus, scope, design, and timing of policy interventions is similarly challenging. Many logistic and methodological barriers for testing policy changes exist, such as finding appropriate control groups. For optimal effect, policies need be consistent and coherent with each other and with coexisting community and other **environmental interventions** so as to support additive, even synergistic, beneficial outcomes. As always, funding can be elusive, and a long time often elapses between the initiation of a policy and the development of tangible results, often limiting social will for costly policies. Finally, as chapter 21 will show, any large-scale policy intervention tends to be governed by complex, nonlinear dynamics. As a result, simple predictions are difficult to make and often the outcomes are counterintuitive.

For these reasons and a host of others, few large-scale policy interventions for obesity have been rigorously conducted and systematically evaluated. As yet, no large-scale, population-wide policy intervention addressing the broad range of factors related to obesity has been attempted. Among those that have been tested are fairly narrow policies that have not necessarily made an impact on population obesity rates. For example, as described earlier in this chapter, breastfeeding is associated with numerous health benefits, including a decreased risk for childhood obesity. Several policies have been enacted to increase breastfeeding rates, including laws requiring large companies to make reasonable accommodations and break times for breastfeeding employees. While the policies have not yet been fully evaluated, studies suggest that these policies can lead to both increased rates of breastfeeding and benefits to the companies in the form of improved employee retention, lower health care costs, and increased work attendance (USDHHS 2008). Restricting the advertising of junk food to children is an area of much opportunity, as well. As described earlier in the chapter, food advertising—particularly to children—is a key factor in the quality and quantity of food consumption. While little policy movement has occurred in the United States, dozens of other countries regulate such advertising, including Australia, which limits food advertising to children under age 14, and Sweden, which bans cartoon characters in food advertising to children under age 12 (Nestle 2006). Still, while the rates of childhood obesity are lower in these countries than in the United States, and estimates suggest that banning fast food advertising to children could reduce obesity rates by nearly 20%, we do not yet have sufficient evidence of effectiveness for these policies (Cawley 2010).

Instead, we can look to validated studies from other areas of chronic disease prevention for insight into what models and policy interventions might be possible to address obesity in the future. One example of successful health behavior change policy is smoking restrictions and tobacco taxation in New York City during the era of Mayor Michael Bloomberg and health commissioner Thomas Frieden (see chapter 10). Initiated shortly after they came to office in 2001-2, these regulations banned smoking in most workplaces, including restaurants and bars, and levied steep taxes on cigarettes. Opposition to the smoking restriction policy primarily focused on potential economic consequences (reduced patronage of restaurants and bars), which did not materialize. Since the initiation of these policies, rates of tobacco use by NYC adults decreased by nearly 30%, and smoking by high school students decreased by more than 50%. Evaluation studies show a concomitant decrease of nearly 20% in the risk of dying

from premature heart disease. Proving that these policies definitively caused the beneficial outcomes is impossible, in part because the policies were initiated in a coordinated fashion alongside other interventions, including education, social media outreach, and increased access to treatment modalities (such as quit lines and tobacco replacement therapy). However, these policies clearly contributed to a substantial improvement in the public's health.

Translating policies such as these to obesity has borne some benefit, but not as significant as in the tobacco case. Restrictions on obesity-related factors are more challenging than simply restricting smoking. Nonetheless, evidence of benefit does exist. For example, restricting competitive foods in schools (i.e., foods that compete with USDA-regulated school lunches that are mandated to adhere to the Dietary Guidelines) has been shown to improve the quality of food eaten by school children. Also, restricting the availability of junk foods in school vending machines has been shown to decrease unhealthful food patterns (Cawley 2010). While suggestions have been made to "ban" sugar or high-fructose corn syrup or other unhealthful nutrients, they are unlikely to garner sufficient social and political will anytime soon, nor does current evidence support such bans. Similarly, changes in food taxation are more complex than simply taxing tobacco products. The most researched option is levying taxes on soft drinks. While a clear relationship between the amount of additional cost (via taxation) and a decrease in consumption of soft drinks appears to exist, the magnitude of this relationship is quite small: a 1% increase in state soft drink tax rate leads to a decrease in BMI of 0.003 points and a decrease in obesity rates of 0.01% (Fletcher et al. 2010). Further, as above, the political and social will for such taxation policies has been difficult to achieve enough to overcome the soft-drink industry's lobbying and campaign financing against such tax initiatives.

Another example of impressive policy changes in an area of health behavior is the North Karelia Project, aimed at reducing levels of heart disease and conducted in Finland over two decades in the 1970s–1980s (see chapter 25). More than a policy intervention alone, this project worked across many sectors of the community. It included health education, media campaigns, training of health professionals, and collaborations with food producers and retailers. Policy changes included restricting smoking and promoting vegetable growing. From 1972 to 1992, risk factors for heart disease (such as smoking) improved dramatically, mortality from heart disease fell nearly 60% in men, rates of stroke and cancer deaths fell significantly, and life expectancy rose dramatically. Results as impressive as these with obesity could lead to impressive improvements in the public's health. Continuing to learn from other areas of health behavior change and rigorously testing future policy interventions to determine what works and how to scale it up have clear value to address this widespread epidemic.

Roles for Key Stakeholders

As described in this chapter, obesity is a complex and multidimensional condition that requires concerted efforts on a range of influences and contributions from a variety of **key stakeholders** throughout society. We describe below some key roles that stakeholders should undertake, although we caution that this discussion is not comprehensive. However, one consideration cuts across all stakeholder groups: We should all strive to question and combat implicit assumptions about and stigmas toward persons who carry excess weight. After learning about the complexity of this fascinating condition and the multitude of factors—many outside the control of individual action—we find it hard to believe that anyone could still feel that obesity simply suggests a lack of self-control. Stigmatizing and shaming people does

not help them, and we now have mounting evidence that such stigma worsens health outcomes and likely causes weight gain and obesity (Sutin and Terracciano 2013). We believe that future generations will see the prejudice now shown toward persons with obesity as similar to prejudices relating to race, ethnicity, or gender.

Researchers

Though we have learned an immense amount about the determinants, contributors, and causes of obesity, and options for obesity prevention and treatment, much, much more needs investigation. Many opportunities exist for novel research across the spectrum of bio-psycho-social aspects of obesity risk and interventions. Additional funding for, and participation in, such research is a central component to generate the knowledge necessary for improved understanding of obesity and how to address it at individual and population levels.

Federal Agencies

While continued and increased investment in research to understand and address obesity is an important role for the federal government, we see a key role for the federal government that is perhaps more valuable than any other. Obesity affects more Americans and leads to more lives lost than any other health behavior condition (perhaps except tobacco use, although recent numbers suggest that obesity may be overtaking tobacco as the number one killer in America), but no centralized federal agency, other than a division within a center within the CDC, is charged with leading and coordinating research, training, education, and intervention for the prevention and treatment of obesity, unlike most other health conditions. In contrast, the National Heart, Lung, and Blood Institute (NHLBI) promotes the prevention and treatment of heart disease; the National Institute for

Occupational Safety and Health coordinates the research and funding aimed at improving worker safety and health; and the National Institute on Drug Abuse leads the nation's research and science on drug abuse and addiction. Obesity research at NIH, for example, is spread widely and thinly among numerous institutes and centers, including the NHLBI, the National Cancer Institute, the National Institute on Aging, and many others. This lack of centralized leadership and coordination limits the federal government's ability to create a powerful and sustained push to understand and address the obesity epidemic and leads to fragmented and inefficient use of our limited resources. We can think of few strategies that would be more valuable than establishing a federally funded coordinating center for obesity research, training, and education, which would be charged with strategic support and conduct of obesity research across a broad range of disciplines. Such a center could ensure effective translation and dissemination of research to improve obesity prevention and treatment and inform obesity policy, and it could coordinate the numerous hubs of obesity study throughout federal and local governments and nongovernmental and academic organizations.

An Institute of Medicine (2013) committee on evaluation of national progress on obesity control recommended, as a prerequisite to its other recommendations, the appointment of a centralized steering body at the federal level. This is essential to forge the necessary agreement and coordination among the multiple departments (e.g., Agriculture, Health and Human Services, the armed services, and others) to establish a common set of measures for surveillance and monitoring of national and community progress on obesity control.

Clinicians

Health professionals have the opportunity to play key roles in obesity prevention and treat-

ment. They have traditionally been limited by lack of training in obesity; for example, until recently there were no classes on obesity in medical schools, and even now, such classes are relatively rare. Because health professionals, especially physicians, are looked upon with extreme respect and have opportunities to strongly influence their patients, building their understanding of the obesity condition and their skills for helping patients prevent and address obesity is important. Further, many reports show that physicians, compared to the general public, show similar, if not greater, stigma toward patients with obesity and treat heavier patients with less respect and concern (Huizinga et al. 2009). Physicians and other health care professionals must make obesity a more central piece of their clinical practice and must support their patients in the same productive and compassionate ways that they would support patients suffering from other conditions. Nationally, expanding health professional training in obesity is essential. This should include standard courses in graduate schools as well as increased access to relevant continuing education opportunities.

Health Insurance Plans and Insurance Companies

For persons already affected by obesity, prevention is not enough. Just as patients who have existing heart disease or cancer require more than messages aimed at prevention—they need explicit treatment modalities—so, too, do patients with obesity need effective, evidence-based treatments. While there are many barriers that limit the availability of such treatments, minimal insurance coverage may be the foremost barrier in our experience. Traditionally, obesity treatment is explicitly excluded from insurance plans, including Medicare (it is notable that Medicare policy was changed in 2012 to provide access for some obesity counseling). In recent years, bariatric surgery has become more commonly covered by insurance plans. Still, we find that often a patient must choose between bariatric surgery or no treatment at all, simply because other treatments are not covered. In many cases, an economic case can be made for coverage: since obesity is an underlying or contributing condition to many costly conditions and chronic diseases, such as high blood pressure, high cholesterol, heart disease, and diabetes, treating obesity may save significant costs by decreasing the levels of these secondary conditions. However, even in the absence of economic benefits, with the current evidence for numerous effective treatments for obesity, we believe it clinically unethical to exclude coverage for obesity, just as it would be for any other addressable health condition.

Conclusion

Despite epidemic levels of obesity and obesity-related health conditions, our rapidly expanding understanding of the multitude of factors involved in obesity bodes well for addressing this epidemic. Though obesity rates have increased steadily over the past few decades, recent data provides optimism that rates will level off and turn downward in the near future. While the public health approach to obesity will need to be intensive and sustained for many decades to come, we believe that many successes are within our reach. Further research, improved funding, improved coordination among stakeholders, and access to treatments will be important to continue to move the needle forward on this core health-behavior-related condition.

NOTES

1. Standard practice in medicine is to avoid defining patients by their condition. That is, it is inappropriate, and possibly stigmatizing, to use *diabetic* to refer to a person who has diabetes, or *a depressive* to refer to a patient with clinical depression, or *cancerous* to refer to someone who has cancer. Similarly, we recommend avoiding the term *obese* to refer to a person who has a diagnosis of obesity.

2. U.S. Department of Agriculture Economic Research Service, www.ers.usda.gov/briefing /CPIFoodAndExpenditures/Data/.

3. See the Environmental Working Group farm subsidy database, www.ewg.org/farm.

REFERENCES

Advertising Age. 2007. 2007 marketer profiles yearbook. AdAge Datacenter, http://adage.com/datacenter.

Anderson PM et al. 2003. Maternal employment and overweight children. *J Health Econ* 22:477–504.

Anderson SE, Whitaker RC. 2009. Prevalence of obesity among US preschool children in different racial and ethnic groups. *Arch Pediatr Adolesc Med* 163:344–48.

Auld MC, Powell LM. 2009. Economics of food energy density and adolescent body weight. *Economica* 76:719–40.

Avenell A, Broom J, Brown TJ, et al. 2004. Systematic review of long-term effects and economic consequences of treatments for obesity and implications for health improvement. *Health Technol Assess* 8 (21): iii–iv, 1–182.

Baker C, Little TD, Brownell KD. 2003. Predicting adolescent eating and activity behaviors. *Health Psychol* 22:189–98.

Baker C, Whisman MA, Brownell KD. 2000. Studying intergenerational transmission of eating attitudes and behaviors. *Health Psychol* 19:376–81.

Baranowski T, Cullen KW, Baranowski J. 1999. Psychosocial correlates of dietary intake: Advancing dietary intervention. *Annu Rev Nutr* 19:17–40.

Barba G et al. 2005. Inverse association between body mass and frequency of milk consumption in children. *Br J Nutr* 93:15–19.

Barker DJP. 2007. Obesity and early life. *Obesity Rev* 8 (suppl. 1): 45–49.

Barker DJP, Osmond C, et al. 2005. Trajectories of growth among children who have coronary events as adults. *N Engl J Med* 353:1802–9.

Beach MC, Roter DL, et al. 2006. Are physicians' attitudes of respect accurately perceived by patients and associated with more positive communication behaviors? *Patient Educ Couns* 62 (3): 347–54.

Berg C, Rosengren A, Aires N, et al. 2005. Trends in overweight and obesity from 1985 to 2002 in Goteborg, West Sweden. *Int J Obes Relat Metab Disord* 29 (8): 916–24.

Berkowitz RI et al. 2003. Behavior therapy and sibutramine for the treatment of adolescent obesity. *JAMA* 289:1805–12.

Black DR et al. 1990. A meta-analytic evaluation of couples weight-loss programs. *Health Psychol* 9:330–47.

Block JP, Scribner RA, DeSalvo KB. 2004. Fast food, race/ethnicity, and income. *Am J Prev Med* 27:211-17.

Bobroff EM, Kissileff HR. 1986. Effects of changes in palatability on food intake and the cumulative food intake curve in man. *Appetite* 7:85-96.

Brown PJ, Konner M. 1987. An anthropological perspective on obesity. *Ann NY Acad Sciences* 499:29-46.

Brownell KD et al. 1978. Effect of couples training and partner cooperativeness in the behavioral treatment of obesity. *Behav Res Ther* 16:323-33.

Brownson RC, Colditz GA, Proctor EK., Eds. 2012. *Dissemination and Implementation Research in Health: Translating Science to Practice.* New York: Oxford University Press.

Butland B, Jebb S, Kopelman K, et al. 2007. Foresight: Tackling obesities: Future choices. Government Office for Science, London, UK. Available at www.bis.gov.uk/assets/foresight/docs/obesity/17.pdf.

Buzby JC, JF Guthrie, LS Kantor. 2003. *Evaluation of the USDA Fruit and Vegetable Pilot Program: Report to Congress.* E-FAN No. EFAN-03-006, April. Washington, DC: U.S. Dept. of Agriculture.

Caballero B, Clay T, Davis SM, et al. 2003. Pathways: A school-based, randomized controlled trial for the prevention of obesity in American Indian schoolchildren. *Am J Clin Nutr* 78 (5): 1030-38.

Callahan P, Manier J, Alexander D. 2006. Where there's smoke, there might be food research, too. *Chicago Tribune,* Jan. 29.

Cawley J. 2010. The economics of childhood obesity. *Health Affairs* 29:364-71.

Cawley J, Liu F. 2007. Maternal employment and childhood obesity: A search for mechanisms in time use data. NBER working paper N. 13600. National Bureau of Economic Research, Cambridge, MA.

Cawley J, Meyerhoefer C. 2012. The medical care costs of obesity: An instrumental variables approach. *J Health Econ* 31 (1): 219-230.

Centers for Disease Control and Prevention (CDC). 1997. Guidelines for school health programs to promote lifelong healthy eating. *J Sch Health* 67:9-26.

———. 2003. Prevalence of diabetes and impaired fasting glucose in adults—United States, 1999-2000. *MMWR* 52 (35) (Sept. 5): 833-37.

———. 2009-10. National Health and Nutrition Examination Survey. National Center for Health Statistics, www.cdc.gov/nchs/nhanes.htm.

Chang VW, Lauderdale DS. 2005. Income disparities in BMI and obesity in the US. *Arch Int Med* 165:2122-28.

Christakis NA, Fowler JH. 2007. The spread of obesity in a large social network over 32 years. *N Engl J Med* 357 (4): 370-79.

Christian T, Rashad I. 2009. Trends in US food prices, 1950-2007. *Econ Hum Biol* 7:113-20.

Darmon N et al. 2002. A cost constraint alone has adverse effects on food selection and nutrient density. *J Nutr* 132:3764-71.

Daviglus ML, Liu K, Yan LL, et al. 2004. Relation of body mass index in young adulthood and middle age to Medicare expenditures in older age. *JAMA* 292 (22): 2743-49.

Digenio AG et al. 2009. Comparison of methods for delivering a lifestyle modification program for obese patients. *Ann Intern Med* 150:255-62.

Drewnowski A. 1997. Taste preferences and food intake. *Annu Rev Nutr* 17:237-53.

Drewnowski A, Darmon N. 2005. The economics of obesity: Dietary entery density and energy cost. *Am J Clin Nutr* 82:265s-273s.

Drewnowski A, Henderson S, et al. 1999. Taste and food preferences as predictors of dietary practices in young women. *Pub Health Nutr* 2:513-19.

Economos CD, Hyatt RR, Goldberg JP, et al. 2007. A community intervention reduces BMI z-score in children: Shape Up Somerville first year results. *Obesity* 15 (5): 1325-36.

Ellaway A, Macintyre S. 2000. Shopping for food in socially contrasting localities. *Br Food J* 102:52-59.

Ello-Martin JA, Ledikwe JH, Rolls BJ. 2005. The influence of food portion size and energy density on energy intake: Implications for weight management. *Am J Clin Nutr* 82:236S-241S.

Epstein LH et al. 1998. Treatment of pediatric obesity. *Pediatrics* 101:554-70.

Fagot-Campagna A. 2000. Emergence of type 2 diabetes mellitus in children: Epidemiological evidence. *J Pediatr Endocrinol Metab* 13 (suppl. 6): 1395-402.

Fertig A et al. 2009. The connection between maternal employment and childhood obesity. *Rev Econ Household* 7:227-55.

Finkelstein EA, Fiebelkorn IC, Wang G. 2003. National medical spending attributable to overweight and obesity: How much, and who's paying? *Health Aff (Millwood),* Jan.-June, W3-219-26.

Finnegan JR Jr., Viswanath K. 2002. Communication theory and health behavior change: The media studies framework. In *Health Behavior and Health Education: Theory, Research, and Practice,* ed. K Glanz, BK Rimer, FM Lewis, 361-88. 3rd ed. San Francisco: Jossey-Bass.

Flegal KM, Troiano RP. 2000. Changes in the distribution of body mass index of adults and children in the US population. *Int J Obes Relat Metab Disord* 24 (7): 807-18.

Fletcher JM, Frisvold D, Tefft N. 2010. Can soft drink taxes reduce population weight? *Contemp Econ Policy* 28 (1) (Jan.): 23-35.

Foster GD, Sherman S, Borradaile KE, et al. 2008. A policy-based school intervention to prevent overweight and obesity. *Pediatrics* 121 (4) (April): e794-802.

Freedman DS, Khan LK, Serdula MK, Deitz WH, Srinivasan SR, Berenson GS. 2005. The relation of childhood BMI to adult adiposity. *Pediatrics* 115:22-27.

Freedman DS, Mei Z, Srinivasan SR, Berenson GS, Dietz WH. 2007. Cardiovascular risk factors and excess adiposity among overweight children and adolescents. *J Pediatr* 150:12-17.

French SA, Story M, et al. 1999. Cognitive and demographic correlates of low-fat vending snack choices among adolescents and adults. *J Am Diet Assoc* 99:471-75.

Furst T et al. 1996. Food choice: A conceptual model of the process. *Appetite* 26:247-65.

Gallagher D, Heymsfield SB, Heo M, Jebb SA, Murgatroyd PR, Sakamoto Y. 2000. Healthy percentage body fat ranges: An approach for developing guidelines based on body mass index. *Am J Clin Nutr.* Available at http://ajcn.nutrition.org/content/72/3/694.full.pdf.

Galuska DA, Will JC, Serdula MK, Ford ES. 1999. Are health care professionals advising obese patients to lose weight? *JAMA* 282 (16): 1576-78.

Garfield SA, Malozowski S, Chin MH, et al. 2003. Considerations for diabetes translational research in real-world settings. *Diabetes Care* 26 (9): 2670-74.

Garvey WT, Ryan DH, et al. 2012. Two-year sustained weight loss and metabolic benefits with controlled-release phentermine/topiramate in obese and overweight adults. *Am J Clin Nutr* 95:297-308.

Gilman MW. 2008. The first months of life: A critical period for development of obesity. *Am J Clin Nutr* 87:1587-89.

Golan M, Crow S. 2004. Targeting parents exclusively in the treatment of childhood obesity: Long-term results. *Obesity Res* 12:357-61.

Gonzalez-Suarez C et al. 2009. School-based interventions on childhood obesity. *Am J Prev Med* 37:418-27.

Green LW. 2001. From research to "best practices" in other settings and populations. *Am J Health Behav* 25 (3) (April-May): 165-78.

Green LW, Ottoson JM. 2004. From efficacy to effectiveness to community and back: Evidence-based practice vs. practice-based evidence. In *From Clinical Trials to Community: The Science of Translating Diabetes and Obesity Research,* ed. R Hiss, L Green, R Glasgow, et al., 15-18. Bethesda: National Institutes of Health.

Gudzune KA, Beach MC, Roter DL, Cooper LA. 2013. Obesity 2013. Available at www.ncbi.nlm.nih.gov/pubmed/23512862.

Gutierrez-Fisac JL, Banegas J, Banegas R, Artalejo FR, Regidor E. 2000. Increasing prevalence of overweight and obesity among Spanish adults, 1987-1997. *Int J Obes Relat Metab Disord* 24 (12) (Dec.): 1677-82.

Halford JC et al. 2004. Effect of television advertisements for foods on food consumption in children. *Appetite* 42:221-25.

Harris JL et al. 2009. Priming effects of television food advertising on eating behavior. *Health Psychol* 28:404-13.

Harris MI, Flegal KM, Cowie CC, et al. 1998. Prevalence of diabetes, impaired fasting glucose, and impaired glucose tolerance in U.S. adults. The Third National Health and Nutrition Examination Survey, 1988-1994. *Diabetes Care* 21 (4): 518-24.

He K, Hu F, Colditz GA, et al. 2004. Changes in intake of fruits and vegetables in relation to risk of obesity and weight gain among middle-aged women. *Int J Obes* 28: 1569-74.

HEALTHY Study Group, Foster GD, Linder B, Baranowski T, et al. 2010. A school-based intervention for diabetes risk reduction. *N Engl J Med* 363 (5): 443-53.

Heitmann BL. 2000. Ten-year trends in overweight and obesity among Danish men and women aged 30-60 years. *Int J Obes Relat Metab Disord* 24 (10): 1347-52.

Hill-Briggs F, Gemmell L. 2007. Problem solving in diabetes self-management and control. *Diabetes Educ* 33:1032-50.

Howard B, Manson J, et al. 2006. Low-fat dietary pattern and weight change over 7 years. *JAMA* 295:39-49.

Howarth N, Saltzman E, Roberts SB. 2001. Dietary fiber and weight regulation. *Nutr Rev* 59:129-139.

Huang TT, Drewnowski A, Kumanyika SK, Glass TA. 2009. A systems-oriented multilevel framework for addressing obesity in the 21st century. *Prev Chronic Disease* 6 (3): A82.

Huizinga MM, Cooper LA, et al. 2009. Physician respect for patients with obesity. *J Gen Intern Med* 24 (11): 1236-39.

Institute of Medicine (IOM). 2010. *Bridging the Evidence Gap in Obesity Prevention: A Framework to Inform Decision Making.* Washington, DC: National Academy Press.

———. 2012. *Accelerating Progress in Obesity Prevention.* Washington, DC: National Academy Press.

———. 2013. *Evaluating Obesity Prevention Efforts: A Plan for Measuring Progress.* Washington, DC: National Academy Press.

International Food Information Council (IFIC). 2010. 2010 Food and Health Survey: Consumer Attitudes toward Food Safety, Nutrition, and Health. International Food Information Council, Washington, DC. Available at www.foodinsight.org/Resources/Detail .aspx?topic=2010_Food_Health_Survey_Consumer _Attitudes_Toward_Food_Safety_Nutrition_Health.

James WP. 2008. The epidemiology of obesity: The size of the problem. *J Intern Med* 263 (4): 336-52.

Jeffery RW et al. 1993. Strengthening behavioral interventions for weight loss: A randomized trial of food provision and monetary incentives. *J Consult Clin Psychol* 61 (6): 1038-45.

Johnson RK, Nicklas TA. 1999. Position of the American Dietetic Association: Dietary guidance for healthy children aged 2 to 11 years. *J Am Diet Assoc* 99:93-101.

Kautiainen S, Rimpela A, Vikat A, Virtanen SM. 2002. Secular trends in overweight and obesity among Finnish adolescents in 1977-1999. *Int J Obes Relat Metab Disord* 26 (4):544-52.

Knowler WC, Barrett-Connor E, Fowler SE, et al. 2002. Reduction in the incidence of type 2 diabetes with lifestyle intervention or metformin. *N Engl J Med* 346 (6): 393-403.

Kopelman P. 2007. Health risks associated with overweight and obesity. *Obesity Rev* 8 (suppl. 1): 13-17.

Lakdawalla D, Philipson T. 2002. The growth of obesity and technological change. NBER working paper no. 8946, National Bureau of Economic Research, Cambridge, MA.

Leibowitz SF. 2002. Central physiological determinants of eating behavior and body weight. In *Eating Disorders and Obesity,* ed. CG Fairburn, KD Brownell. New York: Guilford Press.

Levin BE. 2005. Factors promoting and ameliorating the development of obesity. *Physiol Behav* 86:633-39.

Lindstrom M, Isacsson SO, Merlo J. 2003. Increasing prevalence of overweight, obesity, and physical inactivity: Two population-based studies, 1986 and 1994. *Eur J Public Health* 13 (4) (Dec.): 306-12.

Linn S, Novosat CL. 2008. Calories for sale: Food marketing to children in the twenty-first century. *Ann Am Acad Polit Soc Sci* 615 (1): 133-55.

Livingstone M, Black AE. 2003. Markers of the validity of reported energy intake. *J Nutr* 133 (suppl. 3): 895-920.

Look AHEAD Research Group. 2007. Reduction in weight and cardiovascular disease risk factors in individuals with type 2 diabetes. *Diabetes Care* 30 (6) 1374-83.

———. 2013. Cardiovascular effects of intensive lifestyle intervention in type 2 diabetes. *N Engl J Med* 369:145-54.

Maio G et al. 2007. Lifestyle change: Evidence review: Foresight tackling obesities: Future choices—lifestyle change—evidence review. Government Office for Science, London, UK. Available at www.bis.gov.uk /assets/foresight/docs/obesity/05.pdf.

Mattes RD. 1997. Physiologic responses to sensory stimulation by food: Nutritional implications. *J Am Diet Assoc* 97:406-13.

Maximova K et al. 2008. Do you see what I see? Weight status misperceptions and exposure to obesity among children and adolescents. *Int J Obesity* 32:1008-15.

McClure SM et al. 2004. Neural correlates of behavioral preference for culturally familiar drinks. *Neuron* 44:379-87.

McFarlane T et al. 1988. The effects of false feedback about weight on restrained and unrestrained eaters. *J Abnorm Psychol* 107:312-18.

McGinnis JM et al. 2006. *Food Marketing to Children and Youth: Threat or Opportunity.* Institute of Medicine. Washington, DC: National Academies Press.

McTigue KM et al. 2003. Screening and interventions for obesity in adults: Summary of the evidence for the U.S. Preventive Services Task Force. *Ann Intern Med* 139:933-49.

Menella JA et al. 2001. Prenatal and postnatal flavor learning by human infants. *Pediatrics* 107:E88.

Miller W, Rollnick S. 2002. *Motivational Interviewing: Preparing People for Change.* New York: Guilford Press.

Mink M et al. 2010. Nutritional imbalance endorsed by televised food advertisements. *J Am Diet Assoc* 110:904-10.

Mokdad AH, Marks JS, Stroup DF, Gerberding JL. 2004. Actual causes of death in the United States, 2000. *JAMA* 291 (10): 1238-45.

Mooney C. 1990. Cost and availability of healthy food choices in a London health district. *J Hum Nutr Diet* 3:111-20.

Morland K, Diez Roux AV, Wing S. 2006. Supermarkets, other food stores, and obesity: The atherosclerosis risk in communities study. *Am J Prev Med* 30 (4): 333-39.

Moyer VA et al. 2012. Screening for and management of obesity in adults: US Preventive Services Task Force recommendation statement. *Ann Intern Med* 157:373-8.

Myers KP, Sclafani A. 2006. Development of learned flavor preferences. *Dev Psychobiol* 48:380-88.

Narayan KMV et al. 2003. Lifetime risk for diabetes mellitus in the U.S. *JAMA* 290: 1884-90.

Nestle M. 2006. Food marketing and childhood obesity—A matter of policy. *N Engl J Med* 354 (24): 2527-29.

———. 2013. *Food Politics: How the Food Industry Influences Nutrition and Health.* Berkeley: University of California Press.

NHLBI Expert Panel on the Identification, Evaluation, and Treatment of Overweight and Obesity in Adults (NHLBI). 1998. Clinical guidelines on the identification, evaluation, and treatment of overweight and obesity in adults—the evidence report. *Obesity Res* 6 (suppl. 2): 51S-209S. Available at www.nhlbi.nih.gov/guidelines/obesity/ob_gdlns.htm.

Nielsen SJ, Popkin BM. 2004. Changes in beverage intake between 1977 and 2001. *Am J Prev Med* 27:205-10.

Nielson SJ, Siega-Riz AM, Popkin BM. 2002. Trends in food locations and sources among adolescents and young adults. *Prev Med* 35:107-13.

O'Dea JA. 2003. Why do kids eat healthful food? Perceived benefits of and barriers to healthful eating and physical activity among children and adolescents. *J Am Diet Assoc* 103:497-501.

Ogden CL, Flegal KM, Carroll MD, Johnson CL. 2002. Prevalence and trends in overweight among U.S. children and adolescents, 1999-2000. *JAMA* 288:1728-32.

Ogden CL, Yanovski SZ, Carroll MD, Flegal KM. 2007. The epidemiology of obesity. *Gastroenterology* 132:2087-2102.

Otsuka R, Tamakoshi K, et al. 2006. Eating fast leads to obesity: Findings based on self-administered questionnaires among middle-aged Japanese men and women. *J Epidemiol* 16:117-24.

Pereira MA et al. 2005. Fast food habits, weight gain, and insulin resistance: 15-year prospective analysis. *Lancet* 365:36-42.

Plassmann H et al. 2008. Marketing actions can modulate neural representations of experienced pleasantness. *Proc Natl Acad Sci* 105:1050-4.

Pleis JR et al. 2008. Summary health statistics for US adults. National Health Interview Survey, Washington, DC.

Polivy J. 1996. Psychological consequences of food restriction. *J Am Diet Assoc* 96:589-94.

Polivy J, Herman CP. 2005. Mental health and eating behaviours: A bi-directional relation. *Can J Public Health* 96 (suppl. 3): S43-S46.

Potter JD, Finnegan JR Jr, Guinard J-X, et al. 2006. 5 A Day for Better Health program evaluation report. Available at www.scgcorp.com/docs/5_a_Day_Booklet_sm.pdf.

Povey R et al. 1999. A critical examination of the application of transtheroretical model to dietary behaviors. *Health Educ Res* 14:641-51.

Powell LM, Bao Y. 2009. Food prices, access to food outlets, and child weight. *Econ Hum Biol* 7:64-72.

Powell LM, Szczypka G, Chaloupka FJ, Braunschweig CL. 2007. Nutritional content of television food advertisements seen by children and adolescents. *Pediatrics* 120:576-83.

Prentice A. 2007. Are defects in energy expenditure involved in the causation of obesity? *Obesity Rev* 8 (suppl. 1): 89-91.

Prentice AM, Jebb SA. 2003. Fast foods, energy density, and obesity: A possible mechanistic link. *Obesity Rev* 4:187-94.

Prynne CJ et al. 1999. Food and nutrient intake of a national sample of 4-year old children in 1950: Comparison with the 1990s. *Pub Health Nutr* 2:537-47.

Puhl RM, Brownell KD. 2006. Confronting and coping with weight stigma. *Obesity* 14 (10): 1802-15.

Puhl RM, Heuer CA. 2009. The stigma of obesity: A review and update. *Obesity* 17: 941-64.

Renjilian DA et al. 2001. Individual versus group therapy for obesity. *J Consult Clin Psychol* 69:717-21.

Resnicow K, Davis-Hearn M, et al. 1997. Social-cognitive predictors of fruit and vegetable intake in children. *Health Psychol* 16:272-76.

Riley BL et al. 2007. Organizational change for obesity prevention—perspectives, possibilities, and pitfalls. In *Handbook for Obesity Prevention,* ed. S Kumanyika, RC Brownson. New York: Springer.

Roberto CA, Baik J, Harris JL, Brownell KD. 2010. Influence of licensed characters on children's taste and snack preferences. *Pediatrics* 126:88-93.

Rolls BJ. 1985. Experimental analyses of the effects of variety in a meal on human feeding. *Am J Clin Nutr* 42:932-39.

———. 2003. The supersizing of America. *Nutr Today* 38:42-53.

Rolls BJ, Drewnowski A, Ledikwe JH. 2005. Changing the energy density of the diet as a strategy for weight management. *J Am Dent Assoc* 105 (suppl. 1): S98-S103.

Rolls BJ, Van Duijvenvoorde PM, Rowe EA. 1983. Variety in the diet enhances intake in a meal and contributes to the development of obesity in the rat. *Physiol Behav* 31:21-27.

Rolls ET. 2007. Understanding the mechanisms of food intake and obesity. *Obesity Rev* 8 (suppl. 1): 67-72.

Romon M, Lommez A, Tafflet M, et al. 2009 . Downward trends in the prevalence of childhood overweight in the setting of 12-year school- and community-based programmes. *Pub Health Nutr* 12 (10): 1735-42.

Ryan DH, Johnson WD, Myers VH, et al. 2010. Nonsurgical weight loss for extreme obesity in primary care settings. *Arch Intern Med* 170 (2): 146-54.

Sabate J. 2003. Nut consumption and body weight. *Am J Clin Nutr* 78:647S-650S.

Sallis JF, Glanz K. 2006. The role of built environments in physical activity, eating, and obesity in childhood. *Future of Children* 16:89-108.

Sanchez-Villegas A, Bes-Rastrollo M, et al. 2006. Adherence to a Mediterranean dietary pattern and weight gain in a follow-up study: The SUN cohort. *Int J Obesity* 30:350-58.

Schachter S. 1968. Obesity and eating: Internal and external cues differentially affect the eating behavior of obese and normal subjects. *Science* 161:751-56.

Schnoll R, Zimmerman BJ. 2001. Self-regulation training enhances dietary self-efficacy and dietary fiber consumption. *J Am Diet Assoc* 101:1006-11.

Shepherd J, Harden A, et al. 2001. *Young People and Healthy Eating: A Systematic Review of Research on Barriers and Facilitators.* Evidence for Policy and Practice. London, England: EPPI-Centre.

Simpson SJ, Raubenheimer D. 2005. Obesity: The protein leverage hypothesis. *Obesity Rev* 6:133-42.

Singhal A, Lanigan J. 2007. Breastfeeding, early growth, and later obesity. *Obesity Rev* 8 (suppl. 1): 51-54.

Sjostrom et al. 2007. Effects of bariatric surgery on mortality in Swedish obese subjects. *N Engl J Med* 357:741-52.

Skinner JD et al. 2003. Longitudinal calcium intake is negatively related to children's body fat indexes. *J Am Diet Assoc* 103:1626-31.

Stice E et al. 2002. Risk factors for binge eating onset in adolescent girls. *Health Psychol* 21:131-38.

Stubbs J, Ferres S, Horgan G. 2000. Energy density of foods: Effects on energy intake. *Crit Rev Food Sci Nutr* 40:481-515.

Sturm R. 2007. Increases in morbid obesity in the USA: 2000-2005. *Pub Health* 121:492-96.

Sunkard AJ, Sorensen T, et al. 1986. An adoption study of human obesity. *N Engl J Med* 314:193-98.

Sutin AR, Terracciano A. 2013. Perceived weight discrimination and obesity. *PLoS One* 8 (7): e70048.

Taylor JP, Evers S, McKenna M. 2005. Determinants of healthy eating in children and youth. *Can J Publ Health* 96 (suppl. 3): S20-S26.

Thompson O et al. 2004. Food purchased away from home as a predictor of change in BMI Z-score among girls. *Int J Obes Relat Metab Disord* 28:282-89.

Thorpe KE et al. 2004. The impact of obesity on rising medical spending. *Health Affairs* 23:w480-86.

Tillotson J. 2004. America's obesity: Conflicting public policies, industrial economic development, and unintended human consequences. *Annu Rev Nutr* 24:617-43.

U.S. Department of Agriculture Economic Research Service (USDAERS). 2000. A century of change in American's eating patterns. *Food Rev* 23 (1): 8-15.

U.S. Department of Health and Human Services (USDHHS). 2008. Business Case for Breastfeeding.

Available at Womenshealth.gov, www.womenshealth.gov/breastfeeding/government-in-action/business-case.html.

U.S. Federal Trade Commission (USFTC). 2007. Children's exposure to TV advertising in 1977 and 2004: Information for the obesity debate: Bureau of Economics staff report. Available at www.ftc.gov/reports/childrens-exposure-television-advertising-1977-2004-information-obesity-debate-bureau.

Valente TW. 2012. Network interventions. *Science* 337 (6090) (July 6): 49-53.

Vartanian LR et al. 2007. Effects of soft drink consumption on nutrition and health: A systematic review and meta-analysis. *Am J Public Health* 97:667-75.

Volkow ND, O'Brien CP. 2007. Issues for DSM-V: Should obesity be included as a brain disorder? *Am J Psychiatry* 164:708-10.

Wadden TA et al. 2005. Randomized trial of lifestyle modification and pharmacotherapy for obesity. *N Engl J Med* 353:2111-20.

Wang C, Coups EJ. 2010. Causal beliefs about obesity and associated health behaviors. *Int J Behav Nutr Phys Act* 7:19.

Wang, Y, Beydoun MA, Liang L, Caballero B, Kumanyika SK. 2008. Will all Americans become overweight or obese? Estimating the progression and cost of the US obesity epidemic. *Obesity* 16 (10): 2323-30.

Wang Y, Tussing L, Odoms-Young A, et al. 2006. Obesity prevention in low socioeconomic status urban African-American adolescents: Study design and preliminary findings of the HEALTH-KIDS Study. *Eur J Clin Nutr* 60:92-103.

Wardle J. 2007. Eating behavior and obesity. *Obesity Rev* 8 (suppl. 1): 73-75.

Wardle J, Cooke LJ, et al. 2003. Increasing children's acceptance of vegetables: A randomized trial of parent-led exposure. *Appetite* 40:155-62.

Wardle J et al. 2000. Nutrition knowledge and food intake. *Appetite* 34:269-75.

Wardle J, Gibson EL. 2002. Impact of stress on diet: Processes and implications. In *Stress and the Heart*, ed. SA Stansfeld, M Marmot, 124-49. London: BMJ.

Webb TL, Sheeran P. 2006. Does changing behavioral intentions engender behavior change? A meta-analysis of the experimental evidence. *Psychol Bull* 132:249-68.

Weingarten HP. 1983. Conditioned cues elicit feeding in sated rats: A role for learning in meal initiation. *Science* 220:431-33.

White M. 2007. Food access and obesity. *Obesity Rev* 8 (suppl. 1): 99-107.

WHO Expert Committee on Physical Status. 1995. *Physical Status: The Use and Interpretation of Anthropom-*

etry. World Health Organization Technical Report Series, 854. Geneva: World Health Organization.

Wing RR. 2004. Behavioral approaches to the treatment of obesity. In *Handbook of Obesity: Clinical Applications,* ed. GA Gray, C Bouchard. New York: Marcel Dekker.

Wing RR, Hill JO. 2001. Successful weight loss maintenance. *Annu Rev Nutr* 21:323-41.

Wing R et al. 2006. A self-regulation program for the maintenance of weight loss. *N Engl J Med* 355:1563-71.

Wood W et al. 2005. Changing circumstances, disrupting habits. *J Pers Soc Psychol* 88:918-33.

World Health Organization (WHO). 2008. Global strategy on diet, physical activity, and health. Available at www.who.int/dietphysicalactivity /publications/facts/obesity/en/.

Wright JD, Kennedy-Stephenson J, Wang CY, McDowell MA, Johnson CL, National Center for Health Statistics, CDC. 2004. Trends in intake of energy and macronutrients—United States, 1971-2000. *MMWR* 53 (04): 80-82.

Zimmerman FJ, Bell JF. 2010. Associations of television content type and obesity in children. *Am J Public Health* 100:334-40.

CHAPTER 14

Physical Activity and Behavior Change

ABBY C. KING, MATTHEW BUMAN,
AND ERIC HEKLER

LEARNING OBJECTIVES

After completing the chapter, the reader will be able to

* Define the current U.S. national physical activity recommendations for adults.
* Define the key determinants of physical activity participation across multiple levels of impact (i.e., individual, interpersonal, sociocultural, policy levels).
* Recognize the health-related risks of prolonged sedentary behavior.
* Understand the evidence base supporting physical activity interventions across different levels of impact.

Introduction

Humans evolved to be regularly physically active, and the available evidence indicates that throughout the vast majority of mankind's history we achieved this biological imperative. Hippocrates recognized its importance: "All parts of the body which have a function," he said, "if used in moderation and exercised in labors in which each is accustomed, become thereby healthy, well-developed and age more slowly, but if unused and left idle they become liable to disease, defective in growth, and age quickly." Remarkably, however, as a consequence of human cultural evolution and technological advances, humans have essentially "outrun" their genetic ability to adapt to the far different environments that we find ourselves in today (Eaton et al. 2009). The result has been a biological-environmental disconnect that has set the stage for the plethora of 20th-century public health challenges created or exacerbated by a largely inactive lifestyle.

This chapter provides an overview of the population-wide physical inactivity problem, the **key determinants** associated with inactive versus more active lifestyles, and the evidence-based **interventions** that hold promise for positively influencing this key **health behavior**. We also explore the implications of current evidence for **key stakeholders** and the development of relevant initiatives, programs, and policies (WHO 2006). We apply the standard definition of physical activity, that is, "any bodily movement produced by skeletal muscles that results in energy expenditure," in contrast to exercise, which typically has been defined as a subset of physical activity that involves "planned, structured, and repetitive bodily movements done to improve or maintain one or more components of physical fitness" (Caspersen et al. 1985). Much of the evidence provided by exercise scientists has focused on higher-intensity exercise and sport activity, but the gradual development of an increased public health focus has expanded research in the field to broader dimensions of physical activity behavior. The current interest in health-enhancing physical activity includes a range of physical activity types (e.g., endurance, strengthening, flexibility, balance exercises), intensities (light, moderate, vigorous), and purposes (e.g., for leisure, transport, household and yard maintenance, caretaking, work).

Magnitude

Physical inactivity is recognized as one of the three key health behaviors (alongside tobacco use and dietary patterns) contributing to the chronic diseases responsible for 50% of global **mortality** (Oxford Health Alliance 2009). Among the chronic diseases and conditions strongly linked with inactivity are cardiovascular disease, stroke, some forms of cancer (i.e., colon, breast), type 2 diabetes, depression, loss of physical function, weight gain, cognitive decline in

older adults, and all-cause mortality (PAG 2008; USDHHS 1996). Regular physical activity, by contrast, is associated with lower risk of hip fracture and increased bone density, improved sleep quality, reduced abdominal obesity, lower risk of lung and endometrial cancers, weight maintenance following weight loss, and better functional health among older adults. Among children and adolescents, regular physical activity is strongly associated with improved cardiorespiratory endurance and muscular fitness, body composition, bone health, and cardiovascular health. There is also evidence that regular physical activity reduces symptoms of anxiety and depression (PAG 2008).

The increased health risks associated with physical inactivity occur in a **dose-response** fashion, so those who are least active and unfit are at the greatest risk. Health risks incurred through a physically inactive lifestyle, while generally increasing with age, are independent of other demographic characteristics (e.g., race or ethnicity, gender, education, income, body size). Numerous biological markers of chronic disease risk are affected by physical activity, including body weight, blood pressure, cholesterol, blood-clotting factors, insulin sensitivity, autonomic nervous system regulation, bone and muscle strength, inflammatory processes, and brain vascularization (Hamer 2007; Hamer and Chida 2009; PAG 2008).

Despite this extensive body of scientific evidence, national **surveillance** data indicate that most Americans do not meet national physical activity recommendations (CDC 2007; USDHHS 1996); 20% to 30% of adults report no leisure-time physical activity (CDC 2005). The most current physical activity recommendations for U.S. adults are to participate in at least 150 minutes per week of moderate-intensity aerobic physical activity (i.e., sufficient to increase their heart rate and breathing to some degree) or 75 minutes per week of vigorous-intensity aerobic activity (i.e., sufficient to increase heart rate and breathing to a large extent). Aerobic activity should be performed in episodes of at least 10 minutes, preferably spread throughout the week (PAG 2008). Because the preponderance of U.S. adults fall short of these recommended levels and because of the numerous risks of being physically inactive or unfit, the public health burden associated with a physically inactive lifestyle is similar to or exceeds the burden of other major chronic disease risk factors (Haskell et al. 2009).

Key Determinants

Determinants in this **context** are variables that are associated with, or predictive of, a behavior or outcome. The majority of the evidence published to date has focused on leisure forms of aerobic physical activity (e.g., jogging, bicycling, swimming, walking for exercise), measured via **self-report**; much less attention has been paid to other forms of physical activity (e.g., transport- or work-related physical activity or physical activity aimed at improving strength, flexibility, or balance) (PAG 2008). Although observational evidence may not lend itself to causal inferences, such associative relationships may be instructive in identifying useful pathways for further exploration and intervention development (Bauman et al. 2002; King, Bauman, and Calfas 2002).

Individual-Level Determinants

To date, **individual-level determinants** have received the most study and attention (King, Bauman, and Calfas 2002). Among the individual-level determinants that have consistently been associated with lower levels of physical activity across diverse populations are increased age, female sex, lower levels of education, lower household income levels, lower-rated health, unemployment status, increased body weight, cigarette smoking, depression, living in certain regions of the country (e.g., the southern region), and belonging to certain ethnic minority

groups (i.e., African American, Hispanic) (Dowda et al. 2003; USDHHS 1996). Along with behavioral **self-regulation skills** such as self-monitoring, the most robust cognitive variable associated with higher physical activity levels is physical-activity-specific **self-efficacy** (i.e., an individual's confidence in being able to engage in physical activity across a specified time period) (McAuley and Blissmer 2000). Among other reported beliefs, **expectations** of positive (e.g., benefits) and negative outcomes associated with physical activity have been associated with adult physical activity levels (Brassington et al. 2002; Carels et al. 2005; Neff and King 1995; Wilcox, Castro, and King 2006). Physical activity enjoyment also has been linked with activity levels (Salmon et al. 2003; USHHS 1996).

Among children and adolescents, additional physical activity determinants include parental expectations related to physical activity (Hume et al. 2009; Jago and Baranowski 2004) and perceived competence, expectations of success, and self-worth (Weiss and Ferrer-Caja 2002). Among female adolescents, Caucasian ethnicity and participation in organized sports have been positively associated with physical activity, whereas TV-viewing has been negatively associated with physical activity in some studies (Bungum and Vincent 1997). Evidence also shows that physical activity experiences occurring in childhood or adolescence can set the stage for physical activity participation in adulthood (Taylor et al. 1999; Trudeau et al. 1999) and old age (Cousins 1997).

Older adults represent a population group for which there is a growing determinants literature. Determinants such as physician advice, physical function, and the individual's belief that physical activity is important to his health may be particularly important (Burton et al. 1999; King 2001). For ethnic minority and low-income groups of adults, perceived lack of safety, perceptions of multiple role demands (e.g., wife, mother, daughter, active community member, worker), increased body weight, and lack of (or negative) experiences with exercise or other forms of physical activity may be particularly detrimental (Ball et al. 2006; Eyler et al. 2002). Cost may also be a barrier to physical activity participation in some population groups (Salmon et al. 2003).

Interpersonal-Level Determinants

Family **influences** as well as influences of friends, co-workers, and others in a person's environment are consistently related to physical activity levels across diverse populations, age groups, and measurement instruments (Booth et al. 2000; Smith 1999). Such influences include accompanying an individual during a physical activity episode and supplying verbal support and encouragement for physical activity (Dowda et al. 2003).

Being married is associated with increased physical activity levels in some studies, but decreased physical activity in others (King et al. 1998; Schmitz et al. 1997). These contrasting results may be partially explained by theories of **marital concordance** (i.e., spouses share similar health and behavioral patterns, both positive and negative) (Meyler et al. 2007). Specifically, if spouses share similar behaviors, then marital status may promote increased physical activity for some couples but decrease physical activity for others. Although there is some evidence to support marital concordance in relation to eating behaviors, little research has examined marital concordance for physical activity (Meyler et al. 2007; Pettee et al. 2006).

Marital *transitions*, as well as other life role transitions (such as changes in student or employment status [Calfas et al. 2000], children in the home, or other caretaking activities) also have been associated with changes in physical activity levels, though not always in the direction that we might expect. For example, a 10-year study of the relationship between marital transitions and physical activity levels found that while the transition from a married to a single state did not affect physical activity levels relative to remaining married, the transition from a single to a married state resulted in significant positive changes in physical activity relative to remaining single (King et al. 1998). In contrast, in the Australian Longitudinal Study of Women's Health, a four-year follow-up revealed that women of ages 18-23 at baseline who reported getting married, having a first or subsequent child, or beginning paid work during the four-year time period were more likely to be inactive at follow-up than those who did not report these events (Brown and Trost 2003). Similarly, a prospective study of 32 U.S. work sites found that remaining single across the two-year study period was associated with increased physical activity levels in both sexes relative to other marital contexts (Schmitz et al. 1997).

In addition to human sources of support, pets—in particular, dogs—are recognized as a potentially positive source of **"social capital"** for increased physical activity levels and other health promoting behaviors (Pachana et al. 2005; Wood et al. 2005).

Sociocultural Determinants

In addition to the interpersonal forms of **social support** and influence described above, the more general sociocultural context within which people live can also influence their physical activity. Such determinants include broader **social networks**, life roles and role expectations, and **social norms** and cultural standards. For example, research exploring the often-reported gender differences in physical activity suggests that women may be exposed to societal messages indicating that physical activity is less appropriate or less important for them and may receive less social support for adopting or maintaining a physically active lifestyle (Eyler et al. 2002; Fallon et al. 2005; Vrazel et al. 2008). Similar types of **cultural norms**, beliefs, and expectations may play a role in the lower levels of physical activity often reported in ethnic minority and low-income groups (Eyler 2002; Eyler et al. 1998; Eyler et al. 1999; Fallon et al. 2005). For example, low-income women participating in the Women's Cardiovascular Health Network Project (Eyler 2002) reported having fewer appropriate role models for physical activity, having language and acculturation issues that hindered participation in community exercise programs, and having family and caregiving responsibilities that left little time for physical activity; they also said there was a lack of culturally appropriate programs involving physical activity (e.g., traditional dance) (Eyler et al. 2002). Similar limitations to engaging in adequate physical activity, such as increased caregiving duties or lack of social support have been reported in rural women (Wilcox et al. 2000).

Environment-Level Determinants

Over the past two decades, a burgeoning literature has developed aimed at better understanding the potential effects of the physical environment and related **structural determinants** (e.g., access to facilities where physical activity can occur) on physical activity in a range of populations (French et al. 2001; Saelens et al. 2003). Although the majority of investigations are cross-sectional in design, they nonetheless shed light on the ways in which the physical environment can influence habitual levels of physical activity. For example, both climate and season are associated with physical activity in the United States; those U.S. counties with the highest percentage of dry, moderate conditions also have the greatest proportion of persons meeting national physical activity recommendations (Merrill et al. 2005). Weather and climate alone, however, while potentially influencing acute decisions related to physical activity participation (King et al. 2008; Stetson et al. 2005), likely play a less important role in determining overall physical activity levels than other personal, social, and environmental factors (Humpel et al. 2002; Shumway-Cook et al. 2002).

Features of the **built environment** appear in general to be more stable and robust factors influencing physical activity levels. The literature includes perceived, as well as objectively measured, aspects of the built environment (Boehmer et al. 2006). It increasingly recognizes that different built environmental features may be linked with specific physical activity types or contexts (e.g., physical activity undertaken for transport as opposed to for leisure or recreation) (Giles-Corti, Timperio, et al. 2005; Hoehner et al. 2005). For example, a recent review of the built environment correlates of walking noted the often-reported finding that walking for transportation is consistently associated with residential density, distance to nonresidential destinations, and land-use mix (e.g., commercial versus residential land uses), with less consistent relationships found for route or network connectivity (i.e., presence of street grid patterns, reflecting higher route connectivity, versus cul-de-sacs, reflecting lower route connectivity), parks and open space, and personal safety. Built environment relationships with recreational walking were less clear (Saelens and Handy 2008).

Among the objectively measured built environmental features that have been consistently associated with greater physical activity are increased land-use mix (i.e., presence of residential along with commercial and other land uses), street connectivity (e.g., grid-based street layouts as opposed to cul-de-sacs or dead-end streets), residential density, and neighborhood-level **socioeconomic status** (**SES**) (Frank et al. 2005; King et al. 2005). Ready access to attractive, large public open space also has been found to be associated with higher levels of walking in some locales (Giles-Corti, Broomhall, et al. 2005).

Among the perceived built environmental features that people associate repeatedly with greater levels of physical activity are proximity to destinations; presence of sidewalks, streetlights, and attractive neighborhood aesthetics (e.g., gardens, foliage); lower traffic volumes and speeds; the presence of intersection safety features; social features including the presence of others walking in the neighborhood; and the absence of stray or loose dogs (King et al. 2000; King et al. 2006; Sallis et al. 2007). Perceived neighborhood crime level has shown inconsistent relationships with physical activity; however, a recent review concluded that perceived safety adversely affects subgroups that are more likely to exhibit higher levels of anxiety about crime (e.g., older adults, ethnic minorities) (Foster and Giles-Corti 2008).

For certain ethnic minority and low-income groups as well as older adults, built environment barriers to regular physical activity may be particularly pronounced, including the lack of sidewalks, lighting, intersection safety measures (e.g., marked crosswalks, pedestrian crossing lights), or attractive aesthetic elements (e.g., foliage); increased traffic congestion and speed; greater crime; and less overall access (e.g., longer distances, cost-prohibitive facilities or programs) to community exercise facilities and programs (Eyler et al. 2002; Garcia et al. 2009; Griffin et al. 2008; King et al. 2000). At least one cross-sectional study evaluating perceptions of the neighborhood environment in adults living in Geographic Information System (GIS)–derived higher versus lower SES stratified neighborhoods found that those living in lower SES areas perceived their neighborhoods as busier with traffic, less attractive, and less supportive of walking (Giles-Corti and Donovan 2002b).

Modifying environments to have a positive impact on physical activity for one particular population segment may have unintended consequences for other population subgroups (Giles-Corti and King 2009). For example, although the transportation literature is replete with evidence that enhanced street connectivity (as opposed to cul-de-sacs) is associated with greater levels of transport-oriented physical activity among the working-age populations of adults, some groups of children and teenagers are more active in cul-de-sac-oriented street designs (i.e.,

those with less street connectivity) (Carver et al. 2008). Given that children, including those from inner-city neighborhoods, have been reported to be more active when they are outdoors, one reasonably simple public health message is to encourage children to play outdoors more regularly (Martin and McCaughtry 2008). Additional built environmental factors have been found to come into play when children are being targeted. For instance, both Mexican American and non-Hispanic white parents rated the availability of toilets, safety, drinking water, lighting, and shade as important factors in selecting play spaces for their young children (Sallis et al. 1997). Parental perceptions of traffic on local roads and concern about traffic safety also may be associated with children's recreational physical activity levels, active commuting to school, and body weight (Timperio et al. 2005; Timperio et al. 2006). Although, in some cases, the presence of a steep incline or grade has been an apparent barrier to children's active commuting-to-school behavior, some studies of midlife and older adults have found the reported presence of neighborhood hills or grades to be related to higher levels of physical activity (King et al. 2000; Sallis et al. 2007).

With the growth of this area of study in the physical activity field have come questions related to the role that **self-selection** factors may play in understanding the relations observed between built environment factors and physical activity. That is, regularly active individuals may seek out more "walkable" neighborhoods in which to live; it may not be that the **walkability** of the neighborhood has a causal influence on the people living there. Currently there is little experimental evidence clarifying the directionality of the built environment-physical activity association. However, the available observational evidence suggests that people's choices concerning their neighborhoods cannot fully explain the physical activity–built environment relationship (Handy et al. 2006; Sallis, Saelens, et al. 2009).

Policy-Level Determinants

Public policies, laws, and regulations can also influence the types of, amounts of, and locations for physical activity in a community, both directly (e.g., policies that prevent the use of school grounds or playing fields outside of school hours) and indirectly (e.g., transportation policies that place the automobile, rather than the pedestrian, at the center of urban planning and land use decisions affecting communities) (Heath et al. 2006; Solomon et al. 2009). The differential distribution of amenities and services influencing active transport and recreational physical activity is an area of increasing focus and concern (Garcia et al. 2009). For example, inequities that potentially could be amenable to regulatory oversight or policy-level control have been found to exist in some locales relating to the quality of parks and other public local spaces situated in higher versus lower SES neighborhoods (Crawford et al. 2008).

Considering Combinations of Physical Activity Determinants

The growing use of new research methods, such as multifactorial decision tree analysis and other risk classification methods, has allowed for greater exploration of the interactions among variables in identifying population subgroups at greater or lesser risk of inactivity (Agurs-Collins et al. 1997). For example, in a recent investigation of correlates of physical inactivity in a nationally representative sample, the subgroup with the highest proportion of inactive adults (50% were inactive) consisted of individuals with at least some college education who were in fair to poor health *and* watched more than four hours of television on a typical weekday. The subgroup with the lowest proportion of inactive adults (13% were inactive) consisted of college-educated individuals who were in good to excellent general health, believed that exercise can lower cancer risk, and had a reported **body mass index (BMI)**

of less than 29 (Atienza et al. 2006). Identification of behaviorally at-risk subgroups may set the stage for the development of interventions targeted specifically to the needs and lifestyles of the specific subgroups.

Interestingly, when variables from different levels of impact (personal, interpersonal or social, and environmental) have been evaluated together, environmental variables are not necessarily the primary correlates of physical activity. In one community survey of Australian adults, the influence of physical environmental factors was found to be secondary to individual and social determinants, suggesting that though a supportive physical environment may be necessary, it is not sufficient, to increase physical activity levels (Giles-Corti and Donovan 2002a).

The Evolving Literature Aimed at Sedentary Behaviors

The potentially deleterious health effects of sedentary behaviors, such as sitting and television viewing, independent of physical activity level, are being increasingly recognized (Owen et al. 2000). Among the factors that have been linked with increased sedentary behavior are poor weather, overweight or obesity, older age, lower levels of education and income, unemployment, financial costs related to physical activity, family and work commitments, feeling tired, and poorer health (Bowman 2006; CDC 1997; Salmon et al. 2003). Television viewing also has been found to be a good indicator of other sedentary behaviors among adult women, though not necessarily among men (Sugiyama et al. 2008). Among adolescents and children, lower SES, being male (Fairclough et al. 2009), and increased interpersonal problems and feelings of ineffectiveness (Anton et al. 2006) were all linked with increased sedentary behaviors.

Television viewing is the most frequently studied sedentary activity to date, and among the correlates of high U.S. population levels of viewing (i.e., more than 14 hours per week) are lower household income, greater age, being divorced or separated, lower-rated health, smoking, higher BMI, fewer average minutes per week in leisure-time physical activity, more depression, lower fruit and vegetable intake, reports of unsupportive neighborhood environments for walking (e.g., crime, traffic congestion, poor lighting, lack of aesthetics or scenery), and regularly eating dinner in front of the television (King et al. 2010).

A Conceptual Framework for Intervention Development

Over the past two decades, physical activity researchers have increasingly applied multilevel **social ecological frameworks** in identifying predictors and potential mediators of physical activity intervention success (King, Stokols, et al. 2002). Figure 14.1 reflects a social ecological framework, based on work undertaken by the

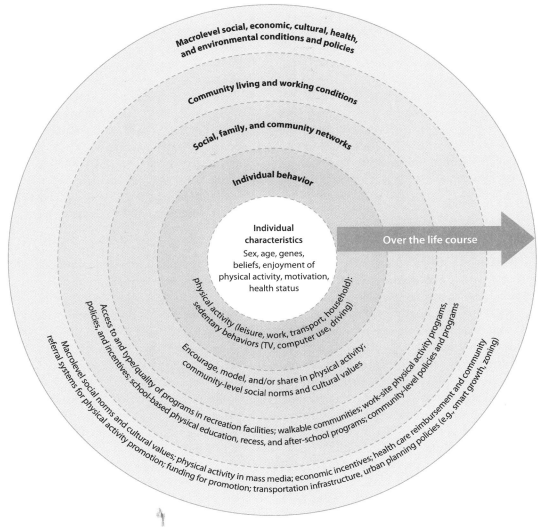

FIGURE 14.1. A social ecological framework for population physical activity promotion.
Source: adapted from IM 2001; King and Sallis 2009.

Institute of Medicine (2001), which has been adapted to include factors of particular relevance to physical activity promotion (King and Sallis 2009). Although efforts to change specific correlates serving as possible mediators of physical activity change have been limited, by and large, to individual-level cognitive and social variables, increased attention to higher-level variables (e.g., physical, social, and cultural environmental contexts) sets the stage for higher-level intervention work that could occur in the future.

This trend notwithstanding, much of the scientific evidence related to physical activity intervention remains targeted at individual-level or interpersonal variables in working-age adults. A number of studies report generally moderate effects, albeit for reasonably limited time periods (i.e., one year or less) (Marcus et al. 2006). Intervention areas that reflect extensive scientific interest or hold particular promise for improving population-wide physical activity levels are highlighted below.

Evidence-Based Interventions

As previously noted, increases in regular physical activity are linked with myriad beneficial physical and mental health outcomes across age, sex, and ethnic groups (PAG 2008). The pervasiveness of the potential positive impacts of regular physical activity across major physical systems, as well as in other behavioral, psychological, and social domains, argues strongly for a population approach to promoting physical activity. In addition, growing evidence indicates that even low levels (e.g., once per week) of moderate-intensity physical activities (such as walking) are healthful, particularly as people age (Sundquist et al. 2004). Such research results set the stage for a wide range of intervention approaches and strategies.

Interventions Aimed at Individual-Level Factors

Among the targets of interventions at the individual level are changes in physical-activity-relevant knowledge, **attitudes**, beliefs, perceptions (including enjoyment of physical activity), self-efficacy, and self-regulatory behavioral skills that have been shown to be helpful in adopting and maintaining physical activity in the face of common personal, social, cultural, and environmental barriers. Such barriers include weather, time constraints, competing work and family commitments, lack of social support for physical activity, injury or illness, lags in **motivation** to be active, boredom, and difficulties in accessing physical-activity-promoting venues or environments (Carels et al. 2005; Courneya et al. 2005; King et al. 2008). Much of the research in this area has been based on **Social Cognitive Theory (SCT)** and similar behavioral approaches to physical activity change (USDHHS 1996). The following self-regulatory skills, derived from SCT and related behavioral theories, have been associated with successfully increasing physical activity:

- initial structuring of realistic physical-activity-related outcome expectations
- setting realistic physical activity **goals**
- correcting erroneous beliefs related to physical activity
- **tailoring** physical activity advice and counseling to fit the preferences and circumstances of the individual or group
- self-monitoring relevant physical activity behaviors
- obtaining specific, personalized behavioral feedback about progress
- marshaling ongoing social support for physical activity participation
- developing plans for overcoming barriers to physical activity that occur (Brassington et al. 2002; Marcus et al. 2000; Rejeski et al. 2003; Wilcox, Castro, and King 2006)

Behavioral-theory-based physical activity programs are generally effective, especially in the short term, for increasing regular physical activity in initially inactive or underactive individuals across a range of population groups (Hillsdon et al. 2005; TFCPS 2001). Numerous delivery sources have been identified for such programs, including health promotion counselors, health professionals, and effectively trained volunteers (Castro et al. 2011; Jacobson et al. 2005). The majority of interventions aimed at this level of impact have targeted primarily recreational or leisure physical activity. The behavioral intervention components described above also can be delivered effectively in a group format, such as an exercise class (Rejeski and Brawley 1997; Rejeski et al. 2003) or a behavioral instructional group (Collins et al. 2004; Dunn et al. 1999).

Systematic efforts have been made to expand the population impact of evidence-based individually adapted behavioral interventions by expanding the communication sources and channels used to deliver the interventions. Expert-system-tailored print (Marcus et al. 1998; Napolitano and Marcus 2002) and heath-adviser-tailored telephone programs (Castro and King 2002; Eakin et al. 2007; King et al. 1991) can increase physical activity levels across diverse populations. Other promising delivery systems include handheld computer devices (King et al. 2008), e-mail, web (Napolitano et al. 2003; Tate et al. 2003; Verheijden et al. 2007), automated-telephone-linked computer systems (King et al. 2007), and pedometers (Bravata et al. 2007).

To improve population health, evidence-based individually adapted interventions will need to be translated and disseminated effectively throughout a community for more extended periods of time than have typically been studied. Although relatively few systematic translation efforts have occurred to date, those that have been disseminated successfully to ethnically diverse populations include health-adviser-adapted telephone programs and behav-

ioral instructional groups for adults (Hooker et al. 2005; Wilcox et al. 2008).

Interventions Aimed at Social, Family, and Community Networks

Among interventions aimed at social, family, and community **networks** are family-oriented physical activity programs; strategies for obtaining support and encouragement from friends, neighbors, co-workers, and other community members; education and **modeling** of physical activity for diverse population segments through the use of mass media and other relevant channels; and strategies for influencing social norms and cultural values.

Although the potential merits of **targeting** the family for physical activity intervention are apparent (Umberson 1987), studies are inconsistent (CDC 2001; Nader et al. 1996). In contrast, social support interventions in community settings (e.g., developing a "buddy system" or a behavior based contracting system with others) are effective (CDC 2001). One potentially promising approach of this type has involved having mothers and daughters exercise together (Ransdell et al. 2003).

Community-wide and mass media informational campaigns increase awareness and knowledge (CDC 2001) but have produced mixed results related to attitude change and have rarely shown evidence of significantly improving physical activity (Marcus et al. 2006; Marshall et al. 2004). A recent example of a mass media campaign that had a positive impact on physical activity is the Centers for Disease Control and Prevention (CDC)'s national VERB campaign for youth. A **quasi-experimental** one-year **evaluation** of this youth-focused, multiethnic advertising campaign indicated an increase in free-time physical activity levels (Huhman et al. 2005). The VERB campaign combined commercial advertising with school and community promotions and Internet activities; it is a useful example of how combining media-oriented approaches with other interventions may be worthwhile (Marshall et al. 2004).

Point-of-choice signage, especially aimed at using stairs instead of escalators or elevators, is another mediated intervention approach that has been recommended for broader dissemination (CDC 2001). Specific messaging at the point of decision may also have relevance for several forms of physical activity, including stair use (Anderson et al. 1998; Blamey et al. 1995; Brownell et al. 1980) and walking (e.g., signage at bus stops encouraging walking to the next bus stop before boarding the bus). Such relatively short bouts of physical activity, particularly if undertaken at a heightened intensity, may have a positive impact on chronic disease risk factors (Boreham et al. 2000; DeBusk et al. 1990). However, the effects of such activities when evaluated alone may not reflect their additional importance as a complement to, or a catalyst for, other components of a comprehensive program.

In addition to these areas, a community networking approach to enhancing individually aimed interventions has been recommended. This approach involves coordination of efforts to enable local learning and ongoing delivery of evidence-based, individually adapted programs throughout a community (Bauman et al. 2009). Potentially relevant delivery sources for such services include primary care settings, YMCAs and other community physical activity organizations, community colleges, places of worship, and nongovernmental and nonprofit organizations (e.g., the American Heart Association, American Cancer Society, AARP). Other forms of social influence also deserve increased scientific attention and potential policy review: appropriately targeted public service announcements on television, radio, and related media; physical-activity-oriented television programming; and electronic entertainment devices involving physical activity (e.g., Xbox Kinect, Playstation Move, Wii-Sport, Dance Dance Revolution).

Interventions Aimed at Living and Working Conditions

Strategies for influencing living and working conditions to improve physical activity and reduce sedentary behavior include increasing access and decreasing other barriers to using recreational facilities (e.g., cost) and optimizing the types and quality of programs and policies offered in community settings. Such settings include work sites (e.g., **incentives** aimed at regular use of stairs, parking policies that encourage more walking, active commuting), health care settings (e.g., regular use of **health risk appraisals** that include physical activity, training health professionals to deliver physical activity advice, patient referral strategies linking health providers with relevant community programs), and schools (e.g., policies and programs related to regular physical education, active recess, after-school recreational programs, physically active commuting to school).

Other intervention targets involve increasing community walkability via specific structural improvements (e.g., sidewalks, bicycle lanes, safe intersection crossing schemes, traffic calming devices) and policies (e.g., urban planning and development policies to increase and protect public green space; pedestrian malls).

Although some interventions delivered in health care settings (e.g., targeted counseling, physical activity prescriptions) increase short- and intermediate-term physical activity levels (Elley et al. 2003), the overall evidence base in this area remains inconclusive (Eden et al. 2002; Marcus et al. 2006). Similar uncertainty exists for physical activity interventions in work sites (Proper et al. 2003), which, with few exceptions (Blair et al. 1986; Heirich et al. 1993), have often involved individually tailored motivational programs or strategically placed environmental prompts (e.g., reminders to use the stairs) (Katz et al. 2005; Marcus et al. 2006). The number of rigorously designed and controlled investigations with extended follow-up remains relatively small. Future investigations would benefit from higher-level organizational and environmental strategies, including the targeting of organization-specific **norms** and policies, organizational communication channels, relevant built environment amenities (e.g., bike racks, shower facilities, walking paths, stairway enhancements), and incentive systems for physical activity promotion.

Greater attention has been aimed at school-based interventions for physical activity promotion (Timperio et al. 2004). Those interventions that incorporate a combination of organizational (e.g., enhanced physical education classes), policy, and environmental approaches have typically been more effective than those targeting classroom curriculum-only approaches (Luepker et al. 1996; Timperio et al. 2004). One study indicated that the physical activity changes initiated during elementary school years persisted into early adolescence (Nader et al. 1999). Similarly, a health-related physical education program for elementary school children was successfully sustained for four years following the original program initiation (Dowda et al. 2005). Research on after-school and active-travel-to-school programs suggests that changes to address specific barriers (e.g., traffic congestion, parental fears for safety) could be useful (Jago and Baranowski 2004).

Encouraging evidence suggests that incorporating physical activity and physical education into the school day may have academic benefits in addition to health benefits. For example, adding short (e.g., 10-minute) activity breaks throughout the school day has been shown to increase on-task behavior during classroom instruction for elementary school children (Mahar et al. 2006).

Studies suggest that targeting a reduction in children's sedentary behaviors may increase physical activity (Roemmich et al. 2004; Simon et al. 2004), whereas interventions targeting only reductions in children's television viewing and computer screen activities may not necessarily

increase physical activity . However, such programs may benefit other health behaviors, such as dietary patterns and body weight (Robinson 1999), and nonhealth behaviors, such as aggression at school (Robinson et al. 2001).

Finally, interventions aimed at the built environment may improve recreational and transportation forms of physical activity in large groups of people (Frank and Kavage 2009; NIHCE 2008). Of the relatively few strategies that have been sufficiently evaluated, strategies that create or improve access to places for physical activity have received a "strongly recommended" rating by the U.S. Task Force on Community Preventive Services (Kahn et al. 2002). These results notwithstanding, at least one prospective study has reported that the building of a multi-use trail was not associated with a discernible increase in physical activity among adults living near the trail (Evenson et al. 2005). The results point to the likely need for multicomponent interventions aimed at both personal and environmental factors.

Interventions Aimed at Societal Conditions and Policies at Local, Regional, National, and International Levels

Interventions, programs, and broader **systems approaches** aimed at societal conditions and policies across different sectors and levels (local, regional, national, international) include the following strategies: economic incentives to be active versus sedentary (e.g., tax rebates for physical activity equipment and programs; tariffs on purchases that encourage sedentary behavior, such as televisions); reimbursement for physical activity counseling undertaken by health care providers and similar health "gatekeepers"; integrated community referral systems for physical activity; integration of relevant physical activity promotion information across local, regional, and national media sources; broader surveillance systems for physical activity that provide benchmark information at local, regional, and national levels; incorporation of physical activity promotion information and community resource identification into health professional training curricula (e.g., physicians, pharmacists, dietitians, nurses, psychologists, physical and occupational therapists); and governmental funding for increasing the physical activity infrastructure and for physical activity promotion. Such broad strategies remain, for the most part, lacking (Bauman et al. 2009).

Implementation Considerations for Special Populations

Although an array of populations merit special consideration, we have singled out two that we believe are particularly deserving of attention. The first is the older adult population, in light of their growing numbers, their heightened risk of both inactivity and the chronic diseases of aging on which regular physical activity can have a positive impact, and the relatively few studies specifically targeting them (Marcus et al. 2006). "Older adult" has often been designated as age 50 and above, in light of the increasing risk of chronic diseases accompanying this and older ages. As noted earlier, although older adults share a number of similar determinants with younger populations, other factors (e.g., physician advice, medication effects and side effects, functional limitations) may be particularly germane to older age groups and bear further investigation. Similarly, the impacts of aging-related life transitions (e.g., menopause, retirement, bereavement, family caregiving) on physical activity levels, preferences, and barriers are less understood and deserve additional attention. As for younger populations, health education alone does not appear to be an effective approach for promoting physical activity in older age groups, compared with behaviorally oriented, skill-based approaches (King 2001; Van der Bij et al. 2002). Although group- or center-based supervised physical activity programs appear to be a particularly useful format for some

older adults, a growing number of studies has demonstrated that directed home-based programs (i.e., supervision occurring either in a face-to-face fashion or through mediated channels, e.g., telephone, computer) are also effective (Ashworth et al. 2005; Castro and King 2002). For some groups of older adults, home-based programs have yielded better physical activity rates, particularly in the longer term, than center-based programs have (Ashworth et al. 2005; King et al. 1995). Of note, studies evaluating age-related preferences regarding physical activity format have found that older adults, as compared with younger adults, may prefer the convenience and familiarity of home-based over center-based formats (Wilcox et al. 1999).

Despite the growing number of studies targeting older populations (Marcus et al. 2006), the quality and interpretative clarity of this literature have been inconsistent. The field would benefit from further application of rigorous methods and careful interpretation of results.

Emphasis on **health disparities** in disadvantaged segments of the population, including low-income groups, certain ethnic minority groups (e.g., African American, Hispanic, American Indian, Asian immigrant groups), and individuals with disabilities (LaVeist 2005; NCPP 2007), has also been increasing. In addition to vulnerabilities in other health areas, these groups typically have relatively low levels of physical activity (CDC 2005). Unfortunately, relatively few studies have specifically targeted such disadvantaged populations for physical activity intervention, and much of the available intervention literature suffers from weak designs and methods (Banks-Wallace and Conn 2002; Taylor et al. 1998; Yancey et al. 2004). Stronger study designs have more recently shown promising results (Albright et al. 2005; Resnicow et al. 2005; Robinson et al. 2003). The relevance of multilevel, community-based participatory research approaches has been emphasized in this area, including the evaluation of interventions aimed at modifying environmental infrastructure and relevant health policies to support physical activity in disadvantaged communities, where infrastructure and resources are especially lacking (Whitt-Glover et al. 2009). A recent review of interventions for obesity prevention among multi-ethnic and minority participants suggested that interventions tended to work better when they utilized individual (as opposed to group) sessions, family involvement, and multicomponent programs (Seo and Sa 2008).

Roles for Key Stakeholders

The selective review above shows clearly that effective action in promoting regular physical activity across the population at large will require sustained activities that are transdisciplinary, intersectoral, and multilevel (King, Stokols, et al. 2002). This section highlights potential roles and opportunities for different key stakeholders in helping to achieve this goal.

Researchers

A multidisciplinary research community has increasingly embraced the importance of expanding research beyond personal and **interpersonal factors** to higher levels of impact, including organizational, environmental, and policy levels (Sallis, Story, and Lou 2009; Srinivasan et al. 2003; Zimring et al. 2005). Certain research needs have been identified as having the potential to improve population-wide levels of physical activity and related health significantly. They include greater application of prospective designs, evaluations of natural experiments, economic analysis, and measurement development in areas related to policy as well as health impact assessment, investigation of policy adoption and implementation, and training of scientists in multilevel and other **complex** statistical analysis methods as well as interdisciplinary collaborative approaches (Sallis, Story, and Lou 2009). An additional area ripe for training is the effective application of community-

based participatory research methods as a means of optimizing both the relevance and the sustainability of successful evidence-based interventions (Blumenthal 2006; Flicker et al. 2007; Horowitz et al. 2009). Such community participatory methods can also be applied in formulating community-focused assessment and intervention tools (Jilcott et al. 2007; YMCA of the USA 2008).

Researchers in the physical activity field would also benefit from obtaining better knowledge of complementary disciplines. One such area is **behavioral economics**, which applies experimental approaches in gaining a greater understanding of human decision making (Zimmerman 2009). Research drawing upon behavioral economics perspectives has been aimed at understanding physical activity choices and sedentary behaviors in obese and nonobese children (Epstein and Roemmich 2001; Epstein et al. 1997; Epstein et al. 2005; Epstein et al. 2007). Less is currently known about how such perspectives could illuminate adults' decision making with regard to physical activity and being sedentary. In addition, the contributions that behavioral economics research has made concerning the highly malleable nature of human preferences and choices can help set the stage for higher-impact interventions. Among the types of contextual anchors of relevance to physical activity decision making are perceptions of social norms concerning how much physical activity others are engaged in (perceptions which often can be inaccurate), framing physical activity as something that is fun as opposed to obligatory, and disrupting early habits of sitting and other sedentary behaviors, which currently serve as the defaults in our society. One potential way to reduce habit formation around sitting is through environmental interventions (e.g., standing desks in schools, motion-based learning). Based on behavioral economics theory, researchers have argued recently that the major goal in the physical activity field should be changing the social and environmental contexts for physical activity for everyone in society, as opposed to targeting small, at-risk groups (Zimmerman 2009).

Given our economically constrained environment, another issue that researchers should consider is the importance of cost-effectiveness studies (Pratt et al. 2004; Sturm 2005). Although a growing body of literature has underscored the costs attendant on an inactive lifestyle (Garrett et al. 2004; Pratt et al. 2000; Wang et al. 2004), relatively few studies have systematically compared the cost-effectiveness of two or more physical activity interventions (Sevick et al. 2000). Additionally, a compelling case has been made for broadening the potential impact of intervention effectiveness research through systematically documenting the population or organizational **reach**, adoption, implementation, and maintenance of an intervention as a basic part of study design and execution (Brownson et al. 2012; Glasgow et al. 2003). By building in methods for better capturing the potential impact of interventions at multiple levels, research in the field will likely have a greater probability of influencing public health decision making and policy (Glasgow et al. 1999). This has been the emphasis of several Institute of Medicine reports evaluating progress in population-level policies and community interventions on obesity and other chronic diseases (IOM 1997, 2010, 2012, 2013).

National and State or Regional Legislative Bodies

Both national and state or regional legislative bodies can play a powerful role in supporting the promotion of physical activity across the population, and to date that contribution has been minimally harnessed. On the federal level in the United States and Canada, relatively little legislative work has been focused on population-wide physical activity, likely owing, at least in part, to commonly held perspectives that physi-cal activity is a personal choice and thus less relevant for government intervention (Morandi 2009). Some legislative successes can be identified, such as the 1991 Intermodal Surface Transportation Efficiency Act (Public Law 102-240, known as ISTEA; it expired in 1997), which represented a major shift in transportation planning and policy in the United States. One consequence of this legislation was that unused railway routes in various portions of the country were converted to walking and bicycling paths for local citizens. A recent U.S. report noted that investments in pedestrian and bicycle infrastructure have increased substantially since passage of ISTEA. Such investments, however, remain a small share of overall transportation programs, and the proportion of federal funds going toward bicycle or pedestrian infrastructure varies substantially across different regions of the country. The impacts of such expenditures on regional walking and bicycling levels remain unclear, largely because of the scarcity of data (Handy et al. 2009).

Far-reaching national initiatives have been put into place in other countries. For example, the ministry of health promotion in Ontario, Canada, has started some after-school initiatives for promoting increased physical activity among children by providing resources for the development of a physically activity lifestyle. The Canadian federal government also has initiated a Children's Fitness Tax Credit whereby parents can claim a tax credit for any prescribed physical activity program for their child. As part of Building Canada, the Canadian government has committed $25 million to developing new multipurpose trails for walking, biking, and other activities.[1]

Be Active Australia was developed to foster physical activity among the Australian population. Plans have been developed for implementing active transport activities as part of this initiative. Although this policy-level case study has not been fully enacted, it is in line with the types of initiatives that could increase physical activity at the population level. In New Zealand, three important pieces of national legislation were passed supporting pedestrian safety. New Zealand's official transportation strategy also includes setting goals to improve access and mobility (in particular, for walking and cycling), protect and promote public health, and increase safety. A related New Zealand strategic plan, "Getting there—on foot, by bicycle," has four main foci, including strengthening foundations for effective action (e.g., expanded collaboration of efforts for walking and cycling), providing supportive environments (e.g., encouraging better land use, improved existing infrastructure, improved networks for long-distance cycling), influencing individual choice (e.g., promoting perceptions and attitudes aimed at changing travel choices), and improving safety and security (e.g., road safety, crime).

Other examples of national legislative and policy initiatives promoting population-wide regular physical activity exist globally. Among the most impressive is the collection of national transportation policies legislated in the Netherlands. A set of mobility management policy measures has been implemented to optimize the use of existing infrastructure with a focus on improving accessibility by public transportation and bicycle. Both the exact nature of these policies and how they are implemented are determined at the local and regional levels. The primary aims of the policies are (1) to achieve greater integration of traffic and transportation policies in deciding land use (e.g., sites for homes, businesses), with a focus on ensuring appropriate access to public transportation and bicycles; (2) to institute regional programs aimed at integrating cycling, public transportation, and carpool promotion programs with existing corporate programs focused on improving working conditions and environment; (3) to improve the quality of cycling facilities such as bike-garaging; (4) to establish chain-mobility

policies that provide better linkages for "door-to-door" transportation, such as commuting structures that facilitate transfer from high-speed rail travel to private car, bus, cycling, and walking options; and (5) to enforce traffic rules more efficiently (e.g., regulate permissible levels of alcohol for drivers more strictly).

Such national legislative achievements are a cause for cautious optimism and underscore the utility of taking a global perspective in identifying effective strategies. Many of these efforts, however, await further evaluation to better understand the most effective and cost-efficient sets of policies that could be implemented in other nations.

Other separate acts of legislation have benefited the physical-activity-promotion movement *indirectly,* such as national policies in support of public transportation—a travel alternative that seems to promote greater levels of walking and cycling (Coogan et al. 2009; Frank et al. 2003; Solomon et al. 2009). Current U.S. Recovery Act investments aimed at public transit systems have been helpful in this way (Solomon et al. 2009). Local, state, and federal initiatives related to the Americans with Disabilities Act have also yielded some positive outcomes having to do with physical activity. For instance, at the end of 2009, the state of California tentatively arrived at a settlement agreement with disability advocacy and public interest groups on improving sidewalks and pedestrian intersections on state highways, many of which cross through cities and are inaccessible for people with disabilities. Among the improvements stipulated in the tentative agreement are widening sidewalks; updating curbs, crosswalks, over-crossings, and park-and-ride lots; and providing accessibility during temporary construction periods that may block sidewalks.

These achievements notwithstanding, the United States and other countries are a long way from developing an integrated body of federal legislation aimed specifically at physical activity promotion. What *has* grown over the past two decades are federally supported policy statements and initiatives that have comprehensively documented the evidence that a physically active lifestyle is important (PAG 2008; CDC 2001; US-DHHS 1996; USHHS 2000) and have paved the way for collective intersectoral action.

Of perhaps greater promise are the legislative activities of recent years at state or regional and local levels. Part of the incentive for increased legislative activity in this sector is the growing evidence of the deleterious health impacts of inactivity in areas such as productivity and health care costs, a significant portion of which are passed on to taxpayers through Medicare, Medicaid, and similar governmental programs. Based on the alarming increases in public and private health insurance costs along with related expenditures, bodies such as the U.S. National Conference of State Legislatures have begun to track proposed and enacted state legislation aimed at healthful lifestyles (i.e., healthful eating and physical activity) and community design and access (Morandi 2009). One area that has been the target of frequent legislative activity is school-based opportunities and directives for students to be physically active. For example, in 2007, 13 states enacted laws aimed at enhancing school physical education or physical activity programs, and 34 states considered such legislation (Winterfeld et al. 2009). Another policy area that increasingly has become a target for state legislative activity concerns promoting built environments conducive to physically active lifestyles. Among relevant laws in this area are mixed-use legislation and transit-oriented development laws, including Washington State's 2006 Physical Activity Promotion Act and South Carolina's 2007 Priority Investment Act (Morandi 2009). In addition, California and some other states have developed a statewide plan for nonmotorized travel including a statewide complete streets policy that provides safe opportunities for pedestrians to use the streets and have required pedestrian or

bicycle plans as a prerequisite for obtaining some state funds (Handy et al. 2009). Such legislative activities are bolstered by communication that thoroughly acquaints lawmakers with the scientific evidence in a manner that makes such evidence accessible, relevant, timely, and compelling. It also helps to make clear all of the benefits, direct and indirect (e.g., positive impacts on academic achievement, worker productivity, automobile-related air pollution, health care costs), accompanying a physically active lifestyle (Bauman et al. 2009; Morandi 2009).

Although local and regional taxation and pricing policies have been shown to influence choice and behavioral decision making related to other health behaviors (e.g., tobacco use, food choices) (Biener et al. 1998; French et al. 2001), the potential impacts of such policies in the physical activity area have received minimal attention. Perhaps the best-known example currently of a relevant taxation policy is London's congestion charge aimed at driving in central London. This is a daily charge for driving in a specific area of central London between 7:00 a.m. and 5:00 p.m., Monday through Friday. The charge aims to reduce traffic congestion and make journeys quicker by encouraging people to choose other forms of transport. The net revenue raised from the congestion charge is reinvested to improve transport in London. The initial result of the congestion charge was a 21% drop in traffic (about 70,000 cars per day) and a 6% increase in bus passengers. More recent data, however, suggest that traffic has risen again to the precharge level. The Mayor's Office of London has attributed this increase to public works projects that have reduced road capacity and, interestingly, increased traffic management measures to help pedestrians. Such possibilities for unintended consequences associated with taxation or pricing policies in such efforts should be explored further. Examples of unintended consequences in other health areas have at times been reported (e.g., bootlegging of cigarettes in response to tobacco taxation policies) (Shelley et al. 2007).

Public Health Agencies

Local and state health departments are important organizing bodies and catalysts for community-wide physical-activity-promotion efforts (Simon et al. 2009). They also represent well-established health infrastructures upon which academic health centers can build sustainable **partnerships** for health science research. As such, they are well positioned to contribute to community-wide physical activity interventions, including organizational practices, policies, and programs occurring in schools, work sites, and other community organizations; land use and transportation policies and practices occurring throughout their jurisdictions; and educational and training functions in support of physical activity promotion (Simon et al. 2009). In view of health departments' typical roles in support of more disadvantaged areas, they are well placed to advance programs and policies to reduce health disparities. For example, health departments can collaborate with schools to ensure high quality physical education for all students; promote social networks for physical activity throughout the community in partnership with parks and recreation departments and similar organizations (e.g., walking groups); provide technical support and assistance to businesses, along with education pertaining to the value gained from a physically active and fit workforce (e.g., reduction in health care costs, increased worker productivity) (Goetzel et al. 2005; Pratt et al. 2000); partner with public housing authorities, planning departments, transportation departments, and redevelopment agencies to promote land use policies and environmental features in support of physical activity throughout the community; and provide community-relevant surveillance information and health impact assessments of proposed land use and related environmental policies that could affect physical activity (Cole and Fielding 2007; Simon et al. 2001; Simon et al. 2009). Finally, health departments have established nationwide communication and organizational networks that aid in the dissemination of successful programs and practices.

Public health programs face well-known barriers with respect to resource and personnel constraints, particularly in the current economic climate. Relatively few have adequate physical activity expertise among their personnel. Goals in this area include building greater physical activity expertise and capacity as well as developing methods for enhancing cross-disciplinary competencies and partnerships with planning, land use, and transportation experts (see "Accreditation and Training Bodies," below).

Community Organizations and Nonprofit Agencies

Community organizations and nonprofit agencies at the local, state, and national levels (Doyle 2009) have missions and foci conducive to promoting healthful lifestyles, including regular physical activity, and are typically knowledgeable concerning community needs and institutions and concerning other stakeholders (e.g., government agencies, schools, work sites, health care settings); often include a focus on underserved population groups that fits well with the growing national commitment regarding health disparities and achieving health equity; and have organizational structures that provide a network for translating and disseminating practices, policies, and programs throughout the country. Nonprofit and **nongovernmental organizations** also can play an important role in national policy advocacy, and some of them have research funding mechanisms that can support relevant investigations in this area (Doyle et al. 2009). Among the nonprofit organizations that have participated in or led physical activity initiatives or programs are the YMCA (Wilcox, Dowda, et al. 2006; YMCA of the USA 2008), the American College of Sports Medicine (ACSM), the American Heart Association (Nelson et al. 2007; Sallis 2009), the American Cancer Society

(Doyle et al. 2009), and the AARP (2007). These and other nonprofit groups have also joined scientific organizations, for-profit groups, governmental agencies, and other organizations in developing the National Physical Activity Plan—an intersectoral initiative aimed at advancing the public health agenda for physical activity promotion (Pate 2009b).

The Private Sector

Businesses have much to gain from a physically active and fit workforce, including lower health care expenditures, lower absenteeism and sick leave, and improved work performance (Anderson et al. 2000; Pronk 2009; Pronk et al. 1999; Proper and van Mechelen 2008). In addition to the more general conditioning effects that can come from regular physical activity are the benefits of incorporating more movement and less sitting throughout the workday as a means of reducing musculoskeletal problems, pain, and other negative work-related health effects (Berqvist 1995; Owen et al. 2009). A set of best practices for promoting employer-sponsored physical activity programs has been recommended, incorporating a multilevel, comprehensive approach (Sallis and Owen 2002) that emphasizes evidence-based interventions while meeting situational and contextual realities (Kottke and Pronk 2006). Among the large set of recommendations for action that have been described for the workplace setting are the following points:

- engaging leadership and management
- promoting employee participation in all aspects of the program
- tailoring the work site
- offering incentives and awards
- providing adequate resources
- communicating strategically
- building accountability into program implementation

- evaluating and modifying the program to facilitate sustainability (Pronk and Kottke 2009)

Of particular importance is the development of supportive environments for employer-based physical activity promotion, along with ways to network such strategies with policies, programs, and practices occurring in other work sites and in other sectors.

In addition to promotion of physical activity among their own workforces, technology-oriented businesses could serve as partners with academic institutions and other community sectors in continuing to build, test, and disseminate technology-driven interventions aimed at physical activity promotion.

Health Care Plans

Increasingly, published research has demonstrated the significant impact that an inactive lifestyle can have on medical expenditures: costs are incurred by employers, taxpayers, and individuals through increased health insurance premiums and tax-related subsidies for public insurance programs (Garrett et al. 2004; Patrick et al. 2009). These statistics set the stage for the exploration of incentives, in the form of reduced premiums or other cost reductions, to engage regularly in health-promoting behaviors such as physical activity. Although such incentive systems have been used for other types of health behaviors (e.g., smoking) (Volpp et al. 2009), the use of incentives in this manner has created dissonance in some sectors (e.g., nonprofit organizations such as the AARP) as well as among some health professionals. The argument has been made that when some individuals are rewarded through reduced health insurance premiums, no matter how "noble" the cause, others who are not able to meet the criteria being set are implicitly disadvantaged. These tensions may limit the degree to which health insurance premium reductions may be used to incentivize regular physical activity. However, other health plan activities, such as health care coverage for physical activity instruction, advice from health care providers, and physical activity referral sources, are well worth pursuing, given the intersectoral costs accrued from an inactive lifestyle. Continued study of the potential cost-effectiveness of reimbursing physical-activity-specific health care services is in order (Fitzner et al. 2002).

Clinical Care Services

As noted earlier, regular physical activity advice as delivered by physicians and other relevant health professionals is a useful tool in raising patient awareness, although measurable impacts on physical activity behavior are at times difficult to discern (Eden et al. 2002; Elley et al. 2003; Jacobson et al. 2005). This area would benefit generally from more rigorous research designs and methods and greater elucidation of the circumstances under which physicians and other health care providers may serve as potent behavior **change agents** (Elley et al. 2003; Jones et al. 2004). Despite these caveats, the many beneficial effects that regular physical activity can have on a range of chronic diseases and conditions provide the rationale for increasing physicians' knowledge and skills related to prescribing this health behavior to their patients (Patrick et al. 2009). Recognizing this fact, the American Medical Association, together with the ACSM, has recently launched the Exercise Is Medicine (EIM) initiative (Sallis 2009). Among the goals of EIM is to add physical activity to routine care as an additional vital sign, along with prescribing regular physical activity or providing appropriate physical activity referrals to all patients (Doyle et al. 2009). In support of such initiatives, written physical activity standards for health care professionals have been available for some time (Fletcher et al. 1995) and

physician training methods in this health area have been described (Marcus et al. 1997). Proponents hope that EIM and similar initiatives will help to capitalize on the authority and credibility that primary care providers and other health professionals bring to the patient interaction. However, advancing this agenda will likely require the facilitation of organizational and structural changes to address the tremendous number of time, financial, and informational barriers most health care providers face in providing such advice and support on a regular basis. Simple, low-cost exercise prescription tools developed specifically for physicians have been shown to be effective and require further translation (Petrella et al. 2003). One promising exercise prescription scheme is New Zealand's "green prescription" program, a clinician-based initiative in general practice that provides counseling on physical activity (Elley et al. 2003). As part of the intervention, general practitioners are prompted to provide oral and written advice on physical activity during consultations. In a 12-month cluster randomized-controlled trial of 42 rural and urban general practices in one region of New Zealand, exercise specialists continued physical activity support through telephone and mail following the physician consultations. In this trial, significant 12-month increases were observed in total energy expenditure as well as improvements in ratings of general health, vitality, and bodily pain among intervention patients relative to controls (Elley et al. 2003).

Although health care referrals to exercise specialists or programs in the community make sense from a community networking and resources perspective, effective ways of making successful referrals await further investigation (Harrison et al. 2005; Jones et al. 2004). In addition to physicians, health care professionals such as pharmacists, nurses, physical and occupational therapists, psychologists, optometrists, chiropractors, dieticians, and podiatrists can serve as important sources of physical activity information and support and should be tapped to do so.

Funding Institutions

Among federal institutions, the CDC has, since the early 1990s, played a central role in building public recognition of the obesity epidemic and its physical activity component, developing public health tools for physical activity surveillance, and enacting and supporting programs and initiatives aimed at physical activity promotion (Pratt et al. 2009). Among the many and varied physical-activity-promotion activities that it has funded are physical activity training activities for public health researchers and practitioners; **capacity building** activities for state physical activity and nutrition, and for obesity prevention; and community-based participatory research grants. CDC staff supported the development of a National Society of Physical Activity Practitioners in Public Health in 2006 and initiated the development and use of an array of public health tools (e.g., the work of the Task Force on Community Preventive Services in *The Community Guide,* health impact assessment, cost-effectiveness analyses) to advance research and practice in the physical activity field (Pratt et al. 2009; Roux et al. 2008). With sufficient funding, CDC could serve as a key partner for a national physical activity effort involving the nation's state and local health departments and other relevant sectors (e.g., transportation, education, recreation and sports, urban planning, public safety). CDC staff members also are fully involved in the current National Physical Activity Plan initiative (described later in this chapter) (IOM 2013; Pate 2009b; Patrick et al. 2009).

In contrast, the National Institutes of Health (NIH) has demonstrated a level of commitment to physical activity research that has been inconsistent at best. The NIH initiated one of the first federal steps in this area through establishing a National Center for Chronic Disease Con-

trol in 1964 that included the investigation of physical activity, heart disease, and public health (Pratt et al. 2009). Though the NIH funded the vast majority of the U.S. research that has contributed to the extensive evidence base supporting the impacts of physical activity on population health, the physical activity field was inexplicably omitted from a list of 360 NIH funding areas posted on the NIH website in 2008 (Yancey and Sallis 2009). However, the list contained the other seven major health behaviors that have been identified, along with physical inactivity, as the true underlying causes of U.S. deaths (McGinnis and Foege 1993). The omission underscores the lack of full recognition, even in the face of a huge body of evidence, of physical activity's role as a key contributor to population health.

In the national policy and public health practice arenas, important U.S. health promotion and disease prevention initiatives that have targeted physical activity and other **lifestyle behaviors** have included, since 1980, the Healthy People initiative, spearheaded by the Office of Disease Prevention and Health Promotion in the U.S. Department of Health and Human Services (Green and Fielding 2011; USDHHS 2000; USDHHS Advisory Committee 2008), and, as noted earlier, important initiatives directed by the CDC (Pratt et al. 2009; TFCPS 2001). Although such efforts have been considerable, they generally have not received consistent federal funding commensurate with the magnitude of the inactivity and obesity epidemics facing the nation.

In the absence of an integrated and orchestrated federal physical activity effort, other national nonprofit funding bodies have stepped up and funded important public health initiatives supporting physical activity research and translation or dissemination. They include the Robert Wood Johnson Foundation, which funded the Active for Life dissemination and evaluation effort of two evidence-based physical activity promotion programs (Wilcox et al.

2008), in addition to the successful Active Living Research (ALR) initiative. ALR, under the direction of Dr. James Sallis, has been an international leader in funding cutting-edge physical activity research in environmental and policy arenas. Despite these successes, it has become clear that funding activities on the part of public as well as private organizations will require further expansion and collaboration if serious advances are to be realized in the field of physical activity promotion.

Accreditation and Training Bodies

The capacity, resources, and skill set among public health practitioners and researchers to mount an effective response in addressing the physical inactivity burden in the United States have recently been criticized as insufficient (Hooker and Buchner 2009; Yancey et al. 2007). Cost-sensitive, innovative approaches supporting public health training and education in this area will likely be an important component of a national effort to address the public health needs related to physical activity promotion. Among the promising approaches that have been or could be developed include intensive time-limited courses in physical activity and public health practice and research for health professionals (Brown et al. 2001); master of public health (MPH) programs that include education and training on physical activity and public health; establishment of essential competencies and benchmarks in the field for training, evaluation, and credentialing purposes, as has been done by a recently formed organization called the National Society of Physical Activity Practitioners in Public Health (Yancey et al. 2007); and training of the next generation of physical activity researchers in methods for conducting successful multidisciplinary and population-relevant research in the field (Sallis et al. 2002). Expanding the professional development opportunities in the physical activity arena will enhance the possibility of reducing population inactivity levels.

Conclusion

The recognized gap at the federal level in orchestrating an integrated national response to the physical inactivity epidemic has led to the initiation of alternative approaches to meeting the public health challenge in this area. For example, a national blueprint for increasing physical activity among adults of age 50 and older has been developed with sponsorship from the AARP and other federal (e.g., the CDC, the National Institute on Aging) and nonfederal organizations (e.g., ACSM, the American Geriatrics Society, the Robert Wood Johnson Foundation) (Chodzko-Zajko 2001). The aim of this endeavor has been to offer organizations and agencies guidance in planning strategies and programs for this age group (Sheppard et al. 2003). Current intersectoral efforts to facilitate action in the physical activity area for the population as a whole are represented by the National Physical Activity Plan—a **coalition** of dozens of public and **private sector** institutions and organizations aimed at developing a multilevel, integrated, and actionable approach to physical activity promotion in this country (Pate 2009a). The coordinating committee for the plan includes representatives from public health, education, research, business, the media, government, clinical services, volunteer and nonprofit organizations, parks and recreation, and environmental and policy sectors. It is too early to judge how effective such a national coalition will be in the current economically constrained climate, but its comprehensive focus and consensus-building approach hold promise.

Among additional developments and challenges currently facing the physical-activity-promotion field are building cooperation and positive synergies with dietary organizations and agencies that address and resolve current tensions that have arisen between these two complementary health fields (Dorfman and Yancey 2009); continuing to reach out to professionals who represent fields that overlap in a mutually beneficial way with the physical activity public health field, such as parks and recreation (Mowen and Baker 2009), professional sports (Yancey et al. 2009), and the climate change–environmental movement (Maibach et al. 2009); finding ways to more thoroughly integrate public health and economic perspectives as a means to advance a productive and realistic physical activity agenda (Bleich and Sturm 2009); and identifying the most useful strategies to promote regular physical activity, strategies that address the increasing health equity gap in the United States, for example, ensuring an equitable distribution of environmental resources that promote physical activity across the population as a whole (Garcia et al. 2009).

In addition, it is critical to focus more systematic attention on efforts to translate and disseminate those physical activity interventions at all levels of impact for which scientific evidence is promising (Brownson and Jones 2009; Brownson et al. 2012; Green and Glasgow 2006). Through engaging public health practitioners in addition to policymakers early in this process, many more scientifically supported interventions may successfully reach the translation and implementation stage (Glasgow et al. 2003; Green and Glasgow 2006).

Finally, the worldwide spread of physical inactivity, stemming from the globalization of technological advances to virtually all aspects of daily living, increasingly demands a global response (WHO 2006). Although this response is still largely in its infancy, some promising international collaborations are currently being developed, including the Oxford Health Alliance's Vision 2020, aimed at community interventions to promote health and prevent disease (Oxford Health Alliance 2009), and the International Physical Activity and the Environment Network (IPEN). IPEN was begun originally as part of the Robert Wood Johnson Foundation's Active Living Research initiative and is currently being funded in part through an NIH grant. Given the **complexity** of the physical inactivity

problem, only taking such a global, systemwide perspective involving active engagement of virtually all societal sectors will likely result in measurable improvement in this area (Bauman et al. 2009; Leischow et al. 2008). Although the challenge is great, the substantial positive impacts on health and other facets of life garnered by putting regular physical activity back into people's daily lives will be worth the effort.

NOTES
    1. See Building Canada, www.buildingcanada-chantierscanada.gc.ca/ creating-creation/nrt-srn-eng .html.

REFERENCES
AARP. 2007. Community-wide campaign to promote physical activity among midlife and older adults: Lessons learned from AARP's Active for LIFE campaign and a synopsis of evidence-based interventions. AARP and Centers for Disease Control and Prevention, Washington, DC.
Agurs-Collins TD, Kumanyika SK, Ten Have TR, Adams-Campbell LL. 1997. A randomized controlled trial of weight reduction and exercise for diabetes management in older African-American subjects. *Diabetes Care* 20 (10) (Oct.): 1503-11.
Albright CL, Pruitt L, Castro C, Gonzalez A, Woo S, King AC. 2005. Modifying physical activity in a multiethnic sample of low-income women: One-year results from the IMPACT (Increasing Motivation for Physical ACTivity) project. *Ann Behav Med* 30 (3) (Dec.): 191-200.
Anderson DR, Whitmer RW, Goetzel RZ, et al. 2000. The relationship between modifiable health risks and group-level health care expenditures. Health Enhancement Research Organization (HERO) Research Committee. *Am J Health Promot* 15 (1) (Sept.-Oct.): 45-52.
Anderson RE, Franckowiak SC, Snyder J, Bartlett SJ, Fontaine KR. 1998. Can inexpensive signs encourage the use of stairs? Results from a community intervention. *Ann Intern Med* 129:363-69.
Anton SD, Newton RL Jr., Sothern M, Martin CK, Stewart TM, Williamson DA. 2006. Association of depression with Body Mass Index, sedentary behavior, and maladaptive eating attitudes and behaviors in 11 to 13-year old children. *Eat Weight Disord* 11 (3) (Sept.): e102-8.
Ashworth NL, Chad KE, Harrison EL, Reeder BA, Marshall SC. 2005. Home versus center based physical

activity programs in older adults. *Cochrane Database Syst Rev* 1:CD004017.

Atienza AA, Yaroch AL, Masse LC, Moser RP, Hesse BW, King AC. 2006. Identifying sedentary subgroups: The National Cancer Institute's Health Information National Trends Survey. *Am J Prev Med* 31 (5) (Nov.): 383-90.

Ball K, Salmon J, Giles-Corti B, Crawford D. 2006. How can socio-economic differences in physical activity among women be explained? A qualitative study. *Women Health* 43 (1): 93-113.

Banks-Wallace J, Conn V. 2002. Interventions to promote physical activity among African American women. *Pub Health Nurs* 19 (5) (Sept.-Oct.): 321-35.

Bauman A, Finegood DT, Matsudo V. 2009. International perspectives on the physical inactivity crisis— structural solutions over evidence generation? *Prev Med* 49 (4) (Oct.): 309-12.

Bauman AE, Sallis JF, Dzewaltowski DA, Owen N. 2002. Toward a better understanding of the influences on physical activity: The role of determinants, correlates, causal variables, mediators, moderators, and confounders. *Am J Prev Med* 23 (2S): 5-14.

Berqvist U. 1995. *Musculoskeletal Disorders and the Workplace: Low Back and Upper Extremities.* Washington, DC: National Academies Press.

Biener L, Aseltine RH Jr., Cohen B, Anderka M. 1998. Reactions of adult and teenaged smokers to the Massachusetts tobacco tax. *Am J Public Health* 88 (9) (Sept.): 1389-91.

Blair SN, Piserchia PV, Wilbur CS, Crowder JH. 1986. A public health intervention model for worksite health promotion: Impact on exercise and physical fitness in a health promotion plan after 24 months. *JAMA* 255:921-26.

Blamey A, Mutrie N, Aitchison T. 1995. Health promotion by encouraged use of stairs. *Br Med J* 311:289-90.

Bleich SN, Sturm R. 2009. Developing policy solutions for a more active nation: Integrating economic and public health perspectives. *Prev Med* 49 (4) (Oct.): 306-8.

Blumenthal DS. 2006. A community coalition board creates a set of values for community-based research. *Prev Chronic Disease* 3 (1) (Jan.): A16.

Boehmer TK, Hoehner CM, Wyrwich KW, Ramirez LK, Brownson RC. 2006. Correspondence between perceived and observed measures of neighborhood environmental supports for physical activity. *J Phys Activity Health* 3:22-36.

Booth ML, Owen N, Bauman A, Clavisi O, Leslie E. 2000. Social-cognitive and perceived environment influences associated with physical activity in older Australians. *Prev Med* 31:15-22.

Boreham CAG, Wallace WFM, Nevill A. 2000. Training effects of accumulated daily stair-climbing exercise in previously sedentary young women. *Prev Med* 30:277-28.

Bowman SA. 2006. Television-viewing characteristics of adults: Correlations to eating practices and overweight and health status. *Prev Chronic Disease* 3 (2) (April): A38.

Brassington GS, Atienza AA, Perczek RE, DiLorenzo TM, King AC. 2002. Intervention-related cognitive versus social mediators of exercise adherence in the elderly. *Am J Prev Med* 23 (2 suppl.) (Aug.): 80-6.

Bravata DM, Smith-Spangler C, Sundaram V, et al. 2007. Using pedometers to increase physical activity and improve health: A systematic review. *JAMA* 298 (19) (Nov. 21): 2296-2304.

Brown DR, Pate RR, Pratt M, et al. 2001. Physical activity and public health: Training courses for researchers and practitioners. *Public Health Rep* 116 (3) (May-June): 197-202.

Brown WJ, Trost SG. 2003. Life transitions and changing physical activity patterns in young women. *Am J Prev Med* 25 (2) (Aug.): 140-43.

Brownell KD, Stunkard AJ, Albaum JM. 1980. Evaluation and modification of exercise patterns in the natural environment. *Am J Psychiatry* 137:1540-45.

Brownson RC, Jones E. 2009. Bridging the gap: Translating research into policy and practice. *Prev Med* 49 (4) (Oct.): 313-15.

Brownson RC, Colditz GA, Proctor EK, eds. 2012. *Dissemination and Implementation Research in Health: Translating Science to Practice.* New York: Oxford University Press.

Bungum TJ, Vincent ML. 1997. Determinants of physical activity among female adolescents. *Am J Prev Med* 13 (2) (March-April): 115-22.

Burton LC, Shapiro S, German PS. 1999. Determinants of physical activity initiation and maintenance among community-dwelling older persons. *Prev Med* 29 (5) (Nov.): 422-30.

Calfas KJ, Sallis JF, Nichols JF, et al. 2000. Project GRAD: Two-year outcomes of a randomized controlled physical activity intervention among young adults: Graduate Ready for Activity Daily. *Am J Prev Med* 18 (1) (Jan.): 28-37.

Carels RA, Darby LA, Rydin S, Douglass OM, Cacciapaglia HM, O'Brien WH. 2005. The relationship between self-monitoring, outcome expectancies, difficulties with eating and exercise, and physical activity and weight loss treatment outcomes. *Ann Behav Med* 30 (3) (Dec.): 182-90.

Carver A, Timperio AF, Crawford DA. 2008. Neighborhood road environments and physical activity among youth: The CLAN study. *J Urban Health* 85 (4) (July): 532-44.

Caspersen CJ, Powell KE, Christenson GM. 1985. Physical activity, exercise, and physical fitness: Definitions and distinctions for health-related research. *Public Health Rep* 100:126-30.

Castro CM, King AC. 2002. Telephone-assisted counseling for physical activity. *Exerc Sport Sci Rev* 30 (2) (April): 64-68.

Castro CM, Pruitt LA, Buman MP, King AC. 2011. Physical activity program delivery by professionals versus volunteers: The TEAM randomized trial. *Health Psychol* 30 (3) (May): 285-94.

Centers for Disease Control and Prevention (CDC). 1997. Monthly estimates of leisure-time physical activity—United States, 1994. *MMWR* 46:393-97.

——. 2001. Increasing physical activity. A report on recommendations of the Task Force on Community Preventive Services. *MMWR Recomm Rep* 50 (RR-18) (Oct. 26): 1-14.

——. 2005. Trends in leisure-time physical inactivity by age, sex, and race/ethnicity—United States, 1994-2004. *MMWR* 54 (39) (Oct. 7): 991-94.

——. 2007. Prevalence of regular physical activity among adults—United States, 2001 and 2005. *MMWR* 56 (46) (Nov. 23): 1209-12.

Chodzko-Zajko WJe. 2001. National blueprint for increasing physical activity among adults age 50 and older: Creating a strategic framework and enhancing organizational capacity for change. *J Aging Phys Act* 9 (suppl.): S1-S91.

Cole BL, Fielding JE. 2007. Health impact assessment: A tool to help policy makers understand health beyond health care. *Annu Rev Public Health* 28:393-412.

Collins R, Lee RE, Albright CL, King AC. 2004. Ready to be physically active? The effects of a course preparing low income multiethnic women to be more physically active. *Health Educ Behav* 31:47-64.

Coogan PF, White LF, Adler TJ, Hathaway KM, Palmer JR, Rosenberg L. 2009. Prospective study of urban form and physical activity in the Black Women's Health Study. *Am J Epidemiol* 170 (9) (Nov. 1): 1105-17.

Courneya KS, Friedenreich CM, Quinney HA, et al. 2005. A longitudinal study of exercise barriers in colorectal cancer survivors participating in a randomized controlled trial. *Ann Behav Med* 29 (2) (April): 147-53.

Cousins SO. 1997. Elderly tomboys? Sources of self-efficacy for physical activity in later life. *J Aging Phys Act* 5:229-43.

Crawford D, Timperio A, Giles-Corti B, et al. 2008. Do features of public open spaces vary according to

neighbourhood socio-economic status? *Health Place* 14 (4) (Dec.): 889-93.

DeBusk RF, Stenestrand U, Sheehan M, Haskell WL. 1990. Training effects of long versus short bouts of exercise in healthy subjects. *Am J Cardiol* 65 (15) (April 15): 1010-13.

Dorfman L, Yancey AK. 2009. Promoting physical activity and healthy eating: Convergence in framing the role of industry. *Prev Med* 49 (4) (Oct.): 303-5.

Dowda M, Ainsworth BE, Addy CL, Saunders R, Riner W. 2003. Correlates of physical activity among U.S. young adults, 18 to 30 years of age, from NHANES III. *Ann Behav Med* 26 (1) (Aug.): 15-23.

Dowda M, James F, Sallis JF, McKenzie TL, Rosengard P, Kohl HW 3rd. 2005. Evaluating the sustainability of SPARK physical education: A case study of translating research into practice. *Res Q Exerc Sport* 76 (1) (March): 11-19.

Doyle C. 2009. The non-profit sector: Leveraging resources and strengths to promote more physically active lifestyles. *J Phys Activity Health* 6 (suppl. 2): S181-S185.

Doyle C, Hutber A, McCarthy WJ. 2009. Physically active lifestyles for all Americans: A call to action for non-profit organizations. *Prev Med* 49 (4) (Oct.): 328-29.

Dunn AL, Marcus BH, Kampert JB, Garcia ME, Kohl HW 3rd, Blair SN. 1999. Comparison of lifestyle and structured interventions to increase physical activity and cardiorespiratory fitness: A randomized trial. *JAMA* 281 (4) (Jan. 27): 327-34.

Eakin EG, Lawler SP, Vandelanotte C, Owen N. 2007. Telephone interventions for physical activity and dietary behavior change: A systematic review. *Am J Prev Med* 32 (5) (May): 419-34.

Eaton SB, Cordain L, Sparling PB. 2009. Evolution, body composition, insulin receptor competition, and insulin resistance. *Prev Med* 49 (4) (Oct.): 283-85.

Eden KB, Orleans CT, Mulrow CD, Pender NJ, Teutsch SM. 2002. Does counseling by clinicians improve physical activity? A summary of the evidence for the U.S. Preventive Services Task Force. *Ann Intern Med* 137 (3) (Aug. 6): 208-15.

Elley CR, Kerse N, Arroll B, Robinson E. 2003. Effectiveness of counselling patients on physical activity in general practice: Cluster randomised controlled trial. *Br Med J* 326:793-98.

Epstein LH, Beecher MD, Graf JL, Roemmich JN. 2007. Choice of interactive dance and bicycle games in overweight and nonoverweight youth. *Ann Behav Med* 33 (2) (April): 124-31.

Epstein LH, Roemmich JN. 2001. Reducing sedentary behavior: Role in modifying physical activity. *Exerc Sport Sci Rev* 2:103-8.

Epstein LH, Roemmich JN, Paluch RA, Raynor HA. 2005. Physical activity as a substitute for sedentary behavior in youth. *Ann Behav Med* 29 (3) (June): 200-209.

Epstein LH, Saelens BE, Myers MD, Vito D. 1997. Effects of decreasing sedentary behaviors on activity choice in obese children. *Health Psychol* 16:107-13.

Evenson KR, Herring AH, Huston SL. 2005. Evaluating change in physical activity with the building of a multi-use trail. *Am J Prev Med* 28 (2 suppl. 2) (Feb.): 177-85.

Eyler AA, Baker E, Cromer L, King AC, Brownson RC, Donatelle RJ. 1998. Physical activity and minority women: A qualitative study. *Health Educ Behav* 25 (5) (Oct.): 640-52.

Eyler AA, Brownson RC, Donatelle RJ, King AC, Brown D, Sallis JF. 1999. Physical activity social support and middle- and older-aged minority women: Results from a US survey. *Soc Sci Med* 49 (6) (Sept.): 781-99.

Eyler AA, Matson-Koffman D, Vest JR, et al. 2002. Environmental, policy, and cultural factors related to physical activity in a diverse sample of women: The Women's Cardiovascular Health Network Project—Summary and Discussion. *Women Health* 36:123-34.

Fairclough SJ, Boddy LM, Hackett AF, Stratton G. 2009. Associations between children's socioeconomic status, weight status, and sex, with screen-based sedentary behaviours and sport participation. *Int J Pediatr Obes* 4 (4): 299-305.

Fallon EA, Wilcox S, Ainsworth BE. 2005. Correlates of self-efficacy for physical activity in African American women. *Women Health* 41 (3): 47-62.

Fitzner K, Madison M, Caputo N, et al. 2002. Promoting physical activity: A profile of health plan programs and initiatives. *Manag Care Interface* 15 (12) (Dec.): 29-41.

Fletcher GF, Balady G, Froelicher VF, Hartley LH, Haskell WL, Pollock ML. 1995. Exercise standards: A statement for healthcare professionals from the American Heart Association. *Circulation* 91:580-615.

Flicker S, Travers R, Guta A, McDonald S, Meagher A. 2007. Ethical dilemmas in community-based participatory research: Recommendations for institutional review boards. *J Urban Health* 84 (4) (July): 478-93.

Foster S, Giles-Corti B. 2008. The built environment, neighborhood crime, and constrained physical activity: An exploration of inconsistent findings. *Prev Med* 47 (3) (Sept.): 241-51.

Frank LD, Engelke PO, Schmid TL. 2003. *Health and Community Design: The Impact of the Built Environment on Physical Activity.* Washington, DC: Island Press.

Frank L, Kavage S. 2009. A National Plan for physical activity: The enabling role of the built environment. *J Phys Activity Health* 6 (suppl. 2): S186-S195.

Frank LD, Schmid TL, Sallis JF, Chapman J, Saelens BE. 2005. Linking objectively measured physical activity with objectively measured urban form: Findings from SMARTRAQ. *Am J Prev Med* 28 (2 suppl. 2) (Feb.): 117-25.

French SA, Story M, Jeffery RW. 2001. Environmental influences on eating and physical activity. *Annu Rev Public Health* 22:309-35.

Garcia R, Bracho A, Cantero P, Glenn BA. 2009. "Pushing" physical activity, and justice. *Prev Med* 49 (4) (Oct.): 330-33.

Garrett NA, Brasure M, Schmitz KH, Schultz MM, Huber MR. 2004. Physical inactivity: Direct cost to a health plan. *Am J Prev Med* 27 (4) (Nov.): 304-9.

Giles-Corti B, Broomhall MH, Knuiman M, et al. 2005. Increasing walking: How important is distance to, attractiveness, and size of public open space? *Am J Prev Med* 28 (2 suppl. 2) (Feb.): 169-76.

Giles-Corti B, Donovan RJ. 2002a. The relative influence of individual, social, and physical environment determinants of physical activity. *Soc Sci Med* 54:1793-1812.

———. 2002b. Socioeconomic status differences in recreational physical activity levels and real and perceived access to a supportive physical environment. *Prev Med* 35 (6) (Dec.): 601-11.

Giles-Corti B, King A. 2009. Creating active environments across the life course: Thinking outside "the square." *Br J Sports Med,* Jan. 9.

Giles-Corti B, Timperio A, Bull F, Pikora T. 2005. Understanding physical activity environmental correlates: Increased specificity for ecological models. *Exerc Sport Sci Rev* 33 (4) (Oct.): 175-81.

Glasgow RE, Lichtenstein E, Marcus AC. 2003. Why don't we see more translation of health promotion research to practice? Rethinking the efficacy-to-effectiveness transition. *Am J Public Health* 93 (8) (Aug.): 1261-67.

Glasgow RE, Vogt TM, Boles SM. 1999. Evaluating the public health impact of health promotion interventions: The RE-AIM framework. *Am J Public Health* 89 (9):1322-27.

Goetzel RZ, Ozminkowski RJ, Baase CM, Billotti GM. 2005. Estimating the return-on-investment from changes in employee health risks on the Dow Chemical Company's health care costs. *J Occup Environ Med* 47 (8) (Aug.): 759-68.

Green LW, Fielding J. 2011. The Healthy People initiative: Its genesis and its sustainability. *Ann Rev Public Health* 32:451-70.

Green LW, Glasgow RE. 2006. Evaluating the relevance, generalization, and applicability of research: Issues in external validation and translation methodology. *Eval Health Prof* 29 (1): 126-53.

Griffin SF, Wilson DK, Wilcox S, Buck J, Ainsworth BE. 2008. Physical activity influences in a disadvantaged African American community and the communities' proposed solutions. *Health Promot Practice* 9 (2) (April): 180-90.

Hamer M. 2007. The relative influences of fitness and fatness on inflammatory factors. *Prev Med* 44 (1) (Jan.): 3-11.

Hamer M, Chida Y. 2009. Physical activity and risk of neurodegenerative disease: A systematic review of prospective evidence. *Psychol Med* 39 (1) (Jan): 3-11.

Handy SL, Cao X, Mokhtarian PL. 2006. Does self-selection explain the relationship between built environment and walking behavior? Empirical evidence from Northern California. *J Am Planning Assoc* 72:55-74.

Handy S, McCann B, Bailey L, et al. 2009. The regional response to federal funding for bicycle and pedestrian projects. Studies IoT, Contract No. UCD-ITS-RR-09-15. Institute of Transportation Studies, University of California-Davis, Davis, CA.

Harrison RA, Roberts C, Elton PJ. 2005. Does primary care referral to an exercise programme increase physical activity one year later? A randomized controlled trial. *J Public Health (Oxf)* 27 (1) (March): 25-32.

Haskell WL, Blair SN, Hill JO. 2009. Physical activity: Health outcomes and importance for public health policy. *Prev Med* 49 (4) (Oct.): 280-82.

Heath G, Brownson R, Kruger J, et al. 2006. The effectiveness of urban design and land use and transport policies and practices to increase physical activity: A systematic review. *J Phys Activity Health* 3 (suppl. 1): S55-S76.

Heirich MA, Foote A, Konopka B. 1993. Work-site physical fitness programs: Comparing the impact of different program designs on cardiovascular risks. *J Occup Med* 35:510-17.

Hillsdon M, Foster C, Thorogood M. 2005. Interventions for promoting physical activity. *Cochrane Database Syst Rev* 1:CD003180 (Jan 25).

Hoehner CM, Brennan Ramirez LK, Elliott MB, Handy SL, Brownson RC. 2005. Perceived and objective environmental measures and physical activity among urban adults. *Am J Prev Med* 28 (2 suppl. 2) (Feb.): 105-16.

Hooker SP, Buchner DM. 2009. Education and training in physical activity research and practice. *Prev Med* 49 (4) (Oct.): 294-96.

Hooker SP, Seavey W, Weidmer CE, et al. 2005. The California active aging community grant program: Translating science into practice to promote physical activity in older adults. *Ann Behav Med* 29 (3) (June): 155-65.

Horowitz CR, Robinson M, Seifer S. 2009. Community-based participatory research from the margin to the mainstream: Are researchers prepared? *Circulation* 119 (19) (May 19): 2633-42.

Huhman M, Potter LD, Wong FL, Banspach SW, Duke JC, Heitzler CD. 2005. Effects of a mass media campaign to increase physical activity among children: Year-1 results of the VERB campaign. *Pediatrics* 116 (2) (Aug.): e277-84.

Hume C, Timperio A, Salmon J, Carver A, Giles-Corti B, Crawford D. 2009. Walking and cycling to school: Predictors of increases among children and adolescents. *Am J Prev Med* 36 (3) (March): 195-200.

Humpel N, Owen N, Leslie, E. 2002. Environmental factors associated with adults' participation in physical activity. *Am J Prev Med* 22:188-99.

Institute of Medicine (IOM). 1997. *Linking Research and Public Health Practice: A Review of CDC's Program of Centers for Research and Demonstration of Health Promotion and Disease Prevention.* Washington, DC: National Academies Press.

———. 2001. *Health and Behavior: The Interplay of Biological, Behavioral, and Social Influences.* Washington, DC: National Academies Press.

———. 2010. *Bridging the Evidence Gap in Obesity Prevention: A Framework to Inform Decision Making.* Washington, DC: National Academies Press.

———. 2012. *An Integrated Framework for Assessing the Value of Community-Based Prevention.* Washington, DC: National Academies Press.

———. 2013. *Evaluating Obesity Prevention Efforts: A Plan for Measuring Progress.* Washington, DC: National Academies Press.

Jacobson DM, Strohecker L, Compton MT, Katz DL. 2005. Physical activity counseling in the adult primary care setting: Position statement of the American College of Preventive Medicine. *Am J Prev Med* 29 (2) (Aug.): 158-62.

Jago R, Baranowski T. 2004. Non-curricular approaches for increasing physical activity in youth: A review. *Prev Med* 39 (1) (July): 157-63.

Jilcott SB, Laraia BA, Evenson KR, Lowenstein LM, Ammerman AS. 2007. A guide for developing intervention tools addressing environmental factors to improve diet and physical activity. *Health Promot Practice* 8 (2) (April): 192-204.

Jones LW, Courneya KS, Fairey AS, Mackey JR. 2004. Effects of an oncologist's recommendation to exercise on self-reported exercise behavior in newly diagnosed breast cancer survivors: A single-blind, randomized controlled trial. *Ann Behav Med* 28:105-13.

Kahn EB, Ramsey LT, Brownson RC, et al. 2002. The effectiveness of interventions to increase physical activity. A systematic review. *Am J Prev Med* 22 (4 suppl.) (May): 73-107.

Katz DL, O'Connell M, Yeh MC, et al. 2005. Public health strategies for preventing and controlling overweight and obesity in school and worksite settings: A report on recommendations of the Task Force on Community Preventive Services. *MMWR Recomm Rep* 54 (RR-10) (Oct. 7): 1-12.

King AC. 2001. Interventions to promote physical activity in older adults. *J Gerontol A Biol Sci Med Sci* 56A (Special Issue II): 36-46.

King AC, Ahn DK, Oliveira BM, Atienza AA, Castro CM, Gardner CD. 2008. Promoting physical activity through hand-held computer technology. *Am J Prev Med* 34:138-42.

King AC, Bauman A, Calfas K, eds. 2002. Innovative approaches to understanding and Influencing physical activity. *Am J Public Health* 89:66-72.

King AC, Castro C, Wilcox S, Eyler AA, Sallis JF, Brownson RC. 2000. Personal and environmental factors associated with physical inactivity among different racial-ethnic groups of U.S. middle-aged and older-aged women. *Health Psychol* 19 (4) (July): 354-64.

King AC, Friedman RM, Marcus BH, et al. 2007. Ongoing physical activity advice by humans versus computers: The Community Health Advice by Telephone (CHAT) Trial. *Health Psychol* 26:718-27.

King AC, Goldberg JH, Salmon J, et al. 2010. Identifying subgroups of U.S. adults at risk for prolonged television viewing to inform program development. *Am J Prev Med* 38 (1) (Jan.): 17-26.

King AC, Haskell WL, Taylor CB, Kraemer HC, DeBusk RF. 1991. Group- vs home-based exercise training in healthy older men and women. A community-based clinical trial. *JAMA* 266 (11) (Sept. 18): 1535-42.

King AC, Haskell WL, Young DR, Oka RK, Stefanick ML. 1995. Long-term effects of varying intensities and formats of physical activity on participation rates, fitness, and lipoproteins in men and women aged 50 to 65 years. *Circulation* 91 (10) (May 15): 2596-2604.

King AC, Kiernan M, Ahn DK, Wilcox S. 1998. The effects of marital transitions on changes in physical activity: Results from a 10-year community study. *Ann Behav Med* 20 (2) (Spring): 64-69.

King AC, Sallis JF. 2009. Why and how to improve physical activity promotion: Lessons from behavioral science and related fields. *Prev Med* 49 (4) (Oct.): 286-88.

King AC, Stokols D, Talen E, Brassington GS, Killingsworth R. 2002. Theoretical approaches to the promotion of physical activity: Forging a transdisciplinary paradigm. *Am J Prev Med* 23 (2S): 15-25.

King AC, Toobert D, Ahn D, et al. 2006. Perceived environments as physical activity correlates and moderators of interventions in five studies. *Am J Health Promot* 21:24-35.

King WC, Belle SH, Brach JS, Simkin-Silverman LR, Soska T, Kriska AM. 2005. Objective measures of neighborhood environment and physical activity in older women. *Am J Prev Med* 28 (5) (June): 461-69.

Kottke TE, Pronk NP. 2006. Physical activity optimizing practice through research. *Am J Prev Med* 31 (4 suppl.) (Oct.): S8-S10.

LaVeist TA. 2005. *Minority Populations and Health: An Introduction to Health Disparities in the United States.* San Francisco: Jossey-Bass.

Leischow SJ, Best A, Trochim WM, et al. 2008. Systems thinking to improve the public's health. *Am J Prev Med* 35 (2 suppl.) (Aug.): S196-S203.

Luepker RV, Perry CL, McKinlay SM, et al. 1996. Outcomes of a field trial to improve children's dietary patterns and physical activity. The Child and Adolescent Trial for Cardiovascular Health. CATCH collaborative group. *JAMA* 275 (10) (March 13): 768-76.

Mahar MT, Murphy SK, Rowe DA, Golden J, Shields AT, Raedeke TD. 2006. Effects of a classroom-based program on physical activity and on-task behavior. *Med Sci Sports Exerc* 38 (12) (Dec.): 2086-94.

Maibach E, Steg L, Anable J. 2009. Promoting physical activity and reducing climate change: Opportunities to replace short car trips with active transportation. *Prev Med* 49 (4) (Oct.): 326-27.

Marcus BH, Bock BC, Pinto BM, Forsyth LH, Roberts MB, Traficante RM. 1998. Efficacy of an individualized, motivationally-tailored physical activity intervention. *Ann Behav Med* 20:174-80.

Marcus BH, Dubbert PM, Forsyth LH, et al. 2000. Physical activity behavior change: Issues in adoption and maintenance. *Health Psychol* 19:32-41.

Marcus BH, Goldstein MG, Jett A, et al. 1997. Training physicians to conduct physical activity counseling. *Prev Med* 26:382-88.

Marcus BH, Williams DM, Dubbert PM, et al. 2006. Physical activity intervention studies: What we know and what we need to know: A scientific statement from the American Heart Association Council on Nutrition, Physical Activity, and Metabolism (Subcommittee on Physical Activity); Council on Cardiovascular Disease in the Young; and Interdisciplinary Working Group on Quality of Care and Outcomes Research. *Circulation* 114 (24) (Dec. 12): 2739-52.

Marshall AL, Owen N, Bauman AE. 2004. Mediated approaches for influencing physical activity: Update of the evidence on mass media, print, telephone, and website delivery of interventions. *J Sci Med Sport* 7 (1 suppl.) (April): 74-80.

Martin JJ, McCaughtry N. 2008. Using social cognitive theory to predict physical activity in inner-city African American school children. *J Sport Exerc Psychol* 30 (4) (Aug.): 378-91.

McAuley E, Blissmer B. 2000. Self-efficacy determinants and consequences of physical activity. *Exerc Sport Sci Rev* 28:85-88.

McGinnis JM, Foege WH. 1993. Actual causes of death in the United States. *JAMA* 270:2207-12.

Merrill RM, Shields EC, White GL Jr., Druce D. 2005. Climate conditions and physical activity in the United States. *Am J Health Behav* 29 (4) (July-Aug.): 371-81.

Meyler D, Stimpson JP, Peek MK. 2007. Health concordance within couples: A systematic review. *Soc Sci Med* 64 (11) (June): 2297-2310.

Morandi L. 2009. The role of state policy in promoting physical activity. *Prev Med* 49 (4) (Oct.): 299-300.

Mowen AJ, Baker B. 2009. Park, recreation, fitness, and sport sector recommendations for a more physically active America: A white paper for the United States National Physical Activity Plan. *J Phys Activity Health* 6 (suppl. 2): S236-S244.

Nader PR, Sellers DE, Johnson CC, et al. 1996. The effect of adult participation in a school-based family intervention to improve children's diet and physical activity: The child and adolescent trial for cardiovascular health. *Prev Med* 25:455-64.

Nader PR, Stone EJ, Lytle LA, et al. 1999. Three-year maintenance of improved diet and physical activity: The CATCH cohort. Child and Adolescent Trial for Cardiovascular Health. *Arch Pediatr Adolesc Med* 153 (7) (July): 695-704.

Napolitano MA, Fotheringham M, Tate D, et al. 2003. Evaluation of an Internet-based physical activity intervention: A preliminary investigation. *Ann Behav Med* 25:92-99.

Napolitano MA, Marcus BH. 2002. Targeting and tailoring physical activity information using print and information technologies. *Exerc Sport Sci Rev* 30:122-28.

National Commission on Prevention Priorities (NCPP). 2007. *Preventive Care: A National Profile on Use, Disparities, and Health Benefits.* Washington, DC: Partnership for Prevention.

National Institute for Health and Clinical Excellence (NIHCE). 2008. *Promoting or Creating Built or Natural Environments That Encourage and Support Physical Activity.* London: National Institute for Health and Clinical Excellence.

Neff KL, King AC. 1995. Exercise program adherence in older adults: The importance of achieving one's expected benefits. *Med Exerc Nutr Health* 4:355-62.

Nelson ME, Rejeski WJ, Blair SN, et al. 2007. Physical activity and public health in older adults: Recommendation from the American College of Sports Medicine and the American Heart Association. *Circulation* 116 (Aug. 28): 1-12.

Owen N, Bauman A, Brown W. 2009. Too much sitting: A novel and important predictor of chronic disease risk? *Br J Sports Med* 43 (2) (Feb.): 81-83.

Owen N, Leslie E, Salmon J, Fotheringham MJ. 2000. Environmental determinants of physical activity and sedentary behavior. *Exerc Sport Sci Rev* 28 (4) (Oct.): 153-58.

Oxford Health Alliance. 2009. *Oxford Vision 2020: Community Interventions for Health.* Oxford, UK: Oxford Health Alliance.

Pachana NA, Ford JH, Andrew B, Dobson AJ. 2005. Relations between companion animals and self-reported health in older women: Cause, effect or artifact? *Int J Behav Med* 12 (2): 103-10.

Pate RR. 2009a. A National Physical Activity Plan for the United States. *J Phys Activity Health* 6 (suppl. 2): S157-S158.

———. 2009b. A National Physical Activity Plan for the United States. Special issue, *J Phys Activity Health* 6 (suppl. 2) (Nov.): S167-S264.

Patrick K, Pratt M, Sallis R. 2009. The healthcare sector's role in the U.S. National Physical Activity Plan. *J Phys Activity Health* 6 (suppl. 2): S211-S219.

Petrella RJ, Koval JJ, Cunningham DA, Paterson DH. 2003. Can primary care doctors prescribe exercise to improve fitness? The Step Test Exercise Prescription (STEP) project. *Am J Prev Med* 24 (4) (May): 316-22.

Pettee KK, Brach JS, Kriska AM, et al. 2006. Influence of marital status on physical activity levels among older adults. *Med Sci Sports Exerc* 38 (3) (March): 541-46.

Physical Activity Guidelines Advisory Committee (PAG). 2008. *Report of the Physical Activity Guidelines Advisory Committee, 2008.* Washington, DC: U.S. Department of Health and Human Services.

Pratt M, Epping JN, Dietz WH. 2009. Putting physical activity into public health: A historical perspective from the CDC. *Prev Med* 49 (4) (Oct.): 301-2.

Pratt M, Macera CA, Sallis JF, O'Donnell M, Frank LD. 2004. Economic interventions to promote physical activity: Application of the SLOTH model. *Am J Prev Med* 27 (3 suppl.) (Oct.): 136-45.

Pratt M, Macera CA, Wang G. 2000. Higher direct medical costs associated with physical inactivity. *Phys Sportsmed* 28:63-70.

Pronk N. 2009. Physical activity promotion in business and industry: Evidence, context, and recommendations for a National Plan. *J Phys Activity Health* 6 (suppl. 2): S220-S235.

Pronk NP, Kottke TE. 2009. Physical activity promotion as a strategic corporate priority to improve worker health and business performance. *Prev Med* 49 (4) (Oct.): 316-21.

Pronk NP, Tan AW, O'Connor P. 1999. Obesity, fitness, willingness to communicate, and health care costs. *Med Sci Sports Exerc* 31 (11) (Nov.): 1535-43.

Proper KI, Koning M, van der Beek AJ, Hildebrandt VH, Bosscher RJ, van Mechelen W. 2003. The effectiveness of worksite physical activity programs on physical activity, physical fitness, and health. *Clin J Sport Med* 13 (2) (March): 106-17.

Proper K, van Mechelen W. 2008. *Effectiveness and Economic Impact of Worksite Interventions to Promote Physical Activity and Healthy Diet.* Geneva, Switzerland: World Health Organization.

Ransdell LB, Taylor A, Oakland D, Schmidt J. 2003. Daughters and mothers exercising together: Effects of home- and community-based programs. *Med Sci Sports Exerc* 35:286-96.

Rejeski WJ, Brawley LR. 1997. Shaping active lifestyles in older adults: A group-facilitated behavior change intervention. *Ann Behav Med* 19 (suppl.): S106.

Rejeski WJ, Brawley LR, Ambrosius WT, et al. 2003. Older adults with chronic disease: Benefits of group-mediated counseling in the promotion of physically active lifestyles. *Health Psychol* 22 (4) (July): 414-23.

Resnicow K, Jackson A, Blissett D, et al. 2005. Results of the healthy body healthy spirit trial. *Health Psychol* 24 (4) (July): 339-48.

Robinson TN. 1999. Reducing children's television viewing to prevent obesity: A randomized controlled trial. *JAMA* 282 (16) (Oct. 27): 1561-67.

Robinson TN, Killen JD, Kraemer HC, et al. 2003. Dance and reducing television viewing to prevent weight gain in African-American girls: The Stanford GEMS pilot study. *Ethn Dis* 13 (1 suppl. 1) (Winter): S65-S77.

Robinson TN, Wilde ML, Navracruz LC, Haydel KF, Varady A. 2001. Effects of reducing children's television and video game use on aggressive behavior: A randomized controlled trial. *Arch Pediatr Adolesc Med* 155 (1) (Jan.): 17-23.

Roemmich JN, Gurgol CM, Epstein LH. 2004. Open-loop feedback increases physical activity of youth. *Med Sci Sports Exerc* 36 (4) (April): 668-73.

Roux L, Pratt M, Tengs TO, et al. 2008. Cost effectiveness of community-based physical activity interventions. *Am J Prev Med* 35 (6) (Dec.): 578-88.

Saelens BE, Handy SL. 2008. Built environment correlates of walking: A review. *Med Sci Sports Exerc* 40 (7 suppl.) (July): S550-S566.

Saelens BE, Sallis JF, Frank LD. 2003. Environmental correlates of walking and cycling: Findings from the transportation, urban design, and planning literatures. *Ann Behav Med* 25:80-91.

Sallis JF, King AC, Sirard JR, Albright CL. 2007. Perceived environmental predictors of physical activity over 6 months in adults: Activity counseling trial. *Health Psychol* 26 (6) (Nov.): 701-9.

Sallis JF, Kraft K, Linton LS. 2002. How the environment shapes physical activity: A transdisciplinary research agenda. *Am J Prev Med* 22 (3) (April): 208.

Sallis JF, McKenzie TL, Elder JP, Broyles SL, Nader PR. 1997. Factors parents use in selecting play spaces for young children. *Arch Pediatr Adolesc Med* 151 (4) (April): 414-17.

Sallis JF, Owen N. 2002. Ecological models of health behavior. In *Health Behavior and Health Education: Theory, Research, and Practice,* ed. K Glanz, FM Lewis, BK Rimer, 462-84. 3rd ed. San Francisco: Jossey-Bass.

Sallis JF, Saelens BE, Frank LD, et al. 2009. Neighborhood built environment and income: Examining multiple health outcomes. *Soc Sci Med* 68 (7) (April): 1285-93.

Sallis JF, Story M, Lou D. 2009. Study designs and analytic strategies for environmental and policy research on obesity, physical activity, and diet: Recommendations from a meeting of experts. *Am J Prev Med* 36 (2 suppl.) (Feb.): S72-S77.

Sallis RE. 2009. Exercise is medicine and physicians need to prescribe it! *Br J Sports Med* 43 (1) (Jan.): 3-4.

Salmon J, Owen N, Crawford D, Bauman A, Sallis JF. 2003. Physical activity and sedentary behavior: A population-based study of barriers, enjoyment, and preference. *Health Psychol* 22 (2) (March): 178-88.

Schmitz K, French SA, Jeffery RW. 1997. Correlates of changes in leisure time physical activity over 2 years: The Healthy Worker Project. *Prev Med* 26 (4) (July-Aug.): 570-79.

Seo DC, Sa J. 2008. A meta-analysis of psycho-behavioral obesity interventions among US multiethnic and minority adults. *Prev Med* 47 (6) (Dec.): 573-82.

Sevick MA, Dunn AL, Morrow MS, Marcus BH, Chen GJ, Blair SN. 2000. Cost-effectiveness of lifestyle and structured exercise interventions in sedentary adults: Results of project ACTIVE. *Am J Prev Med* 19 (1) (July): 1-8.

Shelley D, Cantrell MJ, Moon-Howard J, Ramjohn DQ, VanDevanter N. 2007. The $5 man: The underground economic response to a large cigarette tax increase in New York City. *Am J Public Health* 97 (8) (Aug.): 1483-88.

Sheppard L, Senior J, Park CH, Mockenhaupt R, Chodzko-Zajko W, Bazzarre T. 2003. The National

Blueprint Consensus Conference Summary Report: Strategic priorities for increasing physical activity among adults aged ≥ 50. *Am J Prev Med* 25 (3 suppl. 2): 209-13.

Shumway-Cook A, Patla AE, Stewart A, Ferrucci L, Ciol MA, Guralnik JM. 2002. Environmental demands associated with community mobility in older adults with and without mobility disabilities. *Phys Ther* 82 (7) (July): 670-81.

Simon C, Wagner A, DiVita C, et al. 2004. Intervention centred on adolescents' physical activity and sedentary behaviour (ICAPS): Concept and 6-month results. *Int J Obes Relat Metab Disord* 28 (suppl. 3) (Nov.): S96-S103.

Simon P, Gonzalez E, Ginsburg D, Abrams J, Fielding J. 2009. Physical activity promotion: A local and state health department perspective. *Prev Med* 49 (4) (Oct.): 297-98.

Simon PA, Wold CM, Cousineau MR, Fielding JE. 2001. Meeting the data needs of a local health department: The Los Angeles County Health Survey. *Am J Public Health* 91 (12) (Dec.): 1950-52.

Smith AL. 1999. Perceptions of peer relationships and physical activity participation in early adolescence. *J Sport Exerc Psychol* 21:329-50.

Solomon LS, Standish MB, Orleans CT. 2009. Creating physical activity-promoting community environments: Time for a breakthrough. *Prev Med* 49 (4) (Oct.): 334-35.

Srinivasan S, O'Fallon LR, Dearry A. 2003. Creating healthy communities, healthy homes, healthy people: Initiating a research agenda on the built environment and public health. *Am J Public Health* 93 (9) (Sept.): 1446-50.

Stetson BA, Beacham AO, Frommelt SJ, et al. 2005. Exercise slips in high-risk situations and activity patterns in long-term exercisers: An application of the relapse prevention model. *Ann Behav Med* 30 (1) (Aug.): 25-35.

Sturm R. 2005. Economics and physical activity: A research agenda. *Am J Prev Med* 28 (2 suppl. 2) (Feb.): 141-49.

Sugiyama T, Healy GN, Dunstan DW, Salmon J, Owen N. 2008. Is television viewing time a marker of a broader pattern of sedentary behavior? *Ann Behav Med* 35 (2) (April): 245-50.

Sundquist K, Qvist J, Sundquist J, Johansson SE. 2004. Frequent and occasional physical activity in the elderly: A 12-year follow-up study of mortality. *Am J Prev Med* 27 (1) (July): 22-27.

Task Force on Community Preventive Services (TFCPS). 2001. Increasing physical activity: A report on recommendations of the Task Force on Community Preventive Services. *MMWR* 50:1-14.

Tate DF, Jackvony EH, Wing RR. 2003. Effects of Internet behavioral counseling on weight loss in adults at risk for type 2 diabetes: A randomized trial. *JAMA* 289 (14) (April 9): 1833-36.

Taylor WC, Baranowski T, Young DR. 1998. Physical activity interventions in low-income, ethnic minority, and populations with disability. *Am J Prev Med* 15 (4) (Nov.): 334-43.

Taylor WC, Blair SN, Cummings SS, Wun CC, Malina RM. 1999. Childhood and adolescent physical activity patterns and adult physical activity. *Med Sci Sports Exerc* 31 (1) (Jan.): 118-23.

Timperio A, Ball K, Salmon J, et al. 2006. Personal, family, social, and environmental correlates of active commuting to school. *Am J Prev Med* 30 (1) (Jan.): 45-51.

Timperio A, Salmon J, Ball K. 2004. Evidence-based strategies to promote physical activity among children, adolescents, and young adults: Review and update. *J Sci Med Sport* 7 (1 suppl.) (April): 20-29.

Timperio A, Salmon J, Telford A, Crawford D. 2005. Perceptions of local neighbourhood environments and their relationship to childhood overweight and obesity. *Int J Obesity (Lond)* 29 (2) (Feb.): 170-75.

Trudeau F, Laurencelle L, Tremblay J, Rajic M, Shephard RJ. 1999. Daily primary school physical education: Effects on physical activity during adult life. *Med Sci Sports Exerc* 31:111-17.

Umberson D. 1987. Family status and health behaviors: Social control as a dimension of social integration. *J Health Soc Behav* 28 (3): 306-19.

U.S. Department of Health and Human Services (USDHHS). 1996. *Physical Activity and Health: A Report of the Surgeon General.* Atlanta, GA: U.S. Department of Health and Human Services, Centers for Disease Control and Prevention, National Center for Chronic Disease Prevention and Health Promotion.

———. 2000. *Healthy People 2010: Understanding and Improving Health.* November. Washington, DC: U.S Department of Health and Human Services.

U.S. Department of Health and Human Services, Secretary's Advisory Committee on National Health Promotion and Disease Prevention Objectives for 2020 (USDHHS Advisory Committee). 2008. *Phase I Report: Recommendations for the Framework and Format of Healthy People 2020.* Oct. 10, 2008. Washington, DC: US Department of Health and Human Services.

Van der Bij AK, Laurant MG, Wensing M. 2002. Effectiveness of physical activity interventions for older adults: A review. *Am J Prev Med* 22 (2) (Feb.): 120-33.

Verheijden MW, Jans MP, Hildebrandt VH, Hopman-Rock M. 2007. Rates and determinants of repeated participation in a web-based behavior change program for healthy body weight and healthy lifestyle. *J Med Internet Res* 9 (1): e1.

Volpp KG, Troxel AB, Pauly MV, et al. 2009. A randomized, controlled trial of financial incentives for smoking cessation. *N Engl J Med* 360 (7) (Feb. 12): 699-709.

Vrazel J, Saunders RP, Wilcox S. 2008. An overview and proposed framework of social-environmental influences on the physical-activity behavior of women. *Am J Health Promot* 23 (1) (Sept.-Oct.): 2-12.

Wang G, Pratt M, Macera CA, Zheng Z-J, Heath G. 2004. Physical activity, cardiovascular disease, and medical expenditures in U.S. adults. *Ann Behav Med* 28:88-94.

Weiss MR, Ferrer-Caja E. 2002. Motivational orientations and sport behavior. In *Advances in Sport Psychology,* ed. TSE Horn, 101-83. 2nd ed. Champaign, IL: Human Kinetics.

Whitt-Glover MC, Crespo CJ, Joe J. 2009. Recommendations for advancing opportunities to increase physical activity in racial/ethnic minority communities. *Prev Med* 49 (4) (Oct.): 292-93.

Wilcox S, Castro C, King AC. 2006. Outcome expectations and physical activity participation in caregiving and non-caregiving women. *J Health Psychol* 11 (1): 65-77.

Wilcox S, Castro C, King AC, Housemann R, Brownson RC. 2000. Determinants of leisure time physical activity in rural compared with urban older and ethnically diverse women in the United States. *J Epidemiol Commun Health* 54 (9) (Sept.): 667-72.

Wilcox S, Dowda M, Griffin SF, et al. 2006. Results of the first year of Active for Life: Translation of two evidence-based physical activity programs for older adults into community settings. *Am J Public Health* 96:1201-9.

Wilcox S, Dowda M, Leviton LC, et al. 2008. Active for Life: Final results from the translation of two physical activity programs. *Am J Prev Med* 35 (4) (Oct.): 340-51.

Wilcox S, King AC, Brassington G, Ahn D. 1999. Physical activity preferences of middle-aged and older adults: A community analysis. *J Aging Phys Act* 7:386-99.

Winterfeld A, Shinkle D, Morandi L. 2009. Promoting healthy communities and reducing childhood obesity: Legislative options. March 2009. National Conference of State Legislatures, Denver.

Wood L, Giles-Corti B, Bulsara M. 2005. The pet connection: Pets as a conduit for social capital? *Soc Sci Med* 61 (6) (Sept.): 1159-73.

World Health Organization (WHO). 2006. *Global Strategy on Diet, Physical Activity, and Health: A Framework to Monitor and Evaluate Implementation.* Geneva: WHO.

Yancey AK, Fielding JE, Flores GR, Sallis JF, McCarthy WJ, Breslow L. 2007. Creating a robust public health infrastructure for physical activity promotion. *Am J Prev Med* 32 (1) (Jan.): 68-78.

Yancey AK, Kumanyika SK, Ponce NA, et al. 2004. Population-based interventions engaging communities of color in healthy eating and active living: A review. *Prev Chronic Disease* 1 (1) (Jan.): A09.

Yancey AK, Sallis JF. 2009. Physical activity: Cinderella or Rodney Dangerfield? *Prev Med* 49 (4) (Oct.): 277-79.

Yancey A, Winfield D, Larsen J, et al. 2009. "Live, Learn and Play": Building strategic alliances between professional sports and public health. *Prev Med* 49 (4) (Oct.): 322-25.

YMCA of the USA. 2008. *Activate America—Community Healthy Living Index.* Report No. 9-08. Chicago: YMCA of the USA,

Zimmerman FJ. 2009. Using behavioral economics to promote physical activity. *Prev Med* 49 (4) (Oct.): 289-91.

Zimring C, Joseph A, Nicoll GL, Tsepas S. 2005. Influences of building design and site design on physical activity: Research and intervention opportunities. *Am J Prev Med* 28 (2 suppl. 2) (Feb.): 186-93.

chapter 15

Unintentional Injury and Behavior Change

ANDREA C. GIELEN, DAVID A. SLEET,
AND ELIZABETH M. PARKER

LEARNING OBJECTIVES

After completing the chapter, the reader will be able to

* Describe the burden of unintentional injury in the United States.
* Identify examples of successful efforts to reduce injury.
* Define educational, engineering, and enforcement strategies for injury prevention.
* Describe the relationship between levels of an ecological framework and injury prevention strategies.

Introduction

The burden of injury in the United States is immense. Many people, including health professionals, do not yet fully grasp the burden of injuries, their costs, and their devastating impact on public health and health care (Ikeda 2010). Injuries are the leading cause of death for Americans of ages 1 to 44 and a leading cause of disability for all ages, regardless of sex, race or ethnicity, or **socioeconomic status**. Nearly 180,000 people die each year as a result of unintentional injuries or acts of violence, and 1 in 10 sustain a nonfatal injury serious enough to be treated in a hospital emergency department (CDC 2013a, 2013b). Lifetime costs associated with the 50 million injuries Americans suffer every year are estimated at $406 billion, of which 20% is due directly to medical care expenses (Corso et al. 2006). These injuries may be the result of intentional acts, such as assaults and suicides, or the result of unintentional or accidental causes.

This chapter focuses on unintentional injuries, which make up 67% of all fatal injuries and 93% of all emergency department injury visits (CDC 2013c). Unintentional injuries are most commonly caused by falls, fires and burns, poisoning, drowning, choking, and transportation-related injuries (e.g., injuries to motor vehicle occupants, pedestrians, cyclists) (CDC 2013c).

The Science of Injury Prevention

Prior to the mid-20th century, the perception was that injuries resulted from inevitable, random, or unavoidable events, termed *accidents*. Most public health officials felt that injury prevention was outside the realm of scientific inquiry (Sleet, Dahlberg, et al. 2011). Since then, however, a robust science of injury prevention has developed. The science of injury prevention encompasses activities from **primary prevention** through treatment and rehabilitation. Important progress has been made in taking a scientific approach to injury prevention through the creation of **surveillance** systems that capture injury mechanisms and intent and establishing a scientific framework to address prevention and treatment.

In the last half of the 20th century, scientists identified important risk and protective factors for injuries. Surveillance tools and epidemiological studies identified groups at risk and mutable factors (NCenIPC 2006; NComIPC 1989). Building on this knowledge, researchers and practitioners have produced a wealth of information about effective strategies to prevent unintentional injuries or minimize their **consequences** (Doll et al. 2007).

Examples of proven measures include policies and programs that increase the use of seat belts and child safety seats, alcohol checkpoints, graduated driver licensing systems, smoke alarms and fire sprinkler systems, community-based fall prevention programs, helmet use by bicyclists and motorcyclists, comprehensive trauma care systems, screening and brief **interventions** for alcohol problems, and many more (Doll et al. 2007; Gielen, Sleet, and DiClemente 2006; McClure et al. 2004; Zaza et al. 2005).[1] These policies and practices save lives when public health professionals work closely with those in law enforcement, product safety, and advocacy to protect whole populations. Intervention options are numerous, and public health professionals take a multidisciplinary approach to addressing these problems. Interventions may include education and behavior change, but also environmental supports such as legislation and enforcement, technology and engineering, and changes in the **built environment**.

This chapter surveys the unintentional-injury problem, drawing on examples from specific types of injuries to illustrate the concepts of an **ecological approach** and to provide evidence on the preventability of unintentional injuries. We first define the magnitude of the problem in the United States. We then provide an overview of an ecological approach to the problem with specific illustrations of **key determinants** at each of the different levels. Finally, and consistent with the theme of the book, we focus on the evidence for behavior changes that can reduce injury risks and the roles for **key stakeholders** in achieving these changes in large populations in the United States.

Defining the Problem

Injuries do not happen by accident. The *Oxford English Dictionary* defines the term *accident* as "an unfortunate incident that happens unexpectedly and unintentionally, typically resulting in damage or injury"; or "an event that happens by chance or that is without apparent or deliberate cause."[2] The word *injury* has its root in the Latin term *injurie*, which literally means "unjust" or "not right." Because *accident* implies an (unexpected or unintended) event, it should not be used when referring to an injury, which is a predictable medical or surgical outcome of such an event.

The science of injury prevention teaches that injuries are not accidental or random events—

they are predictable, and many are preventable through changes in consumer products, human behavior, and environments. Using terms such as *injury prevention,* rather than *accident prevention,* helps make clear the potential for preventing these adverse medical outcomes (Sleet and Gielen 2006).

Professionals in the injury prevention field should be encouraged by findings that most people believe that accidents and injuries are preventable (Girasek 1999). Focusing on prevention of both the injury event and its medical, social, and economic consequences helps place the issue of injury within a disease prevention-health promotion framework.

Injuries occur when damage to the body results from acute exposure to thermal, mechanical, radiant, electrical, or chemical energy or from the absence of such essentials as heat or oxygen (NComIPC 1989). Kinetic or mechanical energy, such as in a fall or a crash, contributes substantially to the injury problem overall. Conceptualizing energy as the causal agent in producing injury was a significant advance in the field and led to numerous successful prevention strategies that either separate the potentially dangerous energy source from the human (e.g., fencing around a work zone) or mitigate the impact of an energy transfer (e.g., air bags).

Understanding the role of human behavior and the **social environment** in injury **causation** and prevention can enrich this conceptualization of the injury problem. As an example, airbags, once touted as the "passive prevention" alternative to seat belt use, require individuals to also buckle their seat belts for maximum protection. After the deaths of children and small-statured adults who were in front of an airbag when it deployed in a low-speed crash, parents are now encouraged to put their children in the backseat, *away* from the airbag. Changing the social environment through policies that mandate such preventive behaviors helps to complete the picture of what it often takes to reduce the likelihood of a harmful

transfer of energy and ultimately an injury. Thus, it is appropriate and helpful to define the injury problem broadly from an ecological perspective, as we describe in detail later in the chapter.

The Magnitude and the Burden

Unintentional injury is not only costly, but it is also the leading cause of death in the United States for people of ages 1 to 44, and 120,859 deaths occurred because of it in 2010 (figure 15.1). Table 15.1 shows the number and rate of unintentional injury deaths for the most recently available period, 2006–10. Death rates are higher for children younger than age 5 and older than age 14 compared to those of ages 5 to 9. Adults age 65 and over have the highest death rate, males have a higher rate than females, and American Indian or Alaskan Natives have higher rates than other racial groups.

In addition to deaths, there were 29.3 million emergency department visits resulting from unintentional injury in 2010. Table 15.2 shows the rank ordering of the leading mechanisms of unintentional injury deaths and emergency department visits in 2010. Motor vehicle related injuries and falls are ranked among the top three causes of both fatal and nonfatal injury, making these especially high-priority injury problems for prevention efforts. Clear differences in lethality exist across the causes of injury; for instance, drowning, suffocation, and fires and burns rank high in fatal injury but not in the ranking of nonfatal injury. Conversely, although millions of emergency department visits are caused by being struck by or against an object, cut and pierce injuries, and overexertion, the number of fatalities is low.

The Ecological Model Applied to Unintentional Injury

William Haddon, the father of modern injury epidemiology, introduced the concept of an

FIGURE 15.1. The ten leading causes of death in the United States, 2010, all races, both sexes. *Source:* National Vital Statistics System, National Center for Health Statistics, CDC. Produced by the Office of Statistics and Programming, National Center for Injury Prevention and Control, CDC, using WISQARS.

Rank	<1	1–4	5–9	10–14	15–24	25–34	35–44	45–54	55–64	65+	Total
Age Groups											
1	Congenital Anomalies 5,107	Unintentional Injury 1,394	Unintentional Injury 758	Unintentional Injury 885	Unintentional Injury 12,341	Unintentional Injury 14,573	Unintentional Injury 14,792	Malignant Neoplasms 50,211	Malignant Neoplasms 109,501	Heart Disease 477,338	Heart Disease 597,689
2	Short Gestation 4,148	Congenital Anomalies 507	Malignant Neoplasms 439	Malignant Neoplasms 477	Homicide 4,678	Suicide 5,735	Malignant Neoplasms 11,809	Heart Disease 36,729	Heart Disease 68,077	Malignant Neoplasms 396,670	Malignant Neoplasms 574,743
3	SIDS 2,063	Homicide 385	Congenital Anomalies 163	Suicide 267	Suicide 4,600	Homicide 4,258	Heart Disease 10,594	Unintentional Injury 19,667	Chronic Low. Respiratory Disease 14,242	Chronic Low. Respiratory Disease 118,031	Chronic Low. Respiratory Disease 138,080
4	Maternal Pregnancy Comp. 1,561	Malignant Neoplasms 346	Heart Disease 68	Homicide 150	Malignant Neoplasms 1,604	Malignant Neoplasms 3,619	Suicide 6,571	Suicide 8,799	Unintentional Injury 14,023	Cerebrovascular 109,990	Cerebrovascular 129,476
5	Unintentional Injury 1,110	Heart Disease 159	Homicide 111	Congenital Anomalies 135	Heart Disease 1,028	Heart Disease 3,222	Homicide 2,473	Liver Disease 8,651	Diabetes Mellitus 11,677	Alzheimer's Disease 82,616	Unintentional Injury 120,859
6	Placenta Cord. Membranes 1,030	Influenza & Pneumonia 91	Chronic Low. Respiratory Disease 60	Heart Disease 117	Congenital Anomalies 412	HIV 741	Liver Disease 2,423	Cerebrovascular 5,910	Cerebrovascular 10,693	Diabetes Mellitus 49,191	Alzheimer's Disease 83,494
7	Bacterial Sepsis 583	Septicemia 62	Cerebrovascular 47	Chronic Low. Respiratory Disease 73	Cerebrovascular 190	Diabetes Mellitus 606	Cerebrovascular 1,904	Diabetes Mellitus 5,610	Liver Disease 9,764	Influenza & Pneumonia 42,846	Diabetes Mellitus 69,071
8	Respiratory Distress 514	Benign Neoplasms 59	Benign Neoplasms 37	Benign Neoplasms 45	Influenza & Pneumonia 181	Cerebrovascular 517	HIV 1,898	Chronic Low. Respiratory Disease 4,452	Suicide 6,384	Nephritis 41,994	Nephritis 50,476
9	Circulatory System Disease 507	Perinatal Period 52	Influenza & Pneumonia 37	Cerebrovascular 43	Diabetes Mellitus 165	Liver Disease 487	Diabetes Mellitus 1,789	HIV 3,123	Nephritis 5,082	Unintentional Injury 41,300	Influenza & Pneumonia 50,097
10	Necrotizing Enterocolitis 472	Chronic Low. Respiratory Disease 51	Septicemia 32	Septicemia 35	Complicated Pregnancy 163	Congenital Anomalies 397	Influenza & Pneumonia 773	Viral Hepatitis 2,376	Septicemia 4,604	Septicemia 26,310	Suicide 38,364

TABLE 15.1. Unintentional injury deaths and rates per 100,000, United States, 2006–2010

Characteristics	Number	Rate
Age		
0–4	13,565	13.46
5–14	9,643	4.74
15–24	71,014	32.79
25–54	253,563	40.03
55–64	63,377	37.04
65+	194,751	100.56
Gender		
Males	388,089	53.74
Females	217,998	25.43
Race		
White	522,935	40.88
Black	64,066	34.11
Am Indian/AK Native	8,521	49.67
Asian/Pacific Islander	10,565	15.82
Hispanic origin		
Hispanic	55,985	28.51
Non-Hispanic	548,069	40.33

Source: Centers for Disease Control and Prevention, WISQARS, www.cdc.gov/injury

ecological approach to injury prevention with publication of his seminal paper "On the Escape of Tigers: An Ecological Note" (Haddon 1970). His ecological approach acknowledged that injuries occur when there is an interaction among the **host** (person), an agent (energy), and the environment (physical or social), a concept first introduced by Gordon in 1949 (Sleet et al. 2012). The **Haddon matrix** refined the concept by adding three phases to injury: pre-event (i.e., before the crash), event (i.e., during the crash), and post-event (i.e., after the crash). At each phase, there are opportunities to prevent and control injury-related damage. Freire and Runyan (2006) updated the Haddon Matrix and integrated it with the widely used **PRECEDE-PROCEED** planning model demonstrating how to apply epidemiological analyses and health promotion **planning** methods to injury prevention.

To be effective, injury prevention efforts need to address the most important and most changeable risk factor, which is not necessarily the most obvious, or proximal, one (Baker 1992). For instance, drinking alcohol may be the most

TABLE 15.2. Unintentional injury deaths and emergency department visits: number and ranking by injury cause, United States, 2010

Rank fatal	Number fatal	Unintentional injury cause	Number nonfatal	Rank nonfatal
1	37,236	motor vehicle[a]	4,354,337	4
2	33,041	poisoning	831,295	8
3	26,009	falls	9,146,026	1
4	6,165	suffocation	42,341	19
6	3,782	drowning[b]		>20
7	2,845	fire/burn	400,599	13
14	788	struck by/against	4,565,133	2
18	105	cut/pierce	2,143,400	5
19	10	overexertion	3,430,040	3

Source: Centers for Disease Control and Prevention, WISQARS, www.cdc.gov/injury.
[a]Includes traffic, occupant, pedal cyclist, pedestrian, motorcyclist other transport, other land transport.
[b]Only the top 20 leading causes of fatal unintentional injury and nonfatal unintentional injury are reported by WISQARS.

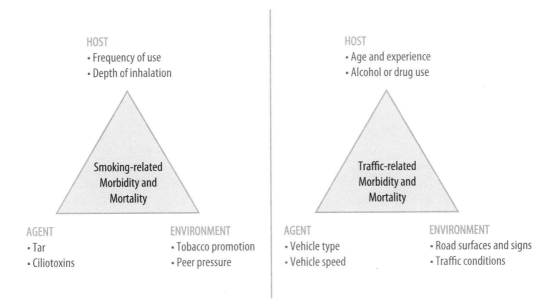

FIGURE 15.2. The interaction of factors in the epidemiological triad related to smoking and traffic safety.
Source: Sleet and Gielen 1998, figs. 10.1 and 10.2.

proximal cause of a motorcycle crash, but the most effective injury prevention strategy may be to require motorcyclists to wear helmets. Wearing a helmet is considered an event-phase behavior because it prevents an injury once the event (i.e., the crash) has occurred. In this example, we see the importance of behavior, whether it is trying to modify the pre-event drinking behavior of a driver or to modify the event behavior of wearing a helmet. From an ecological perspective, this example also illustrates the multifaceted nature of injury problems and multiple options for solutions (Allegrante et al. 2010).

Public health can effectively use its tools and national infrastructure to identify, track, and monitor traffic injuries and deaths and to design short- and long-term solutions to help counter the rising exposure to injuries. One important tool in the fight against injuries has been the **classic epidemiological triad** used to characterize the causal nexus of disease. This basic **ecological model** incorporates aspects of the individual and the environment to understand the **complexity** of changing injury risks and outcomes.

We know that injury results from the interaction between injury-producing **agents** (e.g., kinetic energy transferred to the host when a speeding car crashes), host factors (a young, inexperienced driver or a drinking driver), and the environment (road surfaces, signs, weather). This triad of host (the person affected), agent (the causative element and the vehicle or **vector** carrying it), and the environment (conditions in which the host and agent find themselves) can be applied to the factors contributing to traffic-related injury as well as the more classic use, to explain the development of diseases, such as those related to smoking (figure 15.2).

Intervening on the host (changing behaviors to reduce risk), on the agent (changes in vehicle design to reduce energy transfer), and environments (installing dividing barriers and guardrails) can singly, or in combination, reduce the likelihood both of a crash and of the injuries that result. This approach is a useful means to identify where the causal chain may be interrupted to reduce or prevent injuries.

The success in the United States in reducing injuries resulting from alcohol-impaired driving provides another useful example of ecological approaches, tapping into all phases (pre-event, event, and post-event) as well as multiple **levels of influence**. The proportion of motor vehicle crash deaths that are attributable to alcohol has been reduced from 48% in 1982 to 32% in 2009 (NHTSA 2010), despite the increase in vehicle miles traveled. Numerous factors operating at multiple levels of the ecological model have been credited with contributing to this improvement. Two parents (Doris Aiken and Cindy Lightner) who brought media attention to the problem after their daughters were killed by drunk drivers elevated the visibility of victims, heightened public awareness, and organized at the grassroots community level by creating RID (Remove Intoxicated Drivers) and MADD (Mothers Against Drunk Driving) (Isaacs and Schroeder 2001). **Targeting** the public and policymakers paid off in the passage of numerous state laws deterring drunk driving as well as federal legislation requiring states to pass laws establishing the minimum drinking age at 21 years or risk losing a portion of their federal highway safety funds (Bonnie et al. 1999). Raising the minimum legal drinking age has demonstrated its **effectiveness** in reducing underage alcohol-related motor vehicle fatalities (Shults et al. 2001). Engineering solutions that have been developed include more sophisticated alcohol-sensing devices, Breathalyzer and roadside testing devices, and vehicle lockout devices for convicted drunken drivers (Elder et al. 2011; Evans 2004).

Key Determinants

Although each injury mechanism has its own unique risk and protective factors, the ecological model offers a **conceptual framework** that can be useful for addressing any specific cause of injury (Simons-Morton et al. 2012). McLeroy

and colleagues (1988) suggested the following five levels of influence in an ecological model for health promotion in which the focus is on patterns of behavior as the outcome of interest:

1. Intrapersonal factors: characteristics of the individual such as knowledge, **attitudes**, behavior, self-concept, skills, and so forth. The developmental history of the individual is included.
2. Interpersonal processes and primary groups: formal and informal **social network** and **social support** systems, including the family, the work group, and friendship **networks**.
3. Institutional factors: social institutions with organizational characteristics and with formal (and informal) rules and regulations for operation.
4. Community factors: relationships among organizations, institutions, and informal networks within defined boundaries.
5. Public policy: local, state, and national laws and policies.

The Intrapersonal Level

The **intrapersonal level** refers to characteristics of the individuals at risk and their knowledge, beliefs, skills, and resources to adopt protective actions. Some individual risk factors are more modifiable than others. For instance, risk factors for falls among older adults include advancing age, prior falls, weakness, gait and balance disorders, vision problems, low blood pressure, chronic disease such as arthritis or Parkinson's, and the use of multiple medications (especially psychotropic medications). To identify high priority audiences for intervention, it is necessary to understand the broad array of individual-level risk factors, even those that are not modifiable. To reach those high priority audiences, it is equally important to understand the intrapersonal factors that influence the likelihood of preventive action.

Our ability to effectively communicate about injury hazards and precautions depends in large part on understanding our audience's **risk perceptions** and beliefs (Girasek 2006). A national survey of 943 adults evaluated the extent to which the public perceived unintentional injury as preventable. Results indicated that 83% of respondents thought that accidents were usually preventable, 71% thought that they were usually unpredictable, and 96% associated accidents with the idea that they did not happen on purpose (Girasek 1999). In the same survey, when respondents were asked about how to prevent injuries, 87% could name a prevention strategy for fatal fires or burns, 86% for motor vehicle and drowning deaths, 80% for poisoning deaths, and 55% for fatal falls (Girasek and Gielen 2003). When respondents were asked about the perceived effectiveness of professionally recommended prevention strategies, ratings were generally high across all the causes of injury deaths. For example, requiring the use of life jackets on boats was rated as 86% effective for reducing drowning deaths, and requiring smoke alarms in all residential building was rated as 90% effective.

In addition to risk and preventability beliefs, other research has found correlations between constructs from a variety of intrapersonal theories and injury prevention behaviors (Sleet et al. 2006; Trifiletti et al. 2005). For instance, Peterson, Farmer, and Kashani (1990) examined the relationship between the **Health Belief Model** (**HBM**) and safety practices of 198 parents. Beliefs about the effectiveness of their actions (benefits), a realistic assessment of costs, and high **self-efficacy** were most strongly associated with safety behaviors. Lajunen and Rasanen (2004) examined intentions to use bicycle helmets in 965 Finnish youth ages 12 to 19, using **structural equation** modeling to compare constructs from the three **intrapersonal-level** theories: the **Theory of Planned Behavior** (**TPB**), the HBM, and the **Locus of Control Theory** (**LCT**). Both the TPB and the LCT offered good

fit models for the data, whereas the HBM did not (even though some of its individual constructs were associated with intention). Beliefs about negative peer opinions, the inconveniences of helmet use, not having a helmet visible at home, and the belief that individuals cannot improve their own riding safety were associated with lower intention to use a helmet. The TPB has also recently been used to understand storage of household firearms (Johnson et al. 2008), safe swimming practices (White and Hyde 2010), and the use of safety gear by in-line skaters (Deroche et al. 2009).

The Interpersonal Level

At the **interpersonal level**, injury risk is influenced by significant others, such as friends and family. **Social Cognitive Theory** (**SCT**) is particularly relevant at this level of the ecological model (Simons-Morton and Nansel 2006). The central tenet of SCT is the concept of **reciprocal determinism**, which posits that the environment, behavior, and the person are dynamically interrelated. The physical and social environments are both considered potentially important in SCT. The behavior is the outcome of interest, and "the person" refers to the individual cognitive, affective, and biological self. There are similarities between the constructs of the SCT and ecological models, especially with regard to the role of the physical and social environments and the notion that the multiple factors interact dynamically.

The increased risk of additional passengers in fatal teen-driver crashes dramatically illustrates this level of influence. Chen, Baker, Braver, and Li (2000) found that for both 16- and 17-year-old drivers, those with passengers had a significantly higher **relative risk** of death than those without passengers; the risk increased with the number of passengers, even after controlling for time of day and gender of the driver. The authors reason that this effect is likely caused by more risky driving behaviors (e.g., speeding) and distractions in the presence of other passengers, causes that other literature also supports (Farrow 1987; Williams and Ferguson 2002). These findings, along with the overall elevated risk of motor vehicle crashes and deaths among young people, provide a strong rationale for graduated driver licensing policies, which have demonstrated their lifesaving potential (Chen et al. 2006; Hartling et al. 2004; Vanlaar et al. 2009).

Graduated driver licensing (GDL) policies (see chapter 3) exist in most jurisdictions in the United States. They are designed to phase in full driving privileges gradually over time so that teens gain driving experience in supervised and lower-risk circumstances. Although GDL policies reflect a policy-level intervention in terms of an ecological model (discussed below), their successful implementation depends on **compliance** by teen drivers. Therefore, *parents* play an important role in assuring compliance and helping their teens become safe drivers (Simons-Morton 2007; Simons-Morton and Ouimet 2006). Parent management of teen driving is an area of research that is illustrative of how the interpersonal level of an ecological model helps to address key determinants of the leading cause of death among teens.

The Checkpoints Program was developed to facilitate parental management of teen driving (Simons-Morton and Nansel 2006). It is based on constructs from **Protection Motivation Theory** and SCT and uses a persuasive communication approach. The program was designed to increase parent-teen communication and parental restrictions on teen driving privileges. The program demonstrated significant positive effects on increasing restrictions and decreasing risky driving in the first month after licensure in a Maryland study, although these latter effects declined over time (Simons-Morton et al. 2003, 2004). In a larger study in Connecticut, researchers found that the program resulted in greater limits on teen driving at the time of licensure as well as at three- and six-month

follow-ups and that stricter parental limits were associated with fewer traffic violations and crashes over the 12-month postlicensure period (Simons-Morton et al. 2005, 2006).

The Institutional Level

Organizational policies, procedures, and customs can have substantial influence on individuals' injury risk. For instance, evidence shows that brief alcohol interventions delivered in trauma centers after an alcohol-related trauma significantly reduce the rate of a repeat alcohol-related trauma (Sommers et al. 2006). Based on this evidence, Level 1 and 2 Trauma Centers are now mandated by their accrediting body to provide these Screening, Brief Intervention, Referral, and Treatment programs. This example illustrates how change at the organizational or institutional level can ultimately benefit the individual whose risk behavior is at issue.

Another example comes from fire prevention. The fire service in the United States has had a long tradition of providing Fire and Life Safety Education (FLSE) in the communities it serves. A national survey of fire departments found that 86% reported conducting FLSE (Gielen et al. 2007). The organizational structure influenced whether they conducted FLSE, with volunteer departments being less likely than career departments to provide it (82% versus 99%). Only 12% of fire departments had staff exclusively assigned to this responsibility, and only 33% required staff training for conducting FLSE. Significant barriers to conducting FLSE included not enough funding, lack of time, and too many competing priorities. The ability of FLSE programs to reach their full potential is organizational in nature, as indicated by these findings on staff availability and training and resource constraints. Organizational change theories and methods may be helpful for strengthening the infrastructure needed for prevention in the fire service (Butterfoss et al. 2008).

The Community Level

The social networks, **norms**, and interactions among groups and organizations in a community (e.g., neighborhood, schools, county) can have a powerful influence on individual behavior as well as on the riskiness or safety of the environment. Injury prevention has had a long tradition of using community-wide approaches to protect whole populations. Community-mobilizing theories and principles of practice apply when working at this level (Gielen, Sleet, and Green 2006).

The Injury Free Coalition for Kids initiative that started with the Harlem Hospital Injury Prevention Program in New York (Durkin et al. 1999) is a good example of work focused on the community level to protect children living in the neighborhood around the hospital. Injury surveillance data were used to demonstrate the magnitude of the child injury problem, and a multidisciplinary lay-professional **coalition** was formed to find solutions. The interventions that were established included new educational programs; safe play areas; and supervised activities for children, specifically playground renovations, a Safety City, window guard legislation for high-rise apartments, recreational programs (art, dance, and sports), and free bicycle helmets. Analyses of hospital admission over time in the intervention community compared to an untreated comparison community found that from 1983 to 1995, hospital admissions owing to injury decreased by 55% overall, 46% for pedestrian injury, 50% for playground injuries, and 46% for violence-related injuries (www.IFCK.org). Total injuries also declined in the comparison community, but the reductions in the intervention community were most noticeable in the specific injuries and age groups that were targeted by the program (Davidson et al. 1994).

A second example comes from the Community Trials Project (Treno and Holder 1997), which used community mobilizing as a way to purposely organize the community to support and implement evidence-based policies to reduce alcohol-related trauma. With the emphasis on policy solutions, this example also illustrates how community-level approaches can influence the policy environment as well as the individual. A community-science **partnership** was formed and the decision was made to address the alcohol-injury connection through environmental change. According to Holder and colleagues (1997), the program focused on changing individual behavior by changing the **contexts**— both social and structural—in which alcohol use occurred. Research evidence was used to identify potentially effective policies and programmatic activities. Communities selected the activities that were priorities for them, given local concerns and interests. The mobilization effort included components focused on responsible beverage service, drinking and driving, underage drinking, and alcohol access to raise awareness and support among the public and decision makers, coalitions, task forces, and the media (Holder et al. 1997; Holder et al. 2000). Holder and colleagues (2000) compared intervention communities with control communities on multiple alcohol and injury outcomes. They found significant reductions in the following indicators: 6% in the reported quantity of alcohol consumed, 51% in driving with a blood alcohol level over the legal limit, 10% in nighttime injury crashes, 6% in alcohol-related crashes, and 43% in alcohol-related assault injuries seen in emergency departments (Holder et al. 2000).

The Policy Level

Local, state, and federal laws have been a mainstay in injury prevention because of their important influence on (1) **social norms**, (2) the physical environment, and (3) individual behavior (Shaw and Ogolla 2006). There are numerous examples of each of these policy-level impacts in injury prevention, and many involve elements of community mobilizing as just described. MADD's reduction in drunk driving fatalities is one such example in which the effects on social norms and individual behavior are noteworthy. Isaacs and Schroeder (2001) called the effect of this movement on public policy "stunning," noting that between 1981 and 1985, state legislatures passed 478 laws to deter drunk driving. In 1984 Congress required states to pass the minimum drinking age of 21 or risk losing a portion of their federal highway safety funds. Most recently, Congress used the same approach to encourage states to lower their blood alcohol concentration (BAC) limit for drunk driving from 0.10 to 0.08g/dL, based on evidence that changing the policy would save 500–700 lives annually (Sleet, Mercer, et al. 2011). As Graham describes it, "changes in social norms, in part spurred by such citizen activist groups as MADD, have apparently achieved what many traffic safety professionals believed was virtually impossible: a meaningful change in driver attitudes and behaviors resulting in a reduction of traffic fatalities" (1993, 524).

Product redesign provides an example of how the law, through regulation, can change the physical environment to reduce injury risk. The work of the Consumer Product Safety Commission (CPSC) (www.cpsc.gov) has repeatedly illustrated the power of mandatory standards in protecting consumers from unreasonable risk. For instance, disposable cigarette lighters at one time were responsible for many childhood deaths every year because children could easily ignite themselves. In 1994 the CPSC required manufacturers to develop child-resistant features on lighters. According to Smith, Greene, and Singh (2002), deaths related to disposable lighters have been cut by 58%. Notably, the impetus for this policy change was stimulated by an advocate working at the community level, as described in this excerpt:

> After seeing many children suffering from burns, Diane Denton, a nurse in the Louisville, Kentucky community, began asking the

children's parents how their tragic injuries occurred. She learned that a large number of cases were the result of children playing with disposable cigarette lighters. The lighters are small enough to fit in the palm of the child's hand, are brightly colored, and become "sparking toys" when moved rapidly along a carpet or mattress. Ms. Denton documented these findings and petitioned the U.S. Consumer Product Safety Commission (CPSC) to investigate the risks posed by disposable cigarette lighters. Others in the burn prevention community joined her effort.

> Impressed with the data, Ms. Denton and others in her community examined cases in which children had been badly burned while playing with disposable cigarette lighters. They found that children playing with lighters started residential fires that caused an annual average of 150 fatalities and 1,100 injuries. As many as 200 burn-related deaths among children younger than 3 years could be prevented by a simple and inexpensive childproof device. Ten years after Denton's efforts, with CPSC prompting, the major cigarette lighter manufacturers complied with a request to make childproof disposable lighters, and they marketed them to the public as safer for the protection of children. CPSC finally set a standard (effective in 1994) requiring disposable and novelty lighters to be child-resistant. (Sleet and Gielen 2006, 384)

This example, and many others like it, illustrates the importance of data and broad community support when trying to make change at the policy level.

Prevention Strategies and Methods

Knowing the levels of influence on injury risk and safety behaviors is a helpful first step in building evidence-based prevention initiatives, but how to translate the assessment of influencing factors into effective interventions requires additional effort.

TABLE 15.3. Three injury prevention strategies and the key factors needed for the strategies to work.

Strategy	Key factors
Education and behavior change	Key factors for education and behavior change strategies to work: • The audience must be exposed to the information. • The audience must understand and believe the information. • The audience must have the resources and skills to make the proposed change. • The audience must derive benefit (or perceive a benefit) from the change. • The audience must be reinforced to maintain the change over time.
Legislation and enforcement	Key factors in assuring legislation enforcement strategies work: • The legislation must be widely known and understood. • The public must accept the legislation and its enforcement provisions. • The probability, or perceived probability, of being caught if one breaks the law must be high. • The punishment must be perceived as swift and severe.
Engineering and technology	Requirements to successfully implement engineering and technology solutions that protect large populations: • The technology must be effective and reliable. • The technology must be acceptable to the public and compatible with the environment. • The technology must result in products that dominate the marketplace. • The technology must be easily understood and properly used by the public.

Source: Adapted from Sleet and Gielen 2006.

Strategies in injury prevention (general plans of action used to reduce injuries) are distinct from *methods* (tactics used to implement the strategies). Whereas education is one strategy for preventing burns, clinical counseling is one method of implementing that strategy; another method is using mass media campaigns to make the public aware of a burn-related hazard. There are three generally accepted strategies in injury prevention and many distinct methods for implementing each (table 15.3):

1. Education and behavior change
2. Legislation and enforcement
3. Engineering and technology

A combination of strategies should be selected after an analysis of the situation, including a needs assessment for the population being served. The strategy mix should also take into consideration local standards and the public ac- ceptability of various behavioral, environmental, or engineering and infrastructural changes necessary to reduce injuries.

Education and Behavior Change

Education and behavior change strategies are directed toward decreasing the susceptibility of the host to injury by teaching or motivating persons to behave differently (see table 15.3). Some methods used to implement this strategy (e.g., **social marketing**) may also affect social norms in the environment. For example, the designated-driver campaigns aimed at modifying host drinking behaviors also affect attitudes in the community environment, so that drinking and driving becomes socially unacceptable behavior.

Although the **structural intervention** paradigm might seem straightforward, environmental or technological changes almost always require a corresponding change in human behavior. Children need to wear helmets while bicycling; parents need to correctly install child safety seats and booster seats; homeowners need to check their smoke alarms and change the batteries; parents need four-sided fences around their backyard pools and also need to make sure the gate to the pool is always closed; occupants alerted by a smoke alarm still need to find their way to safety. Even the more passive approach to poison prevention through the use of child-resistant closures—one of the great successes in injury control—requires active individual effort in replacing lids correctly (DiLillo et al. 2002; Shield 1997).

Education and behavior change approaches can also produce effects on those who make laws and design products, such as legislators and engineers, in ways that ultimately protect whole populations (Gielen, et al. 2012). For instance, if engineers are educated about injury prevention as part of their training, when they design products in the future, they may be less likely to design something hazardous. Similarly, when legislators are educated about the benefits of prevention, their beliefs can change, ultimately maximizing the potential that they will make decisions that benefit injury prevention (Tung et al. 2012).

Legislation and Law Enforcement

Legislation and law enforcement strategies have their greatest effect by enhancing safety in both the physical environment (e.g., installing speed bumps on high risk neighborhood roads) and the sociocultural environment (e.g., social attitudes and policies supporting restrictions on drunk driving) (see table 15.3). Laws and regulations can be made to require changes in individual behavior or product design or to alter the environment to reduce hazards or their consequences. In each case, there is an opportunity for the legislation and law enforcement strategies to work synergistically with other strate-

gies. Laws to discourage individuals from drinking and driving (e.g., laws that limit the BAC to of drivers to .08 g/dL may also make persons less tolerant of drinking and boating. Changing the price of alcoholic beverages may also result in fewer alcohol-related injuries.

Legislation can also be aimed at changing the environment, making it less hazardous for everyone. Regulations requiring residential pool fencing, safeguards against workplace hazards, and comprehensive trauma care systems are examples of how these strategies can benefit whole communities. Product safety regulations, such as those affecting toys, home appliances, sports equipment, and playgrounds, are other examples of the application of legislation and law enforcement to benefit multiple targets (Sleet and Gielen 2006).

Engineering and Technology

Engineering and technology strategies have their greatest impact on the agent (vector or vehicle) of energy transfer, but they may also affect environmental factors contributing to injury (see table 15.3). Hip pads designed to reduce hip fractures among older adults by reducing the amount of energy transferred to the host during a fall led to the design of soft flooring materials to reduce environmental risks where risks for falls are high (e.g., nursing homes). Technology and engineering contribute to injury reduction by developing products that reduce the likelihood of sudden energy release. These strategies can affect the safety of environments as well and may even lead to safer behavior on the part of the host (e.g., occupants may increase the use of safety belts while riding in an air-bag-equipped car).

Some of the many technological and engineering advances that reduce personal injuries and have also led to improved environmental safety include reflective clothing, bridged pedestrian paths, child-resistant cigarette lighters, household smoke alarms, institutional sprinkler systems, electrical insulation, swimming pool alarms, household fuses, machine guards, break-away bases, tractor rollover protection, and soft playground surfaces.

Despite advances in technology, however, many protective devices (e.g., swimming pool fences, automotive ignition interlocks to control drinking and driving, and antilock brakes) have had limited success because one or more of the factors previously listed were ignored (e.g., swimming pool fences were not environmentally aesthetic, interlocks were removed from the car after the probationary period, the public did not know how to operate antilock brakes).

Combining Strategies

The importance of using a mix of strategies to prevent and control injuries cannot be overemphasized. The examples above underscore the necessity of combining behavioral and environmental approaches to injury prevention (Sleet and Gielen 1998). This is the approach used in most other areas of disease prevention and health promotion (Green and Kreuter 2005). Successes in both tobacco control and motor vehicle safety (see chapter 3) have taught us that an informed and supportive electorate facilitates the process by which legislative and other environmental strategies are adopted.

An example of combining strategies in an ecological approach to preventing falls among older adults would include any efforts to modify the individual and environmental risk factors. There are several individual risk factors, such as medication use, visual acuity, gait, and balance as well as environmental risk factors, such as unsafe surfaces (slippery or uneven), poorly designed or maintained homes and stairways, and lack of safety devices such as grab bars in showers and handrails on stairways (Michael et al. 2010; Rubenstein 2006; Rubenstein and Josephson 2006). The most effective interventions evaluated to date are multicomponent interventions that couple falls risk

assessment with management programs (Chang et al. 2004). Physical therapy and exercise, including Tai Chi and other programs to improve gait, balance, and strength, have demonstrated effectiveness when used alone or as part of a multicomponent strategy (Michael et al. 2010). Vitamin D supplementation has been found to reduce the risk of falling specifically among community-dwelling older adults (Michael et al. 2010; Johnson et al. 2010). Most of the systematic reviews have focused on community-dwelling older adults, but for those who live in nursing or residential care facilities with high rates of falls, the use of hip protectors has been associated with a reduced risk of hip fractures (Parker et al. 2005).

The Rand Corporation estimated the potential cost-effectiveness of a new Medicare benefit, a falls-prevention rehabilitation program, that combines multifactorial assessment of falls risk with individually tailored recommendations and a supervised exercise program, and determined that such a strategy would be highly cost-effective (even cost-*saving* in persons older than age 75) by preventing Medicare costs from injuries due to falls (Wu et al. 2010). Tinetti and colleagues (2008) recently demonstrated some success in reducing fall-related injuries by disseminating this prevention strategy (i.e., clinical assessment of risk and risk reduction strategies) to clinical practices in Connecticut.

Building Comprehensive Programs

An ecologically focused program planning framework that has been used successfully in unintentional injury prevention is the PRECEDE-PROCEED framework (see chapter 5). This framework includes methods and strategies to address the individual and environmental determinants of a health behavior. The model has been used in conjunction with the Haddon matrix to both identify key determinants and develop comprehensive interventions (Freire and

Runyan 2006). Hendrickson and Becker (1998) used the PRECEDE model as a framework to guide their development of a classroom-based head injury prevention program aimed at increasing bicycle helmet use in low-income rural children. Two interventions were compared against a **control group**: a classroom-only intervention, a classroom intervention with a parental telephone intervention, and a control group that received neither intervention. School nurses were trained to deliver the program; in the first session students viewed a video featuring interviews of young brain-injured adults followed by a discussion and distribution of helmets, and in the second session, nurses referred back to the video and held another brief discussion. Analyses of the pretest and posttest questionnaires revealed that participation in either educational intervention, participation in the parent intervention, and the belief that helmets protect heads were predictive of helmet use after controlling for helmet ownership.

A second example is the Safe Home Project, which used the PRECEDE-PROCEED model as a framework for the planning, implementation, and **evaluation** of a clinic-based intervention focused on reducing in-home child injury risk among low-income urban families (Gielen et al. 2001; Gielen et al. 2008). Residents at a pediatric continuity clinic were randomly assigned to the intervention or the control group. Both groups participated in a one-hour seminar on injury prevention and received materials from the American Academy of Pediatrics Injury Prevention Program, while the intervention group received an additional five hours of experiential instruction on injury prevention content and counseling skills. Also enrolled in the study were families with infants of ages birth to 6 months; they were followed until the child was 12 to 18 months old. Analyses of the baseline and follow-up data showed that parents seen by residents in the intervention group received significantly more injury prevention counseling

on five of the six safety practices and that they were significantly more satisfied with the assistance the residents provided on safety topics.

The Roles of Key Stakeholders

Individual choices, **motivation**, knowledge, skills, and attitudes as well as organizational, economic, environmental, and social factors influence injury prevention behavior (Ross 1984). Therefore, the opportunity to prevent or reduce injury through interventions or policies can be shared among several groups. The key stakeholders who need to be involved in efforts to address the issue are described here.

Clinicians

Health care providers, including pediatricians, can incorporate injury prevention education into routine visits for adults and well-care visits for children and adolescents. To encourage the delivery of these services, health plans should reimburse for them and the National Committee for Quality Assurance should make injury prevention counseling a measured indicator of the quality of health plans. Clinicians can screen for alcohol problems, using one of many brief screening tools, and provide brief interventions designed to reduce problem drinking.

Safety centers can be established in health care settings serving children. Safety centers housed in settings such as hospitals work with parents and health care providers to answer questions, provide advice, and offer services and safety products (to test and to purchase at a low cost) in an effort to reduce unintentional injuries. Currently, there are approximately 40 safety centers around the country, such as the Johns Hopkins Children's Safety Center; therefore, health care settings need **incentives** to encourage the establishment of additional safety centers nationwide.[3]

Finally, clinicians can provide data to be used to monitor progress. For this to be feasible, the External Cause of Injury codes, or e-codes, need to be adopted universally and consistently. Clinicians can keep injury records and chart notes and follow up with patients who exhibit high injury risks.

Employers

Employers play a major a role in injury prevention through education and policies that affect their employees. Employers can, for instance, enforce strict policies against drinking and driving on the job, cell phone use and texting while driving, and workplace safety training. They can encourage a culture of safety and provide a safe place for their employees to work. Employers can have a comprehensive injury prevention plan that focuses on the injuries most common in their specific work environment. Employers must also know what to do if an injury occurs. This will give employees assurance that they will be cared for properly. Employers should also engage the health plan(s) offered to employees and evaluate current coverage for preventive health services, paying particular attention to injury prevention counseling.

Health Plans

Health plans are in a unique position to provide injury prevention education and activities for their members. They can require injury prevention counseling as part of routine visits for adults and well-care visits for children and adolescents; this can be accomplished by providing adequate reimbursement for counseling. Health plans can also focus efforts on physician compliance with counseling requirements. Injury prevention counseling can be a required component of child and adolescent well-care visits, yet it only takes place in about 15% of these visits (Rand et al. 2005).

Health plans can also address unintentional injury with a program similar to the disease management program, which would help to prevent or minimize the effect of injuries and to reduce health care service use and costs for preventable injuries. Disease management has become an increasingly popular method for addressing the needs of individuals with chronic diseases such as diabetes, asthma, coronary heart disease, hypertension, high risk pregnancy, and arthritis. The program is based on the idea that individuals who are educated on how to manage and control their conditions receive better care.

Health plans can also provide or subsidize the purchase of safety products and devices. This can be done by offering discounts or vouchers to their members for items including bicycle helmets and car safety seats. For instance, a health plan in a midwestern state offers to its members, as part of its injury prevention program, a 20% discount on safety items including helmets and padding for bicycles, inline skates, and scooters; athletic braces and supports; and life jackets at a particular sporting goods store. Similarly, in another midwestern state, a health plan offers a falls prevention and safety program, which includes a home risk assessment, follow-up support services, and up to $750 per year to be put toward home safety items that promote safety and injury prevention and encourage increased functioning.

Health plans can provide data to be used in monitoring and evaluation. Data can be used to monitor changes over time, with a focus specifically on the burden of unintentional injury (i.e., injury-related **morbidity** and **mortality**), quality of care, and health care costs.

Health Departments

Health departments are well positioned to build the support and develop the partnerships required for change (Frieden 2010; Friel et al. 2009). Health departments, at both state and local levels, can foster injury prevention by making injury a focal point in the public health and prevention programs in the community. Because injuries are the leading cause of preventable deaths from ages 1 to 44, health departments can play a critical role in establishing injury prevention programs as a regular part of the activities within noncommunicable disease prevention. Injury prevalence and risk factors should be a part of the health department's routine surveillance systems, and programs to reduce injuries can become a regular and expected function. Health departments, in collaboration with community partners, can sponsor fall prevention classes that feature exercise, balance training, medication review, and vision screening.

Policymakers

Epidemiology has shown us that injuries do not occur in isolation. The choices people make, the quality and design of environments, social interactions and family dynamics, alcohol, vehicles (and the roads they are driven on), housing construction, legislation and policy, and social norms contribute as determinants of injury and violence. Since risk taking is an important part of human development, our **goal** is not to eliminate risk, but rather to manage it and control it better. Individuals have some responsibility for this, but so do governments and society.

Policymakers are in a position to provide or support injury prevention legislation for their constituents and the broader community. Given their roles, policymakers can be educated about injury prevention so they can make wise decisions about proposed safety laws, policies, programs, and regulations or for strengthening the enforcement of existing laws. More specifically, legislation can be strengthened in many states to provide maximum safety for the public related to bicycle and motorcycle helmets, swimming pool fencing, prescription drug monitoring programs, and smoke alarms that use lithium batteries or are hardwired.

Conclusion: The Future of Injury Prevention and Behavioral Science

As the 21st century unfolds, public health is placing greater emphasis on the dissemination and implementation of effective injury prevention programs and policies, and on problem behaviors associated with motor vehicle travel, alcohol impaired and distracted driving, falls among older adults, drowning, and prescription drug overdose. Effective trauma care coverage will need to expand into rural and underserved areas to enhance trauma system care and coverage there.

One of the biggest challenges in the future will be to use behavioral science approaches to complement structural approaches and environmental change efforts that will facilitate the work of lawmakers and product designers to protect the public from unreasonable hazards. Behavioral science in the service of injury prevention has the same potential for impact as seen in the successful efforts to prevent tobacco use, increase exercise, and reduce risky sexual behavior. Unintentional injuries can no longer be considered "accidents." Evidence-based strategies to prevent injury that have been uncovered in the past half century need to be disseminated and widely adopted in the next half century. These are issues central to the behavioral sciences. If we can accept the fact that injuries are preventable, then we can apply effective policies and deliver effective programs that can save many more lives.

The burden of injury in the United States is great, yet it has only recently been recognized as an important public health problem. Most unintentional injuries have a strong behavioral component and can therefore be prevented. An ecological model can be used as a conceptual framework to address specific causes of injury. Although each injury mechanism has its own distinctive risk and protective factors, the levels of influence are **generalizable** across multiple injury causes and can be used to identify key determinants of individual injury problems. Identifying the levels of influence on injury risk and safety behaviors is a useful first step in building evidence-based prevention initiatives. Because the factors that contribute to the prevalence of injuries are numerous, multiple groups of stakeholders are necessary to implement interventions or policies for unintentional-injury prevention at the individual, family, and population levels.

Behavioral science can be used to encourage individual behavior change, engineer environments to make safer choices more likely, and contribute in major ways to changing social norms, such as decreasing public acceptance of texting and driving. Behavioral health can also contribute to changing policy that will save lives, such as strengthening regulations for the packaging of caustic substances, requiring helmet use for every cyclist, and shutting down "pill-mills" that contribute to prescription drug overdose. These opportunities to save lives result when behavioral science and public health work with those in law enforcement, product safety, and advocacy toward a common goal of community safety.

The challenges are many. First, we recognize that the injury crisis cannot be solved by public health alone. In order to address the problem comprehensively, we need parents, educators, governments, and **nongovernmental organizations** to assist. We also need to involve engineers, social workers, pediatricians, and developmental psychologists in our work and in our research to uncover everyday solutions. Playground and pool manufacturers, city planners, and architects can take an active interest in injury prevention, since prevention makes it less likely that victims will sue over an injury. Multiple key stakeholders must work together to widely disseminate the proven effective prevention strategies, assuring that we continue to evaluate their implementation and effectiveness under different conditions and with different populations. Second, we must continue advancing our basic understanding of injury causes where questions still remain and when new threats emerge. And finally, we must attend to surveillance needs at local, state, and national levels because routine, systematic data collection and monitoring remains a key to future reductions in injury.

NOTES

This chapter was supported by the Cooperative Agreement Number 5R49CE001507 from the Centers for Disease Control and Prevention. Its contents are solely the responsibility of the authors and do not necessarily represent the official views of the National Center for Injury Prevention and Control, or the U.S. Centers for Disease Control and Prevention.

1. For comprehensive reviews of evidence, see *The Guide to Community Preventive Services,* www.the communityguide.org (accessed Feb. 13, 2014); and Cochrane Collaboration reviews, http://injuries.cochrane .org/injuries-group-reviews (accessed Feb. 13, 2014).

2. *Oxford English Dictionary,* www.oxforddictionaries .com/us/definition/american_english/accident?q= accident, (accessed Feb. 13, 2014).

3. For more information on Johns Hopkins Children's Safety Centers, see www.jhsph.edu/injurycenter/practice /safety_centers/centers/safety_center (accessed Feb. 13, 2014).

REFERENCES

Allegrante JP, Hanson DW, Sleet DA, Marks R. 2010. Ecological approaches to the prevention of unintentional injuries. *Ital J Public Health* 7 (2): 24–31.

Baker S. 1992. *The Injury Fact Book.* New York: Oxford University Press.

Bonnie RJ, Fulco CE, Liverman CT, eds. 1999. *Reducing the Burden of Injury: Advancing Prevention and Treatment.* Institute of Medicine. Washington, DC: National Academy Press.

Butterfoss FD, Kegler MC, Francisco VT. 2008. Mobilizing organizations for health promotion: Theories of organizational change. In *Health Behavior and Health Education: Theory, Research, and Practice,* ed. K Glanz, BK Rimer, K Viswanath. 4th ed. San Francisco: Jossey-Bass.

Centers for Disease Control and Prevention (CDC). 2013a. Web-Based Injury Statistics Query and Reporting System (WISQARS). National Center for Injury Prevention and Control, www.cdc.gov/ncipc/ wisqars (accessed July 30, 2013).

———. 2013b. Web-Based Injury Statistics Query and Reporting System (WISQARS)—non-fatal injury report. National Center for Injury Prevention and Control. Available at www.cdc.gov/ncipc/wisqars (accessed July 30, 2013).

———. 2013c. Fast stats accidents or unintentional injuries. National Center for Health Statistics, www.cdc.gov/nchs/fastats/acc-inj.htm (accessed July 30, 2013).

Chang JT, Morton SC, Rubenstein L, et al. 2004. Interventions for the prevention of falls in older adults: Systematic review and meta-analysis of randomized clinical trials. *Br Med J* 328 (7441): 680-86.

Chen L, Baker S, Braver E, Li G. 2000. Carrying passengers as a risk factor for crashes fatal to 16- and 17-year-old drivers. *JAMA* 283 (12): 1578-82.

Chen L-H, Baker SP, Li G. 2006. Graduated driver licensing programs and fatal crashes of 16-year-old drivers: A national evaluation. *Pediatrics* 118 (1): 56-62.

Corso P, Finkelstein E, Miller T, Fiebelkorn I, Zaloshnja E. 2006. Incidence and lifetime costs of injuries in the United States. *Inj Prev* 12 (4): 212-18.

Davidson LL, Durkin MS, Kuhn L, O'Connor P, Barlow B, Heagarty MC. 1994. The impact of Safe Kids / Healthy Neighborhoods Injury Prevention Program in Harlem, 1988-1991. *Am J Public Health* 84 (4): 580-86.

Deroche T, Stephan Y, Castanier C, Brewer B, Le Scanff C. 2009. Social cognitive determinants of the intention to wear safety gear among adult in-line skaters. *Accident Anal Prev* 41 (5): 1064-69.

DiLillo D, Peterson L, Farmer JE. 2002. Injury and poisoning. In *Handbook of Clinical Health Psychology,* ed. T Boll. Washington, DC: American Psychological Association.

Doll LS, Bonzo S, Mercy JA, Sleet DA, eds. 2007. *Handbook of Injury and Violence Prevention.* New York: Springer.

Durkin M, Laraque D, Lubman I, Barlow B. 1999. Epidemiology and prevention of traffic injuries to urban children and adolescents. *Pediatrics* 103 (6): e74.

Elder RW, Voas R, Beirness D, et al. 2011. Task Force on Community Preventive services. Effectiveness of Ignition Interlocks for preventing alcohol-impaired driving and alcohol-related crashes. *Am J Prev Med* 40 (3) (March): 362-76.

Evans L. 2004. *Traffic Safety.* Bloomfield Hills, MI: Science Serving Society.

Farrow J. 1987. Young driver risk taking: A description of dangerous driving situations among 16-19-year-old drivers. *Int J Addiction* 22:1255-67.

Freire K, Runyan CW. 2006. Planning models: PRECEDE-PROCEED and Haddon Matrix. In *Injury and Violence Prevention: Behavioral Science Theories, Methods, and Applications,* ed. AC Gielen, DA Sleet, RJ DiClemente, 127-58. San Francisco: Jossey-Bass.

Frieden TR. 2010. A framework for public health action: The health impact pyramid. *Am J Public Health* 100 (4): 590-95.

Friel S, Bell R, Houweling T, Marmot M. 2009. Calling all Don Quixotes and Sancho Panzas 2009: Achieving the dream of global health equity through practical action on the social determinants of health. *Glob Health Promot* (suppl. 1), 9-13.

Gielen AC, McDonald EM, Gary TL, Bone LR. 2008. Using the PRECEDE-PROCEED model to apply health behavior theories. In *Health Behavior and Health Education: Theory, Research, and Practice,* ed. K Glanz, BK Rimer, K Viswanath, 407-33. 4th ed. San Francisco: Jossey-Bass.

Gielen AC, McDonald EM, McKenzie LB. 2012. Behavioral approaches. In *Injury Research,* ed. G Li, S Baker, chap. 39. New York: Springer.

Gielen A, McDonald E, Piver J. 2007. Fire and life safety education in US Fire Departments: Results of a national survey, final report to the home safety council. Johns Hopkins Center for Injury Research and Policy, Baltimore, MD.

Gielen AC, Sleet DA, DiClemente RJ, eds. 2006. *Injury and Violence Prevention: Behavioral Science Theories, Methods, and Applications.* San Francisco: Jossey-Bass.

Gielen AC, Sleet DA, Green LW. 2006. Community models and approaches for interventions. In *Injury and Violence Prevention: Behavioral Science Theories, Methods, and Applications,* ed. A Gielen, DA Sleet, RJ DiClemente, 65-82. San Francisco: Jossey-Bass.

Gielen A, Wilson M, McDonald E, et al. 2001. Randomized trial of enhanced anticipatory guidance for injury prevention. *Arch Pediatr Adolesc Med* 155 (1): 42-49.

Girasek D. 1999. How members of the public interpret the word accident. *Inj Prev* 5 (1): 19-25.

———. 2006. Health risk communication and injury prevention. In *Injury and Violence Prevention: Behavioral Science Theories, Methods, and Applications,* ed. A Gielen, DA Sleet, RJ DiClemente, 83-104. San Francisco: Jossey-Bass.

Girasek DC, Gielen AC. 2003. The effectiveness of injury prevention strategies: What does the public believe? *Health Educ Behav* 30 (3): 287-304.

Graham J. 1993. Injuries from traffic crashes: Meeting the challenge. *Annu Rev Public Health* 14 (1): 515-43.

Green LW, Kreuter M. 2005. *Health Program Planning: An Educational and Ecological Approach.* 4th ed. New York: McGraw-Hill.

Haddon W Jr. 1970. On the escape of tigers: An ecologic note. *Am J Public Health* 60 (12): 2229-34.

Hartling L, Wiebe N, Russell K, Petruk J, Spinola C, Klassen T. 2004. Graduated driver licensing for reducing motor vehicle crashes among young drivers. *Cochrane Database Syst Rev* 2:CD003300.

Hendrickson S, Becker H. 1998. Impact of a theory based intervention to increase bicycle helmet use in low income children. *Inj Prev* 4 (2): 126-31.

Holder H, Gruenewald P, Ponicki W, et al. 2000. Effect of community-based interventions on high-risk drinking and alcohol-related injuries. *JAMA* 284 (18): 2341-47.

Holder HD, Saltz RF, Grube JW, Voas RB, Gruenewald PJ, Treno AJ. 1997. A community prevention trial to reduce alcohol involved accidental injury and death: Overview. *Addiction* 92:S155-S171.

Ikeda, RM. 2010. Injury prevention and lifestyle medicine. *Am J Lifestyle Med* 4 (1): 5.

Isaacs SL, Schroeder SA. 2001. Where the public good prevailed: Lessons from success stories in health. *Am Prospect* 12 (10) (June 4): 26-30.

Johnson MA, Kimlin MG, Porter K. 2010. Vitamin D and injury prevention. *Am J Lifestyle Med* 4 (1): 21-24.

Johnson RM, Runyan CW, Coyne-Beasley T, Lewis MA, Bowling JM. 2008. Storage of household firearms: An examination of the attitudes and beliefs of married women with children. *Health Educ Res* 23 (4): 592-602.

Lajunen T, Rasanen M. 2004. Can social psychological models be used to promote bicycle helmet use among teenagers? A comparison of the Health Belief Model, Theory of Planned Behavior, and the Locus of Control. *J Safety Res* 35 (1): 115-23.

McClure RJ, Stevenson M, McEvoy S, eds. 2004. *The Scientific Basis of Injury Prevention and Control.* Melbourne, Australia: IP Communications.

McLeroy KR, Bibeau D, Steckler A, Glanz K. 1988. An ecological perspective on health promotion programs. *Health Educ Behav* 15 (4): 351-77.

Michael YL, Whitlock EP, Lin JS, Fu R, O'Connor EA, Gold R. 2010. Primary care-relevant interventions to prevent falling in older adults: A systematic evidence review for the US Preventive Services Task Force. *Ann Intern Med* 153 (12): 815-25.

National Center for Injury Prevention and Control (NCenIPC). 2006. *CDC Injury Fact Book.* Atlanta: Centers for Disease Control and Prevention.

National Committee for Injury Prevention and Control (NComIPC). 1989. *Injury Prevention: Meeting the Challenge.* New York: Oxford University Press.

National Highway Traffic Safety Administration, Fatality Analysis Reporting System (NHTSA). 2010. Traffic safety facts 2009. Available at www-nrd.nhtsa.dot.gov/Pubs/811402.pdf (accessed Feb. 13, 2014).

Parker MJ, Gillespie WJ, Gillespie LD. 2005. Hip protectors for preventing hip fractures in older people. *Cochrane Database Syst Rev* 3:CD001255.

Peterson L, Farmer J, Kashani J. 1990. Parental injury prevention endeavors: A function of health beliefs? *Health Psychol* 9 (2): 177-91.

Rand C, Auinger P, Klein J, Weitzman M. 2005. Preventive counseling at adolescent ambulatory visits. *J Adolesc Health* 37 (2): 87-93.

Ross H. 1984. *Deterring the Drinking Driver: Legal Policy and Social Control.* Lexington, MA: Health.

Rubenstein L. 2006. Falls in older people: Epidemiology, risk factors, and strategies for prevention. *Age Ageing* 35 (suppl. 2): ii37-ii41.

Rubenstein LZ, Josephson KR. 2006. Falls and their prevention in elderly people: What does the evidence show? *Med Clinics N Am* 90 (5): 807-24.

Shaw FE, Ogolla CP. 2006. Law, behavior, and injury prevention. In *Injury and Violence Prevention: Behavioral Science Theories, Methods, and Applications,* ed. A Gielen, DA Sleet, RJ DiClemente, 442-66. San Francisco: Jossey-Bass.

Shield J. 1997. Have we become so accustomed to being passive that we've forgotten how to be active? *Inj Prev* 3:243-44.

Shults RA, Elder RW, Sleet DA, et al. 2001. Reviews of evidence regarding interventions to reduce alcohol-impaired driving. *Am J Prev Med* 21 (4S): 66-88.

Simons-Morton B. 2007. Parent involvement in novice teen driving: Rationale, evidence of effects, and potential for enhancing graduated driver licensing effectiveness. *J Safety Res* 38 (2): 193-202.

Simons-Morton B, Hartos J, Beck K. 2003. Persistence of effects of a brief intervention on parental restrictions of teen driving privileges. *Inj Prev* 9 (2): 142-46.

———. 2004. Increased parent limits on teen driving: Positive effects from a brief intervention administered at the Motor Vehicle Administration. *Prev Science* 5 (2): 101-11.

Simons-Morton B, Hartos J, Leaf W, Preusser D. 2005. Persistence of effects of the Checkpoints program on parental restrictions of teen driving privileges. *Am J Public Health* 95 (3): 447-52.

———. 2006. The effects of the checkpoints program on parent-imposed driving limits and crash outcomes among Connecticut novice teen drivers at 6-months post-licensure. *J Safety Res* 37 (1): 9-15.

Simons-Morton B, McLeroy KR, Wendel ML 2012. *Behavior Theory in Health Promotion Practice and Research.* Burlington, MA: Jones & Bartnett Learning.

Simons-Morton B, Nansel T. 2006. The application of social cognitive theory to injury prevention. In *Injury and Violence Prevention: Behavioral Science Theories, Methods, and Applications,* ed. A Gielen, DA Sleet, RJ DiClemente, 41-64. San Francisco: Jossey-Bass.

Simons-Morton B, Ouimet M. 2006. Parent involvement in novice teen driving: A review of the literature. *Br Med J* 12 (suppl. 1): i30-i37.

Sleet DA, Baldwin G, Maar A, et al. 2012. History of injury and violence as public health problems and emergence of the National Center for Injury Prevention and Control at CDC. *J Safety Res* 43 (4): 233-48.

Sleet DA, Dahlberg L, Basavaraju SV, Mercy J, McGuire L, Greenspan A. 2011. Injury prevention, violence prevention, and trauma care: Building the scientific base in public health. *MMWR* 60, Oct. 7.

Sleet DA, Gielen AC. 1998. Injury prevention. In *Health Promotion Handbook,* ed. S Sheinfeld Gorin, J Arnold. St. Louis, MO: Mosby.

Sleet DA, Gielen AC. 2006. Injury prevention. In *Health Promotion in Practice*, ed. SS Gorin, J Arnold, 361-91. San Francisco: Jossey-Bass.

Sleet DA, Mercer S, Cole KH, Shults R, Elder R. 2011. Scientific evidence and policy change: Lowering the legal limit to .08 % in the USA. *Glob Health Promot* 18 (1): 23-26.

Sleet DA, Trifiletti LB, Gielen AC, Simons-Morton B. 2006. Individual-level behavior change models: Applications to injury prevention. In *Injury and Violence Prevention: Behavioral Science Theories, Methods, and Applications,* ed. A Gielen, DA Sleet, RJ DiClemente, 19-40. San Francisco: Jossey-Bass.

Smith L, Greene M, Singh H. 2002. Study of the effectiveness of the US safety standard for child resistant cigarette lighters. *Inj Prev* 8 (3): 192-96.

Sommers MS, Dyehouse JM, Howe SR, Fleming M, Fargo JD, Schafer JC. 2006. Effectiveness of brief interventions after alcohol-related vehicular injury: A randomized controlled trial. *J Trauma* 61 (3) (Sept.): 523-31.

Tinetti M, Baker D, King M, et al. 2008. Effect of dissemination of evidence in reducing injuries from falls. *N Engl J Med* 359 (3): 252-61.

Treno A, Holder H. 1997. Community mobilization: Evaluation of an environmental approach to local action. *Addiction* 92 (6s1): 173-88.

Trifiletti L, Gielen A, Sleet D, Hopkins K. 2005. Behavioral and social sciences theories and models: Are they used in unintentional injury prevention research? *Health Educ Res* 20 (3): 298-307.

Tung G, Vernick J, Reiney EV, Gielen AC. 2012. Legislator voting and behavioral science theory: A systematic review. *Am J Health Behav* 36 (6): 823-33.

Vanlaar W, Mayhew D, Marcoux K, Wets G, Brijs T, Shope J. 2009. An evaluation of graduated driver licensing programs in North America using a meta-analytic approach. *Accident Anal Prev* 41 (5): 1104-11.

White K, Hyde M. 2010. Swimming between the flags: A preliminary exploration of the influences on Australians' intentions to swim between the flags at patrolled beaches. *Accident Anal Prev* 42 (6): 1831-38.

Williams A, Ferguson S. 2002. Rationale for graduated licensing and the risks it should address. *Inj Prev* 8 (suppl. 2): ii9-ii16.

Wu S, Keeler EB, Rubenstein L, Maglione MA, Shekelle PG. 2010. A cost-effectiveness analysis of a proposed national falls prevention program. *Clin Geriatr Med* 26 (4) (Nov.): 751-66.

Zaza S, Sleet DA, Shults RA, et al. 2005. Reducing injuries to motor vehicle occupants. In *The Guide to Community Preventive Services: What Works to Promote Health?* ed. S Zaza, P Briss, K Harris, 329-84. New York: Oxford University Press.

CHAPTER 16

Workplace Injury
and Behavior Change

KESHIA POLLACK AND MARIA BULZACCHELLI

LEARNING OBJECTIVES

After completing the chapter, the reader will be able to

* Review the epidemiology and costs of the leading fatal and nonfatal occupational injuries in the United States.
* Define the key determinants of occupational injury within the framework of an ecological model.
* Recognize common theoretical approaches to preventing occupational injury, and provide examples of effective interventions.
* Describe the behavioral aspects of engineering and technological interventions and of administrative or policy interventions.
* Identify key stakeholders and explain how each plays a role in preventing occupational injuries.

Introduction

Workplace, or occupational, safety calls for a multidisciplinary approach to the recognition, diagnosis, treatment, and prevention of adverse health effects resulting from hazardous conditions in the workplace (Levy et al. 2006). The field of occupational safety is broad and includes perspectives from occupational medicine and nursing, occupational health psychology, epidemiology, injury prevention and control, health education, ergonomics, sociology, economics, and engineering. Each of these disciplines has an integral role in ensuring safe workplaces, and together they provide the foundation for a comprehensive approach to workplace safety.

The Centers for Disease Control and Prevention (CDC) cited improvements in workplace safety as one of the "ten great public health achievements" in the period 1900 to 1999 (CDC 1999). Through epidemiological research, behavioral analysis, development of safety programs, employee training, enforcement, and policy formulation and implementation, workplaces became safer and fewer workers were injured or killed. These improvements were accomplished in large part by modifying the work environment through comprehensive strategies that included well-implemented policies and programs. Modifying the workplace to foster safe working conditions can allow employees to exercise safe behaviors more readily during work activities.

One of the major **goals** in the field of occupational safety is protecting and improving the health and safety of workers by preventing fatal and disabling traumatic injuries (Brunette 2006). Workplace safety hazards result in traumatic injury through the sudden uncontrolled transfer of energy (kinetic, electrical, thermal, chemical, or nuclear) to the human body. Examples include working with unprotected electrical sources, working at certain elevations without fall protection, and working in highway construction zones. These safety risks are common and contribute to the estimated 3 million work-related injuries that occur annually in the United States. The **consequences** of occupational injuries are significant and include death and disability, lost productivity and wages, costs to the medical system, and psychological distress. Workers in all industries and occupations are at risk of sustaining work-related injuries; however, certain segments of the workforce, including women, older adults, and Hispanics are disproportionately affected by occupational injury.

Although injuries occur in many settings outside the workplace (e.g., home, community, schools), workplaces are a key environment for injury prevention. Based on data from the 2011 American Time Use Survey, Americans spend on average more waking hours working than doing any other activity in a given 24-hour period (USDL 2011, table A.1). Therefore, while understanding the full spectrum of settings

where injuries occur is important, equally important is **targeting** workplaces, owing to the significant time that is spent there. Moreover, workers are assured safe working conditions as established by the Occupational Safety and Health Act of 1970, which created a "statutory general duty [for employers] to provide a safe and healthful workplace" (OSHA 1970).

Workplace safety extends beyond an injury-free job setting. It also includes the identification, **evaluation**, and control of hazardous work situations, as well as mitigating risks related to developing work-related illnesses. However, as described by Brunette, a scholar in the workplace safety field, data on injuries provide a clear understanding of outcomes of hazardous or unsafe workplaces (Brunette 2006). Therefore, an investigation of occupational injuries is a good indicator of a workplace's level of safety, insofar as injuries are unlikely to occur in safe settings.

Magnitude

Each year in the United States, nearly 3 million workers are injured and approximately 4,700 workers die as a result of work-related incidents (BLS 2008-11a, 2008-11b). The social and economic costs associated with occupational injuries are staggering. The most comprehensive study of the cost of both fatal and nonfatal occupational injuries estimates that these injuries carry a total cost of $132.8 billion, including direct costs of $38.4 billion and indirect costs of $94.3 billion (Leigh et al. 2000). **Direct costs** include medical expenses, such as those incurred for hospital and physician care and for drugs, along with health insurance administration costs. **Indirect costs** include lost wages, the cost of fringe benefits, lost home production, and the costs of retraining and workplace disruption. These direct and indirect impacts affect workers who are injured, their family members, and their employers, as well as consumers via higher prices for commercial products and taxpayers via higher Medicare, Medicaid, and Social Security costs.

The distribution of injuries across industries differs for fatal and nonfatal incidents (tables 16.1 and 16.2). According to the U.S. Bureau of Labor Statistics (BLS), transportation and warehousing; construction; and agriculture, forestry, fishing, and hunting account for the largest numbers of occupational fatalities, whereas, health care and social assistance, manufacturing, and retail trade account for the largest numbers of nonfatal injuries (BLS 2008-11a, 2008-11b). The risk of work-related death also differs by industry. For example, the risk of death in 2011 in the agriculture, forestry, fishing, and hunting industry was seven times as high as the overall rate for all workers, and the risk of death was almost five times as high in the mining industry as for workers overall. Most occupational fatalities in private industry result from transportation incidents (41% of all deaths), contact with objects and equipment (16%), falls (15%), and assaults and violent acts (15%) (BLS 2008-11a). As displayed in table 16.3, different industries have different types of hazards; in construction, the leading hazard is falls; in manufacturing, it is contact with objects and equipment; and in retail trade, assaults and violent acts cause the most deaths.

Nonfatal injuries are more frequent than fatal injuries and may lead to costly medical care, lost work time, and disability. Nearly 34% of all workers who sustain an occupational injury are treated in emergency departments. Most of these injuries result from sprains or strains, lacerations, and contusions. Among all occupational injuries that lead to lost workdays, workers lose an average of six days after sustaining a nonfatal injury (Castillo et al. 2006). This lost work time affects workers, who may lose salary during that time, and employers, who may have to train another employee to replace the injured worker or lose income the injured worker might have generated.

Key Determinants

An **ecological model** displaying the specific factors that influence the risk of occupational injury is presented in figure 16.1, which highlights the numerous factors, at multiple **levels of influence**, affecting workplace safety.

Individual

The first level of influence, the **individual level**, identifies biological and personal history factors that increase the likelihood of experiencing a workplace injury. Some of these factors, including age and experience, gender, race and ethnicity, and health status, are discussed below.

AGE AND EXPERIENCE

The risk of any occupational injury generally decreases with increasing age; however, the risk of fatal injuries is significantly elevated for older workers as compared with younger workers (BLS 2008-11a; Layne and Pollack 2004). This pattern is thought to reflect both the decreasing injury risk associated with increasing experience and time on the job and the decreased ability of older workers to survive an injury. In contrast, younger workers are most at risk for nonfatal injury. Nonfatal injury rates are highest for teen workers and generally decrease with increasing age. However, injury prevalence among older workers is increasing as they are remaining in the workforce for longer periods of time (Castillo et al. 2006).

Separating the influence of age from that of experience is difficult. Most injuries occur among employees with less than one year of service with a particular employer (Castillo et al. 2006). Being new in a job is a risk for injury regardless of the total time that a worker is employed with a company (Pollack, Agnew, et al. 2007). Seasonal employment, such as commercial fishing, agriculture, and construction, introduces additional risks related to experience, further complicating this issue. For example,

TABLE 16.1. Fatal occupational injuries, U.S., 2011

Rank	Industry	Total fatalities	Rate per 100,000 full-time workers
1	Transportation and warehousing	749	15.3
2	Construction	738	9.1
3	Agriculture, forestry, fishing and hunting	566	24.9
4	Management, administrative, and waste services	359	6.4
5	Manufacturing	327	2.2
6	Retail trade	268	1.9
7	Wholesale trade	190	4.9
8	Other services, except public administration	183	3.0
9	Mining, quarrying, and oil and gas extraction	155	15.9
10	Accommodation and food services	138	1.7
11	Health care and social assistance	117	0.7
12	Arts, entertainment, and recreation	93	3.9
13	Professional, scientific, and technical services	74	0.8
14	Real estate and rental and leasing	62	2.5
15	Information	56	1.9
16	Utilities	39	4.2
17	Educational services	37	1.0
18	Finance and insurance	36	0.6
	Total private industry[a]	4,188	3.7
	Government	505	2.2
	All Workers	4,693	3.5

Sources: BLS 2008-11a, 2008-11b.

[a]Total private industry is greater than the sum of the individual industry totals due to rounding.

[b]Of these 3 million cases, 94.8% are injuries, 5.2% are illnesses.

during the commercial fishing season, nonresidents of Alaska travel to the state for lucrative, high-risk work opportunities, thereby increasing rates of injury during these times.

GENDER

Over the past few decades, the participation of women in the paid workforce has increased steadily and dramatically; women currently

TABLE 16.2. Nonfatal occupational injuries and illnesses, U.S., 2011

Rank	Industry	Total recordable cases	Rate per 100 full-time workers
1	Health care and social assistance	631,100	5.0
2	Manufacturing	502,700	4.4
3	Retail trade	424,600	3.9
4	Accommodation and food services	278,600	3.9
5	Transportation and warehousing	193,200	5.0
6	Construction	190,200	3.9
7	Wholesale trade	171,200	3.2
8	Administrative and support and waste management and remediation services	121,900	2.7
9	Other services, except public administration	73,800	2.6
10	Professional, scientific, and technical services	70,000	1.0
11	Arts, entertainment, and recreation	54,500	4.5
12	Real estate and rental and leasing	48,700	3.0
13	Agriculture, forestry, fishing and hunting	48,300	5.5
14	Finance and insurance	41,200	0.8
15	Information	37,900	1.6
16	Educational services	37,500	2.1
17	Management of companies and enterprises	24,400	1.4
18	Utilities	19,300	3.5
19	Mining	17,200	2.2
	Total private industry[b]	2,986,500	3.5
	State and local government	820,900	5.7

account for 47% of the paid labor force in the United States (BLS 2009). Although earlier studies found that women sustained fewer and less severe injuries at work than did men, studies that account for the differential participation of women and men across occupations and industries actually show higher injury rates for women than for men (Berkowitz 1979; BLS

TABLE 16.3. Fatal occupational injuries by industry and event or exposure, in private industry, United States, 2011

	Total fatalities	Violence and other injuries by persons or animals	Transportation incidents	Fires and explosions	Falls, slips, trips	Exposure to harmful substances or environments	Contact with objects and equipment
Transportation and warehousing	749	57	576	5	27	26	58
Construction	738	32	197	11	262	112	122
Agriculture, forestry, fishing and hunting	566	34	278	14	37	45	154
Management, administrative, and waste services	359	39	107	7	96	48	62
Manufacturing	327	34	83	30	49	40	91
Retail trade	268	135	70	5	24	12	21
Wholesale trade	190	17	88	15	18	10	42
Other services, except public administration	183	61	38	9	17	15	43
Mining, quarrying, and oil and gas extraction	155	7	66	13	13	10	46
Accommodation and food services	138	80	24	2	13	11	8
Health care and social assistance	117	37	37	—	18	19	4
Arts, entertainment, and recreation	93	14	43	—	13	10	13
Professional, scientific, and technical services	74	20	31	6	8	5	4
Real estate and rental and leasing	62	29	20	—	6	3	4
Information	56	9	23	—	15	4	5
Utilities	39	5	10	—	7	10	6
Educational services	37	8	22	—	4	—	1
Finance and insurance	36	20	12	—	3	—	—
Totals	4,187	638	1,725	117	630	380	684
Overall Percentage		15.2	41.2	2.8	15.0	9.1	16.3

Source: U.S. Department of Labor, Bureau of Labor Statistics, in cooperation with state, New York City, District of Columbia, and Federal agencies, Census of Fatal Occupational Injuries, April 25, 2013.

2008-11a, 2008-11b, 2009; Casteel and Peek-Asa 2000; Castillo et al. 2006; Chelius 1979; Cox and Cox 1991; Faulkner et al. 2001; IOM and Committee 2000; Islam et al. 2001; Layne and Pollack 2004; Leigh et al. 2000; Lincoln and Lucas 2010; Mearns and Flin 1999; NIOSH 1993, 2009-10a; OSHA 1970; Pollack et al. 2007; Saleh et al. 2001; Smitha et al. 2001; Taiwo et al. 2009; Thomas et al. 2001; Warner et al. 1998; Welch et al. 2000).

There are also specific injury risks to women in industries that historically have been female-dominated. By far, the leading causes of injuries to health care workers, where most employees are women, are back injury and violence. Among all occupations, hospital and nursing home workers have the highest number of occupational back injuries resulting in lost workdays. According to Castillo and co-workers (2006), the health care industry also has the highest inci-

dence of nonfatal workplace assaults, and the patient was the perpetrator in 51% of cases.

RACE AND ETHNICITY

Data on race and ethnicity is limited because these descriptors are not regularly captured in many injury **surveillance** systems. Among the studies that have explored racial and ethnic differences in injury rates, white workers generally have the highest injury rate, though the reason for this is unclear, and Hispanic workers in the United States have a higher injury-related fatality rate (Castillo et al. 2006; Friedman and Forst 2008). This higher fatality rate among Hispanics may be explained by their employment in high risk jobs, such as construction, and inadequate training and knowledge of safety hazards because of language barriers and low literacy levels (Castillo et al. 2006).

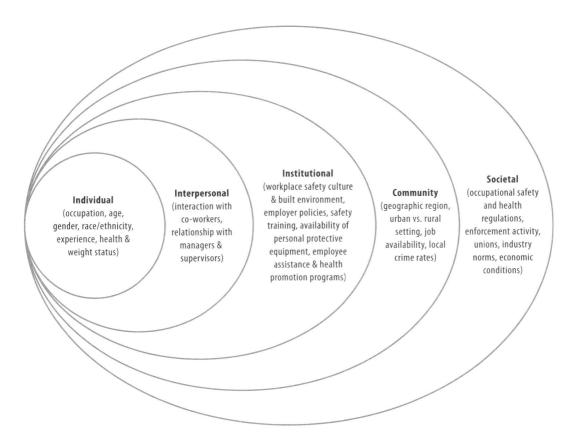

FIGURE 16.1. A conceptual framework of the factors influencing worker safety behavior

FOREIGN BIRTH

Some researchers have found that, compared to U.S.-born workers, foreign-born workers tend to work in industries and occupations with higher rates of fatal and nonfatal injury, probably because of lower levels of education and English-language ability (Orrenius and Zavodny 2009). Three occupation groups in the United States— transportation, construction, and agriculture— have both the highest rates of occupational fatalities *and* the highest proportions of immigrant workers (Schenker 2010). Other researchers have found that regardless of health insurance status, foreign-born workers report lower rates of non-fatal work-related injuries than do U.S.-born workers, possibly related to the tendency for foreign-born workers to have lower education levels or to avoid reporting nonfatal injuries (Zhang et al. 2009). Underreporting of injuries is believed to be very high in immigrant workers because of fears of deportation.

HEALTH STATUS

Several **health behaviors** and health conditions affect occupational injury rates (Pollack and Cheskin 2007; Pollack, Sorock, et al. 2007; Schulte et al. 2008). Research has also supported an increased risk of injury related to medication use, in particular, some specific medications (e.g., antihistamines, antibiotics) (Gilmore et al. 1996; Voaklander et al. 2009). Increased risk of injury related to medication use is alarming especially because an estimated 34% of U.S. adults are obese (Wang et al. 2008). Likely, many of these obese individuals may be taking medications for obesity-related **comorbidities**, which may also increase the risk of occupational injury.

Institutional and Organizational Factors

Institutional and **organizational factors** affect injury risk primarily through the workplace safety culture and climate, which are two distinct but related terms. *Safety climate* reflects employees' perceptions, **attitudes**, and beliefs about risk and safety (Cox and Cox 1991; Mearns and Flin 1999). *Safety culture,* a broader concept, has to do with the values, **norms**, assumptions, and **expectations** regarding safety. A company's safety culture "can be seen though management safety practices . . . reflected in the workplace safety climate" (Mearns and Flin 1999, 5).

A positive safety culture or climate is thought to influence safety behaviors by maximizing employee **motivation** and improving safety knowledge, which, in turn, improves employee **compliance**, thereby resulting in safer behaviors and fewer injuries. Workplace safety policies may also create a strong workplace safety culture or climate. For instance, workplace policies that affect production design and make work less hazardous from the beginning may create a positive safety climate, which may reduce the risk and occurrence of injury.

Community Factors

This next level explores how settings including the social and physical environment and employment opportunities affect injury risk.

SOCIAL ENVIRONMENT

Certain community factors are correlated with the risk of occupational injuries. For instance, several studies have explored the influence of the social and physical environment on injuries related to convenience store robbery. Research supports a strong association of the environment surrounding convenience stores (e.g., degree of social disorder and urbanization, property value of adjacent buildings, presence of vacant structures) with robbery and risk of injury (Casteel and Peek-Asa 2000; Faulkner et al. 2001; NIOSH 1993).

EMPLOYMENT OPPORTUNITIES

Community conditions may also influence access to job choices. In certain parts of the country, where a particular industry is the dominant employer, the risks of workplace injury associated with that industry might be increased. In Alaska, for instance, fishing is one of the biggest industries and many individuals are employed as crew members, deckhands, and fish processors; work-related injury rates are particularly high there because those occupations are quite dangerous (Lincoln and Lucas 2010; NIOSH 2009–10a; Thomas et al. 2001).

Societal Factors

Finally, broad social factors, such as policies and economic conditions, may also contribute to an increased risk of occupational injury.

LAWS AND REGULATIONS

Federal and state occupational safety and health (OSH) regulations aim to prevent injury by setting standards for workplace environments and equipment; by requiring employers to establish safety programs, install protective devices, and provide training; and by requiring workers to follow safety precautions. State workers' compensation insurance laws can create **incentives** for safety by increasing the costs to employers when workers are injured. For example, states can structure their workers' compensation systems in such a way that firms with more injury claims pay higher insurance premiums.

ENFORCEMENT ACTIVITY

Enforcement of OSH regulations through inspections, citations for violations, and penalties is necessary for these regulations to prevent injuries. If safety measures always resulted in a cost savings for employers, there would be little need for enforcement activity. Because compliance with OSH regulations often means higher costs for firms, the threat of being penalized for safety violations can motivate employers to comply with the regulations. In addition to issuing citations for violations, regulatory agencies may also reduce occupational injury rates by providing compliance assistance and consultation.

ECONOMIC CONDITIONS

Fluctuations in the economy may affect occupational injury rates by changing production pressures and trends in worker characteristics (Chelius 1979; Smitha et al. 2001). Workers under production pressures may work longer hours than usual. In addition, if safer work practices take more time than riskier practices do, workers under pressure may be more likely to take risks to save time. During economic upswings, the unemployment rate tends to be low, which may increase production pressures and bring younger, more inexperienced workers into the workforce, increasing the injury rate (Berkowitz 1979; Chelius 1979; Smitha et al. 2001). On the other hand, higher wages and the difficulty of replacing or substituting for injured workers during times of low unemployment may increase the true cost of injury, providing employers with an incentive to invest in safety (Smitha et al. 2001).

Long-term economic shifts also affect employment in ways that could have implications for occupational injury. In the middle to late 20th century, the U.S. economy shifted from manufacturing toward the service sector, which led to the loss of millions of manufacturing jobs and reductions in wages (IOM and Committee 2000). This transition resulted in more individuals working multiple jobs and an increase in independent contractors, contingent workers, and part-time workers. It is difficult to characterize exposure to workplace hazards for these employment categories, because they are inadequately captured by our current data systems.

Evidence-Based Interventions

Because the factors that influence the risk of workplace injury involve many different aspects of the job, including characteristics of the worker, the workplace, the broader community, and the policy **context**, **interventions** addressing any of these factors could potentially prevent workplace injuries. Ideally, interventions should focus on the factors with the greatest promise of prevention. Theories on workplace safety and evidence of **effectiveness** from empirically tested interventions guide the development of new interventions. This section presents some common theoretical approaches to preventing occupational injury and discusses the effectiveness of several specific interventions.

Theoretical Approaches to Occupational Injury Prevention

Perhaps the most commonly used theoretical approach to workplace safety is the Hierarchical Approach to Occupational Injury Prevention, also known as the safety hierarchy (Barnett and Brickman 1986). This safety hierarchy prioritizes the most passive interventions that have the greatest potential to reduce exposure to a hazard. Purely **passive interventions** do not rely on individual workers to protect themselves. In contrast, active interventions require individuals to actively *do something* in order to protect themselves (most interventions are neither purely active nor passive, but lie on a continuum with some aspects of both). Ideal interventions eliminate the hazard altogether. For example, redesigning production processes to use less hazardous material or fewer hazardous methods is the preferred approach, because it eliminates the hazard rather than asking workers to avoid it or protect themselves against it. When a hazard cannot be eliminated completely, minimizing worker exposure to the hazard via engineering controls—a relatively passive intervention—is the next-best option. Training workers and providing them with personal protective equipment are active interventions that rely on individual workers to protect themselves and are the strategies that are *least likely* to afford the needed protection.

Although focusing on worker behavior is the lowest level of the safety hierarchy, it is often necessary, because eliminating hazards from work processes and reducing exposure to haz-

ards through engineering are not always possible. Many theoretical models are useful for explaining health and safety behavior and could therefore be helpful in developing occupational injury prevention interventions (Gielen et al. 2006). One general approach to behavior change that has been used in occupational safety is applied behavior analysis, known as behavior-based safety (BBS) when it is applied to injury prevention (Geller 2006). BBS is based on the idea that people perform a particular behavior because of the consequences they expect will result from that behavior. According to this **theory**, behavior can be motivated by using rewards or punishments that consistently follow an activator, or *signal,* to perform a certain behavior. Worker behavior can then be influenced by making the consequences of that behavior predictable and using activators that prompt safe behavior. The **PRECEDE-PROCEED** model (see chapter 5) has been used widely in workplace injury prevention to identify **determinants** that predispose, enable, and reinforce safe behavior (e.g., Bertera, 1991; Brosseau et al. 2002; Dedobbeleer et al. 1990; Dejoy et al. 1995).

Just as general approaches to influencing worker behavior exist, so do general approaches to identifying workplace hazards in the first place. Systems Safety Analysis is an approach derived from the field of safety engineering. Relevant to this discussion is the job safety analysis (JSA). In a JSA, a team consisting of the worker, the supervisor, and workplace safety specialists performs an in-depth examination of the job, scrutinizing each element to identify hazards (Keyserling 2006). This approach has the potential to identify and address hazards before injuries occur. As with BBS, this approach can be applied to any type of job in any industry.

Effectiveness of Tested Occupational Injury Prevention Interventions

Occupational injury prevention interventions are often grouped into four categories: engineering and technological interventions that target the physical work environment, administrative and policy interventions, educational and behavioral interventions, and multifaceted interventions combining two or more of these approaches (Zwerling et al. 1997). Each of these approaches involves a behavioral element in some way. Engineering solutions require that employers, and sometimes workers, adopt the solutions and use them appropriately. Policy interventions aim to influence employer and worker behavior either directly, by requiring use of certain types of equipment or protocols, or indirectly, by creating incentives for safety. Educational interventions aim to increase safety knowledge, improve attitudes about safety, and ultimately influence safety behavior. Therefore, the benefits of policy changes and new technologies will be realized only if employers adopt them and if workers use safety equipment properly and comply with safety policies and practices.

Numerous interventions of all types—engineering, administrative, educational, and multifaceted—have been developed and implemented, but few of them have been rigorously evaluated for their effectiveness in preventing occupational injury. Nevertheless, some trends are apparent. The remainder of this section presents select evidence of effectiveness of interventions from each of these four categories.

ENGINEERING AND TECHNOLOGICAL INTERVENTIONS

Environmental modifications and engineering solutions are widely accepted as being among the most effective ways to prevent occupational injuries. However, surprisingly few of these interventions have been studied carefully.

One of the best examples of a proven effective engineering intervention is rollover protective structures (ROPS) on tractors. Reynolds and Groves (2000) looked at 14 studies that evaluated the effectiveness of ROPS. They concluded that most fatalities occurred from rollovers of tractors without ROPS and that when

fatalities did involve tractors with ROPS, the farmers operating the tractors were not wearing seatbelts. Furthermore, they reported that in Europe, rollover fatalities have decreased to almost zero as implementation of ROPS has increased. In this review, Reynolds and Groves also discussed eight studies of ROPS implementation. Surveys of ROPS use indicated that a low percentage (about 50%) of tractors in the United States had ROPS and that older tractors and tractors used in low-clearance areas were especially likely to be without ROPS. Even among tractors built after 1985, 38%-45% did not have ROPS, either because they never were installed or because they had been removed. This example highlights not only the importance of developing effective technologies and the potential impact of passive interventions, but also the need for behavioral interventions aimed at swaying employers to adopt these technologies and to reinforce the use of complementary safety precautions, such as wearing seatbelts in this case.

Promising technologies have also been developed for preventing needlestick injuries in health care workers. These technologies generally take the form of safety devices. Needle protective devices and specialized needles can substantially reduce the risk of needlestick injuries that occur during certain health care procedures (Rogers and Goodno 2000; Trim and Elliott 2003). As with ROPS, the overall effectiveness of these types of interventions will depend on the degree to which health care workers adopt the technologies, and this may depend largely on policies set by health care administrators.

Not all engineering interventions have been effective in preventing occupational injury. The degree of effectiveness of an engineering intervention depends on its ease of use. For example, the evidence consistently indicates that back belts have no effect on the incidence of episodes of back pain (Tveito et al. 2004). The evidence also indicates that lumbar supports are not effective in preventing back pain (Linton and van Tulder 2001), with the possible exception of a subgroup of workers at high risk for low back pain who may benefit from lumbar supports (van Poppel et al. 2004). The lack of effectiveness of these interventions may be due in part to incorrect or inconsistent use of these devices. In contrast, some evidence shows that ergonomic interventions such as new chairs, arm supports, and alternative-design keyboards and pointing devices can improve musculoskeletal symptoms (Dejoy et al. 1995; Driessen et al. 2010; Kennedy et al. 2010). Perhaps these products are used correctly more consistently because, once they are in place, the worker doesn't have to remember to use them.

ADMINISTRATIVE AND POLICY INTERVENTIONS

Administrative interventions may be regulatory actions by federal, state, or local governments or workplace-level policies set by employers. Any of these interventions may prescribe certain equipment specifications and safety behaviors or may create incentives for safety. Enforcement of policies is essential for their effectiveness.

Evidence of the effectiveness of merely introducing a new OSH regulation is mixed (Tompa et al. 2007). In evaluations of specific OSH standards, some studies show reductions in injuries after introduction of a new standard (Lipscomb et al. 2003; Suruda et al. 2002), but other studies show no effect (Bulzacchelli et al. 2007). Similarly, evidence is mixed on the general deterrence effect of the *threat* of being inspected by regulators. However, in firms that have *actually* been cited or penalized for safety violations, strong evidence supports a specific deterrence effect, meaning that inspections significantly reduce injury frequency or severity if enforced (Tompa et al. 2007). Thus, regulations without direct enforcement are unlikely to bring about substantial reductions in injuries. Enhancing enforcement efforts to increase the number of firms actually inspected may help in reducing injury rates.

Regulatory agencies may also attempt to reduce occupational injury rates through voluntary means such as providing compliance assistance and consultation to firms to help them improve safety. However, little research has examined the effectiveness of this approach, and the existing evidence is mixed (Baggs et al. 2003; Conway and Svenson 1998; Tompa et al. 2007). State workers' compensation laws appear to be a more promising way to encourage employers to voluntarily improve safety. Evidence shows that workers' compensation insurance systems that use experience rating (setting a firm's insurance premium based on its past claims activity or injury experience) are associated with lower accident rates and injury frequency (Tompa et al. 2007).

Whereas the kinds of occupational safety and health policies described above are commonly directed at employer behavior, workplace-level policies aim to influence the behavior of individual workers. As with all of the types of interventions discussed above, few studies have evaluated the effectiveness of workplace-level safety policies. Some evidence shows that workplace policies requiring the use of particular types of eye protection reduce the frequency of occupational eye injuries, but serious methodological limitations of the studies evaluating these policies make their results questionable (Lipscomb 2000; Wong 1997). Another example is the zero-lift policy, which is common in many hospitals and nursing homes. A zero-lift policy is designed to reduce the risk of injury by promoting mechanical lifting instead of manual lifting, transferring, and repositioning of patients. Evaluations of these policies have shown significant declines in traumatic back injury events and injury claims after the policies were implemented (Charney et al. 2006; Collins et al. 2004).

Although controversial because of privacy concerns, workplace drug-testing programs may be effective in reducing occupational injury rates. Workplace drug and alcohol testing may be accomplished randomly or nonrandomly. Nonrandom testing may include periodic, "for cause," or postaccident testing. Some evidence shows that various types of drug or alcohol testing programs can reduce injuries both in the short term and in the long term, with perhaps the strongest evidence supporting the effectiveness of mandatory random testing (Brady et al. 2009; Cashman et al. 2009; Kraus 2001; van der Molen et al. 2007; Wickizer et al. 2004). Such drug-testing policies have the potential to reduce injuries in a wide range of occupational settings, because alcohol and drug use are risk factors for all types of injuries.

EDUCATIONAL AND BEHAVIORAL INTERVENTIONS

One of the most commonly used educational interventions in the workplace is safety training. Training methods range from lectures, videos, and written materials, to interactive computer-based instruction, to more engaging methods including simulation and hands-on practice. Evidence shows that each of these methods can improve safety behaviors in some work settings; safety knowledge and injury rates tend to improve with increasingly engaging training methods (Burke et al. 2006; DeRoo and Rautiainen 2000; Hartling et al. 2004; Johnston et al. 1994).

The effectiveness of training seems to be more limited in certain work settings and for preventing certain types of injuries. For example, the effectiveness of training is uncertain in agricultural settings. Although some evidence shows that general farm safety education programs can increase knowledge and improve attitudes and **self-reported** behavior of farm workers (DeRoo and Rautiainen RH. 2000; Hartling et al. 2004), other studies have found no evidence that educational interventions in the form of training by occupational safety and health professionals or peers actually reduce injury rates on farms (Rautiainen et al. 2008). One specific area where the results have been mixed is in tractor safety training (Hartling et al. 2004), possibly because engineering solutions are more effective in preventing tractor-related injuries. Educational interventions aimed at increasing the use of engineering measures, such as ROPS on tractors, may be effective if farmers can afford the cost of adopting the technology.

Evidence consistently shows that education and training alone are not effective in preventing low back pain, despite some trainings involving as many as five sessions (Kennedy et al. 2010; Linton and van Tulder 2001; Tullar et al. 2010; Tveito et al. 2004; van Poppel et al. 2004). Although education alone may not work, other behavioral interventions can be effective in preventing low back pain. Some evidence shows that exercise (specifically to strengthen the back muscles) may reduce low back pain when done regularly for several weeks (Barnett and Brickman 1986; Linton and van Tulder 2001; Tullar et al. 2010; Tveito et al. 2004).

Incentives can enhance the effectiveness of educational interventions. Interventions that include incentives (**reinforcement**), which may be financial or other types of rewards, can motivate workers to perform certain safety behaviors. For example, **positive reinforcement** in the form of praise from a supervisor for wearing eye protection can reduce the rate of workplace eye injuries (Lipscomb 2000). Similarly, a review of workplace-based interventions to increase safety belt use found that while all of the interventions reviewed (most of them educational) increased safety belt use, interventions with incentives had a larger effect on safety belt use than those without incentives (Segui-Gomez 2000).

Another workplace intervention that incorporates an educational and behavioral approach is an **Employee Assistance Program (EAP)**. EAPs typically provide screening, assessments, and referrals for brief intervention and outpatient counseling to assist employees and their family members with a variety of personal issues (USDHHS 2000). Issues such as stress, substance abuse, mental health problems, financial strain, and family troubles may negatively affect job performance and may also create hazardous situations in the workplace. For example, women and men who are experiencing intimate partner violence (IPV), which is usually considered a domestic problem, have described being harassed or stalked at work (CAEPV 2002-11). Such **"spillover"** of personal problems into the workplace can put both the affected employee and the employee's co-workers at risk for injury. Many companies rely heavily on EAPs to address IPV among their employees (Lindquist et al. 2010). Thus, EAPs may help prevent injury related to IPV and other personal issues. Approximately 58% of all U.S. employers currently provide EAP services, which women utilize more often than men (Galinsky et al. 2008). Increased implementation of EAPs, along with efforts to make this resource known to all workers, may increase worker EAP utilization rates and prevent some types of injuries in the workplace (Pollack, Austin, et al. 2010; Pollack, McKay, et al. 2010).

MULTIFACETED INTERVENTIONS

Given the inherent limitations of each type of intervention—engineering, administrative, and educational—multifaceted interventions that combine two or more of these approaches may have the best chance of reducing occupational injury rates. The small body of work evaluating the effectiveness of such multifaceted interventions seems to support this idea. In a review of evaluations of farm safety interventions, DeRoo and Rautiainen (2000) found that multifaceted interventions combining safety audits and environmental modifications, with or without financial incentives or education, improved injury incidence, workers' compensation claims, safety behavior (including making engineering or equipment changes), or training provided for workers. Similarly, some evidence supports the effectiveness of multifaceted programs to prevent occupational eye injuries. Interventions combining elements such as education, policy change, vision screening or personal fittings for safety glasses, and provision of eye protection resulted in increased use of eye protection and reduction in eye injuries (Lipscomb 2000). Multicomponent interventions for safe patient handling have also improved musculoskeletal health among workers in health care settings. Interventions that include a policy establishing an organizational commitment to reducing injuries related to patient handling, combined with the purchase of lift equipment and training on either proper lift equipment use or patient handling, have a positive effect on musculoskeletal symptoms (Tullar et al. 2010).

In some examples, especially in the health care industry, an intervention was designed specifically to influence workplace safety culture. In one study, a multifaceted safety program at a rural hospital involving administrative support, creation of an employee safety committee, ergonomic analysis, and marketing that promoted a safe workplace resulted in declines in injury-related claims, needlestick injuries, and injuries resulting in lost workdays (Hooper and Charney 2005).

Discerning which specific elements are essential for an intervention's effectiveness can be difficult, or even impossible in some cases. Ideally, various combinations of elements should be tested to help develop the most efficient multifaceted interventions. In designing interventions to prevent occupational injury, remember that engineering and policy interventions often require some educational component for maximum effect; for example, new technologies often require training in their proper use, and education is essential to create awareness of policy requirements and of the consequences of noncompliance.

We offer one final comment on interventions for this section. The importance of ensuring that safety interventions are implemented, monitored, and evaluated cannot be adequately emphasized. Simply having policies or some intervention "on the books" is not sufficient to reduce workplace injury risks. Workers must be aware of the interventions and should be aware of the rationale for a particular intervention in order to buy in to the approach.

Roles for Key Stakeholders

Although the rates of fatal and nonfatal work-related injuries have declined since the passage of the Occupational Safety and Health Act of 1970, occupational injuries continue to exact a significant toll. Preventing workplace injuries is not the sole responsibility of any single person or organization; **stakeholder** participation is essential to improve workplace safety. We describe here several **key stakeholders** who play a role in injury prevention.

Organizations and Employers

Employers are crucial in efforts to reduce occupational injury risk. They can establish the culture, promote safety, and invest in interventions that will establish a safe working environment. They can also create workplaces where safety and injury prevention is a priority and where employees are encouraged to report injury without fear of retribution or discipline. Each year, the National Safety Council's *Safety*+Health magazine publishes a list of chief executive officers (CEOs) who "get it" when it comes to keeping their employees safe. These CEOs are chosen because they have "made safety a core value of their organization." They were selected for being leaders in ensuring "that best practices for safety and health are adopted consistently" and for "creating systems that measure and reward employees for their safety performance to drive the desired behavior" (NSC 2011).

Federal Agencies

The National Institute for Occupational Safety and Health (NIOSH), housed within the CDC, is the leading federal public health agency charged with generating and funding research aimed at improving worker safety and health. NIOSH is the largest funder of occupational injury research. In fiscal year 2005, the total NIOSH budget was $286 million (the total CDC budget was over $4 billion). The intramural research budget for NIOSH's Traumatic Injury Research Program was roughly $11.8 million dollars, and the extramural research budget was approximately $5.4 million (IOM and NRC 2009). Relative to NIOSH, the National Institutes of Health (NIH) has funded few studies on occupational injury. Since the NIH has a disease-focused organizational structure, this is not surprising; however, in recognizing the strong connection between health conditions and injury, the need for NIH and other federal agencies to fund more research in occupational injury likewise becomes clear. Moreover, the National Center for Injury Prevention and Control (NCIPC) does not support research in occupational injury. Because risk factors for injuries at work and outside of work overlap, an opportunity emerges for interagency collaboration between NIOSH and NCIPC to jointly fund research.

In addition to funding, federal agencies are instrumental in developing regulations and legislative policies relevant to occupational injury. In the United States two primary federal regulatory bodies specifically focused on occupational injury are the Occupational Safety and Health Administration (OSHA) and the Mine Safety and Health Administration (MSHA). The Occupational Safety and Health Act of 1970 established OSHA in the Department of Labor (DOL). OSHA inspects workplaces for violations of safety standards, holds hearings, sets new or revised safety standards, and enforces these standards. The MSHA was created in 1977 when the Federal Coal Mine Health and Safety Act of 1969 was amended (Weeks 2006). MSHA also became structurally located in the DOL and was given authority to write and enforce regulations to protect mine workers. OSHA and MSHA both have developed standards that have significantly reduced worker exposure to serious hazards and the resulting injuries; however, some important differences exist between the two agencies, especially in their enforcement capabilities. For example, an MSHA inspector who decides that danger is imminent can close all or part of a mine, whereas an OSHA inspector has to seek a judicial ruling to close all or part of a private workplace. Also, MSHA requires annual inspections of underground mines, whereas OSHA workplace inspections are discretionary (Weeks 2006). Despite some notable differences between OSHA and MSHA, both agencies must be provided with sufficient resources to inspect work sites, enforce regulations, and hold employers accountable when they have poor safety records.

State and Local Agencies

State and local agencies also have roles in addressing workplace injury. Many states have an occupational health department (often combined with environmental health) that is responsible for occupational health and safety. Recognizing a need to expand the capacity of states to engage in occupational health surveillance, NIOSH released a call for proposals for cooperative agreements (NIOSH 2005). The program provided state agencies with resources to "collect data from existing systems that capture information on occupational safety and health hazards and effects on workers, to identify new sources of occupational safety and health data, to perform occupational health and safety surveillance, and to develop interven-

tions for reducing worker injuries and illnesses in the state." This emphasis on surveillance needs to continue, because it is essential for national, state, and local efforts to illuminate the burden of workplace injuries and to target resources for prevention.

Local agencies are in a unique position to respond to the particular needs of industries and businesses operating within their jurisdiction. For certain types of workplaces, local health inspectors may have more opportunities to observe hazards than do state or federal regulators. Local agencies can also act on issues for which no political will to do so exists at the state level. For example, some states and localities have banned smoking in bars and restaurants to protect the employees working in those establishments from secondhand smoke.

Unions

Unions historically have been key advocates for promoting worker safety, among many other issues. But the percentage of the U.S. workforce that is unionized has declined significantly over many decades. Recently, in order to regain their political strength and collective bargaining prowess, unions have been increasing their efforts to organize workers, especially in health care and among temporary and contractual workers (IOM and Committee 2000). The right to organize at work has been the subject of policy and legislative debates in recent years. Creating an environment where it is easier for workers to form unions may help provide opportunities for safety improvements.

Unionized workplaces are more likely than nonunionized workplaces to have health and safety committees and to have had regular safety audits (Hawke and Wooden 1997). Therefore, some believe that unionized plants are safer than nonunionized plants. Few studies have explored the impact of unions' safety initiatives on occupational injury. The results of one study suggest that unionized workers are more likely to be informed about the health and safety hazards of a job, and thus have lower injury rates, than nonunionized workers (Kriebel 1982). If so, unions should consider advocating for specific safety measures, in addition to their more frequent activities related to collective bargaining for salary and benefits. In addition, unions may partner with employers and be directly involved in developing and implementing workplace safety programs.

One of the largest unions in the United States is the American Federation of Labor and Congress of Industrial Organizations (AFL-CIO), a voluntary federation of 57 national and international labor unions (AFL-CIO 2010). The AFL-CIO represents approximately 11.5 million members. Its mission is to improve the lives of working families through political action, organizing at the grassroots level, and promoting the growth of unions. The AFL-CIO is a strong advocate for legislation aimed at worker safety and health. Many other unions also actively engage in advocating for safer practices, including the United Steelworkers, the United Auto Workers, the National Union of Healthcare Workers, the American Federation of Teachers, the International Association of Machinists and Aerospace Workers, and the International Association of Fire Fighters. Unions have an important role in advocating and holding employers accountable for the safety of working conditions. Allowing workers to form and join a union when one is desired is important.

Clinics and Clinicians

Occupational medicine physicians and occupational health nurses provide clinical care and lead programs aimed at workplace health promotion and disease and injury prevention. They also are responsible for preplacement, periodic, and return-to-work examinations. These clinical services are rendered in work site clinics, in hospital and outpatient clinics, or in academic occupational medicine clinics. Only about 20% of physicians practicing in the field of occupational medicine are actually board certified in occupational medicine. Similarly, only about 25% of the members of the professional society for occupational health nurses are certified in occupational health nursing (IOM and Committee 2000). In the long term, understanding the supply and demand for these professionals, as well as the barriers to board certification in these specialties, may help ensure the availability of well-trained professionals able to contribute to the prevention of occupational injuries and improve the treatment of injured workers.

Insurers

Workers' compensation is often the sole source of income and medical and rehabilitation payments to workers injured on the job (Boden et al. 2006). The United States does not have a unified workers' compensation law; instead, each state (along with three federal workers' compensation jurisdictions) has its own statute and regulations regarding eligibility and coverage. It is important to recognize that, for the injured worker, this financial benefit may be critical for restoring the worker's health and functioning and returning the person to work in a reasonable amount of time.

Insurance companies can prevent loss by engaging in research on the prevention and treatment of workplace injuries and on rehabilitation following injury. Some insurance companies are actively engaged in such research. For example, the Liberty Mutual Research Institute for Safety, part of the Liberty Mutual Insurance Company, has conducted occupational safety and health research on an array of topics, including the economic costs of injury and worker disability. One other example of this type of **partnership** is the Injured Insurance Workers

Fund, which has partnered on research with the Johns Hopkins Bloomberg School of Public Health to develop a screening tool for delayed return to work following low back injuries. Not all insurance companies will have the resources to conduct research in-house or support a research partnership, but for insurance companies that are in a position to do so, such work can lead to new strategies for preventing occupational injuries and new practices that return employees to work as safely and quickly as possible.

Associations and Advocacy Groups

Several national associations and advocacy groups are integral to ensuring a safe workplace for every worker. In this section we mention just a few of these associations. According to its mission statement, the National Safety Council (NSC) "saves lives by preventing injuries and deaths at work, in homes and communities, and on the roads, through leadership, research, education and advocacy" (NSC 1995–2010). It conducts trainings around the country on important workplace safety issues (e.g., preventing "slips, trips, and falls"), collaborates with advocacy groups and other agencies to promote worker safety, and disseminates injury research by publishing the *Journal of Safety Research*. Finally, as previously mentioned, the NSC's *Safety+ Health* annually recognizes CEOs who are leaders in workplace safety (NSC 2011).

Several field-specific associations also exist, such as the National Association of Manufacturers, the American Industrial Hygiene Association, the American Association of Occupational Health Nurses, and the American Society of Safety Engineers. These associations disseminate research and raise awareness of safety issues by sponsoring professional meetings, participating in advocacy, and publishing newsletters. Continued involvement of these and other advocacy groups is essential because of their ability to mobilize around the safety is-

sues that are most important to their respective industries.

Researchers

Researchers possess the skills to conduct studies that generate new knowledge, evaluate existing efforts that might be continued, discontinued, or taken to scale, and translate and disseminate known information. They can collaborate with other stakeholders and provide the necessary scientific data on the modifiable risk factors for occupational injury, and they can make recommendations on policy and programs to reduce injury risk. Although significant understanding regarding occupational injury has already been achieved, several areas warrant additional research.

In 1994, NIOSH, in partnership with many external stakeholders, began a process to identify research priorities for the next decade. This effort resulted in the National Occupational Research Agenda (NORA) (NIOSH 2009-10b). NORA initially included 21 priority areas for research, some focusing on specific vulnerable populations, some focusing on specific injuries and illnesses, and some focusing on cross-cutting themes such as work organization. In recognition of the fact that hazards differ by industry, in 2006 NORA was reorganized. Now NORA takes a sector-based approach, so that a group of stakeholders for each of 10 industry sectors develops industry-specific priorities for research. In addition to these 10 NORA industry sectors, NORA will continue to prioritize research on cross-cutting issues.

One example of a cross-cutting issue is surveillance. A 2009 report by the Government Accountability Office documents the inability of existing surveillance systems to capture the true burden of workplace injury in the United States (GAO 2009). The total *recorded* number of workers who experience nonfatal injuries is believed to underestimate the actual magnitude of nonfatal workplace injury because of underreporting (Wolfe and Fairchild 2010). Accurately quantifying exposures to workplace hazards using individual-level measures of hours worked is critically important. The ability to link databases that contain data relevant to understanding workers' jobs and work experiences and to allow further exploration of the association between health and injury is also important.

The updated NORA also emphasizes the need for increased translation of research into practice (NIOSH 2009-10b). This r2p initiative encourages researchers to consider up front how their research is going to prevent injuries in practice. Under this framework, researchers need to involve stakeholders from the beginning. When they do so, researchers will be asking the questions that are most relevant to individuals who will use the information generated. Additionally, early involvement of stakeholders may facilitate dissemination of research findings.

Conclusions

Workplace injuries cause a substantial health and economic burden. The ecological model highlights how individual workers are nested within institutional, organizational, and community contexts, all of which are influenced by public policies at the local, state, and national levels. This model helps us understand how interventions targeting key factors can reduce the risk of injury. Theory tells us that passive interventions, such as design and engineering changes, hold the greatest promise for preventing injuries. However, passive interventions are not always possible and, even when possible, they often require an educational component for their adoption and appropriate use. Research provides examples of several successful interventions and suggests that multifaceted interventions, using a combination of engineering, policy or administrative, and educational approaches, may have the best chance of reducing occupational injury rates. Preventing work-place injuries requires the participation of several stakeholders, including employers, unions, clinicians, insurers, government agencies, industry associations, and researchers. Occupational injuries have declined over the past several decades, but the 3 million nonfatal injuries and nearly 4,700 deaths suffered by workers each year in the United States are still far too many. Continued attention to and innovation in workplace safety is essential.

REFERENCES

American Federation of Labor and Congress of Industrial Organizations (AFL-CIO).About the AFL-CIO. 2010. Washington, DC: AFL-CIO; Sept. 1, 2006, updated Jan. 1, 2010. Available at www.aflcio.org /about/ (accessed Nov. 1, 2010).

Baggs J, Silverstein B, Foley M. 2003. Workplace health and safety regulations: Impact of enforcement and consultation on workers' compensation claims rates in Washington State. *Am J Ind Med* 43 (5) (May): 483-94.

Barnett RL, Brickman DB. 1986. Safety hierarchy. *J Safety Res* 17 (2) (June): 49-55.

Berkowitz M. 1979. Occupational safety and health. *Annals AAPSS* 443 (1) (May 1): 41-53.

Bertera RL. 1991. The effects of behavioral risks on absenteeism and health-care costs in the workplace. *J Occup Med* 33 (11): 1119-24.

Boden LI, Leifer NT, Strouss DC, Spieler EA. 2006. Legal remedies. In *Occupational and Environmental Health: Recognizing and Preventing Disease and Injury,* ed. BS Levy, DH Wegman, SL Baron, RK Sokas, 74-104. 5th ed. Philadelphia: Lippincott Williams & Wilkins.

Brady JE, Baker SP, DiMaggio C, McCarthy ML, Rebok GW, Li G. 2009. Effectiveness of mandatory alcohol testing programs in reducing alcohol involvement in fatal motor carrier crashes. *Am J Epidemiol* 170 (6) (Aug. 1): 775-82.

Brosseau LM, Parker DL, Lazovich D, Milton T, Dugan S. 2002. Designing intervention effectiveness studies for occupational health and safety: The Minnesota wood dust study. *Am J Ind Med* 41 (1): 54-61.

Brunette MJ. 2006. Safety. In *Occupational and Environmental Health: Recognizing and Preventing Disease and Injury,* ed. BS Levy, DH Wegman, SL Baron, RK Sokas, chap. 10. 5th ed. Philadelphia: Lippincott Williams & Wilkins.

Bulzacchelli MT, Vernick JS, Webster DW, Lees PSJ. 2007. Effects of the Occupational Safety and Health Administration's Control of Hazardous Energy

(Lockout/Tagout) Standard on rates of machinery-related fatal occupational injury. *Inj Prev* 13 (5) (Oct 1): 334–38.

Bureau of Labor Statistics, U.S. Department of Labor (BLS). 2008–11a. Census of fatal occupational injuries 2011; Jan. 2012. U.S. Department of Labor, Washington DC. Available at www.bls.gov/news.release/cfoi.nr0.htm (accessed June 8, 2013).

———. 2008–11b. Industry injury and illness data 2011; Oct. 25, 2012. U.S. Department of Labor, Washington DC. Available at www.bls.gov/news.release/archives/osh_10252012.pdf (accessed June 8, 2013).

———. 2009. Annual averages and the monthly labor review, November. U.S. Department of Labor, Washington DC. Available at www.bls.gov/opub/ee/empearn200911.pdf (accessed Oct. 30, 2010).

Burke MJ, Sarpy SA, Smith-Crowe K, Chan-Serafin S, Salvador RO, Islam G. 2006. Relative effectiveness of worker safety and health training methods. *Am J Public Health* 96 (2) (Feb.): 315–24.

Cashman CM, Ruotsalainen JH, Greiner BA, Beirne PV, Verbeek JH. 2009. Alcohol and drug screening of occupational drivers for preventing injury. *Cochrane Database Syst Rev* 2 (April 15). Available at http://onlinelibrary.wiley.com/o/cochrane/clsysrev/articles/CD006566/frame.html (accessed Feb. 19, 2011.

Casteel C, Peek-Asa C. 2000. The effectiveness of Crime Prevention Through Environmental Design (CPTED) in reducing robberies. *Am J Prev Med* 18 (suppl. 4): 99–115.

Castillo DN, Pizaella TJ, Stout NA. 2006. Injuries. In *Occupational and Environmental Health: Recognizing and Preventing Disease and Injury,* ed. BS Levy, DH Wegman, SL Baron, RK Sokas, chap. 22. 5th ed. Philadelphia: Lippincott Williams & Wilkins.

Centers for Disease Control and Prevention (CDC). 1999. Ten Great Public Health Achievements—United States, 1900–1999. MMWR 48 (12): 241–43.

Charney W, Simmons B, Lary M, Metz S. 2006. Zero lift programs in small rural hospitals in Washington state: Reducing back injuries among health care workers. *AAOHN J* 54 (8): 355–58.

Chelius JR. 1979. Economic and demographic aspects of the occupational injury problem. *Q Rev Econ Bus* 19 (2): 65–70.

Collins JW, Wolf J, Bell J, Evanoff B. 2004. An evaluation of a "best practices" musculoskeletal injury prevention program in nursing homes. *Inj Prev* 10 (4): 206–11.

Conway H, Svenson J. 1998. Occupational injury and illness rates, 1992–96: Why they fell. *Month Labor Rev* 121 (11) (Nov. 1): 36–58.

Corporate Alliance to End Partner Violence (CAEPV). 2002–11. Know the facts. CAEPV, Bloomington, IL.

Available at www.caepv.org/getinfo/ (accessed March 25, 2009).

Cox S, Cox T. 1991. The structure of employee attitudes to safety—a European example. *Work Stress* 5 (2): 93–106.

Dedobbeleer N, Champagne F, German P. 1990. Safety performance among union and nonunion workers in the construction industry. *J Occup Med* 32 (11): 1099–1103.

DeJoy DM, Murphy LR, Gershon RM. 1995. The influence of employee, job/task, and organizational factors on adherence to universal precautions among nurses. *Int J Industr Ergonom* 16 (1): 43–55.69.

DeRoo LA, Rautiainen RH. 2000. A systematic review of farm safety interventions. *Am J Prev Med* 18 (4 suppl.) (May): 51–62.

Driessen MT, Proper KI, van Tulder MW, Anema JR, Bongers PM, van der Beek AJ. 2010. The effectiveness of physical and organizational ergonomic interventions on low back pain and neck pain: A systematic review. *Occup Environ Med* 67 (4) (April): 277–85.

Faulkner K, Landslittle DP, Hendricks S. 2001. Robbery characteristics and employee injuries in convenience stores. *Am J Ind Med* 40 (6): 703–9.

Friedman LS, Forst L. 2008. Ethnic disparities in traumatic occupational injury. *J Occup Environ Med* 50 (3) (March): 350–58.

Galinsky E, Bond JT, Sakai K, Kim SS, Giuntoli N. 2008. 2008 national study of employers. Families and Work Institute, New York.

Geller ES. 2006. Occupational injury prevention and applied behavior analysis. In *Injury and Violence Prevention: Behavioral Science Theories, Methods, and Applications,* ed. AC Gielen, DA Sleet, RJ DiClemente, 297–322. San Francisco: Jossey-Bass.

Gielen AC, Sleet DA, DiClemente RJ, eds. 2006. *Injury and Violence Prevention: Behavioral Science Theories, Methods, and Applications.* San Francisco: Jossey-Bass.

Gilmore TM, Alexander BH, Mueller BA, Rivara FP. 1996. Occupational injuries and medication use. *Am J Ind Med* 30 (2) (Aug.): 234–39.

Government Accountability Office (GAO). 2009. Workplace safety and health: Enhancing OSHA's records audit process could improve the accuracy of worker injury and illness data. GAO-10-10. U.S. Government Accountability Office, Washington DC.

Hartling L, Brison RJ, Crumley ET, Klassen TP, Pickett W. 2004. A systematic review of interventions to prevent childhood farm injuries. *Pediatrics* 114 (4): e483–96.

Hawke A, Wooden M. 1997. The 1995 Australian workplace industrial relations survey. *Aust Econ Rev* 30 (3) (Sept): 323–28.

Hooper J, Charney W. 2005. Creation of a safety culture: Reducing workplace injuries in a rural hospital. *AAOHN J* 53 (9): 394-98.

Institute of Medicine (IOM) and Committee to Assess Training Needs for Occupational Safety and Health Personnel in the United States. 2000. *Safe Work in the 21st Century: Education and Training Needs for the Next Decade's Occupational Safety and Health Personnel.* Washington, DC: National Academies Press.

Institute of Medicine (IOM) and National Research Council (NRC). 2009. *Traumatic Injury Research at NIOSH: Reviews of Research Programs of the National Institute for Occupational Safety and Health.* Washington, DC: National Academies Press.

Islam SS, Velilla AM, Doyle EJ, Ducatman AM. 2001. Gender differences in work-related injury/illness: Analysis of workers compensation claims. *Am J Ind Med* 39 (1): 84-91.

Johnston JJ, Cattledge GTH, Collins JW. 1994. The efficacy of training for occupational injury control. *Occup Med* 9 (2) (April-June): 147-58.

Kennedy CA, Amick BC III, Dennerlein JT, et al. 2010. Systematic review of the role of occupational health and safety interventions in the prevention of upper extremity musculoskeletal symptoms, signs, disorders, injuries, claims, and lost time. *J Occup Rehab* 20 (2) (June): 127-62.

Keyserling WM. 2006. Occupational safety: Preventing accidents and overt trauma. In *Occupational and Environmental Health: Recognizing and Preventing Disease and Injury,* ed. BS Levy, DH Wegman, SL Baron, RK Sokas, chap. 8. 5th ed. Philadelphia: Lippincott Williams & Wilkins.

Kraus JF. 2001. The effects of certain drug-testing programs on injury reduction in the workplace: An evidence-based review. *Int J Occup Environ Health* 7 (2): 103-8.

Kriebel D. 1982. Occupational injuries: Factors associated with frequency and severity. *Int Arch Occup Environ Health* 50 (3) (April 1): 209-18.

Layne L, Pollack KM. 2004. Nonfatal occupational injuries from slips, trips, and falls among older workers treated in hospital emergency departments, United States, 1998. *Am J Ind Med* 46 (1) (July): 32-41.

Leigh JP, Markowitz S, Fahs M, Landrigan P. 2000. *Costs of Occupational Injuries and Illnesses.* Ann Arbor: University of Michigan Press.

Levy BS, Wegman DH, Baron SL, Sokas RK. 2006. Occupational and environmental health: An overview. In *Occupational and Environmental Health: Recognizing and Preventing Disease and Injury,* ed. BS Levy, DH Wegman, SL Baron, RK Sokas, chap. 1. 5th ed. Philadelphia: Lippincott Williams & Wilkins.

Lincoln JM, Lucas DL. 2010. Occupational fatalities in the United States commercial fishing industry, 2000-2009. *J Agromed* 15 (4): 343-50.

Lindquist C, McKay T, Clinton-Sherrod M, Pollack KM, Lasater B, Hardison Walters J. 2010. The role of employee assistance programs in workplace-based intimate partner violence intervention and prevention activities. *J Workplace Behav Health* 25 (1): 46-64.

Linton SJ, van Tulder MW. 2001. Preventive interventions for back and neck pain problems: What is the evidence? *Spine* 26 (7) (April 1): 778-87.

Lipscomb HJ. 2000. Effectiveness of interventions to prevent work-related eye injuries. *Am J Prev Med* 18 (4 suppl.) (May): 27-32.

Lipscomb HJ, Li L, Dement J. 2003. Work-related falls among union carpenters in Washington State before and after the Vertical Fall Arrest Standard. *Am J Ind Med* 44 (2) (Aug.): 157-65.

Mearns K, Flin R. 1999. Assessing the state of organizational safety—culture or climate? *Curr Psychol* 18:5-17.

National Institute for Occupational Safety and Health (NIOSH). 1993. *Preventing Homicide in the Workplace: CDC NIOSH Alert.* Publication 93-109. Washington, DC: US Department of Health and Human Services.

———. 2005. State-based occupational and safety and health surveillance cooperative agreement. Announcement PAR-04-106, Oct. Available at www.cdc .gov/niosh/oep/pdfs/State-Based-Surv-FY05-v.2.pdf (accessed Feb. 19, 2011).

———. 2009-10a. Commercial Fishing Safety, June. Centers for Disease Control, Atlanta. Available at www .cdc.gov/niosh/topics/fishing/ (accessed Feb. 19, 2011).

———. 2009-10b. The National Occupational Research Agenda (NORA), 2008 June. Centers for Disease Control, Atlanta. Available at www.cdc.gov/niosh /nora/ (accessed Jan. 18, 2011).

National Safety Council (NSC). 1995-2010. Safety at work. National Safety Council, Syracuse, NY. Available at www.nsc.org/safety_work/ (accessed Feb. 6, 2011).

———. 2011. Safety + Health 2011: CEOs who "get it." National Safety Council, Syracuse, NY. Available at www.nsc.org/safety_work/Leadership/Pages /CEOsWhoGetIt.aspx (accessed Feb. 6, 2011).

Occupational Safety and Health Administration (OSHA). 1970. Occupational Safety and Health Act of 1970. 29 U.S.C Title § 651 et seq. 29 of the CFR, Part 1900-1999.

Orrenius PM, Zavodny M. 2009. Do immigrants work in riskier jobs? *Demography* 46 (3) (Aug.): 535-51.

Pollack KM, Agnew J, Slade MD, et al. 2007. Use of employer administrative databases to identify systematic causes of injury in aluminum manufacturing. *Am J Ind Med* 50 (9) (Sept.): 676-86.

Pollack KM, Austin W, Grisso JA. 2010. Employee assistance programs: A workplace resource to address intimate partner violence. *J Womens Health (Larchmt)* 19 (4): 729-33.

Pollack KM, Cheskin L. 2007. Obesity and workplace traumatic injury: Does the science support the link? *Inj Prev* 13 (Oct.): 297-302.

Pollack KM, McKay T, Cummiskey C, et al. 2010. Employee assistance program services for intimate partner violence and client satisfaction with these services. *J Occup Environ Med* 52 (8): 819-26.

Pollack KM, Sorock GS, Slade M, et al. 2007. Association between body mass index and acute traumatic workplace injury in hourly manufacturing employees. *Am J Epidemiol* 166 (2) (June): 204-11.

Rautiainen RH, Lehtola MM, Day LM, et al. 2008. Interventions for preventing injuries in the agricultural industry. *Cochrane Database Syst Rev* 3 (Jan. 23): CD006398. Available at http://onlinelibrary.wiley.com/o/cochrane/clsysrev/articles/CD006398/frame.html (accessed Feb. 19, 2011).

Reynolds SJ, Groves W. 2000. Effectiveness of roll-over protective structures in reducing farm tractor fatalities. *Am J Prev Med* 18 (4 suppl.) (May): 63-69.

Rogers B, Goodno L. 2000. Evaluation of interventions to prevent needlestick injuries in health care occupations. *Am J Prev Med* 18 (4 suppl.) (May): 90-98.

Saleh SS, Fuortes L, Vaughn T, Bauer EP. 2001. Epidemiology of occupational injuries and illnesses in a university population: A focus on age and gender differences. *Am J Ind Med* 39 (6): 581-86.

Schenker MB. 2010. A global perspective of migration and occupational health. *Am J Ind Med* 53 (4) (April): 329-37.

Schulte PA, Wagner GR, Downes A, Miller DB. 2008. A framework for the concurrent consideration of occupational hazards and obesity. *Ann Occup Hyg* 52 (7) (Oct.): 555-66.

Segui-Gomez M. 2000. Evaluating worksite-based interventions that promote safety belt use. *Am J Prev Med* 18 (4 suppl.) (May): 11-22.

Smitha MW, Kirk KA, Oestenstad KR, Brown KC, Lee S. 2001. Effect of state workplace safety laws on occupational injury rates. *J Occup Environ Med* 43 (12) (Dec.): 1001-10.

Suruda A, Whitaker B, Bloswick D, Philips P, Sesek R. 2002. Impact of the OSHA Trench and Excavation Standard on fatal injury in the construction industry. *J Occup Environ Med* 44 (12) (Oct.): 902-5.

Taiwo O, Cantley L, Slade M, et al. 2009. Gender differences in injury patterns among workers in heavy manufacturing. *Am J Epidemiol* 169 (2) (Jan. 15): 161-66.

Thomas TK, Lincoln JM, Husberg BJ, Conway GA. 2001. Is it safe on deck? Fatal and non-fatal workplace injuries among Alaskan commercial fishermen. *Am J Ind Med* 40 (6): 693-702.

Tompa E, Trevithick S, McLeod C. 2007. Systematic review of the prevention incentives of insurance and regulatory mechanisms for occupational health and safety. *Scand J Work Environ Health* 33 (2) (April): 85-95.

Trim JC, Elliott TSJ. 2003. A review of sharps injuries and preventative strategies. *J Hosp Infect* 53 (4) (April): 237-42.

Tullar JM, Brewer S, Amick BC III, et al. 2010. Occupational safety and health interventions to reduce musculoskeletal symptoms in the health care sector. *J Occup Rehab* 20 (2) (June): 199-219.

Tveito TH, Hysing M, Eriksen HR. 2004. Low back pain interventions at the workplace: A systematic literature review. *Occup Med* 54 (1) (Jan.): 3-13.

U.S. Department of Health and Human Services (USDHHS). 2000. Health information network: Employee assistance programs 2000. Substance Abuse and Mental Health Services Administration, Washington DC. Available at http://ncadi.samhsa.gov/workplace/fedagencies/employee_assistance_programs.aspx (accessed Jan. 19, 2009).

U.S. Department of Labor (USDL). 2011. American Time Use Survey summary. US Department of Labor and Statistics, Washington DC. Available at www.bls.gov/tus/tables/a1_2011.pdf (accessed June 8, 2013).

van der Molen HF, Lehtola MM, Lappalainen J, et al. 2007. Interventions for preventing injuries in the construction industry. *Cochrane Database Syst Rev* 4 (Oct. 17): CD006251. Available at http://onlinelibrary.wiley.com/o/cochrane/clsysrev/articles/CD006251/frame.html (accessed Feb. 19, 2011).

van Poppel MNM, Hooftman WE, Koes BW. 2004. An update of a systematic review of controlled clinical trials on the primary prevention of back pain at the workplace. *Occup Med* 54 (4) (Aug.): 345-52.

Voaklander DC, Umbarger-Mackey ML, Wilson ML. 2009. Health, medication use, and agricultural injury: A review. *Am J Ind Med* 52 (11) (Nov.): 876-89.

Wang Y, Beydoun MA, Liang L, Caballero B, Kumanyika SK. 2008. Will all Americans become overweight or obese? Estimating the progression and cost of the US obesity epidemic. *Obesity* 16 (10): 2323-30.

Warner M, Baker SP, Li G, Smith GS. 1998. Acute traumatic injuries in automotive manufacturing. *Am J Ind Med* 34 (4): 351-58.

Weeks JL. 2006. Essential of the Mine Safety and Health Administration, Box 3-1. In *Occupational and Environmental Health: Recognizing and Preventing Disease and Injury,* ed. BS Levy, DH Wegman, SL

Baron, RK Sokas, 40-42. 5th ed. Philadelphia: Lippincott Williams & Wilkins.

Welch LS, Goldenhar LM, Hunting KL. 2000. Women in construction: Occupational health and working conditions. *J Am Med Womens Assoc* 55 (2): 89-92.

Wickizer TM, Kopjar B, Franklin G, Joesch J. 2004. Do drug-free workplace programs prevent occupational injuries? Evidence from Washington State. *Health Serv Res* 39 (1) (Feb.): 91-110.

Wolfe D, Fairchild AL. 2010. The need for improved surveillance of occupational disease and injury. *JAMA* 303 (10) (March 10); 981-82.

Wong TY. 1997. A behavioral analysis of eye protection use by soldiers. *Military Med* 162 (11): 744-48.

Zhang X, Yu S, Wheeler K, Kelleher K, Stallones L, Xiang H. 2009. Work-related non-fatal injuries among foreign-born and US-born workers: Findings from the U.S. National Health Interview Survey, 1997-2005. *Am J Ind Med* 52 (1) (Jan.): 25-36.

Zwerling C, Daltroy LH, Fine LJ, Johnston JJ, Melius J, Silverstein BA. 1997. Design and conduct of occupational injury intervention studies: A review of evaluation strategies. *Am J Ind Med* 32 (2) (Aug.): 164-79.

CHAPTER 17

Violence and Behavior Change

ELAINE DOHERTY, MARGARET ENSMINGER,
AND REBECCA EVANS-POLCE

LEARNING OBJECTIVES

After completing the chapter, the reader will be able to

* Elucidate the advantages of framing violence as a public health issue, such as focusing on both perpetrators and victims of violence and allowing for the participation of multiple stakeholders in a multifaceted approach to violence prevention.
* Identify the challenges inherent in violence prevention, including the difficulties in the design, evaluation, and dissemination of interventions that are both evidence-based and amenable to the culture in which they are being implemented.
* Enumerate the many costs and consequences of violence, including physical, emotional, economic, and societal.
* Apply the social ecological model to the problem of violence, acknowledging that violence occurs within many different contexts (i.e., families, schools, neighborhoods, and the larger society) and emphasizing that consideration of this complexity is vital in developing successful intervention strategies to reduce violence.
* Differentiate between successful and unsuccessful violence prevention programs that have been implemented at the individual, school or peer, and community levels, illuminating the challenges of violence prevention.

Introduction

In the past 20 years, violence has become recognized as a major public health problem. Violent activities are associated with considerable **morbidity** and **mortality**. According to the World Health Organization (1996), violence consists of any act that involves the intentional use of threatened as well as actual physical force or power against oneself, another person, or a group or community. It results in or is likely to result in injury, death, psychological harm, or other damage. This definition encompasses a wide range of behaviors, from violence between intimate partners and child abuse, to assaults during the commission of crimes, to youth gang violence, to terrorist activity, to wars among nation states. Violence can be self-inflicted (against oneself), interpersonal (between at least two individuals), or collective (committed by large groups or states, usually with political or social **motivations**) (Krug et al. 2002). Thus, violent activity can be perpetrated by sole individuals, by groups of people, or by nations or states. Furthermore, the impact may range from very severe injury resulting in death to less severe, nonfatal injury. Although both self-directed harm and such acts as terrorism, wars, and po-

litical violence are considered violent behaviors, we focus this chapter on those violent behaviors that are interpersonal in nature, as opposed to social or political collective violence or self-directed violence (i.e., suicide). Interpersonal violence includes family or partner violence (e.g., against children, against a partner), violence against acquaintances, and violence against strangers.

Violence as a Public Health Problem

Since 1960, the Federal Bureau of Investigation (FBI) has been tracking incidents of interpersonal violent crime reported to police, including homicides, robbery, rape, and aggravated assaults. Figure 17.1 depicts the trends of these violent crimes from 1960 to 2011. This time span includes periods of increasing violence, most

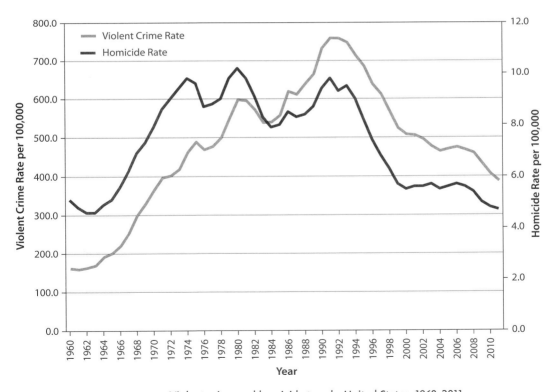

FIGURE 17.1. Violent crime and homicide trends, United States, 1960–2011.
Source: FBI, Uniform Crime Reports.

notably, 1965 to 1980 and 1986 to 1990, and periods of decreasing violence, notably 1980 to 1985 and 1992 to 2000.

Times of increasing violence often warrant a change in conceptualization of the problem or of the response. For example, prior to the 1970s, violence was largely considered solely a criminal justice issue or a psychiatric concern. By the mid-1970s, however, in response to the rising crime rates of the time, as well as discouraging results from **evaluations** of criminal justice rehabilitation programs (e.g., Martinson 1974), the criminal justice system shifted its philosophy of punishment from rehabilitation to crime control (i.e., incapacitation and deterrence). This shift resulted in harsher sentences for violent offenders, a stark increase in imprisonments, and a reduction in correctional programming.

Coinciding with the high crime rates of the 1970s and the shift in the criminal justice approach to violence, a disciplinary shift occurred in the construction of violence as a public health problem. In the 1970s, homicide, especially in younger age groups, was identified by the Centers for Disease Control and Prevention (CDC) as a preventable cause of morbidity, premature mortality, and the loss of years of potential life (Winett 1998). As infectious diseases were being prevented and treated at an increasing rate, injury-related deaths, including homicide and suicide, were becoming more prevalent in comparison (Dahlberg and Mercy 2009). In addition, the success of injury prevention efforts during the 1970s and early 1980s further emphasized the potential for saving lives by focusing not only on unintentional injuries but on intentional injuries as well. Even the change in the CDC language—from "violence" to "intentional injuries"—indicates an increasing adoption of a public health perspective. The implications of this change are dramatic for the definition of violence, the types of behaviors that receive attention, and the recommended **interventions**.

Ideologically, the concepts of individual guilt, blame, and accountability are central to the criminal justice approach, bringing punishment to the forefront. The public health approach places less emphasis on individual culpability and more on the environment that may influence violence, using a **systems approach** (see chapter 21), which emphasizes the interrelatedness of individual and environmental causes (or risk factors), making it more compatible with a focus on prevention (Moore 1993).[1] The focus on social and behavioral factors as precursors to health (e.g., cancer, heart disease) also gained more acceptance within the public health community (Dahlberg and Mercy 2009).

The public health community has been more involved with certain kinds of violence than the criminal justice community has. Domestic violence (e.g., intimate partner violence and child abuse) has received much attention from public health practitioners. The criminal justice community has viewed domestic violence as a difficult arena to address because of the potential danger to police in domestic violence situations, the difficulty in assigning blame, and the reluctance of some victims to cooperate with criminal justice authorities (Glover et al. 2011). Some advocates for women have argued that in rape cases or other domestic violence situations, victims often need to prove to the criminal justice authorities that they were not being provocative or that they resisted the violence. The predominant outcome from a public health perspective revolves around reducing the resulting injuries (Buzawa and Buzawa 2003; Hoyle 1998).

Finally, as implied above, these two perspectives work in concert with each other as to their recommended interventions. At least with regard to the adult criminal justice system, justice is the primary basis of decision making—the system's procedures are intended to provide justice in the determination of guilt or innocence and in the determination of appropriate punishment. In contrast, the public health approach is oriented toward prevention of harm to the victims, providing immediate responses to the victims (e.g., hospital and psychiatric services), and victim reintegration (Krug et al. 2002). Public health programs might target not only victims of violence, but also those who have risk factors for committing violence and those who are potential victims of violence (e.g., children, intimate partners); or the programs might target changing the environment itself. In a 1998 review of public health studies on violence prevention, the most commonly recommended interventions from a public health perspective included changes in gun laws and regulations, public education and awareness programs, behavior modification programs, and clinical services to victims (Winett 1998). More recently, the focus has shifted to **primary prevention** programs at all stages of the life course, but particularly emphasizing early and middle childhood, the period when individuals may start on a trajectory that will influence them throughout their life (Haegerich and Dahlberg 2011). In their review, Haegerich and Dahlberg take an ecologically based view that sees prevention as best operating at all levels, from the individual to society.

The CDC describes four steps in the public health approach to prevention.[2] The first step is to understand the magnitude, the patterns, the sites, and the perpetrators and victims. The second step is to identify risk and protective factors. The third step is to develop and test interventions. The fourth step is the widespread implementation of successful interventions. Further, a public health approach not only focuses on individual behavior change but also examines whether there are policies, environmental factors, or contextual interventions that could influence the likelihood of violence or diminish the harm caused by violence. Mozaffarian and colleagues (2013) add that the public health approach is population-based and focuses on prevention.

We will discuss the major public health steps described above, paying special attention to the key determinants of violent acts, the types of interventions shown to be beneficial in either preventing violence or mitigating the negative health outcomes of violence, the role of public health in combating violence, and the challenges that remain.

Magnitude

Data on violence come from various sources. For instance, death records, records of emergency room visits, police records, and victimization surveys provide vital and unique information, each with strengths and weaknesses. Death records contain data on fatal violent episodes, while hospital records have information regarding both fatal and nonfatal violence-related injury. Still, even hospital records may underestimate the rates of violence, since not all victims of violence are injured to the point of needing medical attention, and patients are not always entirely forthcoming about the source of their injuries. Police records include information about perpetrators of violence and about victims of violence for fatal incidents, yet many violent events are not reported to the police, particularly sexual violence and family violence incidents. Victimization studies are helpful in that they provide information on violent victimizations that do not come to the attention of the police or medical personnel; however, their accuracy relies on recall and honesty and cannot assess victimizations that result in murder. Thus, each of these types of data alone falls short of describing the entire picture of violence, but *together* they help to assess the extent and nature of violence.

In the United States, there are approximately 50,000 violence-related deaths and approximately 5 million violent crimes per year (Karch et. al. 2012; Rand 2009). The extent of violence grows greater when nonfatal injuries due to violent crimes are included. According to Corso and colleagues, more than 2.2 million injuries requiring medical treatment in the United States

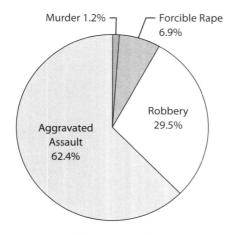

Murder 1.2% ⌐   ⌐ Forcible Rape
6.9%

Robbery
29.5%

Aggravated
Assault
62.4%

FIGURE 17.2. Violent crime by crime type, 2011.
Source: FBI, Uniform Crime Reports.

each year can be attributed to violent incidents (Corso et al. 2007).

According to the FBI's Uniform Crime Report (UCR), there are four major violent crimes: murder, rape, robbery, and aggravated assault. Although robbery may not result in injury, it is considered a crime against a person and involves the physical taking of property by force or threat of force. As shown in figure 17.2, in 2011, although murder was the most serious violent crime, it constituted the smallest proportion of all violent crime reported to the police (1.2%). Aggravated assault was the most common violent crime (62.4%) (FBI 2012).

The Supplemental Homicide Report of the UCR provides an in-depth look at offenders and victims of murder. Overall, offenders and victims tend to be similar with respect to certain demographics such as age, gender, and race. For instance, in 2011, 77.7% of homicide victims were male, the vast majority were age 18 or older (89.8%), and 50.1% were African American. Similarly, the majority of homicide offenders where gender, age, or race was known were male (89.3%), age 18 or older (93.0%), and African American (52.4%). Homicide is largely intraracial, with 92.4% of African American victims killed by African American offenders and 84.5%

of white victims killed by white offenders in 2011 (FBI 2012).

Although the majority of homicide offenders are adults, youth violence (with *youth* defined as younger than age 24) is a major issue for both the criminal justice system and public health. In fact, homicide is the second leading cause of death for youth (ages 10 to 24) and the leading cause of death for African Americans of these ages (CDC 2010a). The increase in the level of violence in the late 1980s and early 1990s (depicted in figure 17.1) was largely due to changes in trends in homicides among those under age 25, with youth violence accounting for 25% of the increase in serious violence (Cook and Laub 1998). School violence is a subset of youth violence that occurs on school property, where children spend most of their day. Isolated incidents of school shootings have a devastating impact, yet these are rare events, constituting less than 1% of homicides (CDC 2010b). Nonfatal violence on school property is more common. According to a 2009 national survey of high school students, 11.1% had been in a physical fight in the previous year while at school and 5.6% reported carrying a weapon to school (CDC 2010a).

Violence within the family is another area of great public health concern. Typically, murder occurs between people who know each other, with 54.7% of homicides in 2008 occurring between acquaintances, 23.3% between family members, and 22.0% between strangers (FBI 2009). Family violence refers to physical and sexual violence as well as threats of violence and emotional abuse to children, spouses, older adults, and other relatives (BJS 2005). In 2005, the Bureau of Justice Statistics published a report that compiled information from the National Crime Victimization Survey and the FBI Supplemental Homicide reports to provide a comprehensive picture of family violence, including reported and unreported acts of violence and homicides (BJS 2005). According to this report, among the 32.2 million victims of violence between 1998 and 2002, 11% were victims of family violence; 49% of these incidents of family violence were against spouses, 11% were parents victimizing their children, and 41% were against other relatives. The majority of victims and perpetrators of family violence were white (74% and 79%, respectively), and the majority of victims were female (73%). One-third of female victims of murder were killed by their husbands or boyfriends, whereas only 3% of male victims were killed by their wives or girlfriends (FBI 2009). Moreover, 22% of murders in 2002 were family murders, with 23% of these being children under age 13 (BJS 2005). Neglect is the leading cause of death among childhood maltreatment fatalities (Douglas and Finkelhor 2005).

Drugs and alcohol also play a role in the perpetration of violence. According to the National Crime Victimization Survey, in 2007, 26% of victims of violence reported that the perpetrator was under the influence of alcohol and/or drugs at the time of the victimization. Similarly, in 2004, 37% and 27% of violent offenders in state prisons and 21% and 24% of violent offenders in federal prisons reported being under the influence of alcohol and drugs, respectively, at the time of their violent offense (Rand et al. 2010).

Costs and Consequences Associated with Violence

One common public health approach to assessing costs to individuals is in estimating the **years of potential life lost** (YPLL), which is the additional number of years a person would have lived, based on normal life expectancy, had the person not died prematurely. Because homicide and suicide are leading causes of death for youth, their YPLL are substantial. Overall, violence-related deaths represent a total of 1.32 million YPLL, which was 11% of potential years lost from all causes of death in 2000 (CDC 2007). Homicide by firearms represented almost one-third of these YPLL. This

burden is by far greater in the United States than in all other First World countries (Richardson and Hemenway 2003). Although the most immediate effect of violence is the physical harm that is sustained by victims, there are several costs associated with violent victimizations beyond the initial physical harm. Most tangible and concrete are the monetary costs such as medical costs, legal expenses, mental health costs, and loss of productivity owing to unpaid workdays (Miller et al. 1996). But there are more intangible costs as well, such as psychological harm, long-term pain and suffering, developmental **consequences**, and reduced **quality of life**.

Significant medical and economic costs are incurred at the societal level also as a result of violence. Beyond the cost of running the criminal justice system, significant productivity loss occurs because of violence. For instance, $64.7 billion was lost nationally in 2000 from loss of work and household productivity caused by interpersonal violence (Corso et al. 2007). Firearm-related violent injuries accounted for the largest share of productivity losses. Moreover, $5.6 billion was spent on medical care for violence-related injuries. When disability-adjusted life years are converted into dollars, this represents $42.6 billion (Brown 2008). Taxpayers pay a large majority of these costs (Wintemute and Wright 1992).

Violent victimization among children and adolescents that does not result in fatality may have long-term consequences. For instance, maltreated children have lower IQ scores and academic performance than others (Rogeness et al. 1986). Abused and neglected children are also more likely to become violent perpetrators themselves; such experiences increase by 30% their likelihood of being arrested for a violent crime (Widom and Maxfield 2001). Violent victimization has also been linked to poor health outcomes such as self-rated health, disabilities, and chronic health problems (Boynton-Jarrett et al. 2008; Plichta and Falik 2001).

Violence exposure is also related to multiple mental health outcomes. This relationship has been studied more closely in female victims but may hold true for male victims as well (Cooker et al. 2002). Generally, increased risk for psychopathology has been found among individuals who have experienced sexual and physical violence. Rates of suicidality, depressive symptoms, posttraumatic stress disorder, and substance-use disorders tend to be higher among those who have experienced violence (Golding 1999). However, since most studies are retrospective, with individuals being assessed after the violence has occurred, a clear causal association remains to be seen.

Victimization has been linked with a **life-course perspective** in order to frame the social and developmental costs of experiencing violence that extend into adulthood (MacMillan 2001). According to the life-course perspective, lives are shaped by multiple trajectories that represent different dimensions of life. Embedded within these long-term trajectories are transitions, which are short-term discrete events (Elder 1985). The short-term events, such as victimization, may have major **influences** on a person's future life course. For instance, exposure to family violence can have detrimental effects on the children in the household, effects that include reduced academic achievement, increased aggression, depression, and psychobiological effects caused by chronic stress (e.g., increased arousal, sleep disturbances) (Margolin and Gordis 2000). Direct and indirect exposure to violence in adolescence can lead to running away, becoming a high-school dropout, teen parenthood, suicide, and arrest (Haynie et al. 2009). Violent victimization as a youth has also been linked to socioeconomic disadvantage in adulthood through reduced educational outcomes (i.e., **self-efficacy**, performance, and attainment) and employment status (MacMillan and Hagan 2004).

Violence can be extremely detrimental to the neighborhoods and communities in which it occurs as well. Half of all homicides occur in just 63 of the largest cities, which house 16% of the U.S. population (Sherman 1997a). Moreover, homicides are concentrated in a handful of communities marked by concentrated poverty, segregation, family disruption, and high gun density (Sherman 1997a; Sherman et al. 1989). These hot spots of violence tend to have residents who are less willing to leave their homes; they experience high levels of stress and anxiety, leading to increased levels of mistrust and decreased levels of community cohesion and **social capital** (Kawachi et al. 1999). Such conditions further exacerbate the problem, allowing more violence to occur in the neighborhood. Recent studies have shown that even residents who only witness violence in their community can experience adverse mental health consequences (Clark et al. 2008). Concentrations of violence can also affect housing prices and can hurt business owners because of fears of violence in the community.

Key Determinants and Evidence-Based Interventions for Preventing Violence

To understand how to best address violence, we must identify and understand the factors that increase or decrease the risk either for perpetration of violence or for a person to become a victim of violence. These influences are best examined in an **ecological** framework (figure 17.3), which considers influences from multiple levels, including the individual, family, school, peer, community, and societal levels. Clusters of risk factors are most likely to place an individual at risk for violence (Satcher 2001).

In this section we will describe different contextual domains and the key determinants of risk within each domain and give some examples of prevention programs that have been developed and evaluated. According to several reviews of primary prevention of physical violence and abuse, there are very few evaluated programs at the societal level (Haegerich and Dahlberg 2011; Joshi et al. 2008).

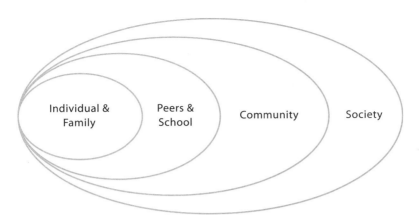

FIGURE 17.3. An ecological framework. *Source:* adapted from LL Dahlberg and EG Krug, Violence—a global public health problem, in Krug et al. 2002, 1–56.

One area in which there have been many attempts to evaluate laws and policies has been that of firearms laws. Hahn and colleagues systematically reviewed the scientific evidence in this area. Using predefined criteria for determining the level of evidence, they concluded, "The evidence available from identified studies was insufficient to determine the **effectiveness** of any of the firearms laws reviewed singly or in combination" (2005, 40). They are careful to point out that there was insufficient evidence, not that there was "no effect."

Following the shootings of 20 children and six adults at Sandy Hook Elementary School in Newtown, Connecticut (Barron 2012; CBC News 2012), there has been renewed interest in and debate about gun control in the United States. In response, a "gun control summit" was held at the Bloomberg School of Public Health, Johns Hopkins University, that featured national experts on guns and violence (Webster and Vernick 2013). They identified seven policy recommendations to reduce gun violence:

1. Institute background checks on gun purchasers.
2. Prohibit high risk individuals from purchasing guns.

3. Implement better control of trafficking of guns and strict dealer licensing.
4. Make guns childproof.
5. Effectively ban assault weapons.
6. Limit high-capacity magazines to 10 rounds of ammunition.
7. Support research funding so that the extent of gun violence and the effectiveness of any programs can be followed. (See Webster and Vernick 2013 for the full background and discussion of these policy recommendations.)

Since these policy recommendations have not been instituted, they have not been evaluated in the United States.

Numerous interventions have been developed at the individual and family level, the peer and school level, and the community level, and we now turn to their description and evaluation. Moreover, we focus on public health interventions rather than those developed in the criminal justice system (for a review of these criminal justice programs see Greenwood 2010).

There are several methods for learning about and evaluating the available intervention programs. With the focus on **evidence-based programs**, recent reviews, meta-analyses, and cost-benefit analyses have summarized the benefits (or lack thereof) of programs. Some reviews assign more "weight" to the evaluations that employ more rigorous methodology; for example, the Maryland Scale gives the greatest weight to randomized designs with no threats to internal validity (Sherman et al. 1997). In other reviews, such as in a meta-analysis, the results of individual study evaluations of similar programs are statistically combined to provide a determination of effectiveness (see Lipsey and Wilson 1998). Several resources list which programs or strategies are most effective, based on stated criteria. For instance, Sherman and colleagues evaluated several interventions regarding crime and delinquency in their report to the U.S. Congress, *Preventing Crime: What Works, What Doesn't, What's Promising* (1997), using the Maryland Scale. The Blueprints for Violence Prevention list has been developed by the Center for the Study and Prevention of Violence at the University of Colorado.[3] This list provides evidence for several programs that are either "model" or "promising" in the area of violence prevention, based on having an **experimental design**, a long-term evaluation, and replications. The CDC Injury Center provides information on violence prevention programs and initiatives with respect to a variety of types of violence, such as child and elder maltreatment and intimate partner and sexual violence (www.cdc .gov/ViolencePrevention/index.html). The British Columbia Injury and Research and Prevention Unit (Joshi et al. 2008) evaluated primary prevention programs for the different ecological levels by life course stage. Recently, the California governor's office published a review of interventions to reduce violence and crime, which consolidates many of these methods and provides a list of effective and ineffective evidence-based programs and strategies (Greenwood 2010).

The following section pulls from several of these lists to provide examples of one ineffective and one effective program for each domain of influence (e.g., individual, school, commu-

nity), as we believe that there is much to be learned from both the unsuccessful programs and the successful ones.

The Individual and Family Level

In the innermost circle of the ecological framework are the individual and family (see figure 17.3). At this level, behavior is influenced by factors such as individual temperament, psychological factors, and **attitudes**, as well as via the family **context**, including the physical context and interactions.

KEY DETERMINANTS

Certain individual characteristics tend to put individuals at risk for becoming violent. For instance, psychological factors, behavioral characteristics, and having beliefs and attitudes favorable to antisocial behavior have been found to differentiate violent individuals from nonviolent individuals (Lipsey and Derzon 1998).

In a meta-analysis of 66 studies, Lipsey and Derzon (1998) find that factors such as hyperactivity, problems with concentrating, restlessness, aggression, and risk-taking behaviors are common characteristics among those who are found to be aggressive and violent as adolescents. These individual characteristics play a vital role in how others interact with such an individual, which may further exacerbate risk. Thus, a difficult temperament may lead to negative interactions with parents, teachers, and peers, and those interactions in turn make it difficult for a child to develop **prosocial skills** (Moffitt 1993) or to do well in school and in peer groups. A low IQ, especially verbal IQ, and low cognitive ability have also been shown to be predictors of violent behavior (e.g., Moffitt 1993). Thus, these negative interactions in early childhood can set a person on a pathway of further aggressive and antisocial behavior in adolescence and a future of violence. For younger children, ages 6 to 11, involvement in antisocial behavior, such as property crime, drugs, smoking, and sex seems to be predictive of later violence. For adolescents, these behaviors are also predictive of violence, along with having antisocial peers and attitudes favorable to violence (Lipsey and Derzon 1998; Satcher 2001).

Contextual factors may also be influential. Violent behavior is more likely for an individual if she grew up in a family with antisocial parents, rejecting parents, parents in conflict, parents who imposed inconsistent punishment, or parents who supervised their children loosely (Sherman 1997b). In fact, one of the most significant predictors that a child will later engage in violence is having antisocial parents, possibly through certain learned behaviors that the parents model rather than through genetic inheritance of violent tendencies (Moffitt 1987). Growing up with poor and dysfunctional parenting can also put one at increased odds to experience violence later in life (Widom 2000). Erratic or harsh disciplinary practices or unclear and lax rules are parenting practices commonly found to increase the risk of violent behavior (Satcher 2001).

EVIDENCE-BASED INTERVENTIONS

Primary prevention is broadly aimed at preventing or delaying the initiation of a behavior. Prevention programs are often aimed at individuals or at a context, such as within the family, a school, or a neighborhood. In the case of violence, such programs might target early aggressive behavior, because there is strong evidence that early aggression often leads to later aggression and violent behavior. From a developmental perspective, interventions at the individual and family levels are designed to prevent the development of criminal potential in individuals at a young age.

Interventions that lie within this domain tend to focus on helping an individual build **social skills** or **life skills**. Particularly early interventions programs may focus on the parent or caregiver of a child, teaching parenting skills individually or in support groups. Some inter-

ventions may be more clinically focused in providing individual or family-level therapy.

One example of an unsuccessful program is the Cambridge-Somerville Youth Study, as described by McCord (1978). In this study, 650 at-risk boys from poor, high-crime areas were matched on a number of characteristics and randomly assigned to treatment or a **control group**. Each boy was assigned a counselor to visit him and offer tailored assistance to the boy and his family and provide mentoring every two months, on average, for five and a half years. The treated boys, in addition, received tutoring and were sent to summer camps. The results showed no significant differences on a variety of outcomes at the end of the treatment. In fact, after 30 years, the treated subjects were more likely to be alcoholics, have mental illness, die early, and have more stress-related behavior (Dishion et al. 1999). Particularly those boys who received a greater amount of the treatment (sent to summer camp for at least two summers), were more likely to have unfavorable outcomes, an outcome that was not explained by baseline differences between the boys who went to summer camp and those who did not. Dishion, McCord, and Poulin (1999) reasoned that the summer camps might have provided an audience and selective attention for their misbehavior. Thus, the delinquent-prone boys received **reinforcement** for their misbehavior. This reinforcement was stronger for those who went to summer camp for at least two years. Overall, this treatment appeared to have a negative effect on long-term delinquent behaviors and crime. Therefore, the authors caution interventionists about aggregating adolescent delinquent peers in this way, as it may have unintended harmful consequences.

Because the family is such a strong influence in the lives of young children, when many risk factors are beginning to develop, the family is an important context for early intervention. The Nurse-Family Partnership program, which includes home visitation to families with young children, has been found to be an effective program both in terms of children's later criminal and antisocial behavior and for child maltreatment (see CSPV 2010; Joshi et al. 2008). David Olds and colleagues (1986) enrolled 400 socially disadvantaged pregnant women with no prior live births in a randomized trial of home visitation by nurses. Families in the intervention groups received home visits during pregnancy and early infancy. Families in the control group received standard prenatal and well-child care in a clinic. Specifically, young, single-parent women of low **socioeconomic status** were randomly assigned to treatment 1 (transportation for prenatal and medical visits), treatment 2 (a nurse home-visitor every two weeks during pregnancy in addition to transportation), treatment 3 (same as 2 but with the visitation continued until the child was two years old), or control (no services).

When the children grew to adolescence, those born to women who had received nurse visits during pregnancy and infancy had a lower incidence of arrest and a lower incidence of convictions and probation violations (Olds et al. 1998). Furthermore, significant differences emerged at the 46-month follow-up for reported child abuse and neglect, infant temperament, behavioral problems, and emergency room visits (Olds et al. 1986). Moreover, using reports from the Child Protective Services, families receiving home visitation had fewer child maltreatment reports involving the mother as perpetrator or the study child as subject (Eckenrode et al. 2000). In an overall evaluation of early childhood home visitation in preventing violence, Bilukha and colleagues (2005) found "strong evidence of effectiveness" for the prevention of child abuse and neglect.

The Peer and School Level

As shown in figure 17.3, as children grow into adolescence, the influence of peers and the context of school become important influences,

while the influence of individual and family level factors continues.

KEY DETERMINANTS

With respect to violent behavior, associating with friends or peers who are violent, antisocial, and delinquent puts children at risk of engaging in violence themselves. Aggressive children or those who are rejected by their peers tend to congregate together, which may reinforce antisocial or aggressive behaviors (Hann and Borek 2001). Having delinquent peers is a long-standing risk factor for increased violence. LaCourse and colleagues (2003) found that being involved in a delinquent group was associated with an increased rate of violence, controlling for past delinquent propensity. Moreover, leaving a delinquent peer group was associated with a decrease in violent behaviors.

Among the most consistent findings in longitudinal studies of children and adolescents is the stability over the life course of levels of aggressive behavior, most often as indicated in school settings and identified by teachers (Ensminger et al. 1983; Gottfredson 1997; Harachi et al. 2006; Hawkins et al. 1992; White et al. 1990). Although aggressive behavior is a big risk for further aggressive and violent behavior, it has also been shown to relate to other undesirable outcomes, such as early initiation of smoking and drug use and school dropout. Therefore, the prevention of early aggression may have benefits for many outcomes, including violence.

EVIDENCE-BASED INTERVENTIONS

Because schools and classrooms provide access to many children, prevention programs for violence and other antisocial behavior often take place in school settings. Children spend a great deal of time during their formative years in school; it is a setting where universal programs (i.e., programs aimed at all children regardless of risk) can most effectively be mounted. The classroom and the playground are often the contexts where aggressive behavior such as bullying is likely to appear, and evidence shows that the context within the school and the classroom may influence the further development or inhibition of aggressive behavior.

Violence interventions in a school setting are prevalent and vary widely. They may range from teacher training and classroom management strategies, to antiviolence education curricula, to educational enrichment, to after-school activities, to attempting to change school **norms** regarding violence. These programs have varied dramatically in the target of the prevention, the implementer, and the theoretical rationale.

Many school-based prevention programs have been aimed at aggressive behavior, but not all have been successful. One common approach used in schools for children already showing signs of aggressive behavior is to remove deviant adolescents from their normal classroom and group them in another place. One meta-analysis of social skills training interventions done in both schools and clinics found that interventions done in groups consisting only of antisocial peers had poorer success in reducing aggressive behavior than when grouping deviant peers together was avoided (Ang and Hughes 2002). Although more research is needed in assessing the behavioral outcomes related to aggregating deviant peers in a school setting, considerable evidence shows the deleterious effect of naturally occurring aggregation of deviant peers in schools. This research suggests that this type of school aggregation can lead to poor outcomes for students, including increased aggressive behavior and later criminality (Dishion et al. Poulin 1999; Gifford-Smith et al. 2005).

In contrast, one type of classroom-based intervention that has shown to be successful is the Good Behavior Game (GBG). The GBG is a universal preventive intervention implemented by teachers and directed at entire regular first- and second-grade classrooms. It focuses on socializing children to the role of student and reducing aggressive, disruptive classroom behavior, a consistently reported early risk factor shared by a broad set of adolescent and adult problem outcomes, particularly those involving externalizing or acting-out behaviors. Appropriate classroom behavior is rewarded for teams of students that do not exceed maladaptive behavior standards, using heterogeneous teams of children to help manage behavior through mutual self-interest (Kellam et al. 2008). Previous research has documented the effectiveness of the GBG in reducing the level and development of aggressive, disruptive behavior, particularly among aggressive, disruptive males (Brown 1993; Dolan et al. 1993; Kellam et al. 1994). In 19 Baltimore public schools, the GBG was implemented in several cohorts of first- and second-grade children. Classrooms, teachers, and students were randomized to the intervention and control conditions. Results from two cohorts of first grade who were followed into young adulthood showed that the aggressive males in the first cohort of intervention classrooms were less likely to be incarcerated for violent (felony) crimes and were less likely to receive a diagnosis of antisocial personality disorder (Petras et al. 2008). Although the direction of these results was similar in the second cohort, the results were not significant. The authors describe the intervention in the second cohort as not being as rigorously monitored or supported. Aggressive males in the treatment classrooms were also more likely to graduate from high school and less likely to have drug abuse problems.

The success of this and other early intervention programs suggests not only that school-based interventions can succeed in reducing later violent behavior, but also that early aggressive behavior can be modified. Moreover, if it is modified, often the observed relationship between early aggressive behavior and later antisocial outcomes is disrupted. These programs also suggest that multiple outcomes may be impacted by these early programs (i.e., benefits are seen not only for violence-related behavior, but also in terms of less alcohol, drug, and cigarette use and higher high school graduation rates).

The Community Level

The third level of influence of behavior, according to the ecological framework depicted in Figure 17.3, is the level of community. Community factors can influence behavior above and beyond the influence of **individual-level factors**, family, peers, and school, both directly and through interaction with the other levels.

KEY DETERMINANTS

Certain characteristics of a community can make its residents more likely to commit acts of violence. High levels of serious crime and violence tend to be concentrated in particular neighborhoods and even often in narrow sections within these neighborhoods (Sherman 1997a). Structurally, areas characterized by **social disorganization** are more likely to be violent (Shaw and McKay 1942). Communities that have physical deterioration, high unemployment, residential instability, and high population density will also be less likely to control their residents informally.

These communities tend to have high proportions of unmarried adult males, teenage males, nonworking adults, poor people, persons with criminal histories, and single parents, all of which result in an inability to maintain adult **networks** of informal control over children (Bursik and Grasmick 1993). The prevalence of unsupervised male teenage groups, local friendship networks, and local participation in formal voluntary association can predict community social disorganization (Hirschfield and Bowers 1997; Rountree and Warner 1999; Sampson and Groves 1989). Closely related to this concept is the idea of a community's level of **collective efficacy**. This refers to the level of trust and willingness of community members to intervene for the public good (Sampson et al. 1997). Collective efficacy helps to promote com-

munity cohesion and trust, which in turn is related to lower levels of violence in the community (Morenoff et al. 2001). Similarly, the "broken windows" thesis posits that areas with deteriorated buildings and public incivility increase the likelihood of violent crimes by giving a visual message that the community members are reluctant to intervene in the welfare of their community (Wilson and Kelling 1982).

Another explanation why certain communities have higher rates of violence than others is that certain communities have higher concentrations of guns than others, thereby increasing the risk of violent crime in those areas. Firearms are the most common weapons present in all types of violent crimes. The increase in violence, especially youth violence, in the late 1980s and early 1990s, and the subsequent decrease, depicted in figure 17.1, was largely a result of the corresponding increase and decrease in the use of handguns among this population (Blumstein 2000). In 2011, 67.8% of homicides involved a firearm, and 72.5% of the firearms were handguns. Although firearms are less common for robbery and aggravated assault, they still play a prominent role. Firearms were used in 41.3% of the robberies and 21.2% of all aggravated assaults known to the police in 2011 (FBI 2012). In fact, firearm-related incidents (including self-directed) resulted in close to 29,000 deaths in the United States in 2000, making firearms one of the leading actual causes of death (Mokdad et al. 2004).

Guns have several attributes that other weapons do not, which can increase the severity of a violent incident. Guns allow the perpetrator to commit an act of violence quickly, at a distance, and without much skill or strength (Cook et al. 2002). Moreover, the presence of guns increases the chances of lethality. As gun ownership and gun violence rise and fall together (Wintemute 2008), the presence of guns clearly has an impact on the likelihood of violence and the severity of violence. Simply having a gun in the home significantly increases the chances of homicide of a family member or intimate partner (Kellermann et al. 1993).

EVIDENCE-BASED INTERVENTIONS

Community-level interventions encompass multiple approaches to reducing violence. They include alternative policing, such as **targeting** hot spots, and modifying the physical environment, for example improving street lighting. Public-health-related strategies also include community empowerment and activism to reduce the number of guns or alcohol outlets in a neighborhood or employing street **outreach** workers in a community.

The current state of science offers no strong evaluations of community programs. In fact, evaluations of community interventions generally employ weak research designs and tend to test programs focused on *symptoms* of community risk factors rather than the root causes themselves. However, at least one community-based program has been consistently shown to be ineffective. Hundreds of gun buy-back programs have been implemented nationwide as a community-based approach to reducing gun violence. The gun buy-back approach provides drop-off locations for firearms that are exchanged for cash or vouchers in neighborhoods that experience high levels of gun-related crime. Overall, these programs have been ineffective for several reasons. For instance, they tend to attract guns with characteristics that differ significantly from those used in firearm-related violence (e.g., type, age, manufacturer), the guns may not be in working order, may come from other areas, or may be guns that were locked up at home (Hahn et al. 2005; Kuhn et al. 2002; Romero et al. 1998; Sherman 1997a). Therefore, the gun buy-back programs are unable to significantly alter the rate of gun violence in a community.

A promising community strategy that has been implemented in various urban environments uses a variety of strategies in the community, including street outreach and mentoring for youth at risk for serious violent offenses, conflict intervention or violence interruption, and media messaging to change norms regarding violence in the community. One such program is CeaseFire, based in Chicago. This program utilizes a **coalition** of community leaders, including clergy, community organizations, city agencies, and police, to develop and implement community-based violence prevention strategies. One of the more novel strategies used in CeaseFire is the hiring of violence interrupters. These individuals are able to establish rapport with the at-risk youth of the community and are intimately involved in what is going on in the community. Thus, they are often able to interrupt and mediate potentially violent situations as they are happening. In a rigorous evaluation of the program, the seven neighborhoods in which CeaseFire was implemented were compared with seven similar communities that received no intervention. The program showed a considerable reduction in violence in the intervention communities. The CeaseFire program was shown to have contributed to a significant (16%-34%) reduction in shootings in six of the seven neighborhoods tested. Retaliatory homicides were also significantly reduced in four of the seven neighborhoods. Qualitatively, participants in the program, including many ex-gang members and violent offenders, said that CeaseFire also helped them considerably through offering help to find jobs and obtain a GED and guidance in leaving a gang (Skogan et al. 2008).

Programs in other urban communities have used similar violence interruption approaches with success. A recent program in Baltimore called Safe Streets, based on the principles of CeaseFire, has shown mixed but promising results in reducing violence. Of the four neighborhoods in which Safe Streets was implemented, two had significantly greater reductions in homicides, and three had significantly greater reductions in nonfatal shootings, compared to similar communities in which no program was implemented (Webster et al. 2013). A similar program in Massachusetts, in which street outreach workers engage local gang members to intervene and prevent violence, has also shown some success. Initial evidence indicates that violence prevention outreach workers are effective both in engaging gang members in peace-making efforts during immediate crises and in connecting gang members to additional services such as employment programs, with the **goal** of preventing future violent incidents (Frattaroli et al. 2010).

One potential reason why community programs such as Safe Streets and CeaseFire have been successful in reducing violence is that these programs have targeted individuals most likely to be involved in the violence. Gun buybacks tend not to attract the guns that would be used for violent acts. The CeaseFire strategy, in contrast, was aimed at the individuals most at risk for committing violence. This strategy may involve more time and energy, to build relationships with the relevant individuals and to anticipate when violent events may occur, but in the end it may have a better payoff for making communities safer. Furthermore, violence interrupters may be seen by at-risk youth as a more credible source than police officers, who are generally the people in charge of gun buyback programs.

Multiple Domains

Ideally, an intervention program would cut across all domains, since individuals do not live in isolation and the risk factors for violence rarely occur singularly or within only one contextual domain. One successful approach that addresses multiple domains is Multisystemic Therapy (MST), a family- and community-based treatment for seriously antisocial youth. The MST approach focuses on intrapersonal (e.g., cognitive) and systemic (e.g., family, peers, and school) factors associated with antisocial

behavior. MST works with existing networks and contexts of high risk youth to promote and enhance the positive relationships and environments of the youth, such as supportive family relationships, and to decrease contact with negative networks such as deviant peer groups. In a randomized trial, high risk youth were assigned to either MST or individual therapy. After four years, there had been a significant reduction in arrests and in the severity of offenses for the experimental group that received MST, compared to the control group that received individual therapy. Furthermore, family relations improved, and parental symptoms improved within the experimental group (Borduin et al. 1995).

Victim-Based Interventions

In any violent situation, at least two parties are involved in a conflict. In the preceding section, we discussed prevention and intervention programs aimed at persons at risk of violent behavior in order to reduce violence overall. Repeat victimization is also a concern of public health professionals. Public health interventions have been aimed at those who are at risk of becoming a victim of violence, both to try to remedy the damage that has been done and to prevent further violence. Prime examples of violence that affects the same victim repeatedly are intimate partner violence, child abuse, and elder abuse.

Several strategies to identify and support victims of violence have been effective. For example, shelters and treatments for victims of domestic violence have been established, where victims of domestic violence may feel protected and where physical and mental health interventions can be based. In a systematic review of the evaluation of interventions aimed at preventing abuse or revictimization of women, Wathen and MacMillan (2003) found evidence that among women who have spent at least one night in a shelter, those who received advocacy and counseling services reported less repeated abuse and an improved quality of life. Still, the authors concluded that information about evidence-based approaches for preventing repeat intimate partner violence is lacking; they argue that the evaluation of interventions to improve the health and well-being of abused women is a key research priority.

Screening and referral services in health care settings are another intervention that is advocated for reducing revictimization, especially among child abuse and neglect cases, cases of elder abuse, and cases of intimate partner violence (Haegerich and Dahlberg 2011; Joshi et al. 2008; Krug et al. 2002). In a recent review of elder mistreatment, Pillemar and colleagues (2007) suggest that there is too little evidence to demonstrate the benefits of interventions such as mandatory reporting, widespread screening, or the education of professionals. Further research is needed to identify the best prevention and intervention practices in this area.

Conclusion

In the past three decades, violence prevention has become a major concern for the public health community in the United States. The public health and criminal justice approaches are complementary, each with its own strengths and challenges. The criminal justice system stresses punishment and retribution, separating offenders and victims. A public health approach focuses on the primary prevention of violence, reparation of the mental and physical harm caused by violence, and addressing the needs of the victim to reduce the risk of revictimization. The public health approach, furthermore, is multifaceted, seeking to gain a better understanding of the causes and risk factors of violence. Intervention strategies focus on multiple **levels of influence**, including the over-all cultural and societal contexts that influence the tolerance of violent behavior and put limits on intervention design.

One major strength of a public health approach is its interdisciplinary nature and the accompanying experience in working with different **key stakeholders** to solve public health problems. Public health draws from multiple fields and areas of expertise, including psychology, epidemiology, sociology, criminology, medicine, education, and economics. Therefore, it can make use of a wide array of resources and tools to address the problem of violence. The public health field is well positioned to implement violence prevention efforts, given its experience in addressing population-wide health challenges. Public health professionals can be instrumental in coordinating a wide array of services, such as child and protective services, hospital and health care services, and the criminal justice system, to reduce violence victimization.

The interdisciplinary **reach** of the public health approach is a particular strength when tragedies of violence such as the mass murders in Newtown, Connecticut, and in Aurora, Colorado, occur. While these acts of violence are rare compared with those occurring in our cities every day, in the wake of such tragedies, public health professionals and academics can draw on mental health service interventions, firearm regulation advocacy groups, and victim services to attempt to prevent such comparatively rare but destructive violent acts.

Furthermore, the prevention framework in public health focuses on understanding risk factors and ways to intervene on these risk factors. The early-prevention work suggests that early intervention is potentially a more effective, cheaper, and easier way to successfully diminish violence than intervening with those who have already become violent offenders. For example, in a review considering the impact of incarceration on crime, Stemen (2007) concludes that several factors have a strong impact on reducing crime rates. He cites Lochner and Moretti (2004), who examine the relationship between crime rates and citizens' education. They argue that a 1% increase in male high school graduation rates would save as much as $1.4 billion nationally through crime reduction.

Despite its strengths, public health faces multiple challenges in addressing the violence problem. First, rates of homicide in developed countries are interconnected with societal and cultural norms (Krug et al. 1998; Reza et al. 2001). For instance, both gender inequity and social inequality in American society increase the likelihood of violence. Mistrust and lack of respect are consequences of inequity that are likely to result in income inequality, and greater income inequality is associated with higher rates of homicide (Fajnzylber et al. 2002).

Second, although societal-level influences clearly need to be addressed, how to intervene effectively at the societal level is not as clear. The **cultural norms** and values of a society are not always in line with what public health science shows is an effective strategy. For example, the value of being able to own firearms is deeply embedded in American culture. Yet, empirically in many situations, the presence of guns is likely to lead to injury and harm. Public health gun control efforts challenge this American value, and as a result, efforts to reduce the presence of guns are difficult. Changing the norms and embedded values of a society can be a difficult endeavor. Creative and innovative strategies are needed to overcome this barrier. Hemenway and Miller (2013) suggest that some social norms that encourage violence might be a target of change efforts (e.g., encouraging those with guns in the home to be aware of how they are stored and handled, making citizens more aware of where guns used in homicides come from [gun trafficking], and changing the view that guns represent power and masculinity).

Third, in several areas research and evaluation of the best practices are needed. Intimate partner violence and elder abuse need increas-

ing attention to program development and evaluation as well as dissemination of these results to practitioners and policymakers.

An additional challenge is the prevailing view that incarceration is the primary way to deal with violence and crime. Prisons and jails are quite costly in resources, and there is not much evidence that they are effective in reducing violence levels. Moreover, they compete with resources for early prevention and intervention. A related challenge is the fragmented way that stakeholders have addressed the issue of violence reduction. These stakeholders include not only the public health community, but also the criminal justice system, primary health care providers, and the educational system. Sharing empirical findings and approaches to violence prevention and reduction would be beneficial to all, yet for the most part this has not happened.

NOTES

1. See also Violence prevention, Centers for Disease Control and Prevention, www.cdc.gov/ncipc/dvp/PublicHealthApproachTo_ViolencePrevention.htm (accessed Feb. 17, 2014).

2. See note 1.

3. See the website of the Center for the Study and Prevention of Violence, www.colorado.edu/cspv/blueprints/.

REFERENCES

Ang RP, Hughes JN. 2002. Differential benefits of skills training with antisocial youth based on group composition: A meta-analytic investigation. *School Psychol Rev* 31:164–85.

Barron J. 2012. Children were all shot multiple times with a semiautomatic, officials say. *New York Times,* Dec. 15.

Bilukha O, Hahn RA, Crosby A, et al. 2005. The effectiveness of early childhood home visitation in preventing violence: A systematic review. *Am J Prev Med* 28 (2S1): 28–39.

Blumstein A. 2000. Disaggregating the violence trends. In *The Crime Drop in America,* ed. A Blumstein, J Wallman, 13–44. Cambridge: Cambridge University Press.

Borduin CM, Mann BJ, Cone LT, et al. 1995. Multisystemic treatment of serious juvenile offenders:

Long-term prevention of criminality and violence. *J Consult Clin Psychol* 63:569-78.

Boynton-Jarrett R, Ryan LM, Berkman LF, Wright RJ. 2008. Cumulative violence exposure and self-rated health: Longitudinal study of adolescents in the United States. *Pediatrics* 122:961-70.

Brown CH. 1993. Statistical methods for preventive trials in mental health. *Stat Med* 12:289-300.

Brown DW. 2008. Economic value of disability-adjusted life years lost to violence: Estimates for WHO member states. *Rev Panam Salud Publica* 24:203-9.

Bureau of Justice Statistics (BJS). 2005. *Family Violence Statistics.* Washington, DC: U.S. Department of Justice.

Bursik RJ Jr., Grasmick H. 1993. *Neighborhoods and Crime: The Dimensions of Effective Community Control.* New York: Lexington.

Buzawa ES, Buzawa CG. 2003. *Domestic Violence: The Criminal Justice Response.* Thousand Oaks, CA: Sage.

CBC News. 2012. 20 children among dead at school shooting in Connecticut. Dec. 14.

Center for the Study and Prevention of Violence (CSPV). 2010. Blueprints for Violence Prevention. Center for the Study and Prevention of Violence, Institute of Behavioral Science, University of Colorado at Boulder. Available at www.colorado.edu/cspv/blueprints (accessed July 30, 2010).

Centers for Disease Control and Prevention (CDC). 2007. Web-based injury statistics query and reporting system (WISQARS). Centers for Disease Control and Prevention, National Center for Injury Prevention and Control, Atlanta GA, http://webappa.cdc.gov/sasweb/ncipc/ypll10.html (accessed Aug. 18, 2009).

———. 2010a. *Youth Violence: Facts at a Glance.* Washington, DC: CDC.

———. 2010b. *Understanding School Violence: Facts at a Glance.* Washington, DC: CDC.

Clark C, Ryan L, Kawachi I, Canner MJ, Berkman L, Wright RJ. 2008. Witnessing community violence in residential neighborhoods: A mental health hazard for urban women. *J Urban Health* 85:22-38.

Cook PJ, Laub JH. 1998. The unprecedented epidemic in youth violence. In *Youth Violence: Crime and Justice: A Review of Research,* ed. M Tonry, MH Moore, 24:27-64. Chicago: University of Chicago Press.

Cook PJ, Moore MH, Braga AA. 2002. Gun control. In *Crime: Public Policies for Crime Control,* ed. JQ Wilson, J Petersilia, 291-329. San Francisco: Institute for Contemporary Studies.

Cooker AL, Smith PH, Bethea L, King MR, McKeown RE. 2002. Physical health consequences of physical and psychological intimate partner violence. *Arch Family Med* 9:451-57.

Corso PS, Mercy JA, Simon TR, Finkelstein EA, Miller TR. 2007. Medical costs and productivity losses due to interpersonal and self-directed violence in the United States. *Am J Prev Med* 32:474-82.

Dahlberg LL, Mercy JA. 2009. History of violence as a public health problem. *Virt Mentor* 11:167-72.

Dishion TJ, McCord J, Poulin F. 1999. When interventions harm: Peer groups and problem behavior. *Am Psychol* 54:775-64.

Dolan LJ, Kellam SG, Brown CH, et al. 1993. The short term impact of two classroom-based preventive interventions on aggressive and shy behaviors and poor achievement. *J Applied Dev Psychol* 14:317-45.

Douglas EM, Finkelhor D. 2005. *Child Maltreatment Fatalities Fact Sheet.* Durham, NH: Crimes Against Children Research Center.

Eckenrode J, Ganzel B, Henderson CR, et al. 2000. Preventing child abuse and neglect with a program of nurse home visitation: The limiting effects of domestic violence. *JAMA* 284:1385-91.

Elder GH Jr. 1985. Perspectives on the life course. In *Life Course Dynamics,* ed. GH Elder Jr., 23-49. Ithaca, NY: Cornell University Press.

Ensminger ME, Kellam SG, Rubin BR. 1983. School and family origins of delinquency: Comparisons by sex. In *Prospective Studies of Crime and Delinquency,* ed. K Van Dusen, S Mednick, 73-97. Hingman, MA: Nijhoff.

Fajnzylber P, Lederman D, Loayza N. 2002. What causes violent crime? *Eur Econ Rev* 46:1323-57.

Federal Bureau of Investigation (FBI). 2009. *Crime in the United States, 2008.* Washington, DC: U.S. Department of Justice.

———. 2012. *Crime in the United States, 2011.* Washington, DC: U.S. Department of Justice.

Frattaroli S, Pollack KM, Jonsberg K, Croteau G, Rivera J, Mendel JS. 2010. Streetworkers, youth violence prevention, and peacemaking in Lowell, Massachusetts: Lessons and voices from the community. *Prog Community Health Partnersh* 4 (3): 171-79.

Gifford-Smith M, Dodge KA, Dishion TJ, McCord J. 2005. Peer influence in children and adolescents: Crossing the bridge from developmental to intervention science. *J Abnorm Child Psychol* 33:255-65.

Glover AR, Paul DP, Dodge M. 2011. Law enforcement officers' attitudes about domestic violence. *Violence Against Women* 17:619.

Golding J. 1999. Intimate partner violence as a risk factor for mental disorders: A meta-analysis. *J Family Violence* 14:99-131.

Gottfredson D. 1997. School-based crime prevention. In *Preventing Crime: What Works, What Doesn't, What's Promising,* ed. LW Sherman, D Gottfredson, D

MacKenzie, J Eck, P Reuter, S Bushway. Report to the U.S. Congress. Washington, DC: U.S. Dept. of Justice.

Greenwood P. 2010. *Preventing and Reducing Youth Crime and Violence: Using Evidence-Based Practices.* Sacramento, CA: Governor's Office of Gang and Youth Violence Policy.

Haegerich T, Dahlberg LL. 2011. Violence as a public health risk. *Am J Lifestyle Med* 5:392.

Hahn RA, Bilukha O, Crosby A, et al. 2005. *Am J Prev Med* 28(2S1) 40-71.

Hann DM, Borek NT, eds. 2001. *NIMH Taking Stock of Risk Factors for Child/Youth Externalizing Behavior Problems.* Washington, DC: U.S. Government Printing Office.

Harachi TW, Fleming CB, White HR, et al. 2006. Aggressive behavior among girls and boys during middle childhood: Predictors and sequelae of trajectory group membership. *Aggress Behav* 32:279-93.

Hawkins JD, Catalano RF, Miller JY. 1992. Risk and protective factors for alcohol and other drug problems in adolescence and early adulthood: Implications for substance abuse prevention. *Psychol Bull* 112 (1) (July): 64-105.

Haynie, DL, Petts RJ, Maimon D, Piquero AR. 2009. Exposure to violence in adolescence and precocious role exits. *J Youth Adolesc* 38:269-86.

Hemenway D, Miller M. 2013. Public health approach to the prevention of gun violence. *N Engl J Med* 368 (May 23): 2033-35.

Hirschfield A, Bowers KJ. 1997. The effect of social cohesion on levels of recorded crime in disadvantaged areas. *Urban Stud* 34:1275-95.

Hoyle C. 1998. *Negotiating Domestic Violence: Police, Criminal Justice, and Victims.* Oxford: Oxford University Press.

Joshi P, Pallaveshi L, Verma P, Pike I. 2008. Primary prevention of physical violence and abuse in British Columbia. BC Injury Research and Prevention Unit, http://injuryresearch.bc.ca/admin/DocUpload/3_20110406_111400Violence_Prevention_Evidence_Paper_071408_Final.pdf.

Karch DL, Logan J, McDaniel D, Parks S, Patel N. 2012. Surveillance for violent deaths—national violent death reporting system, 16 States, 2009. *MMWR* 61 (6): 1.

Kawachi I, Kennedy BP, Glass R. 1999. Social capital and self-rated health: A contextual analysis. *Am J Public Health* 89:1187-93.

Kellam SG, Brown CH, Poduska JM, et al. 2008. Effects of a universal classroom behavior management program in first and second grades on young adult behavioral, psychiatric, and social outcomes. *Drug Alcohol Depend* 95S:S5-S28.

Kellam SG, Rebok GW, Ialongo N, Mayer LS. 1994. The course and malleability of aggressive behavior from early first grade into middle school: Results of a developmental epidemiologically-based preventive trial. *J Child Psychol Psychiatry* 35:259-82.

Kellermann AL, Rivara FP, Rushforth NB. 1993. Gun ownership as a risk factor for homicide in the home. *N Engl J Med* 329:1084-91.

Krug EG, Dahlberg LL, Mercy JA, Zwi AB, Lozano R, eds. 2002. *World Report on Violence and Health.* Geneva: World Health Organization.

Krug EG, Powell KE, Dahlberg LL. 1998. Firearm-related deaths in the United States and 35 other high- and upper-middle-income countries. *Int J Epidemiol* 27:214-21.

Kuhn EM, Nie CL, O'Brien ME, Withers RL, Wintemute GJ, Hargarten SW. 2002. Missing the target: A comparison of buyback and fatality related guns. *Inj Prev* 8:143-46.

LaCourse E, Nagin D, Tremblay RE, Vitaro F, Claes M. 2003. Developmental trajectories of boys' delinquent group membership and facilitation of violent behaviors during adolescence. *Dev Psychopath* 15:183-97.

Lipsey MW, Derzon JH. 1998. Predictors of serious delinquency in adolescence and early adulthood: A synthesis of longitudinal research. In *Serious and Violent Juvenile Offenders: Risk Factors and Successful Interventions,* ed. R Loeber, DP Farrington, 86-105. Thousand Oaks, CA: Sage.

Lipsey MW, Wilson DB. 1998. Effective intervention for serious juvenile offenders: A synthesis of research. In *Serious and Violent Juvenile Offenders: Risk Factors and Successful Interventions,* ed. R Loeber, DP Farrington, 313-45. Thousand Oaks, CA: Sage.

Lochner L, Moretti E. 2004. The effect of education on crime: Evidence from prison inmates, arrests, and self reports. *Am Econ Rev* 94 (1): 155-89.

MacMillan R. 2001. Violence and the life course: The consequences of victimization for personal and social development. *Ann Rev Soc* 27:1-22.

MacMillan R, Hagan J. 2004. Violence in the transition to adulthood: Adolescent victimization, education, and socioeconomic attainment in later life. *J Res Adolesc* 14:127-58.

Margolin G, Gordis EB. 2000. The effects of family and community violence on children. *Annu Rev Psych* 51:445-79.

Martinson R. 1974. What works? Questions and answers about prison reform. *Public Int* Spring: 22-54.

McCord J. 1978. A thirty-year follow-up of treatment effects. *Am Psychol* 33:284-89.

Miller TR, Cohen MA, Wiersma B. 1996. *Victim Costs and Consequences: A New Look.* Washington, DC: National Institute of Justice.

Moffitt TE. 1987. Parental mental disorder and offspring criminal behavior: An adoption study. *Psychiatry* 50:346-60.

———. 1993. Adolescence-limited and life-course persistent antisocial behavior: A developmental taxonomy. *Psychol Rev* 100:674-701.

Mokdad AH, Marks JS, Stroup DF, Gerberding JL. 2004. Actual causes of death in the United States, 2000. *JAMA* 291:1238-45.

Mozaffarian D, Hemenway D, Ludwig DS. 2013. Curbing gun violence: Lessons from public health successes. *JAMA* 309 (6): 551-52.

Moore MH. 1993. Violence prevention: Criminal justice or public health? *Health Affairs* 12:34-45.

Morenoff JD, Sampson RJ, Raudenbush SW. 2001. Neighborhood inequality, collective efficacy, and the spatial dynamics of urban violence. *Criminology* 39:517-59.

Olds D, Henderson C, Chamberlin R, Tatelbaum R. 1986. Preventing child abuse and neglect: A randomized trial of nurse home visitation. *Pediatrics* 78:65-78.

Olds D, Henderson CR Jr., Cole R, et al. 1998. Long-term effects of nurse home visitation on children's criminal and antisocial behavior: 15-year follow-up of a randomized trial. *JAMA* 280:1238-44.

Petras H, Kellam SG, Brown CH, Muthen BO, Ialongo NS, Poduska JM. 2008. Developmental epidemiological courses leading to antisocial personality disorder and violent and criminal behavior: Effects by young adulthood of a universal preventive intervention in first- and second-grade classrooms. *Drug Alcohol Depend* 95S:S45-S59.

Pillemar K, Mueller-Johnson K, Mock S, Suitor J, Lacha M. 2007. Prevention of elder mistreatment. In *Handbook of Injury and Violence Prevention*, ed. L Doll, EN Haas, S Bonzo, D Sleet, J Mercy. New York: Springer.

Plichta SB, Falik M. 2001. Prevalence of violence and its implications for women's health. *Women's Health Issues* 11:244-58.

Rand M. 2009. *Criminal Victimization, 2008.* Washington, DC: Bureau of Justice Statistics.

Rand MR, Sabol WJ, Sinclair M, Snyder HN, U.S. Dept of Justice, Bureau of Justice Statistics. 2010. Alcohol and crime: Data from 2002 to 2008. U.S. Dept of Justice, Bureau of Justice Statistics, Washington, DC.

Reza A, Mercy JA, Krug EG. 2001. Epidemiology of violent deaths in the world. *Inj Prev* 7:104-11.

Richardson EG, Hemenway D. 2003. Homicide, suicide, and unintentional firearm fatality: Comparing the United States with other high-income countries. *J Trauma* 2011 (70): 238.

Rogeness GA, Amrung SA, Macedo CA, Harris WR, Fischer C. 1986. Psychopathology in abused and neglected children. *J Am Acad Child Psychiatry* 25:659-65.

Romero MP, Wintemute GJ, Vernick JS. 1998. Characteristics of a gun exchange program, and an assessment of potential benefits. *Inj Prev* 4:206-10.

Rountree PW, Warner BD. 1999. Social ties and crime: Is the relationship gendered? *Criminology* 37:789-812.

Sampson RJ, Groves WB. 1989. Community structure and crime: Testing social-disorganization theory. *Am J Soc* 94:774-802.

Sampson RJ, Raudenbush S, Earls F. 1997. Neighborhoods and violent crime: A multilevel study of collective efficacy. *Science* 277:918-24.

Satcher D. 2001. *Youth Violence: A Report of the Surgeon General.* Washington, DC: U.S. Department of Health and Human Services.

Shaw C, McKay H. 1942. *Juvenile Delinquency and Urban Areas.* Chicago: University of Chicago Press.

Sherman LW. 1997a. Communities and crime prevention. In *Preventing Crime: What Works, What Doesn't, What's Promising,* ed. LW Sherman, D Gottfredson, D MacKenzie, J Eck, P Reuter, S Bushway. Report to the U.S. Congress. Washington, DC: U.S. Dept. of Justice.

———. 1997b. Family-based crime prevention. In *Preventing Crime: What Works, What Doesn't, What's Promising,* ed. LW Sherman, D Gottfredson, D MacKenzie, J Eck, P Reuter, S Bushway. Report to the U.S. Congress. Washington, DC: U.S. Dept. of Justice.

Sherman LW, Gartin PR, Brueger ME. 1989. Hot spots of predatory crime: Routine activities and the criminology of place. *Criminology* 27:27-56.

Sherman LW, Gottfredson D, MacKenzie D, Eck J, Reuter P, Bushway S., eds. 1997. *Preventing Crime: What Works, What Doesn't, What's Promising.* Report to the U.S. Congress. Washington, DC: U.S. Dept. of Justice.

Skogan WG, Hartnett SM, Bump N, Dubois J. 2008. *Evaluation of CeaseFire—Chicago: Executive Summary.* Evanston, IL: Northwestern University.

Steman D. 2007. Reconsidering incarceration. *Fed Sentenc Rep* 19:221-33.

Wathen CN, MacMillan HL. 2003. Interventions for violence against women. *JAMA* 289:589-600.

Webster DW, Vernick JS. 2013. *Reducing Gun Violence in America: Informing Policy with Evidence and Analysis.* Baltimore: Johns Hopkins University Press.

Webster DW, Whitehill JM, Vernick JS, Curriero FC. 2013. Effects of Baltimore's safe streets program on gun violence: A replication of Chicago's CeaseFire program. *J Urban Health* 90 (1): 27-40.

White JL, Moffitt TE, Earls F, Robins L, Silva PS. 1990. How early can we tell? Predictors of childhood conduct disorder and adolescent delinquency. *Criminology* 28:507.

Widom CS. 2000. Childhood victimization: Early adversity, later psychopathology. *Nat Inst Justice J* January:2-9.

Widom CS, Maxfield MG. 2001. An update on the "cycle of violence." In *National Institute of Justice: Research in Brief.* Washington, DC: U.S. Department of Justice.

Wilson JQ, Kelling G. 1982. The police and neighborhood safety: Broken windows. *Atlantic Monthly* 127:29-38.

Winett LB. 1998. Constructing violence as a public health problem. *Public Health Rep* 114:498-507.

Wintemute GJ. 2008. Guns, fear, the Constitution, and the public's health. *N Engl J Med* 358:1421-24.

Wintemute GJ, Wright MA. 1992. Initial and subsequent hospital costs of firearm injuries. *J Trauma* 33:556-60.

World Health Organization (WHO). 1996. *Global Consultation on Violence and Health: Violence a Public Health Priority.* Geneva: World Health Organization.

———. 2004. *Violence Prevention: The Evidence: Reducing Violence through Victim Identification, Care, and Support Programmes.* Geneva: World Health Organization.

CHAPTER 18

Sexual Risk and Behavior Change

HELEN C. KOENIG AND DAVID HOLTGRAVE

LEARNING OBJECTIVES

After completing the chapter, the reader will be able to

* Define high risk sexual behavior and understand why it is a public health concern.
* Explore how individual, family, sociocultural, and structural or political factors may affect an individual's sexual risk behaviors.
* Understand the difference between evidence-based interventions that (1) seek to affect knowledge and attitudes about safe behaviors by reaching individuals, groups, or communities and (2) attempt to change political, social, or physical structures that either limit individuals' abilities to make safe choices or otherwise act to maintain risk in certain populations.
* Describe the tools available to help determine which interventions can and should be scaled up for greater public health benefit.
* Understand the role of key stakeholders, who are critical in the design and promotion of effective sexual-risk-reduction interventions.

Introduction

Human sexual behavior is governed by social beliefs and **norms** that are culturally specific and vary widely. Although sexual behavior is a very personal way of expressing sexuality and emotional intimacy, it becomes a subject of public health concern when the adverse health **consequences** of risky sexual activities are considered. High risk sexual behavior is associated with an increased incidence of sexually transmitted infections (STIs), including the human immunodeficiency virus (HIV), and unintended pregnancies. These outcomes are a major cause of **morbidity** and **mortality** in adolescents and adults in the United States.

Behavior change has been shown to have significant positive effects on health outcomes and **quality of life** (Koop 1996), and sexual behavior is no exception. Although **interventions** to reduce sexual risk behavior have traditionally been focused on changing individual behavior, sexuality is intrinsically a social behavior that is molded and affected by a much larger array of factors. The purpose of this chapter is to call attention not only to the individual behaviors themselves, but to the social and ecological factors that are critical to understanding the reasons individuals engage in high risk sexual behaviors and to understand how to use this broader view to design and promote effective interventions. Once a **conceptual framework** is in place, we discuss the evidence-based interventions that have been effective in changing sexual behavior and decreasing adverse outcomes, the practical aspects of intervention implementation in real-world settings, and potential roles for **stakeholders**.

Magnitude

High risk sexual behavior consists of engaging in unprotected sex with someone who could be infected with HIV or an STI or engaging in unprotected sex when a pregnancy is not desired. Related high risk behaviors include having unprotected sex with concurrent partners, having unprotected sex with multiple recent or lifetime sex partners, sex while intoxicated, early initiation of sex, and exchanging unprotected sex for drugs or money (Lin et al. 2008). Surveys such as the 2002 National Survey of Family Growth (NSFG) and the 2007 National Youth Risk Behavioral Survey (NYRBS) (CDC 2009f, 2009j) can provide information on the percentage of people having unprotected sex, the proportion who have multiple partners, and the mean age of onset of sexual activity. For example, 60% of men and 78% of women ages 15–44 who had had at least one sexual partner within the preceding 12 months had not used a condom dur-

ing their most recent sex act (NSFG), 35% of high school students had had sex in the most recent 3 months (NYRBS), and 18% of men and 14% of women ages 15–44 had had two or more partners in the preceding year (NSFG).

However, it is difficult to understand the level of riskiness in these behaviors. For example, having unprotected sex is often not a high risk behavior if it occurs in monogamous relationships, between individuals who have tested negative for STIs and are using other means of contraceptives, or between individuals who desire pregnancy. Measuring the consequences of high risk behavior, such as HIV, STIs, and unintended or unwanted pregnancies, is necessary to provide an accurate estimate of the magnitude of the public health problems that are the result of high risk sexual activity.

HIV and STIs, in contrast to other infectious diseases, remain a leading cause of morbidity and mortality in this country. Approximately 20 million new cases of STIs are reported each year, half of which occur in young adults between the ages of 15 and 24 (Owusu-Edusei et al. 2013; Weinstock et al. 2004). These preventable diseases result in serious complications, such as infertility, ectopic pregnancy, chronic liver disease, and in some cases such as HIV/AIDS, hepatitis C, and HSV infection in newborns, even death; they cost the U.S. health care system $15.6 billion annually (in 2010 dollars) (Owusu-Edusei et al. 2013). The major STIs and their incidence rates between 2000 and 2007 are listed in table 18.1 (note that changes in reporting and case definition may affect apparent trends in disease incidence).

Despite significant prevention efforts, the rates of chlamydia and syphilis continue to rise, and the incidence of HIV and gonorrhea remains unchanged at a high level (CDC 2009i). In 2011, there were 1,412,791 chlamydial infections reported to the Centers for Disease Control and Prevention (CDC), and the number of gonorrhea infections was estimated at 321,849; these figures are roughly equivalent to the popula-

TABLE 18.1. HIV and sexually transmitted infection incidence rates per 100,000 population in the United States

	HIV	Chlamydia	Gonorrhea	Syphilis[a]	Hepatitis B
2000	19.5	251.4	128.7	11.2	2.9
2003	19.7	301.7	115.2	11.8	2.6
2007	22.8[b]	370.2	118.9	13.7	1.5[c]
2011	15.8	454.1	104.2	14.9	1.5[d]

Sources: Data are taken from CDC 2004a, 2009i, 2009l; Hall et al. 2008; Centers for Disease Control and Prevention, Sexually transmitted diseases surveillance, 2011, www.cdc.gov/std/stats11/toc.htm (accessed June 4, 2013); Centers for Disease Control and Prevention, Hepatitis B information for health professionals, www.cdc.gov/hepatitis/HBV/HBVfaq.htm #overview (accessed June 5, 2013); Centers for Disease Control and Prevention, HIV surveillance report, 2011, vol. 23, published Feb. 2013, www.cdc.gov/hiv/topics/surveillance/resources/reports/ (accessed June 5, 2013).

[a]Reflects incidence of all stages of syphilis (including primary and secondary, early and late latent, and congenital).

[b]HIV incidence data is from 2006, as 2007 incidence data is not yet available for the U.S. This 2006 incidence estimate was derived using new technology and methodology that more directly measure the number of new HIV infections (Hall et al. 2008), and may not be directly comparable with previous incidence estimates.

[c]Due to significant underreporting of hepatitis B, the CDC estimates that the actual incidence of hepatitis B in 2007 was 10 times higher than the levels reported above.

[d]Hepatitis B data are from 2009 rather than 2011; these are the most updated data from the CDC on hepatitis B surveillance.

tions of San Diego and Saint Louis, respectively. In 2011 there were more than 46,746 cases of syphilis reported, which is comparable to the number of people who die from motor vehicle accidents each year in the United States.[1]

Acquired immune deficiency syndrome (AIDS) was the sixth leading cause of death in Americans ages 25–44, the fourth leading cause of death in African American men ages 25–44, and the third leading cause of death for African American women ages 25–44 in 2009 (CDC 2013b). The CDC estimates that the total number of adolescents and adults living with HIV in the United States at the end of 2010 was 888,921 and that the incidence of HIV, which remained stable at 55,000 new cases per year between 2003 and 2006, went down slightly to 50,000 in 2011 (CDC 2013b; Hall et al. 2008). The transmission rate for HIV in 2008 was 4.06 new cases per 100 patients living with HIV; this rate represents a substantial reduction from the rates in 1980 (92.3) and 1990 (11.7), but the decline has been far slower over the past 10 years (Holtgrave, Hall, et al. 2009). Although treatment of HIV has progressed dramatically, efforts to *prevent* new

cases of HIV have not been adequately **scaled up** (increased in proportion to need). Despite continued efforts to reduce transmission, a new HIV infection occurs on average every 9.5 minutes in this country (CDC 2009e). Therefore, to curb this epidemic it is essential to put effective prevention interventions into practice.

In addition to the direct morbidity and mortality associated with these diseases, STIs can have other devastating public health consequences. For example, individuals with active ulcerative diseases such as syphilis are two to five times more likely to acquire HIV (CDC 2009g). Furthermore, it is estimated that more than 2 million pregnant women are infected with STIs each year. STIs that cross the placenta during pregnancy or are transmitted from the mother to the baby during delivery can increase the chance of stillbirth, low birth weight, neonatal sepsis, neurologic damage, and many other chronic diseases states (CDC 2008).

Finally, unintended pregnancies are another consequence of risky sexual behaviors. In 2001, half of all pregnancies were unintended (CDC 2009k). Teenage birth and pregnancy rates are higher in the United States than in many other developed countries (Ventura et al. 2001). The abortion rate among women ages 15–44 remained fairly stable from 2000 to 2006 at 16.1 per 1,000, and it was down slightly to 15.1 in 2009 (CDC 2013a). Deaths of women from complications of legal abortions continue to slowly decline; in 2008, the last year for which mortality data are known, 12 abortion-related deaths occurred (Pazol et al. 2012). In addition, the negative health and social consequences of childbearing by adolescents, to both the mother and the child, can be significant and long-lasting. Examples include the amount of schooling a young mother is able to complete, compromised physical and intellectual attachment of the child to the parent, economic and social instability for young parents, and financial costs to society (Fielding and Williams 1991; Moore et al. 1979, 19).

In summary, high risk sexual behaviors can result in serious medical and psychological consequences as well as a tremendous cost to society. In order to develop interventions that have a true impact on high risk sexual behaviors, it is critical to understand both the individual **interpersonal factors** and the larger social and contextual factors that shape individual behavior and that lead or predispose people to engage in high risk sexual activities.

Key Determinants

The choices that individuals make about their sexual behavior, and whether or not to engage in behaviors that place them at risk for STIs and unintended pregnancies, are determined by individual, partner, family, community, sociocultural, and political factors (Aral et al. 2007). Knowledge of these **key determinants** can inform intervention strategies that can be focused on general populations or specific at-risk groups. Reviewing all of these factors is beyond the scope of this chapter, but we provide here a sampling of some of the most relevant key determinants to sexual behavior (table 18.2).

Individual Determinants

Condom use varies by whether sex occurs with main partners or casual partners. In one study of adolescent women, consistent condom use was reported by 38% of women in shorter sexual relationships (less than 6 months), as compared to 21% of women in longer sexual relationships (more than 6 months) (Wiemann et al. 2009). Perception of sexual relationships (main versus casual) may differ in adolescents when compared to adults, and these differences in perceived intimacy likely affect condom usage (Foulkes et al. 2009). However, there is still significant risk of acquiring HIV and STIs from a main sex partner. After a study found that most HIV transmissions (between 52% and 74%) between men who have sex with men (MSM) in five U.S. cities were from main sex partners (Sullivan et al. 2009), there has been significant debate on this topic.

Situational factors in a person's life can affect choices about sexual behavior. In women, a personal history of child abuse, substance abuse (including injection drugs, crack cocaine, and alcohol), intimate partner abuse, and mental illness have all been associated with sexual risk behavior to varying degrees (Bensley et al. 2000; El-Bassel et al. 2000; Gielen et al. 2007; Kalichman et al. 1998; NIMH 1998; Orr et al. 1994; Rees et al. 2001; Wingood and DiClemente 1998). For MSM, factors such as substance use, heterosexual self-identification, bisexual experience, history of childhood sexual abuse, having no education beyond high school, and having a partner with unknown HIV status have been found to be associated with increased rates of unprotected anal intercourse (Denning and Campsmith 2005; Goodenow et al. 2002; Kalichman et al. 2004; Waldo et al. 2002). Finally, poor risk-reduction skills (correct condom use, sexual negotiation, and problem-solving skills) and cognitive and **attitude** factors (inaccurate beliefs about risk to self, negative attitudes toward condoms, negative outcome expectancies

TABLE 18.2. Summary of key determinants
by level within an ecological framework

Individual determinants
    History of childhood sexual abuse
    Substance use or abuse
    Mental illness
    Sexual self-identification
    Education
    Having a partner with unknown HIV serostatus
    Poor risk-reduction skills
    Belief about risk to self or others
    Negative attitude toward condoms
    Poor perceived self-efficacy
    Socioeconomic status and race (indirectly)

Family and dyad determinants
    Cohesive family
    Positive family relationships (particularly
    mother-daughter)
    Parental monitoring
    Parental conversations about sex
    Power relationship within a couple
    Age differential within a couple
    Sero-sorting and negotiated safety practices
    "Down low" sexual activity

Sociocultural determinants
    Perceptions of peer sexual activity
    Media portrayal of sex and risk
    Traditional gender roles
    Sex-ratio imbalances
    Cultural norms regarding same-sex couples

Structural and political determinants
    Abstinence-only policies
    Bans on gay marriage
    Parental notification laws
    Access to reproductive and sexual health services
    Condom accessibility
    Housing status
    Neighborhood resources
    Product labeling

of practicing safer sex behaviors, and poor perceived **self-efficacy** to make safe sexual choices) have been found to predict high risk sexual behaviors (Kelly and Kalichman 2002).

Race by itself is not a risk factor for sexual risk behavior, and **socioeconomic status (SES)** is also unlikely to affect risk directly. However, race and SES may be associated with factors such as access to health care and cultural beliefs about contraceptives that place members of a certain racial or sociodemographic group at increased risk of negative behavioral health consequences. For example, several studies have shown racial and ethnic differences in patterns of sexual behavior (Auslander et al. 2009; Halpern et al. 2004). Among American youth ages 15-19 in 2002, the proportion of students engaging in sexual activity was highest among African American males (63.4%) and females (57%), followed by Hispanic males (55.5%) and white females (46.1%), with the lowest rates among white males (41.1%) and Hispanic females (40.4%) (CDC 2009j). However, it is unclear how much these differences are due to other factors. In a multivariate analysis of racial disparities in HIV incidence among young MSM in Baltimore, race by itself was not an independent risk factor for high risk sexual activity. Furthermore, disparate rates of HIV and STIs in different racial groups may be related to underlying racial differences in background prevalence rather than racial differences in risk behaviors (Sifakis et al. 2007).

SES is a total measure of a person's income, education, and occupation, and it is often cited as a marker for high risk sexual activity (Imamura et al. 2007). However, the association between SES and sexual risk behavior is complicated and may be **confounded** by other factors, such as the number of sexual partners, urban versus rural environment, and access to preventive health resources (Wojcicki 2005). For example, homeless youth demonstrate higher sexual risk behaviors, including exchange of sex for money and earlier age of first intercourse. However, these youth are at increased risk probably not owing to their homelessness alone but more likely owing to a lack of personal and social resources, such as trusting relationships with parents and friends, access to health care services, and participation in school and extracurricular activities (Rew et al. 2008).

Family and Dyad Determinants

Partner and family relationships can affect individual behavior. Research with adolescents has shown that cohesive families, positive relationships within families, greater parental monitoring, and parental conversations about sex are associated with delay of onset of sexual activity and an overall decrease in sexual risk behaviors (Holtzman and Rubinson 1995; Karofsky et al. 2001; McNeely, Shew, et al. 2002; Romer et al. 1999). One study showed that young women who were not sexually experienced at baseline were more likely to delay first sex when their mothers had expressed disapproval about them having sex, when the daughter was satisfied with the mother-daughter relationship, and when there was frequent communication between the mother and parents of the daughters' friends (McNeely et al. 2002).

For both adolescents and adults, relationships with partners likely have a powerful effect on sexual behavior. Women are often unable to make independent decisions to use contraceptives if men hold the decision-making power within a relationship, even when sexual or physical abuse is not present (Pulerwitz et al. 2000). Furthermore, young women are more likely to engage in sexual intercourse with older, more sexually experienced partners than with partners of the same age (Kaestle et al. 2002), which may also affect choices about contraception. Finally, adolescents are more likely to use condoms with students from a different racial or ethnic group or students who live in geographically different areas (Ford et al. 2001).

HIV and STIs continue to affect MSM disproportionately in this country (Wolitski et al. 2008). Currently, MSM comprise almost half of the people living with HIV in the United States and report more than half of all new HIV infections each year (CDC 2009d). In a recent meta-analysis, the prevalence of unprotected anal intercourse was found to be 30% with HIV-positive partners and 26% with either a status-unknown or HIV-negative partner (Crepaz et al. 2009). Notions of safety in same-sex relationships are **complex** and are influenced by knowledge of the individual's own and the individual's partner's status, by whether a relationship is perceived to be monogamous, and by agreements about sexual practices within and outside of the primary relationship. The majority of MSM protect their partners during sexual activity (Crepaz et al. 2009), although several studies have shown that some MSM practices, such as serosorting and negotiated safety, can paradoxically increase the risk of infection (Snowden et al. 2009). Serosorting is choosing to engage in sexual activity exclusively with seroconcordant partners (i.e., partners with similar diseases status, such as two HIV-positive partners); negotiated safety involves choosing not to use condoms after negotiating rules about HIV testing, sexual behavior with casual sex partners or other partners outside the primary relationship, or mutual disclosure of rule breaking (Snowden et al. 2009). When men who are in monogamous relationships with women also have sex with other men without the knowledge of their female partners, the risk of STI and HIV transmission can be increased (Whyte et al. 2008). Finally, "barebacking" is an HIV risk behavior generally considered to be intentional unprotected anal sex between men when HIV transmission is a possibility, although this behavior is in itself influenced by a variety of dynamic relationships and perceptions (Berg 2009).

Sociocultural Determinants

The social and cultural **context** in which individuals, couples, and families live influences their perceptions and attitudes toward healthful sexual behaviors. Different groups have their own **social** or **cultural norms** and bodies of information about sexual behavior, risk of STIs, and pregnancy. For example, early research demonstrated that adolescents' behavioral choices are influenced not only by their own curiosity about sexual activity and their pressure from partners, but also by perceptions of peer sexual activity (Romer et al. 1994). These perceptions can be shaped by media portrayal of sex; one longitudinal study showed that the more sexual activity is seen on television by adolescents, the earlier sex is initiated (Collins et al. 2004). Traditional gender roles and sex-ratio imbalances in different regions where there are more women than men have also been shown to limit the ability of women to negotiate safe sex practices and protect themselves from STIs (Logan et al. 2002; Pequegnat and Stover 1999). Risky sexual behavior is also increased in cultures where norms or other social pressures support the exchange of sex for money or drugs (Windle 1997).

Cultural norms also vary by sexual orientation. In heterosexual males, transition to marriage or living with a significant other is associated with a decrease in rates of new sex partners (Johnson et al. 2001; Mosher et al. 2005). However, the effect of domestic partnerships on sexual risk behaviors in MSM may be more complex, as some studies show that high risk behaviors persist into older age groups and do not decrease as significantly upon cohabitation with a partner (CDC 2004b; Fenton et al. 2005), whereas other studies have found an association between same-sex domestic partnerships and lower-risk sexual behaviors (Klausner et al. 2006). Sexual risk behaviors in MSM may be influenced by macrolevel social factors that limit the rights of homosexuals and same-sex couples. Negative media representation of gay men, public criticism of same-sex marriage, and homophobia foster marginalization (particularly in Latino and African American MSM) and have been associated with increased sexual risk-taking (APA Council 2004; Bontempo and D'Augelli 2002; Meyer 2003; Meyers et al. 2003).

As antiretroviral medications have changed HIV from an always-fatal disease to a chronic disease with reasonable life expectancy (Kelly et al. 1998; Vanable et al. 2000), how this changing public perception of HIV has affected sexual risk-taking is still unclear. Advertisements by pharmaceutical companies that relay misleadingly optimistic messages about HIV therapy may affect perception of risk and subsequent risky behaviors (Suarez and Miller 2001). "AIDS burnout" describes the phenomenon whereby years of HIV prevention messages may have dulled people's acuity regarding the severity of the disease and have thus been independently associated with unprotected anal intercourse among HIV-positive MSM, according to one large four-city study (Ostrow et al. 2002). Many theories exist about the complex effect the AIDS epidemic and the improved health outcomes in the past 10 years have had on sexual risk behaviors; however, the extent to which behavior has been affected in different populations in the United States remains unclear.

Structural and Political Determinants

Structural determinants refer to a community's network of available agencies and their policies and procedures that influence the choices available to individuals within that community. For example, access to adequate health care services, particularly prevention services, affects the behaviors of the individuals living in that community (Averett et al. 2002). Having a larger number of health care providers trained in counseling about sexual behavior and risk-reduction strategies has been shown to increase STI screening and counseling rates in a community (Ozer et al. 2005). Several studies have shown that students with access to school-based preventive health services use more contraceptives than students without access to these services (Kirby et al. 1991; Zabin et al. 1996). Programs that make condoms accessible in schools have been found to have a positive effect on condom use among students and have not been found to increase sexual activity (Kirby and Brown 1996; Schuster et al. 1998; Wolk and Rosenbaum 1995). Evidence also shows that school-based STI screening programs can reduce STI prevalence, theoretically by increasing safer sexual behaviors (Cohen et al. 1999). Unfortunately, most schools do not provide reproductive health care services at this time.

Other services available to a community that have been found to influence sexual behavior include social and peer normative supports for risk-reduction behavior change (Kelly and Kalichman 2002). For example, involvement in a faith-based institution has been shown in cross-sectional studies to be associated with delays in sexual initiation (Marsiglio and Mott 1986; Mott et al. 1996). Furthermore, certain geographic regions in several cities have been associated with disproportionately higher rates of repeat gonorrhea infection, which suggests that there are core groups of individuals who cluster together spatially and engage in high risk sexual activity with each other (Bernstein 2004; Bernstein et al. 2004; Ellen et al. 1997). Finally, several observational studies have noted that people living with HIV who have stable housing engage in less high risk behavior and have better health status than those without housing (Aidala et al. 2005; Kidder, Wolitski, Campsmith, and Nakamura 2007). A prospective randomized controlled trial also found that people living with HIV/AIDS required less medical care and reported improved physical and mental health when they were stably housed (Wolitski et al. 2009).

Public policies, either local or national, can also shape the context in which individual behaviors occur. Until recently, national policy allocated a significant amount of funding for abstinence-only sex education, even though these educational programs have repeatedly been found to have little efficacy and to possibly cause harm owing to inaccurate information about risk and safe-sex behaviors (Kirby et al. 2007). Implementation of parental notification and consent laws for contraception and abortion has also been found to negatively impact sexual behaviors in some settings, probably by limiting health care resources available to vulnerable adolescent groups (Jones et al. 2005; Zavodny 2004). Finally, there are data that living in states with policies that reduce discrimination against gays and lesbians including laws that recognize same-sex unions, with hate crime laws that specify sexual orientation as a protected category, and with bans on sexual orientation employment discrimination, was associated with decreased psychiatric morbidity among lesbians, gays, and bisexuals (Hatzenbuehler et al. 2009).

Evidence-Based Interventions

The **determinants** of sexual behavior described above inform the types of interventions that can be designed to facilitate healthful choices. These interventions fall broadly into two main categories, although they are often overlapping in practice: (1) interventions that seek to affect knowledge and attitudes in order to promote the choice of safe behaviors, by reaching individuals, groups, or communities, and (2) interventions that attempt to change political, social, or physical structures that either limit individuals' abilities to make safe choices or otherwise act to maintain risk in certain populations. Figure 18.1 portrays a novel conceptual framework that incorporates the following interventions.

Knowledge and Attitude Interventions

Interventions designed to promote sexual-risk-reduction behaviors can focus on individuals, **dyads**, small groups, or communities. Each of

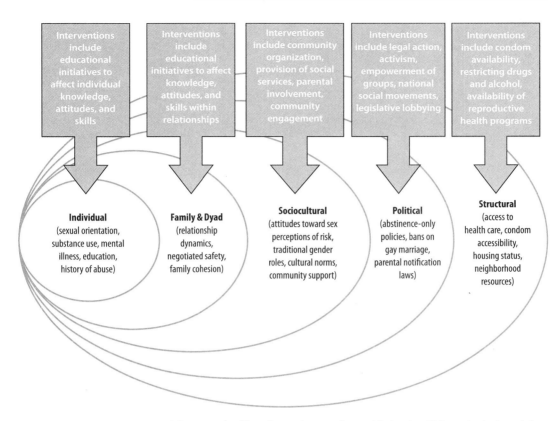

FIGURE 18.1. A conceptual framework of key determinants of sexual behavior. This ecological model demonstrates the different layers of influence that affect individual choices. Interventions can be designed at each of level, as depicted in the boxes above the key determinants.

these approaches has advantages and disadvantages; for example, an education effort that involves a group of three to five individuals may be more time-effective than educating individuals separately, but the success of interventions delivered in small groups may depend on group dynamics (Aral et al. 2007). **Community-level interventions** can require a significant amount of time and effort to initially implement, because they often use **multilevel interventions** to affect **social norms**, but they are more likely to support lasting changes in healthful behavior, by mobilizing resources within a community and encouraging community "ownership" of behavior change efforts.

The CDC recommends that health departments and community-based organizations im-

plement evidence-based interventions for HIV and STI prevention. The CDC's HIV/AIDS Prevention Research Synthesis (PRS) team was created in 1996 to systematically evaluate behavioral interventions using a rigorous set of scientific **selection** criteria, including quality of study design, quality of implementation and analysis, and strength of evidence for behavior change or STI/HIV reduction. Table 18.3 is a compilation of the current "best-evidence" individual, dyad, and small-group interventions identified by the CDC (CDC 2009b).

Although community-level interventions have been very commonly used in STI and HIV prevention efforts, these strategies are difficult to monitor and evaluate in the field. The PRS team has not determined that any

TABLE 18.3. Best-evidence interventions delivered to individuals, dyads, or small groups

Name	Unit of delivery	No. sessions (total hours)	Intervention effects
Interventions for heterosexual adults			
CHOICES	Group	16 (32)	↓ new STI
Communal Effectance–AIDS Prevention	Group	6 (9 to 12)	↑ condom use
Connect	Indiv/group	6 (12)	↑ condom use, ↓ UVI
Female and Culturally Specific Negotiation	Individual	4 (2 to 2.5)	↓ sex with paying sexual partners, ↓ trade sex for money, ↑ condom use
Focus on the Future	Individual	1 (45–50 min)	↓ new STI, ↓ new sex partners, ↑ condom use
Health Improvement Project	Group	10 (10)	↓ UVI, ↓ new sex partners
"light"	Group	7 (10.5 to 14)	↓ UVI/UAI, ↑ condom use, ↑ abstinence, ↓ new STI
Project FIO	Group	9 (18)	↓ UVI/UAI, ↓ VI/AI
Project S.A.F.E.	Indiv/group	3 (9 to 16.5)[a]	↓ USI, ↓ new sex partners, ↓ new STI
Project START	Individual	6 (4 to 7)	↓ UVI/UAI
Project RESPECT (+/− booster)	Individual	2 (0.7) (booster, 0.3)	↓ new STI, ↓ UVI (With booster, also ↓ new sex partners, ↓ USI, ↓ sex with 1-time partner or on day of meeting)
Safe in the City	Group	1 (23 min)	↓ new STI
Sister-to-Sister	Indiv/group	Indiv: 1 (0.3) Group: 1 (3.3)	↓ new STI (indiv); ↑ condom use (group); ↑ condom use, ↓ UVI, ↓ new STI (combined)
VOICES/VOCES	Group	1 (1)	↓ new STI
Women's Co-Op	Indiv/group	4 (3 to 4.3)	↓ USI
Women's Health Project	Group	12 (18 to 24)	↑ condom use
Interventions for high-risk youth			
BART	Group	8 (12 to 16)	↓ SI, ↑ condom use, ↓ UVI
Be Proud! Be Responsible!	Group	1 (5)	↓ risky behavior, ↓ new female sex partners, ↓ SI, ↑ condom use
CLEAR	Individual	18 (27)	↑ condom use, ↑ condom use with HIV+ sexual partners
Cuidate	Group	6 (6)	↓ SI, ↓ USI, ↓ multiple partners, ↑ condom use

Intervention	Format	Sessions (hours)	Outcomes
FOY + ImPACT	Group	9 (~12.5)	↓ USI
SiHLE	Group	4 (16)	↑ condom use, ↓ new sexual partners, ↓ UVI, ↓ new STI
Sisters Saving Sisters	Group	1 (4.2)	↑ condom use, ↓ USI, ↓ USI while high on drugs or alcohol, ↓ new sex partners, ↓ multiple partners
Interventions for men who have sex with men			
Brief Group Counseling	Group	1 (3)	↓ sex partners, ↓ UAI
EXPLORE	Individual	10 (10)[a]	↓ UAI, ↓ URAI
Personalized Cognitive Risk-Reduction Counseling	Individual	1 (1)[a]	↓ UAI
SUMIT Enhanced Peer-led	Group	6 (18)	↓ URAI with HIV or serostatus-unknown sex partners
Interventions for people living with HIV/AIDS			
CLEAR	Individual	18 (27)	↑ condom use, ↑ condom use with HIV+ sex partners
Healthy Living Project	Individual	15 (22.5)	↓ UAI/UVI
Healthy Relationships	Group	5 (10)	↓ UAI/UVI, ↓ AI/VI, ↑ condom use, ↓ non-HIV+ sex partners, ↓ UAI/UVI and AI/VI with non-HIV+ sex partners
LIFT	Group	15 (22.5)	↓ UAI/UVI with all partners and with HIV or serostatus-unknown sex partners
Positive Choice: Interactive Video Doctor	Individual	2 (48 min)	↓ UAI/UVI, ↓ casual sex partners
SUMIT Enhanced Peer-led	Group	6 (18)	↓ URAI with HIV- or serostatus-unknown sexual partners
WiLLOW	Group	4 (16)	↓ UVI, ↑ condom use, ↓ new STI

Sources: The table was modified from Lyles et al. 2007, table 2, with additional references from CDC 2009b.

Notes: MSM = men who have sex with men, ↓ = decrease in, ↑ = increase in, STI = sexually transmitted infections, SI = sexual intercourse, USI = unprotected sexual intercourse, UVI = unprotected vaginal intercourse, C&T = counseling and testing, UAI = unprotected anal intercourse, URAI = unprotected receptive anal intercourse, VI = vaginal intercourse, AI = anal intercourse, IDU = intravenous drug use.

[a] Additional sessions, either counseling and testing or booster sessions, were offered and are not included in time estimates.

community-level interventions meet criteria for "best evidence," but it lists several as "promising-evidence interventions" (Table 18.4) (CDC 2009b). These interventions use a variety of strategies to increase HIV-protective behavior in different communities and have been shown to significantly reduce several sexual risk behaviors as well as the rate of new STIs or HIV. In addition, the Task Force on Community Preventive Services uses systematic evidence reviews to make recommendations about community-level interventions, although only a few community-level interventions regarding sexual behavior have thus far been evaluated by the Task Force. The interventions currently recommended by the Task Force are coordination with community services to reduce sexual risk behaviors in adolescents, a variety of community-level programs to reduce sexual risk behaviors in MSM, and partner counseling and referral services for partners of people living with HIV/AIDS (CDC 2009a).

Health departments and community-based organizations wishing to utilize these evidence-based interventions can choose based on the population of interest, the amount of time an organization or agency has to dedicate to the intervention, and whether an individual- or group-level intervention is preferred. Although it is possible that an intervention carried out with one group, such as heterosexual adults, may also be effective with other at-risk populations such as adolescents, MSM, or people living with HIV/AIDS, additional study is needed to determine whether this crossover effect exists.

Structural Interventions

Structural interventions work by targeting conditions outside the control of an individual and strive to change the political, social, legal, or physical environment in order to improve health outcomes (Cohen and Scribner 2000). These interventions typically aim to affect behavior *directly* by improving the availability and

accessibility of resources as well as *indirectly* by altering the acceptability of behaviors that lower sexual risk. Although structural interventions have increasingly been shown to be effective in HIV-prevention efforts, scientific and political obstacles have limited their adoption (Auerbach 2009). Below are four general categories of structural interventions—product availability, social structures and policies, media and cultural messages, and the physical environment—and examples of structural interventions in each of the categories.

PRODUCT AVAILABILITY

Interventions can seek either to increase or to decrease the availability of products or resources. Internationally, one of the best examples of this type of intervention was the extremely successful 100% condom campaign in Thailand, which made condoms widely available and implemented laws mandating condom use by commercial sex workers (Weniger et al. 1991). In the United States, condom availability has been promoted to a limited degree in schools, clinics, and communities and has often been coupled with **social marketing** campaigns that increase awareness and acceptability of condom use (Calsyn et al. 1992; Cohen et al. 1999). Introduction of the female condom to commercial sex workers in Madagascar was associated with increased use of any type of protection and decreased rates of STIs, whereas it had no effect in an intervention trial in Kenya (Feldblum et al. 2001; Hoke et al. 2007). This suggests that simply supplying the female condom may not be sufficient to improve health outcomes and that perceptions of and education about condom use are likely important as well ("Female condom" 2008). Restricting alcohol through taxation has also been shown to be an effective structural intervention in reducing STIs and HIV, insofar as increased alcohol use has been associated with multiple high risk sexual behaviors (Chesson et al. 2000; Chesson et al. 2003). Finally, availability of school-based

TABLE 18.4. Promising-evidence community-level interventions

Name	Target communities	Delivery methods	Intervention effects
Community Promise	Underserved populations at risk for HIV infection, including IDUs, female sex partners of male IDUs, non-gay-identified MSM, high-risk youth, female sex workers, and residents in areas with high rates of STIs	Outreach, printed materials (brochures, pamphlets, flyers, trading cards), risk reduction supplies (condoms, bleach)	Intervention communities showed greater increase in mean stage-of-change scores for condom use with main partner and non-main partners ($p < 0.05$).
Mpowerment	Young gay men	Demonstration/modeling, discussion, role-playing, social events, performance, printed materials, risk reduction supplies (condoms), video	The intervention community showed a decrease in the proportion of men engaging in UAI compared to the control community ($p < 0.03$) as well as from baseline to follow-up post-intervention ($p < 0.05$).
Popular Opinion Leader	Men who frequent gay bars	Public opinion leader training (goal setting, group discussion, modeling, role play, skill building), casual one-on-one conversations, printed materials (logos, symbols, other devices)	The intervention city participants reported greater reductions in any UAI (all p's < 0.05), greater increases in condom use during anal intercourse (all p's < 0.05), and greater reductions in having multiple sex partners ($p < 0.05$) than participants in control communities.
Real AIDS Prevention Project	Sexually active, low-income women of reproductive age in inner-city communities	Discussion, outreach, printed materials, role-model stories, risk reduction supplies (condoms), safer-sex parties, workshops	Intervention communities showed a significant decrease in the proportion of women who reported never using condoms with main partner ($p = 0.03$)
Teen Health	Adolescents of high risk for HIV who live in urban, low-income housing developments	Performances, risk reduction supplies (condoms), skills building exercises, small media (e.g. brochures, project newsletters, T-shirts), social events	Intervention communities were more likely to have remained abstinent at 18 months post baseline (2 months after intervention completion) ($p = 0.04$), and significantly more likely to report condom use at last sex at 18 months post baseline ($p = 0.05$).

Notes: The table was constructed from promising-evidence community-level interventions listed in CDC 2009b.
IDU = intravenous drug user, MSM = men who have sex with men, STI = sexually transmitted infection, UAI = unprotected anal intercourse.

reproductive health programs has been found to increase use of contraceptives while not increasing sexual activity (Kirby 2002; Kirby et al. 1991).

SOCIAL STRUCTURES AND POLICIES

Interventions that target social structures and policies are implemented by those who wield legislative and administrative power; such interventions can have a powerful effect on the context in which **health behaviors** take place. On a local level, the introduction of supervised activities for youth can reduce incidents of unprotected sex (O'Donnell et al. 1999), and interventions that promote economic empowerment for vulnerable groups such as commercial sex workers can decrease high risk sexual behaviors (Sherman et al. 2006). On a national level, policies that mandate evidence-based prevention interventions or certain standards of care in health care and community-based settings could increase access to and availability of resources for hundreds of thousands of patients annually. For example, "responsible sexual behavior" is a leading indicator in Healthy People 2010, which makes it a focus of national attention and encourages individuals, groups, and businesses to integrate it into plans and programs (USDHHS 2010). In addition, repeal of antisodomy laws in the United States can affect sexual practices by destigmatizing homosexual behavior (Auerbach 2009).

MEDIA AND CULTURAL MESSAGES

Media advocacy—the use of media to advocate for community changes—seeks to alter the social and policy environment in ways that lead to healthier environments and ultimately behaviors (Aral et al. 2007). Media campaign interventions can be facilitated locally through messages in pamphlets, health fairs, and supermarket flyers, or they can be conducted on a regional or national level to reach a larger populace. Social marketing interventions are a type of media advocacy that couples conventional marketing tools with theories of behavior change. Media advocacy can be a powerful way of influencing a large number of people, as messages about safer sexual behaviors can be strategically placed on radios, in newspapers, and on popular television sitcoms and programs (Aral et al. 2007). Just as the Truth campaign that was initiated in 2000 was found to significantly decrease youth smoking in a cost-efficient manner (Holtgrave, Wunderink, et al. 2009), Nine and a Half Minutes is a mass media campaign launched in 2009 to increase awareness of HIV/AIDS in the United States and decrease the **stigma** associated with it (CDC 2009e). However, there are obstacles to mass media social marketing of condoms and HIV prevention messages in the United States, including difficulty reaching marginalized populations because of the fragmentation of media (Price 2001) and political and social opposition to certain types of messages or messaging frequency.

PHYSICAL ENVIRONMENT

Finally, interventions that target physical aspects of the environment involve regulating or closing physical structures and buildings in which unsafe sexual practices are promoted. Examples of these structures are crack houses and shooting galleries (settings that promote unsafe sex as well as illicit drug use) and alcohol outlets. Bathhouses are establishments that serve several purposes, although up to 14% of men who go to bathhouses engage in unprotected anal intercourse (Binson et al. 2009). Although many cities have attempted to close or regulate these facilities, the **effectiveness** of the interventions has not been widely evaluated (Cohen et al. 2004; Wood et al. 2003; Woods and Binson 2003). Interestingly, the legalization of brothels in Nevada, in combination with a mandatory condom program, has been associated with a significantly decreased risk of HIV and STI transmission (O'Leary and Martins 2000).

Implementation Considerations

For those who must choose which intervention or combination of interventions to provide or fund, identifying the interventions that are evidence-based is only the first step in moving from data to action. Providers and policymakers must be able to prioritize interventions that are likely to be both effective and affordable, replicate them in real-world rather than research settings, scale them up to meet local needs, and determine how to make the interventions sustainable over time. Although later chapters will address some of these steps as they apply to behavior change interventions in general, certain aspects may be specific to interventions that promote healthful sexual risk behaviors.

Cost-effectiveness analyses can be extremely useful in allocation of prevention funding and resources. Cost-effectiveness studies of sexual risk behavior interventions are typically based on prevention of disease (STIs and HIV) or conceptions under age 18 as the primary outcomes. However, many intervention studies report intermediate outcomes only (e.g., increased condom use, decreased number of new or concomitant sexual partners, or later initiation of sex), either owing to issues of research design (e.g., choice of primary outcomes, small sample size) or duration of follow-up. Therefore, certain assumptions about efficacy of disease prevention must be made in order to conduct cost-effectiveness analyses of these interventions. Of note, sustainable sexual behavior change may have other health benefits apart from prevention of disease and unintended pregnancies (specifically, long-term emotional and developmental effects) that could also serve as worthwhile primary outcomes but have not yet been well studied.

Several interventions designed to decrease high risk sexual behaviors have been shown to be cost-effective, and sometimes even cost *saving*. A recent systematic review of one-to-one interventions to reduce STIs and conceptions under age 18 included 55 studies and concluded that most were cost-effective (Barham et al. 2007). A 2009 systematic review of U.S.-based cost-utility analyses of a wide variety of HIV/AIDS prevention and management interventions (Hornberger et al. 2007) found that three of the behavioral interventions were cost-saving and three others were cost-effective (defined by a cost per **quality-adjusted life year [QALY]** saved of less than $100,000). The *cost-saving* interventions for HIV prevention included a behavioral intervention in high risk urban women (Holtgrave and Kelly 1996), a counseling and testing intervention in patients in an STI clinic (Varghese et al. 1999), and a counseling and testing intervention for soon-to-be-released prisoners (Varghese and Peterman 2001). The *cost-effective* interventions were an expanded testing program for primary HIV infection (Coco 2005), a skills training and lecture intervention for MSM (Pinkerton et al. 1997), and a sexual behavior intervention for HIV-positive injection drug users (although this intervention did not show greater risk reduction in the experimental group compared to controls) (Tuli et al. 2005). Finally, a review of behavioral interventions that ranked HIV prevention interventions by their cost-effectiveness ratios found 17 behavioral interventions to be cost-saving (defined as costing less than $200,000 per infection averted) and an additional five interventions to be cost-effective (defined as costing less than $750,000 per infection averted) (Pinkerton et al. 2001). These thresholds were based on an estimate of the lifetime cost of medical care for a patient with HIV of approximately $200,000 (Holtgrave and Pinkerton 1997).

Cohen and colleagues used a mathematical model to rank HIV and STI preventions in order of combined cost-effectiveness and potential to prevent the most infections. This procedure demonstrated that funds should be allocated across nine interventions, seven of which were focused on sexual behavior change (Cohen et al. 2005). These seven interventions included instructional videos in STI clinics (O'Donnell et al. 1998), partner notification (Wykoff et al. 1991), community mobilization (Mpowerment) (Kegeles et al. 1996), mass-media campaigns (Dubois-Arber et al. 1997), opinion leader programs (Kelly et al. 1992), and HIV counseling and testing (Kamb et al. 1998).

The CDC has recently developed a model for allocating HIV prevention funds in the United States, using estimates of HIV incidence and prevalence in the general population as well as three high risk groups (high risk heterosexuals, MSM, and injection drug users), rates of movement in and out of each risk population, transmission rates, costs and outcomes of prevention programs (both behavioral interventions and testing to identify positives unaware of their status), current spending patterns, and budgetary constraints. The model simulates multiple possible outcomes when the amount of available funds is fixed and determines the allocation scenario that optimizes cost-effectiveness (Hicks and Wirth 2003; Lasry et al. 2009). Early use of the model has found that cost-effectiveness is optimized on a national level when funding is targeted to behavioral and testing interventions for risk populations rather than the general population (Lasry et al. 2009).

In addition to cost-effectiveness, it is critical to focus attention on the replication, dissemination, and **scale-up** of interventions in real-world settings to achieve a large public health impact. The CDC conducted replication projects between 1997 and 2000 for several of the evidence-based interventions included in tables 18.3 and 18.4, in which the developers of the interventions created kits with instructions and materials and collaborated with the replication site to help implement the intervention. This project revealed that the adoption process of these behavioral interventions was complicated owing to the differences between the research settings and the replication sites and that each intervention could be broken down into core elements (the elements considered to be necessary to have an effect) and key characteristics (the elements that could be modified if necessary) (Gandelman et al. 2006).

Strategies that help service organizations to implement interventions by providing a "package" comprising manuals, training workshops, and follow-up consultations have been found to result in more frequent adoption and use of evidence-based HIV prevention interventions (Kelly et al. 2000). Therefore, to aid in dissemination efforts for HIV and STI prevention interventions, the CDC created a Diffusion of Effective Behavioral Interventions (DEBI) program in 2002. The DEBI program provides intensive support for state and community providers who wish to implement interventions by offering training and continued technical assistance. One of the main training sources is the STI/ HIV Prevention Training Centers (DEBI 2009).[2] Early results of several DEBI initiatives, and the experiences of organizations using them to implement prevention interventions, have begun to be reported (Dworkin et al. 2008; Shea et al. 2006).

Roles for Key Stakeholders

Today, effective HIV and STI prevention requires a combination of biomedical, individual, and structural interventions. Although prevention research has led to the development of multiple behavioral interventions that are effective and cost-effective in reducing high risk sexual behaviors, most of these programs have not been scaled up sufficiently to have a large public health impact. In addition, limited funding restricts the amount of new research being conducted on the spectrum of HIV/STI prevention science. Listing all possible stakeholders that play a role in HIV prevention is beyond the scope of this chapter, but we have highlighted below a few key roles that stakeholders can play

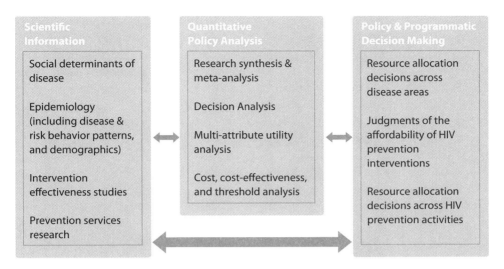

FIGURE 18.2. A framework for the inclusion of quantitative policy analysis in
HIV prevention technology transfer activities. *Source:* Holtgrave 2004, 21.

in promoting effective behavioral interventions. Importantly, in 2010, the National HIV/AIDS Strategy was released by President Obama, following work that was initiated by the Coalition for a National AIDS Strategy in 2007.[3]

Researchers

Even well-done studies, once published, do not automatically change policy and practice. The policymakers and public health practitioners charged with the promotion, funding, and implementation of evidence-based interventions require that the science be translated into information they can use to determine the interventions' affordability and relative public health return on investment. Figure 18.2 describes one framework that can be used to understand the relationship between research and practice. In the leftmost box is the scientific information that requires transfer, and the rightmost box represents the policy and programmatic decision making that occurs. The middle box depicts the quantitative policy analysis tools needed to put research findings into a format

suitable for policymakers as well as to make the researchers aware of the additional information or evidence needs of the policy analysts. The bidirectional arrows depict the dialogue that can and should occur between individuals in these different roles (Holtgrave 2004).

Researchers conducting the scientific work in the leftmost box should attempt to include the information (such as cost and feasibility) that is important for real-time policy and programmatic decisions. Documentation should include details about the intervention that may not be included in the publication itself but will be important for replication in other settings, such as information about staffing, resources, challenges, and stakeholders (Eke et al. 2006). Furthermore, a new generation of researchers is choosing to specialize in the quantitative analysis tools in the middle box, to be effective translators of technology and science. Comparative effectiveness research is a broader title for these "middle box" efforts and has recently received a great deal of political funding and support. This is an ideal time for academic centers and community organizations to initiate studies that help determine which programs are the most effective (and cost-effective) in reducing high risk sexual behaviors in real-world settings.

In addition, researchers are called to work more effectively with communities to plan research interventions, collect and analyze data, and interpret findings. Community-based participatory research (CBPR) is a powerful research tool that can be used to include community voices in behavioral intervention studies, make the research more relevant by informing the purpose and overall framework, and increase the chances of success. A systematic review by the Agency for Healthcare Research and Quality (AHRQ) of published studies that used CBPR revealed that authors felt CBPR increased community participation rates, **generalizability**, and community capacity and decreased rates of **loss to follow-up** (Viswanathan et al. 2004).

Federal Legislative Bodies

Legislative bodies create the overall legal framework in which public health policy can be created and maintained as well as act as a critical source of funding. Federal policymakers (most notably, members of the U.S. Congress and the Cabinet) can promote new policies that expand preventive services such as behavioral interventions, reevaluate potentially harmful policies that restrict safe sex behavior, and continue to make funding a priority for the implementation and scale-up of interventions that have been found to be effective. New federal policies that could promote healthful sexual behaviors could include sexual health counseling and education programs in school clinics, mandatory counseling and behavioral interventions for prisoners with high risk behaviors, and development of reimbursement mechanisms for counseling to encourage clinicians to implement behavioral interventions. Examples of current bills under consideration are the RE-

PEAL HIV Discrimination Act of 2013 (H.R.1843) and the Stop AIDS in Prison Act of 2013 (H.R. 895).[4] Policies that have been shown to be ineffective (and potentially harmful) include abstinence-only education programs, the requirement for parental approval for contraception provision (Aral et al. 2007; Jones et al. 2005; Santelli et al. 2004), and policies such as the Defense of Marriage Act (recently upheld by the Department of Justice) that limit the rights of same-sex partners. Finally, federal funding dollars should be allocated for structural interventions, such as housing initiatives, that have been shown to affect behavior, as a means of HIV/STI prevention (Kidder et al. 2007). The U.S. Congress can also use its tax power to assess taxes on substances such as alcohol that have been linked with high risk sexual behaviors (Chesson et al. 2000; Chesson et al. 2003; Rees et al. 2001; Wingood and DiClemente 1998).

Public Health Agencies

With regard to behavioral interventions to reduce high risk sexual activity, the CDC and the National Institutes of Health (NIH) direct research priorities and drive public health policymaking. As described above, the CDC has supported the development of the Prevention Research Synthesis, a systematic review and ranking of the most effective prevention interventions, and has helped to promote the implementation of these interventions through its DEBI program. The landscape is ripe for national large-scale promotion of these interventions by the CDC as well as a real investment in implementation research across the country by both the CDC and the NIH. CDC **guidelines** on screening and counseling, such as the recent guidelines recommending pre-exposure prophylaxis in persons at high risk, would help further this effort. Because clinics with written or electronic protocols for STI testing are significantly more likely to screen for high risk behaviors (Taylor et al. 2005), protocols for behavioral prevention interventions could also be useful. In addition, media and social marketing campaigns could focus on promoting the acceptability of prevention interventions in diverse settings and maintaining a sense of urgency about the morbidity and mortality of HIV and STIs.

The Food and Drug Administration (FDA), which assures the safety and efficacy of drugs, vaccines, medical devices, and some foods, can also play an important role in promoting safer sexual behaviors. A recent paper demonstrated that the way in which condoms are labeled (information label versus warning label) can be associated with people's beliefs about condom effectiveness in reducing transmission of HIV/STIs and their willingness to recommend condom use to friends (Bleakley et al. 2008). Further exploration of condom labeling, as well as alcohol labeling (because alcohol has been linked with high risk sexual behaviors) (Chesson et al. 2000; Chesson et al. 2003; Rees et al. 2001; Wingood and DiClemente 1998), should be undertaken to more accurately and effectively represent the risks and benefits of these products.

Other agencies entrusted with the public's health, such as local and state health departments, are critical stakeholders in prevention of HIV, STIs, and unintended pregnancies. Local and state health departments offer a wide range of programs that serve to modulate risky behaviors, programs such as individual- and group-level behavioral interventions, **outreach** and HIV/STI testing, condom distribution, and collaborative programs with groups such as schools and faith-based organizations to expand the **reach** of prevention activities. Effective and comprehensive **surveillance** systems are critical for following trends in at-risk groups in order to target prevention interventions where they are most needed. In addition, data from several large federally supported surveys such as the Morbidity Monitoring Project, the National HIV Behavioral Surveillance System, and the HIV Testing Survey are available to lo-cal and state health departments and contain information on sexual behaviors and barriers to access to care (CDC 2009c). Thorough analysis of these data sets can improve our understanding of regional patterns in sexual behavior, factors associated with high risk activities, and the effectiveness of certain prevention interventions. As mentioned above, it is important for these public health agencies to be able to measure the effectiveness of interventions and to coordinate efforts in order to bring about an effective national response.

Community Planning Groups and Community-Based Organizations

Community members and community service providers usually have firsthand information about risk behaviors and high risk groups in their communities; therefore, their input into research and policymaking agendas is critical (Kelly and Kalichman 2002). Communities that implement evidence-based behavioral interventions in their own school, clinic, and faith settings can evaluate these interventions and disseminate their results to build on current implementation research. Alternatively, communities may already be using interventions they have found to be successful but have not appeared in the published literature; dissemination of the success or failure of these efforts is imperative. Finally, communities can proactively seek collaboration with research or funding groups that can help them reach out to specific risk groups or target specific risky behaviors with which they are most concerned.

Communities are major **influences** in shaping norms and behaviors, particularly for adolescents, and neighborhood characteristics can affect sexual risk behaviors. For example, membership in a religious group is associated with a delay in sexual activity (Marsiglio and Mott 1986; Mott et al. 1996), although one study found this to be true only when a child's friends attended the same church (Mott et al. 1996). Religiosity has also been found to decrease high risk sexual behaviors after sexual debut in both HIV-negative (Lefkowitz et al. 2004) and HIV-positive individuals (Galvan et al. 2007). Empowerment strategies that increase **social support** through social interactions and participating in social functions have been shown to significantly impact sexual risk behaviors in developing countries (Kerrigan et al. 2007) and should be considered in HIV-prevention programs in U.S. communities. Youth leaders are also a valuable potential resource for communities: City Year, a youth-led organization that involves children and adolescents in community service and civic leadership experiences, has seen a dramatic rise in popularity and has involved youth in more than 20 million hours of service since it was founded more than 25 years ago.[5] Youth empowerment demonstration projects are being designed to delay onset of sex and reduce drug risk by forging group identity and cohesion and encouraging engagement in community activism (Berg et al. 2009).

Community leaders and organizations can therefore play a critical role in positively affecting sexual behavior change by identifying priorities and making these priorities known to community **opinion leaders** and politicians who rely on their votes for reelection. Furthermore, stakeholders such as bar owners, sex club owners, commercial sex workers, and drug users should be invited to provide their perspectives and to become engaged in positive community solutions. New initiatives such as reverse research day have been initiated, in which city agencies and community-based organizations present their research needs to academic universities through an annual interactive poster session, with the **goal** of connecting the needs of these groups with university research resources (Johns Hopkins 2009).

Managed Care Plans

Managed care organizations (MCOs) can serve several important roles. First, they can promote continuity of care by encouraging use of a single primary care provider and in that way increase the uptake of preventive services. Comprehensive primary care, including sexual health assessments, well care, and counseling, is essential to prevention and reduction of high risk sexual activities, particularly for adolescents (Lafferty et al. 2002). However, a study by Civic and colleagues found that nearly half of adolescent enrollees of MCOs use out-of-plan care, and those who did seek care from another source were more likely to be sexually active, to use alcohol, and to have had STIs (Civic et al. 2001). The most common reasons reported by adolescents for seeking care from someone other than their regular provider were confidentiality and lack of convenience.

MCOs are sometimes unwilling to fund services that prevent long-term complications, as enrollees may change health insurance plans before the health (and cost) benefits can be realized. However, a significant portion of the costs incurred by unsafe sex practices are short-term costs (e.g., treatment of STIs, costs related to prenatal visits and delivery). Reduction of high risk sexual behavior should be an important focus of disease prevention for MCOs, particularly for those such as Medicaid that include beneficiaries with disproportionately higher rates of STIs and HIV (Pourat et al. 2002). Therefore, if MCOs wish to have an impact on the consequences of high risk sexual behaviors, they need to promote continuity of care by educating and informing adolescents about confidentiality and addressing issues of convenience of accessing care (Civic et al. 2001).

Second, most managed care plans in the United States collect data on a set of performance measures called HEDIS (Healthcare Effectiveness Data and Information Set), since it is mandated by the Centers for Medicare and Medicaid Services for MCOs to participate in Medicare managed care programs. HEDIS data allow plans to be compared across multiple measures, including provision of preventive health services targeted toward sexual health and STI prevention. Plans that participate in HEDIS demonstrate higher use of preventive health services than plans that do not (Phillips et al. 2000). This model provides a good framework with potential to improve universal provision of preventive health services. However, greater efforts must be dedicated to understanding the extent to which the HEDIS sexual health performance measures are accurate (Tao et al. 2002).

Furthermore, despite HEDIS performance measures that reflect current CDC or U.S. Preventive Services Task Force (USPSTF) recommendations, providers in a network may not meet HEDIS goals. Several MCOs recommend STI practice guidelines directly to their providers, but a study of Medicaid MCOs found that the proportion of providers who followed STI prevention guidelines was the same whether the guidelines were recommended by the MCO or not (Pourat et al. 2002). Therefore, MCOs must look for different ways of encouraging providers to follow guidelines and incorporate prevention services into their practice, and these efforts will likely require communication and collaboration with providers. For example, one successful intervention increased screening for chlamydia by engaging clinic leadership, demonstrating the gap between best practice and current practice, and assembling a team to champion the screening efforts (Shafer et al. 2002). This would not be possible for every intervention, but it suggests that clinicians must be engaged to some degree in the development and maintenance of successful interventions.

The MCO perspective clearly differs from the societal perspective regarding cost-effectiveness of interventions to prevent STIs and HIV, insofar as it depends on the proportion of high risk individuals that belong to that specific MCO. However, the HIV-prevention services that should be included in performance standards, at a minimum, are basic HIV risk monitoring and HIV testing for persons aged 15 to 65 in accordance with USPSTF recommendations. Collaboration between MCOs and health departments could also help MCOs incorporate

cost-effective interventions at a lower cost by making use of existing infrastructure and resources (Pinkerton and Holtgrave 1998).

Clinics and Clinicians

Currently, most health care is still delivered in formal health care settings, and 92% to 98% of patients in one survey reported that they expected their primary care physician to offer advice on health matters such as diet, exercise, and alcohol use (Vogt et al. 1998). Physician advice has been shown to be effective in changing behavior, most notably for smoking cessation (Fiore et al. 2008), and physicians generally accept and value their role in promoting healthful behavior (Wechsler et al. 1996; Valente et al. 1986). However, clinicians may not appreciate the health benefits of behavior change interventions because these interventions may appear to have limited effectiveness on an individual basis. But small-to-modest benefits achieved on the individual level translate to large decreases in morbidity and mortality when applied to entire populations of at-risk individuals (Abrams et al. 1996).

There are several ways in which busy clinicians can promote reduction in high risk sexual behavior. One way is simply to increase the number of high risk and vulnerable patients who are seen in the clinic as well as to find ways to retain these patients in care. One innovative project piloted by the Family Medical & Counseling Services in Washington, D.C., used a "blitz" approach to recapture patients. Chart review revealed 450 clients **lost to follow-up** in the preceding five years; using an "all-hands-on-board" approach, this clinic incentivized all staff members, from clinicians to secretaries, to make contact with these patients. Although often more than 10 contacts per patient were required, care was reestablished for 70% of these patients.[6] Clinics can also bring in additional high risk patients by forming community **partnerships** and working to lessen community distrust of health care providers.

A second way in which clinicians can promote screening for high risk sex behavior and counseling to encourage behavior change is to incorporate evidence-based interventions into routine care in the presence of office support programs. Busy clinicians will likely not have enough **motivation** and time for multiple preventive interventions in addition to managing other pressing health concerns (Solberg, Kottke, Brekke, et al. 1998). However, office programs have been shown to allow for the effective delivery of preventive services; these programs generally consist of preventive services guidelines, mechanisms that systematically and automatically identify patients in need of a service and remind clinicians during a visit, and resources to provide support and follow-up after the office visit (Solberg, Kottke, and Brekke 1998). For example, written or electronic systems for STI screening were found to significantly increase sexual risk assessment questioning by HIV care providers (Taylor et al. 2005). In a randomized controlled trial of community family practices, practices that received tailored systems support for preventive service delivery were significantly more likely to provide these services after one year (Goodwin et al. 2001).

Funding Institutions

Approximately half of the nation's HIV prevention budget is funded by the CDC ($337 million), with state and local governments supplying more than one-third of the HIV prevention funding ($205 million) administered by U.S. health departments (Kaiser Family Foundation 2009). Other funding institutions include federal agencies mentioned previously, such as the NIH, the AHRQ, and the Health Resources and Services Administration (HRSA), as well as foundations such as the Gates Foundation and the Robert Wood Johnson Foundation and some professional medical organizations.

Funding is one of the biggest driving factors in promoting research, prioritizing health care

interventions, and addressing unmet prevention needs. The CDC's HIV prevention budget would need to increase from its current level to approximately $1.321 billion per year and be sustained at that level to address unmet HIV prevention needs in the United States, according to estimates (Holtgrave 2008). A distinct opportunity exists for all funders to support carefully designed research in the areas highlighted in the "Researchers" section above. Support from federal agencies that fund demonstration projects, such as HRSA and AHRQ, will help answer crucial questions about cost-effectiveness, scale-up, replication, and sustainability. In addition, funders interested in making a difference in HIV transmission might be best served by funding more expansive interventions such as social marketing campaigns that affect norms and behaviors in addition to more traditional research endeavors. Because these types of interventions can take time to lead to changes in behavior, funders who are willing to support projects that span a greater number of years (such as community-based participatory research endeavors) may see larger and more meaningful effects.

Conclusion

High risk sexual behaviors have resulted in tremendous physical, emotional, and monetary cost to society. Sexual behavior, like any other behavior, is complex and multifaceted. The choices that individuals make about their sexual behaviors are shaped by individual, partner, family, community, sociocultural, and political factors. Understanding the determinants of sexual behavior informs the types of interventions—those that affect knowledge and attitudes and those that target political and social structures—that can be designed to facilitate healthful choices. A conceptual framework based on the **ecological** model can help coordinate these different levels of key determinants in order to plan effective behavioral, biomedical, and structural interventions.

NOTES

The authors would like to thank Dr. Carl Latkin and Dr. Ronald Stall for their critical review of this chapter and for the benefit of their wealth of knowledge and thoughtful insight into HIV prevention.

1. 2011 sexually transmitted diseases surveillance, Centers for Disease Control and Prevention, available at www.cdc.gov/std/stats11/toc.htm (accessed June 4, 2013).

2. Also see National network of STD/HIV prevention training centers, Centers for Disease Control and Prevention, http://depts.washington.edu/nnptc/index.html (accessed Aug. 22, 2009).

3. Coalition for a National AIDS Strategy, http://nationalaidsstrategy.org/ (accessed Nov. 7, 2009).

4. Further information can be obtained from the Library of Congress at http://thomas.loc.gov/home/c111query.html (accessed June 6, 2013).

5. See City Year, www.cityyear.org (accessed Sept. 5, 2009). City Year's geographical location is 287 Columbus Ave, Boston MA, 02116.

6. A "modern response" to a "modern epidemic": HIV/AIDS in the District of Columbia," reported at the 16th Conference on Retroviruses and Opportunistic Infections, 2009.

REFERENCES

Abrams DB, Orleans CT, Niaura RS, Goldstein MG, Prochaska JO, Velicer W. 1996. Integrating individual and public health perspectives for treatment of tobacco dependence under managed health care: A combined stepped-care and matching model. *Ann Behav Med* 18 (4) (Fall): 290-304.

Aidala A, Cross JE, Stall R, Harre D, Sumartojo E. 2005. Housing status and HIV risk behaviors: Implications for prevention and policy. *AIDS Behav* 9 (3) (Sept.): 251-65.

APA Council of Representatives. 2004. Resolution of sexual orientation and marriage. American Psychological Association, Washington, DC.

Aral SO, Douglas JM Jr., Lipshutz JA, eds. 2007. *Behavioral Interventions for Prevention and Control of Sexually Transmitted Diseases.* New York: Springer.

Auerbach J. 2009. Transforming social structures and environments to help in HIV prevention. *Health Affairs* 28 (6) (Nov.-Dec.): 1655-65.

Auslander BA, Biro FM, Succop PA, Short MB, Rosenthal SL. 2009. Racial/ethnic differences in patterns of sexual behavior and STI risk among sexually experienced adolescent girls. *J Pediatr Adolesc Gynecol* 22 (1) (Feb.): 33-39.

Averett SL, Rees DI, Argys LM. 2002. The impact of government policies and neighborhood characteristics on teenage sexual activity and contraceptive use. *Am J Public Health* 92 (11) (Nov.): 1773-78.

Barham L, Lewis D, Latimer N. 2007. One to one interventions to reduce sexually transmitted infections and under the age of 18 conceptions: A systematic review of the economic evaluations. *Sex Transm Infect* 83 (6) (Oct.): 441-46.

Bensley LS, Van Eenwyk J, Simmons KW. 2000. Self-reported childhood sexual and physical abuse and adult HIV-risk behaviors and heavy drinking. *Am J Prev Med* 18 (2) (Feb): 151-58.

Berg M, Coman E, Schensul JJ. 2009. Youth Action Research for Prevention: A multi-level intervention designed to increase efficacy and empowerment among urban youth. *Am J Commun Psych* 43 (3-4) (June): 345-59.

Berg RC. 2009. Barebacking: A review of the literature. *Arch Sex Behav* 38 (5) (Oct.): 754-64.

Bernstein KT. 2004. Repeat sexually transmitted diseases and core transmitters. Paper presented at the National STD Prevention Conference, Philadelphia.

Bernstein KT, Curriero FC, Jennings JM, Olthoff G, Erbelding EJ, Zenilman J. 2004. Defining core gonorrhea transmission utilizing spatial data. *Am J Epidemiol* 160 (1) (July 1): 51-58.

Binson D, Pollack LM, Blair J, Woods WJ. 2009. HIV transmission risk at a gay bathhouse. *J Sex Res Sep* 14:1-9.

Bleakley A, Fishbein M, Holtgrave D. 2008. An assessment of the relationship between condom labels and HIV-related beliefs and intentions. *AIDS Behav* 12 (3) (May): 452-58.

Bontempo DE, D'Augelli AR. 2002. Effects of at-school victimization and sexual orientation on lesbian, gay, or bisexual youths' health risk behavior. *J Adolesc Health* 30 (5) (May): 364-74.

Calsyn DA, Meinecke C, Saxon AJ, Stanton V. 1992. Risk reduction in sexual behavior: A condom giveaway program in a drug abuse treatment clinic. *Am J Public Health* 82 (11) (Nov.): 1536-38.

Centers for Disease Control and Prevention (CDC). 2004a. Diagnoses of HIV/AIDS—32 states, 2000-2003. *MMWR* 53 (47) (Dec. 3): 1106-10.

——. 2004b. *Sexually Transmitted Disease Surveillance, 2003.* Atlanta, GA: U.S. Department of Health and Human Services.

——. 2008. STDs and pregnancy—CDC fact sheet. Available at www.cdc.gov/std/STDFact-STDs&Pregnancy.htm (accessed Nov. 29, 2009).

——. 2009a. *The Community Guide.* Available at www.thecommunityguide.org (accessed Aug. 16, 2009).

——. 2009b. HIV/AIDS prevention research synthesis project. Available at www.cdc.gov/hiv/topics/research/prs/ (accessed Aug. 12, 2009).

——. 2009c. HIV/AIDS statistics and surveillance. Available at www.cdc.gov/hiv/topics/surveillance/index.htm (accessed Sept. 20, 2009).

———. 2009d. HIV and AIDS among gay and bisexual men. Available at www.cdc.gov/nchhstp/newsroom /docs/FastFacts-MSM-FINAL508COMP.pdf (accessed Nov. 29, 2009).

———. 2009e. Nine and a half minutes. Available at www.nineandahalfminutes.org (accessed Aug. 22, 2009).

———. 2009f. Sexual and reproductive health of persons aged 10-24 years—United States, 2002-2007. *MMWR* 58 (SS06): 1-58.

———. 2009g. Sexually transmitted diseases. Available at www.cdc.gov (accessed Nov. 29, 2009).

———. 2009h. Slide Set: HIV Mortality (through 2006). Available at www.cdc.gov/hiv/topics/surveillance /resources/slides/mortality/index.htm (accessed Nov. 21, 2010).

———. 2009i. Trends in reportable sexually transmitted diseases in the United States, 2007: National surveillance data for chlamydia, gonorrhea, and syphilis. Available at www.cdc.gov/std/stats07/trends.htm (accessed July 17, 2009).

———. 2009j. 2007 National Youth Risk Behavior Survey overview. Available at www.cdc.gov/HealthyYouth /yrbs/index.htm (accessed July 23, 2009).

———. 2009k. Unintended pregnancy protection. Available at www.cdc.gov/reproductivehealth/Unintended Pregnancy/index.htm (accessed July 23, 2009).

———. 2009l. Viral hepatitis. Available at www.cdc.gov /hepatitis/HBV/HBVfaq.htm#overview (accessed July 17, 2009).

———. 2013a. Reproductive Health: Data and Statistics Division of Reproductive Health, National Center for Chronic Disease Prevention and Health Promotion. Available at www.cdc.gov/reproductivehealth/Data _Stats/ (accessed June 6, 2013).

———. 2013b. Slide Set: HIV Mortality (through 2009). Available at www.cdc.gov/hiv/topics/surveillance /resources/slides/mortality/index.htm (accessed June 6, 2013).

Chesson H, Harrison P, Kassler WJ. 2000. Sex under the influence: The effect of alcohol policy on sexually transmitted disease rates in the United States. *J Law Econ* 43 (1): 215-38.

Chesson HW, Harrison P, Stall R. 2003. Changes in alcohol consumption and in sexually transmitted disease incidence rates in the United States: 1983-1998. *J Stud Alcohol* 64 (5) (Sept.): 623-30.

Civic D, Scholes D, Grothaus L, McBride C. 2001. Adolescent HMO enrollees' utilization of out-of-plan services. *J Adolesc Health* 28 (6) (June): 491-96.

Coco A. 2005. The cost-effectiveness of expanded testing for primary HIV infection. *Ann Fam Med* 3 (5) (Sept.-Oct.): 391-99.

Cohen DA, Ghosh-Dastidar B, Bluthenthal R, et al. 2004. Gonorrhea and the 1992 civil unrest in Los Angeles. Program and abstracts of the XV International Conference on AIDS, Bangkok, Thailand, July.

Cohen DA, Nsuami M, Martin DH, Farley TA. 1999. Repeated school-based screening for sexually transmitted diseases: A feasible strategy for reaching adolescents. *Pediatrics* 104 (6) (Dec.): 1281-85.

Cohen DA, Scribner R. 2000. An STD/HIV prevention intervention framework. *AIDS Patient Care STDS* 14 (1) (Jan.): 37-45.

Cohen DA, Wu SY, Farley TA. 2005. Cost-effective allocation of government funds to prevent HIV infection. *Health Affairs* 24 (4) (July-Aug.): 915-26.

Collins RL, Elliott MN, Berry SH, et al. 2004. Watching sex on television predicts adolescent initiation of sexual behavior. *Pediatrics* 114 (3) (Sept.): e280-89.

Crepaz N, Marks G, Liau A, et al. 2009. Prevalence of unprotected anal intercourse among HIV-diagnosed MSM in the United States: A meta-analysis. *AIDS* 23 (13) (Aug. 24): 1617-29.

Denning PH, Campsmith ML. 2005. Unprotected anal intercourse among HIV-positive men who have a steady male sex partner with negative or unknown HIV serostatus. *Am J Public Health* 95 (1) (Jan.): 152-58.

Diffusion of Effective Behavioral Interventions (DEBI). 2009. Available at www.effectiveinterventions.org/ (accessed Aug. 22, 2009).

Dubois-Arber F, Jeannin A, Konings E, Paccaud F. 1997. Increased condom use without other major changes in sexual behavior among the general population in Switzerland. *Am J Public Health* 87 (4) (April): 558-66.

Dworkin SL, Pinto RM, Hunter J, Rapkin B, Remien RH. 2008. Keeping the spirit of community partnerships alive in the scale up of HIV/AIDS prevention: Critical reflections on the roll out of DEBI (Diffusion of Effective Behavioral Interventions). *Am J Commun Psych* 42 (1-2) (Sept.): 51-59.

Eke AN, Neumann MS, Wilkes AL, Jones PL. 2006. Preparing effective behavioral interventions to be used by prevention providers: The role of researchers during HIV Prevention Research Trials. *AIDS Educ Prev* 18 (4 suppl. A) (Aug.): 44-58.

El-Bassel N, Gilbert L, Rajah V, Foleno A, Frye V. 2000. Fear and violence: Raising the HIV stakes. *AIDS Educ Prev* 12 (2) (April): 154-70.

Ellen JM, Hessol NA, Kohn RP, Bolan GA. 1997. An investigation of geographic clustering of repeat cases of gonorrhea and chlamydial infection in San Francisco, 1989-1993: Evidence for core groups. *J Infect Dis* 175 (6) (June): 1519-22.

Feldblum PJ, Kuyoh MA, Bwayo JJ, et al. 2001. Female condom introduction and sexually transmitted infection prevalence: Results of a community intervention trial in Kenya. *AIDS* 15 (8) (May 25): 1037-44.

The female condom: Still an underused prevention tool. 2008. *Lancet Infect Dis* 8 (6) (June): 343.

Fenton KA, Mercer CM, Johnson AM. 2005. Evolution of sexual risk behaviours and STD transmission risk among MSM. Oral presentation at the 16th Biennial Meeting of the International Society for Sexually Transmitted Diseases Research (ISSTDR), Amsterdam, Netherlands, July 10-13. Abstract Available at www.isstdr.nl/0605%20ISSTDR%20Program%20Book%20DEF.pdf.

Fielding JE, Williams CA. 1991. Adolescent pregnancy in the United States: A review and recommendations for clinicians and research needs. *Am J Prev Med* 7 (1) (Jan.-Feb.): 47-52.

Fiore MC, Bailey WC, Cohen SJ, et al. 2008. *Treating Tobacco Use and Dependence. A Clinical Practice Guideline.* Rockville, MD: U.S. Department of Health and Human Services.

Ford K, Sohn W, Lepkowski J. 2001. Characteristics of adolescents' sexual partners and their association with use of condoms and other contraceptive methods. *Fam Plann Perspect* 33 (3) (May-June): 100.

Foulkes HB, Pettigrew MM, Livingston KA, Niccolai LM. 2009. Comparison of sexual partnership characteristics and associations with inconsistent condom use among a sample of adolescents and adult women diagnosed with Chlamydia trachomatis. *J Womens Health (Larchmt)* 18 (3) (March): 393-99.

Galvan FH, Collins RL, Kanouse DE, Pantoja P, Golinelli D. 2007. Religiosity, denominational affiliation, and sexual behaviors among people with HIV in the United States. *J Sex Res* 44 (1) (Feb.): 49-58.

Gandelman AA, Desantis LM, Rietmeijer CA. 2006. Assessing community needs and agency capacity—an integral part of implementing effective evidence-based interventions. *AIDS Educ Prev* 18 (4 suppl. A) (Aug.): 32-43.

Gielen AC, Ghandour RM, Burke JG, Mahoney P, McDonnell KA, O'Campo P. 2007. HIV/AIDS and intimate partner violence: Intersecting women's health issues in the United States. *Trauma Violence Abuse* 8 (2): 178-98.

Goodenow C, Netherland J, Szalacha L. 2002. AIDS-related risk among adolescent males who have sex with males, females, or both: Evidence from a statewide survey. *Am J Public Health* 92 (2) (Feb.): 203-10.

Goodwin MA, Zyzanski SJ, Zronek S, et al. 2001. A clinical trial of tailored office systems for preventive service delivery: The Study to Enhance Prevention by Understanding Practice (STEP-UP). *Am J Prev Med* 21 (1) (July): 20-28.

Hall HI, Song R, Rhodes P, et al. 2008. Estimation of HIV incidence in the United States. *JAMA* 300 (5) (Aug. 6): 520-29.

Halpern CT, Hallfors D, Bauer DJ, Iritani B, Waller MW, Cho H. 2004. Implications of racial and gender differences in patterns of adolescent risk behavior for HIV and other sexually transmitted diseases. *Perspect Sex Reprod Health* 36 (6) (Nov.-Dec.): 239-47.

Hatzenbuehler ML, Keyes KM, Hasin DS. 2009. State-level policies and psychiatric morbidity in lesbian, gay, and bisexual populations. *Am J Public Health* 99 (12) (Dec.): 2275-81.

Hicks KA, Wirth K. 2003. User's guide to accompany the HIV Prevention Funding Allocation Model (HPFAM). Available at www.cdc.gov/hiv/topics/prev_prog/ce/materials/PDF/HPFAM_Users-Guide.pdf (accessed Nov. 7, 2009).

Hoke TH, Feldblum PJ, Van Damme K, et al. 2007. Temporal trends in sexually transmitted infection prevalence and condom use following introduction of the female condom to Madagascar sex workers. *Int J STD AIDS* 18 (7) (July): 461-66.

Holtgrave DR. 2004. The role of quantitative policy analysis in HIV prevention technology transfer. *Public Health Rep* 119 (1) (Jan.-Feb.): 19-22.

———. 2008. Written testimony on HIV/AIDS incidence and prevention for hearing to be held September 16, 2008. U.S. Congress, Committee on Oversight and Government Reform. Available at www.reform.democrats.house.gov/documents/20080916115223.pdf. Accessed Feb/16, 2010.

Holtgrave D, Hall HI, Rhodes PH, Wolitski R. 2009. Updated annual HIV transmission rates in the United States, 1977-2006. *J Acquir Immune Defic Syndr* 50 (2) (Feb. 1): 236-38.

Holtgrave DR, Kelly JA. 1996. Preventing HIV/AIDS among high-risk urban women: The cost-effectiveness of a behavioral group intervention. *Am J Public Health* 86 (10) (Oct.): 1442-45.

Holtgrave DR, Pinkerton SD. 1997. Updates of cost of illness and quality of life estimates for use in economic evaluations of HIV prevention programs. *J Acquir Immune Defic Syndr Hum Retrovirol* 16 (1) (Sept. 1): 54-62.

Holtgrave DR, Wunderink KA, Vallone DM, Healton CG. 2009. Cost-utility analysis of the national truth campaign to prevent youth smoking. *Am J Prev Med* 36 (5) (May): 385-88.

Holtzman D, Rubinson R. 1995. Parent and peer communication effects on AIDS-related behavior among U.S. high school students. *Fam Plann Perspect* 27 (6) (Nov.-Dec.): 235.

Hornberger J, Holodniy M, Robertus K, Winnike M, Gibson E, Verhulst E. 2007. A systematic review of cost-utility analyses in HIV/AIDS: Implications for public policy. *Med Decis Making* 27:789-821.

Imamura M, Tucker J, Hannaford P, et al. 2007. Factors associated with teenage pregnancy in the European Union countries: A systematic review. *Eur J Public Health* 17 (6) (Dec.): 630-36.

Johns Hopkins Urban Health Institute and Baltimore City Health Department. 2009. REVERSE Research Day. Available at www.jhsph.edu/urbanhealth/events/revresearchday.html (accessed Nov. 7, 2009).

Johnson AM, Mercer CH, Erens B, et al. 2001. Sexual behaviour in Britain: Partnerships, practices, and HIV risk behaviours. *Lancet* 358 (9296) (Dec. 1): 1835-42.

Jones RK, Purcell A, Singh S, Finer LB. 2005. Adolescents' reports of parental knowledge of adolescents' use of sexual health services and their reactions to mandated parental notification for prescription contraception. *JAMA* 293 (3) (Jan. 19): 340-48.

Kaestle CE, Morisky DE, Wiley DJ. 2002. Sexual intercourse and the age difference between adolescent females and their romantic partners. *Perspect Sex Reprod Health* 34 (6) (Nov.-Dec.): 304-9.

Kaiser Family Foundation and National Alliance of State and Territorial AIDS Directors. 2009. National HIV prevention inventory: The state of HIV prevention across the U.S. Available at www.kff.org/hivaids/7932.cfm (accessed Nov. 7, 2009).

Kalichman SC, Gore-Felton C, Benotsch E, Cage M, Rompa D. 2004. Trauma symptoms, sexual behaviors, and substance abuse: Correlates of childhood sexual abuse and HIV risks among men who have sex with men. *J Child Sex Abus* 13 (1): 1-15.

Kalichman SC, Williams EA, Cherry C, Belcher L, Nachimson D. 1998. Sexual coercion, domestic violence, and negotiating condom use among low-income African American women. *J Womens Health* 7 (3) (April): 371-78.

Kamb ML, Fishbein M, Douglas JM Jr., et al. 1998. Efficacy of risk-reduction counseling to prevent human immunodeficiency virus and sexually transmitted diseases: A randomized controlled trial. Project RESPECT Study Group. *JAMA* 280 (13) (Oct. 7): 1161-67.

Karofsky PS, Zeng L, Kosorok MR. 2001. Relationship between adolescent-parental communication and initiation of first intercourse by adolescents. *J Adolesc Health* 28 (1) (Jan.): 41-45.

Kegeles SM, Hays RB, Coates TJ. 1996. The Mpowerment Project: A community-level HIV prevention intervention for young gay men. *Am J Public Health* 86 (8) (Aug.): 1129-36.

Kelly JA, Hoffman RG, Rompa D, Gray M. 1998. Protease inhibitor combination therapies and perceptions of gay men regarding AIDS severity and the need to maintain safer sex. *AIDS* 12 (10) (July 9): F91-95.

Kelly JA, Kalichman SC. 2002. Behavioral research in HIV/AIDS primary and secondary prevention: Recent advances and future directions. *J Consult Clin Psychol* 70 (3) (June): 626-39.

Kelly JA, Somlai AM, DiFranceisco WJ, et al. 2000. Bridging the gap between the science and service of HIV prevention: Transferring effective research-based HIV prevention interventions to community AIDS service providers. *Am J Public Health* 90 (7) (July): 1082-88.

Kelly JA, St Lawrence JS, Stevenson LY, et al. 1992. Community AIDS/HIV risk reduction: The effects of endorsements by popular people in three cities. *Am J Public Health* 82 (11) (Nov): 1483-89.

Kerrigan D, Telles P, Torres H, Overs C, Castle C. 2007. Community development and HIV/STI-related vulnerability among female sex workers in Rio de Janeiro, Brazil. *Health Educ Res,* March 14.

Kidder DP, Wolitski RJ, Campsmith ML, Nakamura GV. 2007. Health status, health care use, medication use, and medication adherence among homeless and housed people living with HIV/AIDS. *Am J Public Health* 97 (12) (Dec.): 2238-45.

Kidder DP, Wolitski RJ, Royal S, et al. 2007. Access to housing as a structural intervention for homeless and unstably housed people living with HIV: Rationale, methods, and implementation of the housing and health study. *AIDS Behav* 11 (6 suppl.) (Nov.): 149-61.

Kirby D. 2002. The impact of schools and school programs upon adolescent sexual behavior. *J Sex Res* 39 (1) (Feb.): 27-33.

Kirby DB, Brown NL. 1996. Condom availability programs in U.S. schools. *Fam Plann Perspect* 28 (5) (Sept.-Oct.): 196-202.

Kirby DB, Laris BA, Rolleri LA. 2007. Sex and HIV education programs: Their impact on sexual behaviors of young people throughout the world. *J Adolesc Health* 40 (3) (March): 206-17.

Kirby D, Waszak C, Ziegler J. 1991. Six school-based clinics: Their reproductive health services and impact on sexual behavior. *Fam Plann Perspect* 23 (1) (Jan.-Feb.): 6-16.

Klausner JD, Pollack LM, Wong W, Katz MH. 2006. Same-sex domestic partnerships and lower-risk behaviors for STDs, including HIV infection. *J Homosex* 51 (4): 137-44.

Koop EC. 1996. Health promotion and disease prevention in clinical practice. In *Health Promotion and Disease Prevention in Clinical Practice,* ed. RS Lawrence, SH Woolf, S Jonas, vii-ix. Baltimore: Williams & Wilkins.

Lafferty WE, Downey L, Holan CM, et al. 2002. Provision of sexual health services to adolescent enrollees in Medicaid managed care. *Am J Public Health* 92 (11) (Nov.): 1779-83.

Lasry A, Sansom S, Hicks K, Uzunangelov V. 2009. Modeling the impact of HIV prevention strategies in the United States. Paper presented at the National HIV Prevention Conference, Atlanta, GA.

Lefkowitz ES, Gillen MM, Shearer CL, Boone TL. 2004. Religiosity, sexual behaviors, and sexual attitudes during emerging adulthood. *J Sex Res* 41 (2) (May): 150-59.

Lin JS, Whitlock E, O'Connor E, Bauer V. 2008. Behavioral counseling to prevent sexually transmitted infections: A systematic review for the U.S. Preventive Services Task Force. *Ann Intern Med* 149 (7) (Oct. 7): 497-508, W96-99.

Logan TK, Cole J, Leukefeld C. 2002. Women, sex, and HIV: Social and contextual factors, meta-analysis of published interventions, and implications for practice and research. *Psychol Bull* 128 (6) (Nov.): 851-85.

Lyles CM, Kay LS, Crepaz N, et al. 2007. Best-evidence interventions: Findings from a systematic review of HIV behavioral interventions for US populations at high risk, 2000-2004. *Am J Public Health* 97 (1) (Jan.): 133-43.

Marsiglio W, Mott FL. 1986. The impact of sex education on sexual activity, contraceptive use, and premarital pregnancy among American teenagers. *Fam Plann Perspect* 18 (4) (July-Aug.): 151-62.

McNeely CA, Nonnemaker JM, Blum RW. 2002. Promoting school connectedness: Evidence from the National Longitudinal Study of Adolescent Health. *J Sch Health* 72 (4) (April): 138-46.

McNeely C, Shew ML, Beuhring T, Sieving R, Miller BC, Blum RW. 2002. Mothers' influence on the timing of first sex among 14- and 15-year-olds. *J Adolesc Health* 31 (3) (Sept.): 256-65.

Meyer IH. 2003. Prejudice, social stress, and mental health in lesbian, gay, and bisexual populations: Conceptual issues and research evidence. *Psychol Bull* 129 (5) (Sept.): 674-97.

Meyers HF, Javanbakht M, Martinez M, Obediah S. 2003. Psychosocial predictors of risky sexual behaviors in African American men: Implications for prevention. *AIDS Educ Prev* 15 (suppl. A): 66-79.

Moore KA, Hofferth SL, Wertheimer R 2nd. 1979. Teenage motherhood: Its social and economic costs. *Child Today* 8 (5) (Sept.-Oct.): 12-16.

Mosher WD, Chandra A, Jones J. 2005. Sexual behavior and selected health measures: Men and women 15-44 years of age, United States, 2002. *Adv Data* (362) (Sept. 15): 1-55.

Mott FL, Fondell MM, Hu PN, Kowaleski-Jones L, Menaghan EG. 1996. The determinants of first sex by age 14 in a high-risk adolescent population. *Fam Plann Perspect* 28 (1) (Jan.-Feb.): 13-18.

National Institute of Mental Health (NIMH). 1998. The NIMH Multisite HIV Prevention Trial: Reducing HIV sexual risk behavior. National Institute of Mental Health (NIMH) Multisite HIV Prevention Trial Group. *Science* 280 (5371) (June 19): 1889-94.

O'Donnell CR, O'Donnell L, San Doval A, Duran R, Labes K. 1998. Reductions in STD infections subsequent to an STD clinic visit: Using video-based patient education to supplement provider interactions. *Sex Transm Dis* 25 (3) (March): 161-68.

O'Donnell L, Stueve A, San Doval A, et al. 1999. The effectiveness of the Reach for Health Community Youth Service learning program in reducing early and unprotected sex among urban middle school students. *Am J Public Health* 89 (2) (Feb.): 176-81.

O'Leary A, Martins P. 2000. Structural factors affecting women's HIV risk: A life-course example. *AIDS* 14 (suppl. 1): S68-S72.

Orr ST, Celentano DD, Santelli J, Burwell L. 1994. Depressive symptoms and risk factors for HIV acquisition among black women attending urban health centers in Baltimore. *AIDS Educ Prev* 6 (3) (June): 230-36.

Ostrow DE, Fox KJ, Chmiel JS, et al. 2002. Attitudes towards highly active antiretroviral therapy are associated with sexual risk taking among HIV-infected and uninfected homosexual men. *AIDS* 16 (5) (March 29): 775-80.

Owusu-Edusei K Jr., Chesson HW, Gift TL, et al. 2013. The estimated direct medical cost of selected sexually transmitted infections in the United States, 2008. *Sex Transm Dis* 40 (3) (March): 197-201.

Ozer EM, Adams SH, Lustig JL, et al. 2005. Increasing the screening and counseling of adolescents for risky health behaviors: A primary care intervention. *Pediatrics* 115 (4) (April): 960-68.

Pazol K, Gamble SB, Parker WY, et al. 2012. Abortion surveillance—United States, 2009. *MMWR Surveill Summ,* Nov. 23. Available at www.cdc.gov/mmwr/preview/mmwrhtml/ss6108a1.htm (accessed June 6, 2013).

Pequegnat W, Stover E. 1999. Considering women's contextual and cultural issues in HIV/STD prevention research. *Cult Divers Ethn Minor Psychol* 5:287-91.

Phillips KA, Fernyak S, Potosky AL, Schauffler HH, Egorin M. 2000. Use of preventive services by managed care enrollees: An updated perspective. *Health Aff (Millwood)* 19 (1) (Jan.-Feb.): 102-16.

Pinkerton SD, Holtgrave DR. 1998. The cost-effectiveness of HIV prevention from a managed care perspective. *J Public Health Man Pract* 4 (1) (Jan.): 59-66.

Pinkerton SD, Holtgrave DR, Valdiserri RO. 1997. Cost-effectiveness of HIV-prevention skills training for men who have sex with men. *AIDS* 11 (3) (March): 347-57.

Pinkerton SD, Johnson-Masotti AP, Holtgrave DR, Farnham PG. 2001. Using cost-effectiveness league tables to compare interventions to prevent sexual transmission of HIV. *AIDS* 15 (7) (May 4): 917-28.

Pourat N, Brown ER, Razack N, Kassler W. 2002. Medicaid managed care and STDs: Missed opportunities to control the epidemic. *Health Aff (Millwood)* 21 (3) (May-June): 228-39.

Price N. 2001. The performance of social marketing in reaching the poor and vulnerable in AIDS control programmes. *Health Policy Plan* 16 (3) (Sept.): 231-39.

Pulerwitz J, Gortmaker S, DeJong W. 2000. Measuring sexual relationship power in HIV/STD research. *Sex Roles* 42 (637): 660.

Rees V, Saitz R, Horton NJ, Samet J. 2001. Association of alcohol consumption with HIV sex- and drug-risk behaviors among drug users. *J Subst Abuse Treat* 21 (3) (Oct.): 129-34.

Rew L, Grady M, Whittaker TA, Bowman K. 2008. Interaction of duration of homelessness and gender on adolescent sexual health indicators. *J Nurs Scholarsh* 40 (2): 109-15.

Romer D, Black M, Ricardo I, et al. 1994. Social influences on the sexual behavior of youth at risk for HIV exposure. *Am J Public Health* 84 (6) (June): 977-85.

Romer D, Stanton B, Galbraith J, Feigelman S, Black MM, Li X. 1999. Parental influence on adolescent sexual behavior in high-poverty settings. *Arch Pediatr Adolesc Med* 153 (10) (Oct.): 1055-62.

Santelli JS, Abma J, Ventura S, et al. 2004. Can changes in sexual behaviors among high school students explain the decline in teen pregnancy rates in the 1990s? *J Adolesc Health* 35 (2) (Aug.): 80-90.

Schuster MA, Bell RM, Berry SH, Kanouse DE. 1998. Impact of a high school condom availability program on sexual attitudes and behaviors. *Fam Plann Perspect* 30 (2) (March-April): 67-72, 88.

Shafer MA, Tebb KP, Pantell RH, et al. 2002. Effect of a clinical practice improvement intervention on chlamydial screening among adolescent girls. *JAMA* 288 (22) (Dec. 11): 2846-52.

Shea MA, Callis BP, Cassidy-Stewart H, Cranston K, Tomoyasu N. 2006. Diffusion of effective HIV prevention interventions—lessons from Maryland and Massachusetts. *AIDS Educ Prev* 18 (4 suppl. A) (Aug.): 96-107.

Sherman SG, German D, Cheng Y, Marks M, Bailey-Kloche M. 2006. The evaluation of the JEWEL project: An innovative economic enhancement and HIV prevention intervention study targeting drug using women involved in prostitution. *AIDS Care* 18 (1) (Jan.): 1-11.

Sifakis F, Hylton JB, Flynn C, et al. 2007. Racial disparities in HIV incidence among young men who have sex with men: The Baltimore Young Men's Survey. *J Acquir Immune Defic Syndr* 46 (3) (Nov. 1): 343-48.

Snowden J, Raymond HF, McFarland W. 2009. Prevalence of seroadaptive behaviors of men who have sex with men, San Francisco, 2004. *Sex Transm Infect,* June 7.

Solberg LI, Kottke TE, Brekke ML. 1998. Will primary care clinics organize themselves to improve the delivery of preventive services? A randomized controlled trial. *Prev Med* 27 (4) (July-Aug.): 623-31.

Solberg LI, Kottke TE, Brekke ML, Conn SA, Magnan S, Amundson G. 1998. The case of the missing clinical preventive services systems. *Eff Clin Pract* 1 (1) (Aug.-Sept.): 33-38.

Suarez T, Miller J. 2001. Negotiating risks in context: A perspective on unprotected anal intercourse and barebacking among men who have sex with men—where do we go from here? *Arch Sex Behav* 30 (3) (June): 287-300.

Sullivan PS, Salazar L, Buchbinder S, Sanchez TH. 2009. Estimating the proportion of HIV transmissions from main sex partners among men who have sex with men in five US cities. *AIDS* 23 (9) (June 1): 1153-62.

Tao G, Walsh CM, Anderson LA, Irwin KL. 2002. Understanding sexual activity defined in the HEDIS measure of screening young women for Chlamydia trachomatis. *Jt Comm J Qual Improv* 28 (8) (Aug.): 435-40.

Taylor MM, McClain T, Javanbakht M, et al. 2005. Sexually transmitted disease testing protocols, sexually transmitted disease testing, and discussion of sexual behaviors in HIV clinics in Los Angeles County. *Sex Transm Dis* 32 (6) (June): 341-45.

Tuli K, Sansom S, Purcell DW, et al. 2005. Economic evaluation of an HIV prevention intervention for seropositive injection drug users. *J Public Health Man Pract* 11 (6) (Nov.-Dec.): 508-15.

U.S. Department of Health and Human Services (USDHHS). 2010. *Healthy People.* Office of Disease Prevention and Health Promotion. Available at www.healthypeople.gov/ (accessed Sept. 20, 2009).

Valente CM, Sobal J, Muncie HL Jr., Levine DM, Antlitz AM. 1986. Health promotion: Physicians' beliefs, attitudes, and practices. *Am J Prev Med* 2 (2) (March–April): 82-88.

Vanable PA, Ostrow DG, McKirnan DJ, Taywaditep KJ, Hope BA. 2000. Impact of combination therapies on HIV risk perceptions and sexual risk among HIV-positive and HIV-negative gay and bisexual men. *Health Psychol* 19 (2) (March): 134-45.

Varghese B, Peterman TA. 2001. Cost-effectiveness of HIV counseling and testing in US prisons. *J Urban Health* 78 (2) (June): 304-12.

Varghese B, Peterman TA, Holtgrave DR. 1999. Cost-effectiveness of counseling and testing and partner notification: A decision analysis. *AIDS* 13 (13) (Sept. 10): 1745-51.

Ventura SJ, Mathews TJ, Hamilton BE. 2001. Births to teenagers in the United States, 1940-2000. *Natl Vital Stat Rep* 49 (10) (Sept. 25): 1-23.

Viswanathan M, Ammerman A, Eng E, et al. 2004. Community-based participatory research: Assessing the evidence. *Evid Rep Technol Assess* (99) (Aug.): 1-8.

Vogt TM, Hollis JF, Lichtenstein E, Stevens VJ, Glasgow R, Whitlock E. 1998. The medical care system and prevention: The need for a new paradigm. *HMO Pract* 12 (1) (March): 5-13.

Waldo CR, McFarland W, Katz MH, MacKellar D, Valleroy LA. 2002. Very young gay and bisexual men are at risk for HIV infection: The San Francisco Bay Area Young Men's Survey II. *J Acquir Immune Defic Syndr* 4:168-74.

Wechsler H, Levine S, Idelson RK, Schor EL, Coakley E. 1996. The physician's role in health promotion revisited—a survey of primary care practitioners. *N Engl J Med* 334 (15) (April 11): 996-98.

Weinstock H, Berman S, Cates W Jr. 2004. Sexually transmitted diseases among American youth: Incidence and prevalence estimates, 2000. *Perspect Sex Reprod Health* 36 (1) (Jan.-Feb.): 6-10.

Weniger BG, Limpakarnjanarat K, Ungchusak K, et al. 1991. The epidemiology of HIV infection and AIDS in Thailand. *AIDS* 5 (suppl. 2): S71-S85.

Whyte J 4th, Whyte MD, Cormier E. 2008. Down low sex, older African American women, and HIV infection. *J Assoc Nurses AIDS Care* 19 (6) (Nov.-Dec.): 423-31.

Wiemann CM, Chacko MR, Kozinetz CA, et al. 2009. Correlates of consistent condom use with main-new and main-old sexual partners. *J Adolesc Health* 45 (3) (Sept.): 296-99.

Windle M. 1997. The trading of sex for money or drugs, sexually transmitted diseases (STDs), and HIV-related risk behaviors among multisubstance using alcoholic inpatients. *Drug Alcohol Depend* 49 (1) (Dec.): 33-38.

Wingood GM, DiClemente RJ. 1998. The influence of psychosocial factors, alcohol, drug use on African-American women's high-risk sexual behavior. *Am J Prev Med* 15 (1) (July): 54-59.

Wojcicki JM. 2005. Socioeconomic status as a risk factor for HIV infection in women in east, central, and southern Africa: A systematic review. *J Biosoc Sci* 37 (1) (Jan.): 1-36.

Wolitski RJ, Kidder DP, Pals SL, et al. 2009. Randomized trial of the effects of housing assistance on the health and risk behaviors of homeless and unstably housed people living with HIV. *AIDS Behav,* Dec. 1.

Wolitski RJ, Stall R, Valdiserri RO, eds. 2008. *Unequal Opportunity: Health Disparities Affecting Gay and Bisexual Men in the United States.* New York: Oxford University Press.

Wolk LI, Rosenbaum R. 1995. The benefits of school-based condom availability: Cross-sectional analysis of a comprehensive high school-based program. *J Adolesc Health* 17 (3) (Sept.): 184-88.

Wood E, Kerr T, Spittal PM, et al. 2003. The potential public health and community impacts of safer injecting facilities: Evidence from a cohort of injection drug users. *J Acquir Immune Defic Syndr* 32 (1) (Jan. 1): 2-8.

Woods WJ, Binson D. 2003. Public health policy and gay bathhouses. *J Homosex* 44 (3-4): 1-21.

Wykoff RF, Jones JL, Longshore ST, et al. 1991. Notification of the sex and needle-sharing partners of individuals with human immunodeficiency virus in rural South Carolina: 30-month experience. *Sex Transm Dis* 18 (4) (Oct.-Dec.): 217-22.

Zabin LS, Emerson MR, Ringers PA, Sedivy V. 1996. Adolescents with negative pregnancy test results: An accessible at-risk group. *JAMA* 275 (2) (Jan. 10): 113-17.

Zavodny M. 2004. Fertility and parental consent for minors to receive contraceptives. *Am J Public Health* 94 (8) (Aug): 1347-51.

CHAPTER 19

Clinicians and Behavior Change

JILL MARSTELLER, AYSE P. GURSES,
YEA-JEN HSU, A. ANT OZOK, SCOTT KAHAN,
AND PETER J. PRONOVOST

LEARNING OBJECTIVES

After completing the chapter, the reader will be able to

* Describe the main factors affecting provider choice in implementing desired behavior changes with respect to health care delivery.
* Explain the path from preexisting system elements through implementation of a behavior change intervention to patient outcomes.
* Describe collaboratives and learning networks as provider behavior change strategies.
* Analyze strengths and weaknesses of collaborative-style behavior change interventions.
* Detail the interests and mechanisms of influence of a range of stakeholders affecting provider behavior change and the kinds of data or arguments they find most convincing.

Introduction

In health care, a wide range of **stakeholders** could benefit from changes in certain aspects of clinician behavior. For example, patients would like their physicians to spend more time with them, to treat them with kindness and respect regardless of their external or cultural characteristics, and to provide them with the highest quality of care to accurately diagnose and treat even the least common problem. As much as physicians would like to accomplish all of these **expectations**, they are also pressured by many other stakeholders and system factors to focus on other priorities, such as seeing more patients and ordering fewer tests. Although everyone, in principle, supports higher quality of care and treating patients equally and with respect, these desired behaviors can sometimes be more difficult to realize than is readily apparent. What affects behavior change among clinicians when the government, society, payers, health care organizations, researchers, and patients seek to encourage a desired clinical behavior?

Accepted, evidence-based guidance for clinician behavior is detailed in numerous practice **guidelines**, defined **interventions**, and new **innovations** (such as decision support tools). We tend to assume that if clinicians all followed these desirable behaviors, patients would receive better care and be more satisfied with their physicians and the health care system, there would be fewer medical errors, and costs would be minimized. Whether all this is true is uncertain—our guidelines and interventions need continuous refinement—but what is clear is that clinicians' **compliance** with many published guidelines and other successful interventions is often poor and inconsistent.

In this chapter, we discuss **key determinants** of clinician behavior, based on several contributing literatures, and offer examples from clinical experience and empirical research that demonstrate these factors. We focus on clinicians' compliance with practice guidelines as a case in point, although this discussion generalizes to virtually any desirable clinician behavior. We will thus use the terms *desired behavior, guideline, evidence-based practice, intervention*, and *innovation* interchangeably in this chapter. In addition, we intend the words *clinician* and *provider* to mean any health care professional or allied staff, including nurses, therapists, dieticians, and medical assistants. We describe two approaches to encouraging behavior change toward compliance with evidence-based medicine. Finally, we consider roles for **key stakeholders** in influencing behavior change.

Magnitude and Public Health Burden

The benefits from investments in biomedical science are awe-inspiring and lifesaving. Since 1955, the average life expectancy in America has increased from 69 to 78 years as a result of many lifesaving advances in medicine. Yet these advances are overshadowed by an estimated 98,000 deaths annually from health-care-acquired infections, diagnostic or other medical errors, and mismanaged care (IOM 1999). Although knowledge of all the pathways of preventable harm is immature, we know that preventable death is a leading cause of death. Moreover, preventable medical errors result in an annual cost of $19.5 billion to the U.S. economy and more than 10 million lost workdays from temporary disability (Shreve et al. 2010).

Consistent use of evidence-based guidelines can significantly increase the extent to which patients receive recommended therapies and can improve the quality and safety of care (Chassin 1990; IOM 1990). However, clinicians' compliance with evidence-based guidelines is often poor and inconsistent (Erasmus et al. 2010; Graham 1990; Rello et al. 2002; Woolf 1993). For example, advice to quit smoking is given to only 63% of current smokers during adult checkups (McGuckin et al. 2009), and the compliance rate of hand hygiene among clinicians in the United States is still below 50% (AHRQ 2010). According to estimates, patients receive only 50% of recommended therapies; that statistic increased a mere 3% during the first decade after 2000 (McGlynn et al. 2003; USDHHS 2008).

Key Determinants

Inadequate guideline compliance and other issues of provider behavior are **complex** and difficult problems to tackle, because behavior is influenced by several factors, some of which the clinician has little control over. The following four broad categories of factors affect clinician behavior in terms of guideline compliance or other desired behaviors:

1. *Clinician characteristics:* personal traits of health care providers, such as their **attitudes** toward guidelines in general.

2. *Guideline, intervention, or innovation charac-teristics:* aspects of the guideline or innovation itself that affect uptake, such as how complex the guideline is and whether compliance can be observed easily.

3. *System characteristics:* structural features of the health care organization, rules, culture, and peer pressure.

4. *Implementation characteristics:* aspects of when and how a guideline or innovation is implemented, including change processes and promotion strategies.

In addition, the presence of environmental pressures, such as government regulation, and of underlying societal expectations can influence the four broad contributing factors to guideline compliance or other behavior change. In this section we describe each of these categories of **determinants**.

Clinician Characteristics

Several clinician characteristics affect guideline compliance. In summary, the literature indicates these include clinician awareness, familiarity, and agreement with the guideline; **self-efficacy** (i.e., a clinician's belief that he can perform the guideline recommendations); **outcome expectancy** (i.e., a clinician's belief that guideline compliance will lead to the desired outcome); **motivation** (e.g., lack of motivation may be due to inertia from **habits** and routines of previous practice), which some theories break into further subconcepts; **normative beliefs** (i.e., perception of colleagues' expectations that the clinician will comply with a particular guideline); and **subjective norms** (i.e., perceived social pressure on clinicians to comply with a guideline).

Cabana and colleagues (1999) published a conceptual model that identifies clinician-related factors affecting guideline compliance. This model posits that three primary factors

affect physicians' compliance with evidence-based guidelines: knowledge, attitudes, and external factors. According to this model, lack of awareness or familiarity with guidelines, because of variables such as high volumes of clinical information to sift through and poor access to guidelines, obstruct physicians' *knowledge* of guidelines. As Cabana and colleagues describe it, physician *attitudes* about guidelines and guideline compliance are affected by lack of agreement with a guideline, lack of self-efficacy, lack of outcome expectancy, and inertia from habits and routines. This model describes appropriate knowledge and attitudes as necessary, but not sufficient, for consistent guideline compliance. Even if knowledge and attitudes are consistent with following a guideline, physicians may still experience *external barriers* that negatively influence their behavior. External barriers, discussed in later sections, may be due to the nature of the guideline itself (e.g., confusing and cumbersome) or environmental factors (e.g., lack of resources).

Another model that describes clinician factors affecting provider behavior is the **Theory of Planned Behavior** (**TPB**), which originated in the field of psychology and was intended to link attitudes to behaviors (Azjen 1991; Whitby et al. 2006). TPB posits that behavior is predicted by the value clinicians place on the behavior (positive or negative), subjective norms (perceived social pressure on clinicians to comply), and **perceived behavioral control** (clinicians' perceptions of their ability to comply with a desired behavior by overcoming constraints and difficulties). These predictors are, in turn, affected by clinicians' behavioral, normative, and **control beliefs**. Specifically, clinicians' attitudes toward complying with a guideline or other desired behavior are affected by their **behavioral beliefs** (the perceived likelihood that complying with the behavior will lead to positive outcomes); the social pressure to undertake the desired behavior is formed by clinicians' *normative* beliefs (perception of colleagues' expectations of their compliance); and clinicians' perceived ability to undertake a desired behavior is formed by their *control* beliefs (the perceived factors that may impede or facilitate compliance).

Few empirical studies have attempted to use TPB to explain clinicians' behavior, and the findings that do exist are contradictory (Whitby et al. 2007). Two recent studies support aspects of the TPB model in explaining compliance with hand hygiene guidelines (see also chapter 9). A cross-sectional survey of physicians and nurses from neonatal intensive and intermediate care units revealed that the intention to comply with hand hygiene guidelines was significantly related to perceived control over the difficulty of performing hand hygiene and a positive perception of superiors' valuation of hand hygiene (Pessoa-Silva et al. 2005). Another cross-sectional survey found that attitudes and subjective norms were also significantly related to intention to wash hands (Whitby et al. 2006). In contrast, a longitudinal study conducted among 120 critical and postcritical care units found that none of the factors from the TPB model significantly predicted observed compliance with hand hygiene guidelines—in this study, only intensity of activity in the unit, measured as a five-item index (i.e., unit type, time of day, hand washing indication frequency, unit census, and nurse-to-patient ratio), predicted compliance rates (O'Boyle et al. 2001). Intensity of activity was negatively associated with compliance.

Both the Cabana (Cabana et al. 1999) and the TPB (Azjen 1991) models place substantial emphasis on the clinicians' characteristics and less emphasis on nonclinical characteristics (characteristics of the desired behavior or intervention, of the system, and of implementation). Furthermore, we found significant overlap in the factors identified by the two models. For example, the construct of outcome expectancy in the Cabana model corresponded to the construct of behav-

ioral beliefs in the TPB model. However, some factors differed between the models. For example, awareness and familiarity with desired behaviors and practice inertia were important clinician-related factors described in the Cabana model but not the TPB model; similarly, normative beliefs and subjective norms were identified in the TBP model but not explicitly in the Cabana model. These findings suggest that no single conceptual model exists that comprehensively identifies clinicians' characteristics affecting compliance with desired behaviors.

Guideline Characteristics

Rogers applied **Diffusion of Innovations Theory (DIT)** (Rogers 1995b.), developed with regard to an individual's adoption of any innovation, to understand how characteristics of a particular behavior can affect clinicians' compliance. In this view, a new **evidence-based practice** guideline, for example, is viewed as an "innovation," and DIT explains its adoption. DIT places substantial emphasis on innovation characteristics and less emphasis on clinician or system characteristics. Based on this theory, the adoption of an innovation (or a desired behavior) is affected by the following five attributes:

1. Relative advantage: whether undertaking the behavior is superior to not complying with it (in terms of effectiveness and cost-effectiveness);
2. Compatibility: whether the behavior is consistent with clinicians' values, norms, and perceived needs;
3. **Complexity**: how easy or hard is it to integrate the behavior into current work practice;
4. **Trialability**: whether the clinician can test or try this behavior with relative ease; and
5. Observability: whether the clinician can easily observe other clinicians who have incorporated the new behavior.

Based on DIT, an innovation or desired behavior with most or all of these attributes will be adopted more rapidly and widely by clinicians.

Beyond the factors described by DIT, two additional innovation characteristics have been reported to significantly affect compliance. One is the strength of research evidence supporting the behavior. In general, the stronger and more consistent the research evidence supporting a particular desired behavior, the more likely that it will be adopted.

The other characteristic has been called "**exception ambiguity**," which refers to the whether the benefits of applying a particular intervention to a specific patient outweigh the potential risks (including patient discomfort) (Gurses et al. 2007; Gurses et al. 2008; Gurses et al. 2009; Michie and Johnston 2004; Stross 1999). As an example, consider a recent recommendation to use leg straps to secure urinary catheters to prevent catheter-associated urinary tract infections. Intensive care unit nurses reportedly questioned whether they should secure catheters in this manner for patients who have significant leg edema, because the leg strap usually gets too tight and might cause blood flow restriction (Gurses et al. 2008). Another example in the area of primary care guidelines is that evidence-based practices most often apply to a single disease and do not consider patients who suffer from multiple coexistent conditions. Boyd and colleagues noted that for a hypothetical 79-year-old woman with chronic obstructive pulmonary disease, type 2 diabetes, osteoporosis, hypertension, and osteoarthritis, following guidelines exactly would result in the patient being prescribed 12 medications and directed to follow a complicated exercise and nutrition plan (Boyd et al. 2005). In such cases, ambiguity arises because the interventions as defined do not clearly specify what to do and how to change practice for all patients and all situations. To increase the probability that a desired behavior will be used, the behavior should be unambiguous to the user (not the developer) as

to who is to do what, where, when, and how, for different patients and in nuanced clinical situations.

System Characteristics

System characteristics that affect desired behaviors can be differentiated from other categories of factors simply by asking whether a noncompliance issue would remain even if we replaced the specific clinician(s) involved, varied the nature of the behavior, or changed the implementation process. If yes, then noncompliance is likely linked to a system characteristic. For example, if two drugs with similar labels are stored near each other, and a nurse under time pressure accidentally takes the wrong one, this is likely a system error because it could happen to anyone.

The fields of organizational theory, organizational behavior, and human factors engineering offer robust conceptual models that characterize how systems affect guideline compliance and compliance with other desired interventions. **Organizational theory** and **organizational behavior** are concerned with the design and structure of organizations, the coordination of work, and how human beings interact with each other and with the system within an organization. **Human factors engineering** is concerned with the "understanding of interactions among humans and other elements of a system . . . to optimize human well-being and overall system performance" (IEA 2009), and it is increasingly being applied in health care (Carayon 2007; Gosbee 2002; Grandjean 1980).

The Systems Engineering Initiative for Patient Safety (SEIPS) model is a human factors framework that helps describe the system in which clinicians work. According to SEIPS (Carayon and Smith 2000; Smith and Carayon-Sainfort 1989), a care system is composed of five main components, four of which are considered systems characteristics. In addition to the person (e.g., the physician or the nurse), the four system characteristics include the following kinds of factors:

1. Task factors: characteristics of tasks or jobs that clinicians perform, such as workflow, time pressure, job autonomy, and workload. For example, heavy workload has been identified as one of the major barriers to hand-washing compliance.
2. Tools or technology factors: quality and quantity of technology or tools in the organization, including type, availability, and location of the technology or tools. For example, a checklist is a simple, cost-effective tool to prevent omission errors in standardized care procedures.
3. Physical environment factors: features of the care delivery environment, such as layout and noise. For example, placing a sink or an alcohol dispenser inside and outside each patient room may make it easier to comply with hand-washing guidelines.
4. Organizational factors: structural and cultural characteristics (e.g., resources, leadership, organizational culture) of the organization. For example, empowering nurses to stop violations of established guidelines can significantly increase compliance rates.

These five components interact with and influence one another, and their interactions affect processes (such as evidence-based practices) and outcomes (Carayon and Smith 2000; Smith and Carayon-Sainfort 1989). Clinician behavior is influenced by a complex interplay of emotional, social, political, cultural, and physical factors, each of which can support or inhibit performance. Knowledge of these characteristics can be used to determine how to intervene in a system to improve compliance with desired behaviors.

Some negative elements in a care environment that cannot feasibly be changed may be "balanced out" by focusing on the positive elements. For example, physicians typically experience competing demands and multiple distractions when performing procedures. Although highly demanding work conditions cannot be changed (at least in the short term), using a checklist as a cognitive aid may reduce the negative impact of high workload and distractions on patient safety.

Another system characteristic that influences clinician behavior is ambiguity (Gosbee 2002). Four system ambiguities negatively affect compliance with desired behaviors: (1) **task ambiguity** (e.g., no good mechanism to clarify and communicate **goals** for a patient to the multiple clinicians providing care), (2) **expectation ambiguity** (e.g., unclear norms and expectations within a unit or organization regarding guideline compliance), (3) **responsibility ambiguity** (e.g., lack of clarity regarding who is responsible for completing a particular step of a guideline), and (4) **method ambiguity** (e.g., confusion over where to find the necessary supplies to comply with a guideline).

These ambiguities contribute to noncompliance and suggest strategies to reduce or eliminate compliance problems. For example, the lens of ambiguities permits a focus on effecting clinician behavior change in such areas as **cultural competence** (the ability to recognize and appropriately respond to major cultural features that affect health care) or patient-centeredness (Betancourt 2006; Paez et al. 2008; Saha et al. 2008). A difficulty in asking clinicians to change the way they interact with patients is that the expectation is ambiguous: first, expectations for these desired behaviors are primarily based on societal preferences for equity or respect, since scientific evidence on the benefits of these behaviors is scarce (expectation ambiguity). Second, the actions that the clinician must take to correctly interact socially are not clear (task ambiguity). Moreover, the science of measuring these characteristics is immature. Thus, a standard must exist for clinicians to be able to comply, unless their personalities or background naturally allow them to do so. Further, *how* to meet expectations must be spelled out in practical steps that can be applied by anyone (to avoid method ambiguity).

Implementation (Change Process) Characteristics

When and how a desired behavior is implemented (as a new innovation) is critical in ensuring high compliance. These factors are called implementation characteristics, or characteristics of the change process. Although some of the change process factors may overlap with characteristics of the desired behavior or systems characteristics and can interact with clinician characteristics, the process of implementing a guideline or intervention, independent of the existing system characteristics, is critical for successful adoption and therefore merits its own category. Two well-known models describe the factors that affect the success of organizational efforts to change clinician behavior: the **Organizational Change Manager Model** (Gustafson et al. 2003; Molfenter et al. 2005) and the **Social Marketing Model** (Andreasen 2002; Mah et al. 2008).

The Organizational Change Manager Model identifies 16 factors associated with successful change (Molfenter et al. 2005), the following 10 of which are applicable to the area of implementation process:

1. *Tension for change.* The degree of dissatisfaction with the status quo is a key predictor of the successful implementation of an innovation (Kotter 1998; Kotter and Schlesinger 1979). Because tension is difficult to create, it is important to consider the existing level of tension for change when deciding what innovation to implement and when to implement it (Gustafson et al. 2003). Both internal factors (e.g., system factors such as leadership focus) and external factors (e.g., payment policies, public reporting)

can create tension for change (Seo et al. 2004). Internally, for example, a leader may attempt to create tension for change by revisiting the mission and goal of the organization, examining the current position of compliance with a specific intervention, offering comparisons to competing peer units or other benchmarks, and identifying what changes are needed to move the unit from the status quo to where it wants to be. An example of an external factor is the Centers for Medicare and Medicaid Services (CMS) policy change regarding reimbursement for hospital-acquired infections (HAIs). Since October 2008, CMS has withheld reimbursement for some HAIs that could reasonably have been prevented through the application of evidence-based guidelines. This change in reimbursement policy has led hospitals to invest resources to achieve better compliance with guidelines for preventing HAIs (Reed and Lissner 1993).

2. *Mandate or preparation and planning.* Implementing a new innovation, such as a guideline, will be more successful if a mandate for change is issued from a high level in the organization that clearly articulates the *need for change.* Yet mandates alone are usually insufficient. Adequate preparation and **planning** are necessary, in which the needs, tasks, and high performance expectations are clearly defined, before launching a new innovation or program (Lee and Steinberg 1980).

3. *Leader and middle manager involvement and support.* Involvement and support of leaders and middle managers is critical for successful implementation of any innovation. Support is more likely to occur if the organizational agenda and goals of leaders and middle managers are aligned with the program and if these individuals are adequately informed about the program. For example, to ensure that teams participating in a new initiative are supported by leaders, many programs require that an executive hospital leader, such as the vice president of nursing, be closely involved in the project (Marsteller et al.

2012; Pronovost, Berenholtz, Goeschel, et al. 2008; Pronovost, Needham, et al. 2006).

4. *Change agents' characteristics.* **Change agents** are people who can demonstrate the need to alter health care processes and policies to improve clinical, operational, and other outcomes (Rogers 1995a; Thompson et al. 2006). Change agents influence values, norms, and skills by sharing ideas, clarifying concepts, and providing encouragement. To have a positive impact on program implementation, change agents should have prestige both inside and outside the organization (Freeman 1982), be committed to the success of the program, be persistent (Schon 1963), and have influence and access to resources in the organization (Kanter 1983). The change agent can be either external or internal to the organization (Thompson et al. 2006). For example, a change agent can call attention to problems in a physician practice or unit that seeks to change, seek to engage clinician interest through anecdotes of past experiences, and encourage clinicians to evaluate their own problems and estimate the associated harm or potential harm (Berenholtz et al. 2009; Pronovost, Berenholtz, Goeschel, et al. 2008; Pronovost, Needham, et al. 2006).

5. *Strong opinion leaders.* Identifying **opinion leaders** in a system and directing any promotional activities about the particular innovation to or through these individuals can increase the rate of innovation adoption (Rogers 1995a). Opinion leaders facilitate transfer of research into practice by raising awareness and spreading new information about an innovation within professional **networks** (Mittman et al. 1992; Rogers 1995a, 1995b; Young et al. 2003). One study found that opinion leaders' tutorials were more effective than the traditional training programs in improving compliance with guidelines (Seto et al. 1991). Yet opinion leaders exist in a Darwinian struggle with opponents of the change. The relative strength of the supporters (opinion leaders) of a new innovation, compared with the strength of opponents of the innovation, is a critical determinant of an innovation's success (Gustafson et al. 2003).

6. *Exploration of problem and customer or staff needs.* Clinicians' needs, and the underlying causes of their resistance to change, should be identified and addressed before a guideline or intervention is implemented (Gustafson et al. 2003). Pretesting of the intervention with a sample of target clinicians is also essential (Andreasen 2002). For example, a new program might start as a pilot in a single physician practice or hospital unit, with regular assessments and input from physicians, nurses, and other stakeholders regarding satisfaction with the program and with the program's relevance and impact (Boult et al. 2008; Boyd et al. 2008; Marsteller et al. 2010; Sylvia et al. 2008). Once the problems faced during the pilot have been sufficiently addressed, the program can be implemented more broadly.

7. *Seeking ideas from outside the organization.* Implementing innovations such as guidelines is more likely to be successful if implementers look to other organizations for ideas and strategies (Gustafson et al. 2003; Molfenter et al. 2005; Utterback 1971). **Boundary spanners** play a critical role in this process. They have significant social connections within and outside the organization and provide a link to the outside world with respect to adoption of a particular innovation. Organizations that support boundary spanning roles adopt innovations more quickly (Barnsley et al. 1998; Ferlie et al. 2001). Often, a focal team member serves this role.

8. *Funding availability.* Implementing an innovation is more likely to be successful if adequate financial and other resources, including time and staff availability, are allocated (Damanpour 1991; Fitzgerald et al. 2002).

9. *Monitoring and feedback mechanisms.* An organization must have adequate and appropriately designed monitoring and feedback mechanisms to assess and report performance both during and after the innovation is implemented (Gustafson et al. 2003; Rogers 1995a).

10. *Clear and simple implementation plan.* An innovation is more likely to be adopted if the implementation plan is simple and the schedule and task assignments are clearly defined, including a clear timeline and explicit instructions regarding what to do (Lee and Steinberg 1980; Marsteller et al. 2012).

Another approach to successfully managing the implementation process is the **Social Marketing Model**, which is "the application of commercial marketing technologies to the analysis, planning, execution, and **evaluation** of programs designed to influence the voluntary behavior of target audiences in order to improve their personal welfare and that of society" (Andreasen 1995, 7). **Social marketing** has been used particularly to improve hand hygiene compliance. It borrows principles from the commercial sector and applies them to social and health care problems. In addition to the 10 implementation factors described above, social marketing argues that the following three factors should be present for a clinician behavior change effort to be successful (Andreasen 2002; Mah et al. 2008):

1. *Segmentation and targeting.* Social marketing argues for dividing the audience (i.e., clinicians) into segments based on common characteristics, such as job type, readiness to change, desired benefits, and values, to efficiently and effectively use scarce resources. Then, one or a few audience segments are targeted, and if possible the intervention is customized for these audiences. For example, an infection control professional may find out from a survey that adherence to hand hygiene is very low in certain patient care units, whereas in other units, reported adherence is high. Because resources are scarce, the infection control professional may decide to target the units with low adherence rates by investigating barriers to hand hygiene in those areas and developing unit-specific, appropriate interventions. **Segmentation** and

targeting have been shown to achieve higher adoption rates and behavior changes while using scarce resources efficiently and effectively (Andreasen 2002; Mah et al. 2006).

2. *Exchange of value.* To improve adoption of a guideline, clinicians should be offered tangible and intangible benefits and reduced costs in exchange for voluntarily participating in the intervention (Bagozzi 1975; Mah et al. 2006). This can be achieved by strategically applying the **"4 Ps"** (product, price, place, promotion) in the design and implementation of intervention, including guideline compliance.

- Product, or *service,* is a bundle of benefits that meets clinicians' needs (Mah et al. 2006).
- Price is the tangible and intangible cost of performing a desired behavior (Kotler and Zaltman 1971).
- Place is the reduction of the location cost of a product or service by increasing accessibility and convenience (Mah et al. 2006).
- Promotion is the use of communication and persuasion strategies to make the product or service familiar, acceptable, and desirable to clinicians (Mah et al. 2008; Kretzer and Larson 1998; Morris and Clarkson 2009).

Mah and colleagues (2006) illustrated the 4 Ps with an example of the installation of antiseptic handrub dispensers in accessible locations to promote hand hygiene. The *product* or benefits include the ease and convenience of handrub use in a septic setting, protection of patients and other health care workers from infections, and perceived pride of working in an institution with low infections. A high *price* is dermatitis owing to frequent hand-washing, especially for health care workers whose skin has low tolerance to alcohol-based antiseptic handrub. Another high *price* is time spent on washing hands in a busy workday. As to *place,* installing the antiseptic handrub dispensers close to the point of care and in highly visible and convenient places can increase hand-washing rates. *Promotion* channels may include small media (e.g., employee newsletters, posters, computer workstation screen savers), social media, special activities (e.g., contests), and interpersonal communication (e.g., face-to-face communication between an infection control professional and a leader of a unit with a low adherence rate).

3. *Attention to behavioral competition.* For every desired behavior that a clinician should perform, alternative behavioral choices exist that are called **competing behaviors** (Morris and Clarkson 2009). For example, placing an intravenous line in a femoral vein (in the groin) is a competitive behavior to placing it in the internal jugular or subclavian veins (in the neck, a location associated with lower infection rates). To increase the probability of changing clinicians' behavior and increasing compliance rates, forces competing with the desired behavior should be identified and analyzed, and strategies and tactics should be developed to eliminate or reduce this competition (Girou and Oppein 2001).

Studies that used social marketing to increase guideline compliance have had conflicting findings (Mah et al. 2008; Rao et al. 2002). Overall, while a social marketing approach has the potential to improve compliance with evidence-based guidelines and other desired clinician behaviors, further research may be needed to fully demonstrate this potential.

An Interdisciplinary Conceptual Framework

We have described several theoretical and conceptual models developed or adapted from different disciplines and many published studies aimed at improving guideline compliance or altering clinician behavior. One main reason for failure to change clinician behavior is the complex and interdisciplinary nature of the problem. Bringing together different disciplin-

ary focuses on the problem can take advantage of the different strengths of their perspectives.

Figure 19.1 offers an interdisciplinary framework to provide a blueprint for efforts to improve guideline compliance and other clinician behavior. Underlying the entire system are societal expectations that affect every individual factor represented in the process, including how the system is set up. In addition, other environmental factors, such as governmental regulation or pressures for change from health plans, affect mainly the preexisting factors of the framework. Preexisting characteristics include clinician, system, and desired behavior characteristics. The system and the desired behavior characteristics each influence clinicians' mutable characteristics, such as self-efficacy in using an intervention. Characteristics of a desired behavior such as guideline compliance can have indirect effects on system characteristics through the implementation characteristics, leading perhaps to the creation of a new or altered routine or process. We suggest that the guideline or desired behavior is largely not modifiable by the system or provider, insofar as it is developed based on the existing scientific evidence or on societal expectations for equality, access to care, and so on.

The three sets of preexisting characteristics influence implementation characteristics (or the change process), and the implementation characteristics may, in turn, change clinician and system characteristics (in a feedback loop). Furthermore, the preexisting characteristics affect clinicians' behavior through their impact on implementation characteristics. Implementation characteristics can have different roles in the movement from preexisting characteristics to outcomes. For example, within clinician characteristics, the negative impact of low self-efficacy on compliance might disappear if implementation is done well enough, including enough education to change self-efficacy assessments. But good implementation might improve self-efficacy only among those with low self-assessments. Ultimately, clinicians' compliance

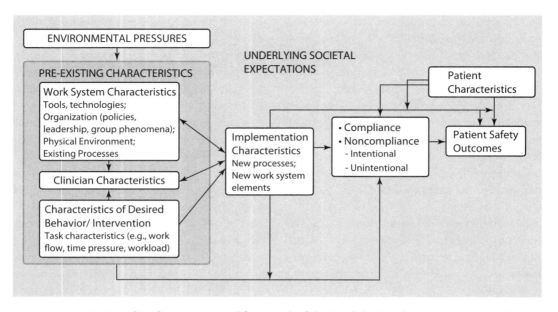

FIGURE 19.1. An interdisciplinary conceptual framework of clinician behavior change. *Source:* adapted from AP Gurses, JA Marsteller, A Ant Ozok, Y Xiao, S Owens, PJ Pronovost, Using an interdisciplinary approach to identify factors that affect clinicians' compliance with evidence-based guidelines, *Critical Care Medicine* 38 (suppl.) (2010): S282–S291.

behavior will affect patient outcomes, with the caveat that patient characteristics may drive clinician behavior independent of the process being considered in this chapter. Also possible is that certain innovations will seek to remove the clinician decision of whether to comply or not (e.g., the introduction of a new kind of tubing that fits only one port and therefore removes any human decision element from a process). Finally, the changes in the patient outcomes, clinician compliance, and implementation characteristics should, in turn, have an impact on the preexisting characteristics. What has been learned in the implementation efforts and through evaluating compliance and patient outcomes should be fed back into the system and may modify the work system, desired behavior, or clinician characteristics as a result.

Evidence-Based Interventions

The key determinants described above suggest opportunities to alter clinician behavior. How-

ever, consistent behavior change remains elusive. A primary reason is the complex and interdisciplinary nature of the problem. It is now well recognized that multifaceted interventions achieve better guideline compliance results than do one-dimensional interventions (e.g., clinician education only) (Cabana et al. 1999; Kretzer and Larson 1998). Each of these approaches has strengths, yet alone is incomplete. Therefore, an integrated model is needed. An effective behavior change attempt should simultaneously address determinants of behavior at multiple **levels of influence** (i.e., individual or clinician level, intervention level, system level, and implementation level).

Behavior change efforts should include learning from the clinical disciplines of medicine, nursing, pharmacy, organizational theory and behavior, human factors and systems engineering, psychology, health services research, management, sociology, marketing, economics, epidemiology, and informatics. The more facilitators and barriers we can identify by tapping into all disciplinary lenses, the higher the probability that performance will improve.

In this section, we consider two general interventions meant to enable clinician behavior change toward guideline compliance or other desired behaviors. One multifaceted, large-scale approach to clinician behavior change is the **collaborative method**, which has been applied to a broad number of topic areas and stages of care. It is large-scale in that it can encompass many behavior changes and many organizations at the same time. The second, smaller-scale approach is the Barrier Identification and Mitigation tool.

The Collaborative Method

Collaboratives are learning networks among health care organizations, convened to improve some aspect of health care services. They have been widely used as a change method that may operate at two levels—first, facilitating change within an organization, and second, inspiring movement in the field of organizations. Collaboratives typically supply participants with the evidence base for the intervention undertaken; quality improvement and measurement training; structure for the improvement process; and a mixture of peer support, applied ideas, and competitive spirit both from collaborative faculty and from other organizations participating in the collaborative.

Although collaboratives vary widely, they may provide a mechanism that is both effective and efficient for improving guideline compliance and patient outcomes. Collaboratives can centralize the summarization of evidence, producing guidelines (if none exist), developing performance measures, and monitoring and feeding back performance—all resource-intensive steps that would be inefficient for individual clinicians or health care organizations to do alone. Yet collaboratives also allow (and encourage) local modification on how the guidelines are implemented, based on local barriers and

context (Pronovost, Berenholtz, and Needham 2008).

The collaborative method has been used to improve a range of health-care-related problems, including medication errors (Leape et al. 2000; Meisel et al. 1998), caesarean section deliveries (Flamm et al. 1998), patient waits and delays (Boushon et al. 2006; Murray and Berwick 2003; Nolan 1996), disparities (Lurie et al. 2008), cancer care (Katlic et al. 2011; Kerr et al. 2002), HIV/AIDS treatment (Landon et al. 2004), asthma care (Homer et al. 2005; Mangione-Smith et al. 2005; Schonlau et al. 2005), hip replacements (Jones and Piterman 2007), patient safety in intensive care units (Marsteller et al. 2012; Pronovost, Needham, et al. 2006), mental health treatment (Katzelnick et al. 2005), and chronic illness care (Cretin et al. 2004; Daniel et al. 2004). Common features of collaboratives include multidisciplinary teams from participating organizations, face-to-face meetings to teach methods and evidence, use of a listserv and telephone conferences for maintaining contact among teams, training in improvement methods, measurable targets for improvement, disease- or problem-specific best practices, follow-up support from faculty, and interaction with other teams in the collaborative (Marsteller et al. 2007; Øvretveit et al. 2002). Collaborative-style quality improvement has been undertaken in numerous countries, including the United States, Australia, France, the Netherlands, Norway, Sweden, the United Kingdom, Russia, Ecuador, Nicaragua, and Peru (Franco and Marquez 2011; Kilo 1998; Wilson et al. 2003).

The evidence of effectiveness for collaboratives is incomplete as yet, insofar as many of those conducted to date have not been reported in the literature or did not collect enough data of sufficient quality to assess success (Øvretveit et al. 2002). A review from nine studies concluded that the evidence for the effectiveness of collaboratives was positive but limited (Schouten et al. 2008). (Most of these studies seem to have tested the effectiveness of collaborative content, without testing the utility of the collaborative approach itself as a vehicle for disseminating clinician behavior change efforts. To properly assess the contribution of the collaborative model would require a study arm featuring the same content but no collaborative features for behavior change.)

One successful collaborative model has been used, with some variations, by the Johns Hopkins Armstrong Institute for Patient Safety and Quality in hospital patient safety programs in the state of Michigan, two Adventist health systems, and the national On the CUSP: Stop BSI program (AHRQ 2012; Marsteller et al. 2012; Pronovost, Needham, et al. 2006). The overall program has three parts: clinical and cultural intervention(s) (including the evidence-based guidelines to improve care), an implementation framework (to implement the intervention), and the collaborative model. Within these parts, this program addresses many of the key determinants described above.

INTERVENTION

The intervention piece features two main components. The first component is an overarching program to improve teamwork, communication, and overall patient safety, called the Comprehensive Unit-Based Safety Program (CUSP) (Pronovost, Berenholtz, Goeschel, et al. 2008; Pronovost et al. 2005). This safety program asks staff to evaluate their culture of safety, undergo training in the science of safety to understand systems and safe design, identify how patients are or could be harmed on the unit, partner with a hospital executive to support safety efforts, regularly learn from identified system defects, and implement tools to improve teamwork and communication. CUSP is an ongoing effort that lasts throughout, and hopefully beyond, the duration of the collaborative intervention period. This behavior change approach emphasizes the context of intervention, because good teamwork, efficient and satisfying communication, and a climate promoting pa-

tient safety are critical to successful interventions to reduce errors. They are also essential to the development of a healthful work environment. The emphasis on developing a positive climate for everyday interaction (as well as for patient safety) is an important difference from some behavior change models that concentrate primarily on a clinical topic without providing analysis of, or tools for, improving teamwork and the work environment.

The second component of the intervention is a patient safety (or quality) issue of focus and a series of evidence-based processes or practices that have been shown to reduce the safety problem. For example, to reduce infection rates, evidence-based practices include handwashing before procedures, using full barrier precautions (e.g., sterile gowns, masks, and gloves) and maintaining a sterile field, avoiding central line placement at high risk sites (such as the femoral vein in the groin area), using chlorhexidine to cleanse the site of procedures, and removing unnecessary central lines promptly (they otherwise pose infection risks). An observer (usually a nurse) uses a checklist to ensure that clinicians follow these evidence-based practices. The clinical part of the intervention includes (1) summarizing the evidence, (2) identifying expected barriers to implementation, (3) measuring baseline performance, and (4) ensuring that all patients receive the intervention, using an implementation framework (discussed below). No matter what patient safety issue is being addressed, teams work on CUSP and the clinical focus simultaneously throughout the length of the collaborative.

THE IMPLEMENTATION FRAMEWORK

As noted in the key determinants section, clinician behavior change efforts sometimes fail not because the intervention is unworthy but because implementation goes astray. The implementation framework is shown in table 19.1. It guides collaborative faculty and quality-

TABLE 19.1. Implementation framework

	Frontline staff	Team leaders	Senior executives
Engage	Ask, *How does this make the world a better place?*		
Educate	*What do I need to do?* Convert evidence to behaviors Evaluate awareness and agreement		
Execute	*How can I do it?* Listen to resisters Standardize, create independent checks, and learn from mistakes		
Evaluate	*How do I know we made a difference?*		
Endure	*Has this become business as usual? How do I know it will last?* Make policies and procedures, train new people, walk the process		
Expand	*Who else needs to know this? What's next?* Pass it on to other units Identify and address your next challenge		

improvement teams as they "roll out" a collaborative. This framework has been informed appropriately by theories of behavior change but is designed to be easily understood by providers unfamiliar with the theories. The collaborative seeks to find the balance between two tensions: how scientifically sound versus feasible to make the work and whether to take a centralized (top down) versus local (bottom up) approach. Our experience is that many collaboratives lack credibility with clinicians because they lack scientific rigor. Therefore, we seek to have interventions based on robust evidence and measures that are valid and reliable, but all guidance for intervention seeks to make compliance the easiest thing for a clinician to do. Moreover, rather than deciding on a top-down versus a bottom-up approach, the collaborative seeks to centralize those components of the work that are most efficient to do once, centrally (e.g., evidence, measures, and methods of collecting and feeding back performance data), yet encourage local modification regarding how that evidence is implemented.

This iterative approach to implementation addresses many of the key determinants discussed above and includes the following elements:

1. *Engagement* of providers, which consists of motivating staff to undertake the intervention and to feel a "tension for change" away from the usual care.

2. The *Education* phase has technical aspects, including what to teach others to do (i.e., the evidence-based practices), but it requires an adaptive communication plan that identifies the best channels for communication and overcomes specific message barriers. In this we convert evidence into explicit behaviors and evaluate the staff's awareness of, and agreement with, the evidence, all with the goal of reducing ambiguity regarding what behaviors are expected and why.

3. *Execution* is the use of the evidence-based practices and is largely technical work. At the same time, however, we try to expose adaptive barriers by listening to staff who

oppose the intervention to better understand what they fear they might lose.

4. The *Evaluation* phase features formative
assessment of what is going well and what
is not, on an ongoing basis, as well as
late-stage assessment of whether a difference has been achieved.

5. *Endurance* refers to sustaining the intervention over time. Even the most effective
changes will have little impact, ultimately,
if they are not sustained. This includes
ensuring that written policies are present
and that new staff orientations include
instruction in the evidence-based practices.

6. *Expansion* refers to spreading the intervention to other units within the hospital or in
other hospitals. Expansion to other units
and sites is not necessarily required for
effective implementation, but it plays an
important role for the team that is the first
to implement and for the larger organization, which has an interest in ensuring
safety in all of its units and methods to
continuously monitor performance. For the
first-to-implement teams, expansion of the
intervention to other units brings recognition among management and peers as well
as the opportunity to solidify and organize
their own knowledge by teaching others
(Pronovost, Berenholtz, et al. 2006).

Each of these activities must be undertaken
at three organizational levels: among frontline
staff, quality-improvement team leaders, and
senior executives. Failures of implementation
that stymie the intervention can occur in any of
these phases and at any organizational level.
The model seeks to create a **chain of accountability** in which senior leaders monitor performance and hold team leaders accountable; team
leaders, in turn, hold frontline staff accountable. Finally, the framework can be thought of
as an **iterative process**—that is, prior implementation phases can be revisited as barriers arise.
For example, if, during the evaluation of a

program, a tool or a process is found to not work
in its first implementation attempt, quality-
improvement teams may need to revisit it and
make adjustments (i.e., return to the engagement, education, or execution phases before re-
implementing an improved process).

THE COLLABORATIVE METHOD

The third part of this behavior change approach
is the use of a collaborative method to communicate and transmit the intervention and implementation framework to the participants. The
primary advantage of collaborative interventions is to introduce the pre-researched evidence
to a large-scale community of teams that are all
working toward the same goal. Compared to
traditional, isolated behavior change initiatives,
the collaborative structure offers the presence
of expert faculty who bring the solid evidence
base for intervention, supportive interaction
with peers, healthy competition among organizations that improves inter-professional cohesion on each team, and better comparability of
performance measures across large numbers of
organizations.

Once the clinical part of the intervention has
been developed, participating sites have been
recruited, and teams have been formed within
the sites, an immersion period educates teams
about the intervention over the course of six to
eight weekly telephone conferences. During this
time, teams gather baseline data and prepare
materials and supplies. After the immersion period, teams begin implementing the intervention, which unfolds at different rates at different
sites over the course of 18 months. Teams are
encouraged to use the implementation framework and to adapt the intervention components
(such as forms for setting daily goals for patient
care) to their own settings. Within the first few
months of activity, teams and faculty come together for a face-to-face meeting for additional
training and social **integration**. Usually, at this
meeting, the teams are asked to identify potential barriers or failure modes they foresee. After

the face-to-face meeting, didactic calls with teams are reduced to once monthly, and open line coaching calls are added once monthly. All teams are asked to participate, and interactions with each other "offline" are encouraged to help them develop a learning community that will contribute to long-term sustainability of the behavior change.

Barrier Identification and Mitigation

We also describe a smaller-scale intervention that could be nested within a collaborative or other behavior change effort. Within a behavior change initiative, success depends heavily on identifying barriers to consistent compliance and developing strategies to eliminate these barriers or mitigate their effects. The Barrier Identification and Mitigation (BIM) tool is an instrument that encourages guideline adherence by analyzing and removing barriers to compliance. The BIM tool provides a systematic, research-based approach to identifying barriers and reducing their effects (Gurses et al. 2009).

This tool requires completing a five-step process. First, an interdisciplinary team is assembled. Second, each team member identifies barriers based on observations, interviews, and "walking the process" (i.e., carrying out a particular guideline), using a barrier identification form to identify possible corrective actions. Third, the data are compiled on a table form. Fourth, the team convenes, reviews the barriers identified, and prioritizes them based on the likelihood of experiencing each particular one and the probability of that barrier leading to noncompliance. Finally, the team develops an action plan for each prioritized barrier. A leader is identified for implementing each action, along with the measures and evaluation methods. Implicit in this approach is the assumption that clinicians want to provide high quality care and that if they do not, their lack of desire is likely due to barriers that need to be identified and mitigated.

It is important to consider possible interactions among groups of characteristics while designing and implementing interventions to mitigate or eliminate barriers, because modifying some factors that affect providers' compliance may not be feasible. For example, complying with a particular guideline may require a considerable and unavoidable amount of effort from care providers (task characteristics) owing to the nature of the guideline. However, this barrier may be overcome if appropriate and well-designed tools and technologies are made available (e.g., use of checklists) and if the organizational structure is modified (e.g., adequate autonomy is provided to nurses to stop line insertion if there is a deviation from the guideline) to facilitate the task. Rather than focusing improvement efforts on factors that are hard or impossible to modify, the focus should be on those that are easier to manipulate and can improve compliance through their interactions with the hard-to-manipulate factors.

A process of "looking forward and backward" in the causal pathway, and looking for **antecedents** and **consequences** of a change in some factor that ultimately influences compliance with a desired behavior, can help identify all the causes and the appropriate intervention point to bring compliance to desired levels. For example, staff complaints about the amount of time needed to enact the new guideline may be considered the compliance problem. However, these complaints might originate from staff not including the new process in their daily routine, and the contributors to that problem might include insufficient practice time during the educational effort or disagreement on the best dissemination techniques among members of the original implementation team. Looking forward in the causal pathway, potential consequences of not standardizing the practice include intentional noncompliance (staff slipping back to old methods and undermining the intervention by their actions and words). Problem-solving efforts must envision whether potential solutions will aggravate the identified compliance problem or its anticipated consequences. Time-intensive retraining, for example, could increase staff impressions that the guideline is not time- or cost-effective.

The BIM tool can help identify barriers to guideline compliance and reduce their effects. It should be used in the pre-implementation phase of an effort to anticipate barriers and mitigate them before a guideline is implemented. It can also be used during the pilot and implementation phases to identify active barriers. After the implementation phase, the BIM tool can be used periodically (e.g., every three to six months) if compliance is below expectations.

Roles for Key Stakeholders

Encouraging health care providers to implement desired behaviors, such as following recommendations and evidence-based guidelines, requires multifaceted interventions that take into account characteristics of the clinician, the system, the intervention, and the implementation. Yet, environmental pressures for change and underlying societal expectations may likewise influence each of these characteristics. Although many interventions encourage guideline compliance and other desired behaviors, many are not themselves based on any theoretical framework, a fair number have not been rigorously evaluated, and most of these programs have not been applied widely enough to have a large impact on provider behavior nationwide. By extension, they rarely have a large public health impact. The proportion of research funding that is devoted to the translation of medical evidence into bedside care is dwarfed by spending on the development of new medical interventions. Nevertheless, stakeholders can play important roles in promoting provider behavior change, especially when their interests are aligned. This section discusses the interests of each stakeholder group, how the group can best be influenced, and the ways each can in

turn influence provider behavior to meet its interests.

Researchers

Researchers' interests tend to revolve around publishing, obtaining grant funding and running a research enterprise, training the researchers of tomorrow, and the general pursuit of knowledge and understanding. In addition, many hope ultimately to influence policy and care provision toward societal benefit, although the path to greatest benefit is not always completely clear. They are most likely to support provider behavior change that has clear supporting evidence emanating from solid research designs and methods. However, sometimes researchers can be so involved in a particular intervention or change that their impartial assessment of the merits of the intervention is impaired.

Researchers may have several roles in promoting change, depending on the stage of development of the science supporting the guideline or other desired behavior. After the basic science stages have discovered effective therapies, evidence-based guidelines must be translated into clinical care interventions (i.e., how do we apply the evidence in actual practice?). Then, successful interventions in a few settings must be applied to improve the health of a population. Too little attention is paid to this end of the bench-to-bedside progression of scientific knowledge. The downfall of many scientific innovations is that they are not translated into actionable behaviors as part of a defined intervention, and then some effective interventions are not widely disseminated because no researcher assessed their capacity for dissemination. Finally, researchers often do not consider themselves in the business of dissemination, so they publish their studies and then hope that legislators or industry will develop useful applications of their research. However, researchers could influence provider behavior by operationalizing research evidence (i.e., translating findings into behaviors); by publicizing research that demonstrates the ability to affect care quality and safety; and by seeking to engage clinicians, health care organizations, patients and families, payers, and policymakers in the importance of their research and its benefits to patients. On the other hand, researchers could also choose to obstruct provider behavior change, which might be in their interests if their research suggested that a change was not cost-efficient, for example, or if their preferred method or model faced a competing one. Finally, if researchers found the evidence supporting an intervention or change to be wanting, they might oppose widespread implementation of a specific intervention in the name of putting the resources to better use elsewhere.

Health Care Foundations

Several important health-care-focused foundations, including the Robert Wood Johnson Foundation (RWJF), the John A. Hartford Foundation, the Commonwealth Fund, and many others, contribute millions of dollars to health care research annually. Their interests are to support safe, equitable, high-quality care for all patients or a specific group of interest (e.g., the John A. Hartford Foundation focuses on care for the elderly population).[1] In addition, foundations must concern themselves with the faithful stewardship of their resources and therefore seek to support high-quality studies that have reportable, policy-relevant outcomes and can bring publicity to the work of the organization. Foundations have an interest in perpetuating themselves, so that they can continue to work to meet their missions into the distant future.

These foundations have important **influences** on the nature of health care delivery as well as on consumer health by setting the program areas in which they will fund research. Some foundations also have programs that fund direct care for patients, often as tests of innovative care models, or work directly with com-munities to set health goals (e.g., RWJF's Healthy Kids, Healthy Communities program).[2] Researchers often must follow the funding, so the development of new practices and refinement of methods to bring best practices to the patient are often driven by foundation priorities. This suggests that foundations may not further certain types of change where they do not focus resources.

State and Federal Legislative Bodies

The interests of state and federal legislators are primarily in promoting societal good and in reelection to their position or election to other positions. They hope to protect patients from harm and obtain the highest quality and efficiency in care, at a nationwide cost that can be supported by the economy and in government programs that can be supported by the government budget. With enough clamor from other stakeholders, legislators can be swayed to encourage provider behavior changes that have sufficient support and little enough opposition. Legislators are highly responsive to the concerns of patients and families, large consumer groups, and influential business and professional associations, because these constituents support them with votes and campaign funds. Often legislative support does not require researchers' endorsement or even much evidence of effectiveness. Legislators may be prone to being influenced by anecdotes in cases where they lack health care expertise, because such case histories are easily understood by the public and are often emotionally engaging. Further, legislators are also highly motivated by the need to conserve government resources and the compelling trade-offs they must face daily.

Legislative bodies create the laws that govern health care organizations, payers, health professional educational institutions, professional societies, and ultimately individual clinicians. Thus, they can openly require or prohibit certain behaviors among clinicians through law. In addition, they legislate payment policies that affect clinicians and health care institutions through the government insurance programs: Medicare; Medicaid; and state and federal government employee, military, and veterans health benefits programs. These payment policies tend to lead other health plans, insurers, and employer health benefits plans to adopt similar rules because the government programs are so large that they have considerable market power. Further, several states and the CMS require public reporting of various quality-of-care measures by hospitals.[3] These ostensibly allow consumers to assess and select hospitals based on the quality of care provided, and they may induce provider organizations to work harder to meet reportable quality indicators.

Legislators can also indirectly influence provider behavior by encouraging research into provider behavior change or quality improvement methods and comparative effectiveness of interventions by allocating funds to government research-granting institutions such as the National Institutes of Health (NIH) and the Agency for Healthcare Quality and Research (AHRQ). In some cases, they may also provide recognition or awards for researchers or industry actors who promote the public good in health care. Legislators primarily influence provider behavior change, however, through legal constraints, payment **incentives**, and funding research.

Although we know that legislators make laws, it is naive to believe that they can "make" health care providers do what they think is best. Individual clinicians, professional societies, and health care organizations often develop "workarounds," or ways to circumvent policies that impinge on current practice or the bottom line. This may happen even with seemingly innocuous policies, because any change in current patterns is costly in some sense. Legislators can thus sometimes obstruct change by attempting to force it through legislation. Furthermore, in cases in which resources are put toward required efforts, they are not available for other worthy innovations, potentially pushing out some desired behavior change.

Public Health Agencies

Public health agencies' interests revolve around protecting the health of the population and ensuring their own survival, growth, and importance relative to other government agencies. They seek to ensure that high-quality, safe, effective, and low-cost care is provided to the people of their jurisdictions. They must do what they can toward this mission within the often-limited resources of their appropriated budgets. Public health agencies are less responsive to needs of individual patients and more concerned with the larger populace or specific populations within the whole. Because these agencies are themselves populated by natural scientists, epidemiologists, clinicians, and researchers, they are persuaded most by research-based evidence of the effectiveness of specific provider behaviors. In addition, they are greatly concerned with meeting their obligations to legislative bodies and their superiors in the executive branches, including the U.S. president and the state governors.

Public health agencies execute the laws of the legislative branch and help create the regulatory environment for health care organizations, private payers or insurers, health professional educational institutions, professional societies, and ultimately individual clinicians. Thus, they may require or prohibit certain behaviors through regulation, where supported by law, and they can encourage behaviors by making recommendations, providing supporting information, or creating incentives for and against behaviors by making some paths more convenient than others (e.g., with respect to paperwork). As an example of their power to make recommendations and provide information, the AHRQ acts as a clearinghouse for best practices and clinical guidelines. In addition, the CDC, the AHRQ, and the state health departments all have roles in encouraging compliance with infection prevention practices as outlined in the national Healthcare Acquired Infections (HAI) Plan.[4] In the same way that health care organizations and clinicians may circumvent laws, they may also seek to get around regulations and may ignore guidelines, as we have already discussed. Surveillance functions of these agencies could conceivably play an important role in solidifying action behind specific health priorities, for example through publications like the National Healthcare Quality and Disparities Reports of AHRQ (AHRQ 2010).

Some of these agencies also have budgets supporting health research. Some portion of such budgets is spent on research into how health services are delivered and how provider behavior change can be encouraged. Public health agencies may fail to support some provider behavior change, however, because their focus is on large populations, disease pathologies, and basic and environmental science. Their focuses are directly responsive to their stated missions, but also to what the agency perceives as desired by legislators who allocate funds and thereby determine the agency's size and power as a research funder. They typically provide less funding support for implementation research and no monetary support for implementation of guidelines within health care organizations.

Health Plans, Employers, and Public Payers

Another key stakeholder group is private health plans (for-profit and not-for-profit); employers providing health benefits to their employees (self-insured and not); and government insurance programs such as Medicare, Medicaid, and state and federal government employee, military, and veterans health benefits programs. Although their interests are not always aligned, in general, members of the payer group seek low-cost health care that meets quality and safety standards. Private health plans must also earn a profit to survive. Public payers such as the CMS author the details of payment policies that are required by law and that affect clinicians and health care institutions directly. In addition, these policies influence clinicians and organizations indirectly through the public payers' considerable influence on other health plans, insurers, and employer health benefits plans. Their interest in cost efficiency (as well as efficacy) may put them at odds with clinicians, professional societies, and patients in regard to provider behavior change issues in which the change does not save money over usual care. Like public health agencies, however, these organizations are concerned with the quality of health care delivered. The CMS, for example, requires reporting of quality measures known as the Healthcare Effectiveness Data and Information Set from all health plans that provide care to Medicare managed care plan enrollees.

Payers are most receptive to arguments for provider behavior change that would balance the issues of cost and high quality. Some provider behavior change might not be supported by payers (such as the provision of all necessary preventive care), insofar as the costs of the services are immediately borne by the health plan, but the potential cost savings from providing these services accrue only after many years. Enrollees may change health care plans before the plan realizes any benefits of the services provided.

Some payers employ health care professionals or own health care provider organizations. These health plans have stronger influences on provider behavior, because provider salaries depend on their compliance with organizational policies and procedures. Among other things, these organizations can require desired provider behaviors. However, providers still have great discretion in how they deliver health care; furthermore, sometimes poorly designed systems or cultural issues constrain provider adherence to desired behaviors, so noncompliance can be common even in these systems.

Standard-Setting Organizations

Another group of organizations does not directly regulate or otherwise control health care providers but has tremendous power in the health care arena by setting standards for care. These include such entities as the Joint Commission, which accredits hospitals and other health care organizations; the National Quality Forum, which creates consensus standards for quality-related measurements; and the National Committee on Quality Assurance, which accredits primary care medical homes. These organizations are interested in promoting the prestige of their accreditation and thereby the use of their services or products, which primarily promote safety, high quality of care, and other desirable provider behaviors. Such organizations are persuaded to encourage a behavior by research evidence or sometimes by theoretical arguments and substantial public interest in a topic. For example, the Joint Commission requires hospitals to measure the culture of safety in their organizations, although the evidence in the literature linking improved patient outcomes to stronger safety culture is still somewhat limited.

Accrediting bodies have considerable influence on what aspects of care health care organizations, and therefore their employed providers, focus efforts toward improving. Organizations seek accreditation and use accepted performance measures in order to send a signal of high quality to the market. Notably, the creation of standards and reporting criteria in specific areas leads organizations to focus on improvement of specific measures of quality. This fact makes the process of selecting measures for tracking progress and for public reporting extremely important and politically sensitive. The measures selected must be "the right" measures, or as close as we can get to the right measures. Otherwise, great effort could be spent chasing a measure that does not really represent high quality care. Also, prioritization processes, though necessary to get people working together in a unified effort, tend to create winners and losers. This may result in discord within an organization, and the scarcity of resources suggests that some worthy efforts may not be pursued because resources are spent on reportable measures.

Patients, Families, and Consumer or Disease Advocacy Groups

The interests of patients and families, and therefore of consumer groups and disease or condition-specific advocacy groups that represent them, are primarily focused on receiving whatever health care services they want or require, at the highest quality and the lowest out-of-pocket cost possible. They would also like to have convenient care, to have access to it when they need it, and to receive equitable treatment as compared to any other patients. These stakeholders are likely to respond most strongly to the experiences of their peers. Research evidence on best practices can also motivate patients (depending on how accessible the information is).

Patients would support most provider behavior changes that conceivably lead to better outcomes. When patients act alone, they are not very influential on the system; when they act as a group, through consumer organizations such as the Consumers Union, they see progress in influencing provider behavior. Patients can use group power better (consciously or unconsciously) when they are better informed on provider outcomes and can make choices among providers based on these data. However, in some egregious cases, the experiences of one patient can bring about monumental change in provider systems, as when Libby Zion's untimely death stimulated a limitation on resident work hours in New York (Lerner 2009).

Disease advocacy or consumer groups respond strongly to the desires of group members. They likely prefer sophisticated evidence to endorse behavior change strategies, but owing to their zeal, they may also be swayed by promising new ideas that need further testing. In fact these groups are often the experts on a given disease or body system and are the source of recommendations for best care. However, disease advocacy groups would only put their weight behind strategies focused on care for their disease or system of focus and may not support other behavior change because it would compete with efforts in the area they support.

Health Care Systems and Organizations

The systems and organizations that provide health care, such as hospitals, clinics, home care agencies, nursing homes, hospices, dialysis agencies, and private physicians' offices, are uniformly interested in both providing good care and surviving financially. Even nonprofit and public health care organizations have to be concerned with earning enough revenues to be viable. The reputation for the quality of the care that a given organization delivers is an important piece of remaining viable in most markets. However, where there are few choices for health care services, there may be less impact of perceived quality on the size of the clientele and on revenues. It is also clear that high quality is not the only determinant of which facility patients choose; they also care about proximity to home and family and ease of use (parking, good food, and so on). Importantly, the quality of care is not easily assessed by patients. Health care organizations must also be concerned with keeping employees happy so as to retain them.

To meet their interests, health care organizations may seek to enhance the quality, safety, and equity of their care by creating systems that bypass provider choice. For example, if a machine can regulate self-delivery of pain medication to patients in a safe way, then there is no need to depend on a nurse to personally hand a pill to a patient and make sure it is taken. The use of such machines avoids accidental failure to deliver medications in a timely way. Oversight of the process is still required, and often self-administered pain medications are not the only pain treatment required to keep patients comfortable, but such automation of the system supports health care providers by removing one task from their long list of things to remember; it also may help prevent errors.

Most interventions to improve care, however, require provider compliance to use the tool or adhere to the guideline. Provider organizations can create policies and protocols within the organization to guide provider behavior, can endorse and provide resources for quality improvement or safety activities, and can have managers set an appropriate tone by role modeling and providing rewards for desired behaviors. Organizations have greater power over the behavior of health care professionals where they employ these individuals (e.g., nurses and some physicians are employed by hospitals, but in many hospitals, physicians are independent entities that use the hospital facilities). Without a concomitant employment relationship, providers are freer to disregard policies of the organization, especially if competing organizations are located nearby. For example, a nonemployed physician might admit his patients to a different hospital if he did not agree with a hospital's policies regarding performing daily interdisciplinary rounds for each patient.

On the other hand, provider organizations themselves may impede desirable provider behavior changes, either purposely or accidentally. For example, some changes may be judged to be too expensive or not to demonstrate savings and therefore to be a potential waste of resources. Sometimes organizations impede change unintentionally by their nature as hierarchical entities, with rules or "red tape" that discourages innovation.

Health Care Providers and Professional Societies

The interests of health care providers, including physicians, nurses, and allied health care professionals, are primarily in providing the highest quality and safest health care possible within the resource constraints they face. In general, we assume that most providers believe they provide equitable care to all groups. We anticipate that most would address differences in care if they were aware of them and if they were given access to tools to reduce disparities. Physicians, in particular, historically have practiced medicine with great autonomy, and protecting that autonomy is a major concern, especially given that physicians are primarily liable in the current system if errors occur and a lawsuit results. Furthermore, many physicians are independent businesspeople who must be concerned with the survival of their business and retaining their employees as well as with the care of patients. Other care providers are primarily concerned with providing the best care possible as well as with opportunities for professional growth and a rewarding career.

Providers are most swayed to make changes that are supported by evidence of clinical impact that meets statistical significance criteria, that do not require extensive reworking of current habits, and that are consistent with their preexisting beliefs and values. In addition, changes that are supported from within an organization can often be made more easily than when all the impetus for change comes from external pressure.

Providers and professional societies obviously have direct impact on the care that is given to patients, and their ability to bring about behavior change among their peers is also great. Some providers have more influence with their peers than others, and recruiting these opinion leaders to act as change agents or champions can have a powerful impact on the success of an intervention to improve care. However, as dis-cussed at length in this chapter, all providers have to work within a system, which features some elements that will support change and some that will constrain change. Successful change is much more likely when the complex elements of this system can be aligned to support a change in a unified fashion.

Conclusion

Clinicians practice medicine to help, rather than harm, patients. Therefore, if clinicians do not comply with a guideline or other desired clinical behavior, there is a reason (or reasons). If we are to improve quality of care, patient safety, patient-centeredness, and cultural competence as well as reduce preventable harm and disparities, we must identify and eliminate reasons for noncompliance with the desired behaviors and proactively implement programs that address clinician behavior change for the benefit of patient care.

NOTES

1. See the John A. Hartford Foundation, www .jhartfound.org/about_us.htm.

2. You can learn more about the Healthy Kids, Healthy Communities program at www.healthykids healthycommunities.org/.

3. See, for example, Medicare.gov, www.medicare. gov/hospitalcompare/.

4. See the Health care-associated infections (HAIs) page at the health.gov website, www.hhs.gov/ash /initiatives/hai/actionplan/.

REFERENCES

Agency for Healthcare Research and Quality (AHRQ). 2010. *National Healthcare Quality Report: 2009.* Washington, DC: U.S. Department of Health and Human Services, AHRQ.

———. 2012. AHRQ report. Available at www.ahrq.gov /news/press/pr2012/pspclabsipr.htm.

Andreasen A. 1995. *Marketing Social Change: Changing Behavior to Promote Health, Social Development, and the Environment.* San Francisco: Jossey-Bass.

———. 2002. Marketing social marketing in the social change marketplace. *J Public Policy Marketing* 21 (3): 13.

Azjen I. 1991. The theory of planned behavior. *Organ Behav Hum Decis Process* 50 (2): 179-211.

Bagozzi RP. 1975. Marketing as exchange. *J Marketing* 39 (4): 32-39.

Barnsley J, Lemieux-Charles L, McKinney MM. 1998. Integrating learning into integrated delivery systems. *Health Care Man Rev* 23 (1): 18-28.

Berenholtz SM, Schumacher K, Hayanga AJ, et al. 2009. Implementing standardized operating room briefings and debriefings at a large regional medical center. *Jt Comm J Qual Patient Saf* 35 (8): 391-97.

Betancourt JR. 2006. Cultural competency: Providing quality care to diverse populations. *Consult Pharm* 21 (12): 988-95.

Boult C, Reider L, Frey K, et al. 2008. Early effects of "Guided Care" on the quality of health care for multimorbid older persons: A cluster-randomized controlled trial. *J Gerontol A Biol Sci Med Sci* 63 (3): 321-27.

Boushon B, Provost L, Gagnon J, Carver, P. 2006. Using a virtual breakthrough series collaborative to improve access in primary care. *Jt Comm J Qual Patient Saf* 32 (10): 573-84.

Boyd CM, Darer J, Boult C, Fried LP, Boult L, Wu AW. 2005. Clinical practice guidelines and quality of care for older patients with multiple comorbid diseases: Implications for pay for performance. *JAMA* 294 (6): 716-24.

Boyd CM, Shadmi E, Conwell LJ, et al. 2008. A pilot test of the effect of guided care on the quality of primary care experiences for multimorbid older adults. *J Gen Intern Med* 23 (5): 536-42.

Cabana MD, Rand CS, Powe NR, et al. 1999. Why don't physicians follow clinical practice guidelines? A framework for improvement. *JAMA* 282 (15): 1458-65.

Carayon P. 2007. *Handbook of Human Factors and Ergonomics in Health Care and Patient Safety.* Hillside, NJ: Erlbaum.

Carayon P, Smith M. 2000. Work organization and ergonomics. *Appl Ergonom* 31 (6): 649-62.

Chassin MR. 1990. Practice guidelines: Best hope for quality improvement in the 1990s. *J Occup Med* 32 (12): 1199-1206.

Cretin S, Shortell SM, Keeler EB. 2004. An evaluation of collaborative interventions to improve chronic illness care: Framework and study design. *Eval Rev* 28:28-51.

Damanpour F. 1991. Organizational innovation: A meta analysis of effects of determinants and moderator. *Acad Man J* 34 (3): 555-90.

Daniel DM, Norman J, Davis C, et al. 2004. A state-level application of the chronic illness breakthrough series: Results from two collaboratives on diabetes in Washington State. *Jt Comm J Qual Saf* 30 (2): 69-79.

Erasmus V, Daha TJ, Brug H, et al. 2010. Systematic review of studies on compliance with hand hygiene guidelines in hospital care. *Infect Control Hosp Epidemiol* 31 (3): 283-94.

Ferlie E, Gabbay J, Fitzgerald L, Lolock L, Dopson S. 2001. Evidence-based medicine and organisational change: An overview of some recent qualitative research. In *Organisational Behaviour and Organisational Studies in Health Care: Reflections on the Future,* ed. L Ashburner. Basingstoke, UK: Palgrave.

Fitzgerald L, Ferlie E, Wood M, Hawkins C. 2002. Interlocking interactions: The diffusion of innovations in health care. *Human Rel* 55 (12): 1429-49.

Flamm BL, Berwick DM, Kabcenell A. 1998. Reducing cesarean section rates safely: Lessons from a "breakthrough series" collaborative. *Birth* 25:117-24.

Franco LM, Marquez L. 2011. Effectiveness of collaborative improvement: Evidence from 27 applications in 12 less-developed and middle-income countries. *BMJ Qual Saf* 20 (8): 658-65.

Freeman C. 1982. *The Economics of Industrial Innovation.* Cambridge, MA: MIT Press.

Girou E, Oppein F. 2001. Handwashing compliance in a French university hospital: New perspective with the introduction of hand-rubbing with a waterless alcohol-based solution. *J Hosp Infect* 48 (suppl. A): S55-S57.

Gosbee J. 2002. Human factors engineering and patient safety. *Qual Saf Health Care* 11 (4): 352-54.

Graham M. 1990. Frequency and duration of handwashing in an intensive care unit. *Am J Infect Control* 18 (2): 77-81.

Grandjean E. 1980. *Fitting the Task to the Man: An Ergonomic Approach.* London: Taylor & Francis.

Gurses A, Murphy D, Martinez E, Berenholtz S, Pronovost P. 2009. A practical tool to identify and eliminate barriers to evidence-based guideline compliance. *Jt Comm J Qual Patient Saf* 35 (10): 526-32.

Gurses AP, Seidl K, Vaidya V, et al. 2008. Systems ambiguity and guideline compliance: A qualitative study of how intensive care units follow evidence-based guidelines to reduce healthcare-associated infections. *Qual Saf Health Care* 17 (5): 351-59.

Gurses AP, Xiao Y, Seidl K, Vaidya V, Bochicchio G. 2007. Systems ambiguity: A framework to assess risks and predict potential system failures. In *Proceedings of the Human Factors and Ergonomics Society 51st Annual Meeting,* 626-30. Santa Monica, CA: Human Factors and Ergonomics Society.

Gustafson DH, Sainfort F, Eichler M, Adams L, Bisognano M, Steudel H. 2003. Developing and testing a model to predict outcomes of organizational change. *Health Serv Res* 38 (2): 751-76.

Homer CJ, Forbes P, Horvitz L, Peterson LE, Wypij D, Heinrich P. 2005. Impact of a quality improvement program on care and outcomes for children with asthma. *Arch Pediatr Adolesc Med* 159 (5): 464-69.

Institute of Medicine (IOM). 1990. *Clinical Practice Guidelines.* Washington, DC: National Academy Press.

———. 1999. *To Err Is Human: Building a Safer Health System.* Washington, DC: National Academy Press.

International Ergonomics Association (IEA). 2009. What is ergonomics? Available at www.iea.cc (accessed Sept. 14, 2009).

Jones K, Piterman L. 2007. Promoting best practice in general practitioner management of osteoarthritis of the hip and knee: Arthritis and Musculoskeletal Quality Improvement (AMQuIP) Program. *Aust J Primary Health* 13 (2): 104-12.

Kanter RM. 1983. *The Change Masters: Corporate Entrepreneurs at Work.* London: Unwin.

Katlic MR, Facktor MA, Berry SA, McKinley KE, Bothe A Jr., Steele GD Jr. 2011. ProvenCare lung cancer: A multi-institutional improvement collaborative. *CA Cancer J Clin,* doi: 10.3322/caac.20119.

Katzelnick DJ, Von Korff M, Chung H, Provost LP, Wagner EH. 2005. Applying depression-specific change concepts in a collaborative breakthrough series. *Jt Comm J Qual Patient Saf* 31 (7): 386-97.

Kerr D, Bevan H, Gowland B, Penny J, Berwick D. 2002. Redesigning cancer care. *Br Med J* 324 (7330): 164-66.

Kilo CM. 1998. A framework for collaborative improvement: Lessons from the Institute for Healthcare Improvement's Breakthrough Series. *Qual Manag Health Care* 6 (4): 1-13.

Kotler P, Zaltman G. 1971. Social marketing: An approach to planned social change. *J Marketing* 35 (3): 3-12.

Kotter JP. 1998. Winning at change. *Leader to Leader* 10:27-33.

Kotter JP, Schlesinger LA. 1979. Choosing strategies for change. *Harvard Bus Rev* 57 (2): 106-14.

Kretzer EK, Larson EL. 1998. Behavioral interventions to improve infection control practices. *Am J Infect Control* 26 (3): 245-53.

Landon BE, Wilson IB, McInnes K, et al. 2004. Effects of a quality improvement collaborative on the outcome of care of patients with HIV infection: The EQHIV study. *Ann Intern Med* 140 (11): 887-96.

Leape LL, Kabcenell AI, Gandhi TK, Carver P, Nolan TW, Berwick DM. 2000. Reducing adverse drugs events: Lessons from a breakthrough series collaborative. *J Qual Improv* 26:321-31.

Lee WB, Steinberg E. 1980. Making implementation a success of failure. *J Systems Man* 3 (4): 19-25.

Lerner BH. 2009. A life-changing case for doctors in training. *New York Times,* March 2, 5D.

Lurie N, Fremont A, Somers SA, et al. 2008. The national health plan collaborative to reduce disparities and improve quality. *Jt Comm J Qual Patient Saf* 34 (5): 256-65.

Mah MW, Deshpande S, Rothschild ML. 2006. Social marketing: A behavior change technology for infection control. *Am J Infect Control* 34 (7): 452-57.

Mah MW, Tam YC, Deshpande S. 2008. Social marketing analysis of 20 [corrected] years of hand hygiene promotion. *Infect Control Hosp Epidemiol* 29 (3): 262-70.

Mangione-Smith R, Schonlau M, Chan KS, et al. 2005. Measuring the effectiveness of a collaborative for quality improvement in pediatric asthma care: Does implementing the chronic care model improve processes and outcomes of care? *Ambul Pediatr* 5 (2): 75-82.

Marsteller JA, Hsu YJ, Reider L, et al. 2010. Physician satisfaction with chronic care processes: A cluster-randomized trial of guided care. *Ann Fam Med* 8 (4): 308-15.

Marsteller JA, Sexton JB, Hsu YJ, et al. 2012. A multi-center, phased, cluster-randomized controlled trial to reduce central line-associated bloodstream infections in intensive care units. *Crit Care Med* 40 (11): 2933-39.

Marsteller JA, Shortell SM, Lin M, et al. 2007. How do teams in quality improvement collaboratives interact? *Jt Comm J Qual Patient Saf* 33 (5): 267-76.

McGlynn EA, Asch SM, Adams J, et al. 2003. The quality of health care delivered to adults in the United States. *N Engl J Med* 348 (26): 2635-45.

McGuckin M, Waterman R, Govednik J. 2009. Hand hygiene compliance rates in the United States—a one-year multicenter collaboration using product/volume usage measurement and feedback. *Am J Med Qual* 24 (3): 205-13.

Meisel S, Sershon L, White D. 1998. Reducing adverse drug events and medication errors using rapid cycle improvement. *Qual Manag Health Care* 6:15-28.

Michie S, Johnston M. 2004. Changing clinical behaviour by making guidelines specific. *Br Med J* 328 (7435): 343-45.

Mittman BS, Tonesk X, Jacobson PD. 1992. Implementing clinical practice guidelines: Social influence strategies and practitioner behavior change. *QRB Qual Rev Bull* 18 (12): 413-22.

Molfenter T, Gustafson D, Kilo C, Bhattacharya A, Olsson J. 2005. Prospective evaluation of a Bayesian model to predict organizational change. *Health Care Man Rev* 30 (3): 270-79.

Morris ZS, Clarkson PJ. 2009. Does social marketing provide a framework for changing healthcare practice? *Health Policy* 91 (2): 135-41.

Murray M., Berwick DM. 2003. Advanced access: Reducing waiting and delays in primary care. *JAMA* 289: 1035-40.

Nolan TW. 1996. *Reducing Delays and Waiting Times throughout the Healthcare System.* Boston: Institute for Healthcare Improvement.

O'Boyle CA, Henly SJ, Larson E. 2001. Understanding adherence to hand hygiene recommendations: The theory of planned behavior. *Am J Infect Control* 29 (6): 352-60.

Øvretveit J, Bate P, Cleary P, et al. 2002. Quality collaboratives: Lessons from research. *Qual Saf Health Care* 11:345-51.

Paez KA, Allen JK, Carson KA, Cooper LA. 2008. Provider and clinic cultural competence in a primary care setting. *Soc Sci Med* 66 (5): 1204-16.

Pessoa-Silva CL, Posfay-Barbe K, Pfister R, Touveneau S, Perneger TV, Pittet D. 2005. Attitudes and perceptions toward hand hygiene among healthcare workers caring for critically ill neonates. *Infect Control Hosp Epidemiol* 26 (3): 305-11.

Pronovost PJ, Berenholtz SM, Goeschel CA, Needham DM, et al. 2006. Creating high reliability in health care organizations. *Health Serv Res* 41 (4 pt 2): 1599-1617.

Pronovost PJ, Berenholtz SM, Goeschel C, Thom I, et al. 2008. Improving patient safety in intensive care units in Michigan. *J Crit Care* 23 (2): 207-21.

Pronovost PJ, Berenholtz SM, Needham DM. 2008. Translating evidence into practice: A model for large scale knowledge translation. *Br Med J* 337:a1714.

Pronovost P, Needham D, Berenholtz S, et al. 2006. An intervention to decrease catheter-related bloodstream infections in the ICU. *N Engl J Med* 355 (26): 2725-32.

Pronovost P, Weast B, Rosenstein B, et al. 2005. Implementing and validating a comprehensive unit-based safety program. *J Patient Safety* 1 (1): 33-40.

Rao GG, Jeanes A, Osman M, Aylott C, Green J. 2002. Marketing hand hygiene in hospitals—a case study. *J Hosp Infect* 50 (1): 42-47.

Reed S, Lissner G. 1993. Clinical study on the effectiveness of tear drainage with a single canalicular system under environmental stress. *Ophthal Plast Reconstr Surg* 9 (1): 27-31.

Rello J, Lorente C, Bodi M, Diaz E, Ricart M, Kollef MH. 2002. Why do physicians not follow evidence-based guidelines for preventing ventilator-associated pneumonia? A survey based on the opinions of an international panel of intensivists. *Chest* 122 (2): 656-61.

Rogers EM. 1995a. *Diffusion of Innovations.* 4th ed. New York: Free Press.

———. 1995b. Lessons for guidelines from the diffusion of innovations. *Jt Comm J Qual Improv* 21 (7): 324-28.

Saha S, Beach MC, Cooper LA. 2008. Patient centeredness, cultural competence, and healthcare quality. *J Natl Med Assoc* 100 (11): 1275-85.

Schon DA. 1963. Champions for radical new inventions. *Harvard Bus Rev* 41 (2): 77-86.

Schonlau M, Mangione-Smith R, Chan KS, et al. 2005. Evaluation of a quality improvement collaborative in asthma care: Does it improve processes and outcomes of care? *Ann Fam Med* 3 (3): 200-208.

Schouten LM, Hulscher ME, van Everdingen JJ, Huijsman R, Grol RP. 2008. Evidence for the impact of quality improvement collaboratives: Systematic review. *Br Med J* 336 (7659): 1491-94.

Seo M, Putnam LL, Bartunek JM. 2004. Dualities and tensions of planned organizational change. In *Handbook of Organizational Change and Innovation,* ed. MS Poole, AH Van de Ven, 73-107. New York: Oxford University Press.

Seto WH, Ching TY, Yuen KY, Chu YB, Seto WL. 1991. The enhancement of infection control in-service education by ward opinion leaders. *Am J Infect Control* 19 (2): 86-91.

Shreve J, Van Den Bos J, Gray T, Halford M, Rustagi K, Ziemkiewicz E. 2010. The economic measurement of medical errors. Society of Actuaries. Available at www.soa.org/research/research-projects/health /research-econ-measurement.aspx (accessed July 5, 2013).

Smith MJ, Carayon-Sainfort P. 1989. A balance theory of job design for stress reduction. *Int J Industr Ergonom* 4:67-79.

Stross JK. 1999. Guidelines have their limits. *Ann Intern Med* 131 (4): 304-6.

Sylvia ML, Griswold M, Dunbar L, Boyd CM, Park M, Boult C. 2008. Guided care: Cost and utilization outcomes in a pilot study. *Dis Manag* 11 (1): 29-36.

Thompson GN, Estabrooks CA, Degner LF. 2006. Clarifying the concepts in knowledge transfer: A literature review. *J Adv Nurs* 53 (6): 691-701.

U.S. Department of Health and Human Services (USDHHS). 2008. *National Healthcare Quality Report.* Report No. 08-0040. Rockville, MD: Agency for Healthcare Research and Quality.

Utterback J. 1971. The process of innovation: A study of the origination and development of ideas for new scientific instruments. *IEEE Trans Engin Manag* 18 (4): 124-31.

Whitby M, McLaws ML, Ross MW. 2006. Why healthcare workers don't wash their hands: A behavioral explanation. *Infect Control Hosp Epidemiol* 27 (5): 484-92.

Whitby M, Pessoa-Silva CL, McLaws ML, et al. 2007. Behavioural considerations for hand hygiene practices: The basic building blocks. *J Hosp Infect* 65 (1): 1-8.

Wilson T, Berwick DM, Cleary PD. 2003. What do collaborative improvement projects do? Experience from seven countries. *Jt Comm J Qual Saf* 29 (2): 85-93.

Woolf SH. 1993. Practice guidelines: A new reality in medicine. III. Impact on patient care. *Arch Intern Med* 153 (23): 2646-55.

Young JM, Hollands MJ, Ward J, Holman CD. 2003. Role for opinion leaders in promoting evidence-based surgery. *Arch Surg* 138 (7): 785-91.

Part III

CROSS-CUTTING ISSUES IN BEHAVIOR CHANGE

Behavioral Economics and Incentives to Promote Health Behavior Change

KEVIN G. VOLPP AND GEORGE LOEWENSTEIN

LEARNING OBJECTIVES

After completing the chapter, the reader will be able to

* Understand decision errors that make people predictably irrational.
* Contrast programs such as value based insurance design, which build on standard economics, with behavioral economics.
* Understand how incentives have been used to change health behaviors.
* Describe how programs based on incentives have been used in areas such as smoking and obesity.

Introduction

Many major health problems in the United States and other developed nations, including lung cancer, hypertension, and diabetes, are caused at least in part by unhealthful behaviors. Modifiable behaviors such as tobacco use, unhealthful eating, physical inactivity, and alcohol abuse account for nearly one-third of all deaths in the United States (Flegal et al. 2005; Mokdad et al. 2004). Experts have estimated that as much as 40% of premature mortality in the United States is due to unhealthful behaviors (Schroeder 2007).

Moreover, the potential benefits of many medical advances, such as medications to control blood pressure and lower cholesterol levels, have been limited by patients not doing their part (Kripalani et al. 2007). For example, by one year after having a myocardial infarction, about half of patients prescribed cholesterol medications have stopped taking them (Jack-evicius et al. 2002). Reducing **morbidity** and **mortality** may depend as much on motivating changes in human behavior as on developing new treatments.

Economics, the social science discipline traditionally most closely tied to public policy, would logically seem to be one of the key disciplines in addressing behaviors that are potentially harmful to health. Yet, conventional economics does not provide satisfactory policy solutions to problems caused by self-harmful behavior, because it is premised on a rational choice perspective. By assuming that individuals make optimal decisions given their information, resources, and preferences, such a perspective in effect assumes away these problem behaviors. Consistent with a rational choice perspective, economists have argued that addiction is the outcome of a rational choice (Becker and Murphy 1988), that people are obese because they have judged that the pleasure of eating is worth the discounted costs (Murphy 2006), and that suicide is a rational choice for those who have decided that "the total discounted lifetime utility . . . reaches zero" (Hamermesh and Soss 1974). The implication of analyses such as these is that **interventions** to reduce addiction, obesity, or suicide are likely to be counterproductive, since the individuals who have chosen these behaviors have done so because they were optimal given their preferences. The main policy tools suggested by conventional economics—providing information or changing prices—will only partially address these problems.

The new field of **behavioral economics** has, over the past few decades, begun to import concepts from psychology to address these limitations (Camerer and Loewenstein 2003). Behavioral economists have identified pitfalls in human decision making—termed **decision errors**—that help explain when and why individuals engage in self-harming behaviors.

Insights from behavioral economics can contribute to solutions for public health problems that have challenged clinicians and public health professionals. In the sections that follow, we describe key decision biases that ordinarily lead to self-harming behavior and then offer examples of how they can be strategically used in interventions to instead promote healthful behaviors.

Decision Errors

Most people are prone to a wide range of common decision errors that lead to suboptimal behavior in certain predictable circumstances. Many of us, for example, have trouble dieting, exercising, and saving money, and many of us tend to procrastinate even when the cumulative **consequences** are severe.

Moreover, people with commercial interests often use decision errors to exploit consumers (Issacharoff and Delaney 2006; Loewenstein and Haisley 2008; Loewenstein and O'Donoghue 2006). Credit card companies and auto manufacturers lure new customers with "$0 down and 0% interest," which appeals to tendencies to focus on the present rather than the future. States market lottery tickets that return just $0.45 on the dollar, worse than any other legal form of gambling, and promote these games of chance using simplistic assessments of probabilities (e.g., "You can't win if you don't play").

However, the same decision errors that typically harm individuals can also be used to help them. By recognizing the existence of decision errors, and in some cases using them to influence individuals' behavior, public health and behavior change interventions can in many cases be designed more effectively.

Present-Biased Preferences

Perhaps the most problematic decision errors from the standpoint of encouraging healthful behaviors are present-biased preferences (Ainslie 1975; Frederick et al. 2002; Loewenstein 1992; Loewenstein and Angner E. 2003; Loewenstein et al. 2003; O'Donoghue and Rabin 1999), also known as **hyperbolic time discount-**

ing. **Present-bias** refers to two important behavioral propensities: (1) the tendency to overweight immediate costs and benefits relative to those occurring at any point in the future and (2) the tendency to take a more evenhanded approach to delayed costs and benefits occurring at different points in time. People are much more willing to begin to diet *tomorrow* for this reason, as the **overweighting** of immediate costs deters the individual from the immediate deprivation of dieting, and the more balanced perspective on future time makes the individual willing to impose these costs on herself in the future.

Although present-biased preferences typically weigh in on the side of unhealthful behaviors, policymakers can exploit them for beneficial effects instead. The tendency to overweight immediate costs and benefits suggests that, first, the motivational impact of costs and benefits (e.g., rewards for good behavior or punishments for bad behavior) can be greatly increased by making them immediate. Ideally, such rewards or punishments should coincide as closely as possible with the timing of the behaviors in question. Second, the more evenhanded **attitude** toward different times in the future suggests that people would be willing to commit to a future self-control approach that they would not be willing to undertake immediately. Indeed, such a strategy has been used successfully to encourage saving in Thaler and Benartzi's "save more tomorrow" scheme in which people can commit to saving money out of future payroll increases (Thaler and Benartzi 2004).

Nonlinear Probability Weighting

This decision error has another two-part effect, in which (1) we tend to put disproportionate weight on outcomes that have a small probability of occurring but (2) tend to be insensitive to variations in probability at the low end of the probability scale, a pattern known as **probability neglect** (Sunstein 2002). Because people draw little distinction between, for example, a 0.00001 versus 0.0000001 chance of winning a prize, even though the probabilities differ by several orders of magnitude, such overweighting is especially extreme for very small probabilities. This overweighting of small probabilities has various negative effects on decision making. For example, at an individual level, it is probably largely responsible for the enormous attraction of lottery tickets. Actuarially, state-run lotteries are unfavorable gambles, in that the average payout rate across states is just 52%, which is lower than the rate for any other form of legal gambling (Clotfelter and Cook 1989). Yet, in 2004, consumers spent $48 billion on state lottery tickets ($166 per person in the United States) (Coughlin et al. 2006). All but eight states have a state-run lottery. More than 50% of adults in lottery states play the lottery at least once per year. The small chance of a large payoff is especially attractive because people tend to overweight small probabilities in making decisions (Kahneman and Tversky 1979; Prelec 1998). The appeal of lottery tickets probably also stems in part from the immediacy of the winnings (see the previous discussion of present-biased preferences). Most lotteries offer a combination of a relatively large chance of a small payout and a very small chance of a larger payout. The frequent small payoffs increase the attractiveness of lotteries by giving lottery players intermittent **positive reinforcement**. Moreover, the feedback is often very rapid or even immediate; most games have daily draws, and more than 40% of state revenues now come from instant scratch-off tickets.

Like present-biased preferences, the overweighting of small probabilities can be used in public health interventions. Many programs provide small **probabilistic** rewards to individuals for engaging in healthful behaviors. The overweighting of small probabilities, and indeed our own specific research employing lottery rewards for **health behavior** change, suggests that lotteries can be used to obtain more "bang for the buck" from such economic **incentives**.

Loss Aversion

This decision error is the tendency to put substantially greater weight on losses than on gains (Kahneman et al. 1991; Tversky and Kahneman 1991). It can produce a variety of suboptimal patterns of behavior, from pathological risk-aversion (as discussed above) to the tendency for people to hold on too long to investments such as houses (Genesove and Mayer 2001) or stocks (O'Dean 1998; Shefrin and Statman 1985; Weber and Chapman 2005). However, the same property that makes **loss aversion** destructive in some situations—its tendency to amplify the weight put on specific outcomes that are framed as losses—can be used to advantage when people's natural tendency is to **underweight** outcomes.

Thus, for example, if people are putting too little weight on delayed outcomes because they discount the future excessively, framing those delayed outcomes as losses can potentially increase their emphasis, thereby correcting one error with another. For example, there could be an incentive plan tied to weight loss in which people are awarded their winnings up front but in which these winnings are subject to being lost if the people are unsuccessful in losing weight. If people (in part owing to over-optimism, described next) are willing to engage in precommitment contracts in which they voluntarily agree to forfeit deposits if they are unable to make intended behavior changes (described more fully below), loss aversion can further augment **motivation** so that they are more successful in changing their behavior.

Over-optimism

Self-predictions of future behavior are usually overly optimistic. For example, research shows that we tend to underestimate task completion times (Buehler et al. 1994, 2002). In the health domain, people prefer paying a flat rate for gym memberships, even though they would spend less if they were to pay on a per-visit basis (Della Vigna and Malmendier 2002); this seems to result, in part, from their tendency to overestimate their future gym usage. Mail-in product rebates are a frequently cited example of this bias. Although such rebates have been shown to promote sales, only a small number (5% to 20% in one study) are actually redeemed. The overly optimistic bias apparent in people's self-predictions of their future behavior is especially important in this context, given that in each of these examples the target behavior is largely under the individual's control. Later in the chapter, we show how over-optimism, when combined with **projection bias** (described below), can be leveraged to facilitate weight loss.

Defaults

The default, or status quo, bias refers to our tendency to take "the path of least resistance"—to continue doing what we have been doing, or to do what comes automatically, even when superior alternatives exist (Johnson and Goldstein 2003; Kahneman et al. 1991; Samuelson and Zeckhauser 1988). Defaults have been blamed for a wide range of suboptimal outcomes, from the failure of employees to put aside retirement funds in companies when the default contribution rate is zero (Gneezy and Potters 1997; Madrian and Shea 2001; Thaler and Benartzi 2004), to suboptimal allocations between investment alternatives (Thaler et al. 1997), to excessive ingestion of fries and large sodas as part of "supersized" meals at McDonald's (Halpern et al. 2007; Loewenstein et al. 2007; Thaler and Sunstein 2003). In Western European countries that have an "opt in" policy for organ donation—that is, the default is nonparticipation (as in the United States), donation rates tend to be close to 10%. But in countries with an "opt out" policy, where citizens are automatically enrolled as organ donors unless they actively choose to opt out, organ donation rates are typically 98%-99% (Johnson and Goldstein 2003). If chosen wisely, defaults can be used to propel people toward self-beneficial behaviors. For example, the defaults on prescription refills could be changed from 30 days to 90 days (or longer) for people with a need for lifelong therapy, to decrease the risk of medication noncompliance owing to running out of pills.

Peanuts Effects

The **peanuts effect** refers to the common tendency to put little weight on very small outcomes—both gains and losses (Markowitz 1952; Prelec and Loewenstein 1991; Weber and Chapman 2005). Generalized, the peanuts effect can encompass the under-weighting of nebulous or amorphous, often delayed, consequences, which helps explain such diverse self-destructive patterns of behavior as cigarette smoking, weight gain, and cell phone use while driving. In each of these cases, the benefits of the activity (e.g., the pleasure of smoking a cigarette or of eating, and the convenience of conducting business or socializing in otherwise "dead" time) are immediate and tangible, but the costs—an infinitesimally small increase in the chance of lung cancer, an imperceptible increase in weight, or a tiny increase in the risk of injury or death—are amorphous. Again, the peanuts effect can be viewed as a form of underweighting, and this mistake can in some situations be channeled to help people rather than hurt them. For example, the same tendency to underweight small outcomes that leads one to spend money over and over can also make it relatively painless for people who might have trouble saving a large chunk of money in one fell swoop to instead make a large number of much smaller deposits.

Projection Bias and Hot-Cold Empathy Gaps

Projection bias (Loewenstein et al. 2003) refers to the tendency to project current preferences onto the future. **Hot-cold empathy gaps**, which often underlie projection bias, refer to the tendency for people in a cold, unemotional state to underestimate the impact of emotions and drives on their own future behavior. People who are not hungry, for example, overestimate the likelihood that they will choose healthful options (Read and van Leeuwen 1998), and they judge other people who fail to show dietary moderation more harshly than they judge themselves when they are hungry (Nordgren et al. 2007). Projection bias leads to diverse suboptimal patterns of behavior, from over-shopping at the grocery store on an empty stomach to excessively seeking wealth and status (because the individual fails to anticipate the extent to which he will adapt to either). However, as we show below, because projection bias can cause people to underappreciate how self-denial will feel in the future, it can be used to encourage people to precommit to self-binding measures that help them to accomplish their long-term **goals**.

Narrow Bracketing

Choice bracketing refers to the process of grouping individual choices together into sets. When making choices, we bracket them either *broadly,* by considering all of the consequences taken together (as standard economic theory assumes), or *narrowly,* by making each decision in isolation (Read et al. 1999). A **bracketing effect** occurs when choice outcomes under narrow bracketing differ from those under broad bracketing. We tend to bracket narrowly; we myopically focus on the local consequence of the most immediately available choices and ignore the aggregated costs and benefits over a long time horizon (Herrnstein and Prelec 1992; Sabini and Silver 1982). This tendency becomes especially pronounced when choices are made sequentially, such as when a person has heightened risk aversion to the extent that she makes investment decisions in isolation (as opposed to in aggregate) (Benartzi and Thaler 1995; Gneezy and Potters 1997). Bracketing effects interact with many other errors and biases and can be used as a tool to induce these other biases. For example, the peanuts effect is more likely to occur when costs or benefits are framed narrowly, so, to the extent that the peanuts effect can be used to help people help themselves, narrow bracketing can be used to increase the likelihood that people will frame outcomes as "peanuts." Thus, for example, an exercise goal could be framed to be less onerous by expressing it as miles per day instead of miles per month or year.

Regret Aversion

Research has found that the desire to avoid regret is a potent force in decision making (Connolly and Butler 2006) and that feedback to nonadherent patients (such as a patient who is not compliant with taking a medication) about how they would have benefited had they been adherent will maximize the impact of regret. This approach has been inspired in our work by the success of the Dutch postal code lottery, in which winning postal codes are selected. People living within the postal code who purchased a ticket receive a prize, and those who failed to purchase a ticket learn that they would have won had they purchased a ticket (Zeelenberg and Pieters 2004). **Anticipated regret** has been shown to affect a variety of preventive behaviors, such as the significant increase in vaccination use among people who have experienced illness after failing to get vaccinated (Chapman and Coups 2006).

Improving Health Behaviors: Decision Errors Applied to Health Behavior Change

As mentioned above, the greatest opportunities for improvement in health involve population-wide changes in health behaviors. It is well

documented that smoking and obesity, despite the reductions in prevalence of smoking over the past several decades, are the two most significant contributors to premature mortality in the United States, with smoking contributing to more than 400,000 deaths per year (Mokdad et al. 2004).

Improving these numbers depends on changing health behaviors. Evidence to date suggests that giving people more information is not going to solve these problems. People are acutely aware of the health hazards of smoking; indeed, some say that smokers tend to *overestimate* the hazards (Slovic 2001; Viscusi 1992). Furthermore, about 70% of smokers say they want to quit smoking, although only about 2%-3% per year succeed (Bartlett et al. 1994; Hughes 2003). The problem is not likely due to poorly informed decision making, but rather not being able to follow through on good intentions in environments that make long-term success difficult.

Behavioral economists have proposed an asymmetric paternalism approach to public policy (Camerer et al. 2003; Thaler and Sunstein 2003). **Asymmetric paternalism** is *paternalistic* in the sense of attempting to help individuals achieve their own goals, in effect protecting them from themselves, as compared to conventional forms of regulation, which are generally designed to prevent individuals from harming others. However, asymmetric paternalism differs from "heavy-handed" **paternalism** in attempting to do so without limiting freedom of choice.

Asymmetric paternalism is *asymmetric* in the sense of helping individuals who are prone to making irrational decisions, while not harming those who make informed, deliberate decisions. For example, arranging the presentation of food in a cafeteria line so that the healthful foods appear first is likely to increase the amount of healthful food chosen, without depriving those who want the unhealthful foods of the opportunity to purchase them (Thaler and Sunstein 2003). Asymmetric paternalism is also asymmetric in the sense that those who believe people behave optimally should not object, because such measures do not limit freedom; at the same time, those who accept the limits of relying on human rationality should endorse such measures.

Rather than focusing on giving individuals information about the long-term consequences of their behavior, an approach that is at best partially effective, many specific interventions proposed by advocates of asymmetric paternalism use a common strategy: they exploit the same biases that otherwise contribute to self-harmful behavior to instead promote healthful behavior.

For instance, there are many ways in which the default, or status quo, option is the unhealthful one. At fast food restaurants, for example, combination meals typically include large sodas, which become even larger if the meal is supersized. Replacing the soft drink with a bottle of water as the default, so that soda is served only on request, would cost restaurants little and preserve freedom of choice, but it could produce a major change in beverage consumption behavior. Defaults could also be used to advantage when it comes to beneficial medical tests. For many types of medical tests, the default is not to get the test; patients and providers are responsible for remembering, for example, that a patient has not had a colonoscopy for five years and is due to get one. An asymmetrically paternalistic policy would change the default such that the next test is automatically scheduled (with provision made for reminders); it would need to be "unscheduled" to be avoided. Another possible policy would establish obtaining a second opinion for certain types of medical procedures as the default, which could be overridden only by making an explicit decision to do so, with an appropriate rationale, for not doing so.

Present-biased preferences can also be exploited to help individuals, rather than harm them, by altering immediate costs and benefits. The key, again consistent with changing the path of least resistance, is to make healthful behaviors more convenient (less immediately costly) and unhealthful behaviors less convenient (more immediately costly). For example, companies could offer free chilled bottles of water within easy access of employees, while soft drinks could be sold in less convenient locations farther away from employee work stations or offices. Positioning the soft drink vending machines in obscure places would also help because individuals would not have to constantly choose whether to consume them, a choice that requires, and thus depletes, willpower each time it is made in favor of the healthier alternative. Similar measures could be introduced in schools. Healthful foods could be served in convenient "grab and go" containers that could be obtained and consumed quickly, leaving the student with free time for desired activities. Less healthful foods could be located in less convenient locations. This subtle change in the path of least resistance could potentially produce a major change in behavior. Rather than requiring individuals to make decisions based on consideration of their long-term best interests, these strategies attempt to change short-term incentives in such a way that the actions that are beneficial to the individual are also easier to choose. Some schools have, in fact, begun to use this approach, banning or making less accessible various products, such as soda and candy from vending machines (Martin 2007).

It is also possible to take advantage of another feature of present-biased preferences. People are often willing to commit themselves to far-sighted behavior (e.g., to saving money or dieting) *in the future* because doing so does not entail immediate costs. This aspect of present-biased preferences can be exploited by giving individuals choices between health-benefiting and health-harming behaviors before the time they will actually have to act on them. For example, individuals could choose to schedule gym visits and lab tests to monitor their cholesterol ahead of time and to voluntarily accept financial penalties for last-minute cancellation. Soft drink machines could be programmed with a personal identification code such that they cannot be accessed on the following day if an individual has not enabled his access or if the individual has disabled his access. A person with a goal of losing weight is much more likely to be willing to deny himself the pleasure of tomorrow's soft drink than today's.

Although the overweighting of immediate and tangible costs and benefits typically works against healthful behavior, these same factors can be used to promote **compliance** by providing tangible but small immediate rewards for beneficial behaviors. Funds to do this could be provided by employers or insurers for whom this might be a cost-effective way to improve health and worker productivity (Warner et al. 1996). Such rewards have been shown to have dramatic effects in the area of drug addiction (Higgins et al. 2000). Many patients with drug addiction experience major adverse consequences, such as loss of their livelihood and disfranchisement from their families, but these costs are often insufficient to motivate abstinence. Small incentives offered on proof of abstinence have succeeded in helping people quit smoking when the far larger (but delayed) incentives for abstinence have failed (Volpp et al. 2006). Such an approach could be used more widely in contexts like weight loss or regularly taking prescribed medications.

Specific Contexts of Behavioral Economics to Promote Health Behavior Change

The concepts of behavioral economics have been applied to numerous areas of public health and health behavior change. We describe below several illustrative examples of these concepts in action.

Smoking Cessation

Smoking cessation interventions have demonstrated that simple direct payment interventions designed to reduce procrastination and, at least in part, respond to present-biased preferences are successful at increasing smoking cessation rates (see chapter 10). Developing effective smoking cessation strategies remains a critical challenge in tobacco control; while 70% of smokers say they want to quit, only 2%-3% of smokers effectively quit each year (Bartlett et al. 1994; Hughes 2003).

Smoking is a good example of a behavior that people have great difficulty changing, despite manifest short- and long-term health and economic benefits. For one, people who quit smoking by age 50 reduce their risk of dying before age 65 by half (USDHHS 2000). Moreover, the excess risk of myocardial infarction ("heart attack") and stroke for smokers relative to nonsmokers falls by nearly 50% within two years after stopping smoking (Lightwood and Glantz 1997). The risk of sudden cardiac death in patients with known coronary artery disease is also no higher among ex-smokers than among people who have never smoked (Goldenberg et al. 2003).

A recent study randomized 179 veterans at the Philadelphia Veterans Affairs Medical Center to receive either a free smoking cessation program (**control group**) or a free smoking cessation program plus incentives of $20 for attending each of five classes (total $100) and $100 for biochemically confirmed smoking cessation 30 days after program completion (intervention group). On average, participants had smoked a mean of 21.9 (minimum of 10) cigarettes per day at baseline and for an average of 30.3 years. In this study, the incentive group had significantly higher rates of program enrollment, completion, and, most importantly, quitting by 30 days after completion (16.3% versus 4.6%) (Volpp et al. 2006). The six-month follow-up after cessation of payments, however, showed a narrowing of the difference in quit rates (6.5% for the incentive group versus 4.6% for the control group). This study highlights the importance of having incentives extend through the period of highest risk of relapse; while this program was highly effective in changing short-term behavior, incentives for longer-term maintenance are also important.

This study was followed by a larger effort conducted among employees at General Electric that involved 878 employees at 85 work sites. Study participants were randomly assigned to receive information about smoking cessation programs (control group) or information about programs plus incentives of $100 for completing a smoking cessation program, $250 for biochemically confirmed cessation six months after study enrollment, and $400 for biochemically confirmed cessation after an additional six months (intervention group). In this study, the incentive group had significantly higher rates of smoking cessation nine and 12 months postenrollment (14.7% versus 5.0%) and at 15 and 18 months postenrollment (9. 4% versus 3.6%). This means that the initial quit rate ratio of 2.9 (14.7% versus 5.0%) at nine or 12 months dropped to 2.6 six months after the incentives were discontinued. As part of this initiative, incentive group participants also had significantly higher rates of enrollment in a smoking cessation program (15.4% versus 5.4%), completion of a smoking cessation program (10.8% versus 2.5%), and smoking cessation within the first six months postenrollment (20.9% versus 11.8%). The fact that the ratio of quit rates is largely sustained after discontinuation of the incentives suggests that this approach has promise in improving long-term cessation rates.

The comparative **effectiveness** of such approaches may be fairly high (figure 20.1). Recent published meta-analyses of medical therapies for smoking cessation, such as Zyban (buproprion), Chantix (varenicline), and nicotine replacement therapies (gum, patches, spray, lozenges, and inhalers) found similar benefits of intervention versus control groups. Such a comparison, however, is no substitute for trials directly comparing the effectiveness of treatments. Although we focused on the ratio of the quit rate in the treatment group compared to that in the control group in each study rather than directly comparing the quit rates between studies, the effectiveness of a given treatment may also vary with the population being studied, and direct, head-to-head comparisons of different approaches are needed. In addition, combining incentives with medical therapies may provide synergistic benefit.

Interestingly, paying rewards much smaller than the amounts smokers would save just by quitting (a pack-a-day smoker would save between $5 and $7 per day, or $1,500-$2,000 per year, depending on which state she lives in) led to significantly higher cessation rates. A few behavioral economics principles may be in effect here:

1. Getting rewards is more salient than not spending money, consistent with research showing that people tend to under-weight opportunity costs (Thaler 1999).
2. One large reward can have greater impact than having small amounts saved each day, consistent with the peanuts effect (Weber and Chapman 2005).
3. Anticipated regret can be a potent motivator (Connolly and Butler 2006; Hoelzl and Loewenstein 2005).

Cocaine Use

Significant work has been done to develop reward programs to help people combat addictions in the settings of drug treatment programs and aftercare programs (Bigelow and Silverman 1999). In controlled settings, financial incentives have been highly effective in modifying behavior and have led to higher rates of program retention and drug abstinence (Higgins 1999). For example, one study randomized

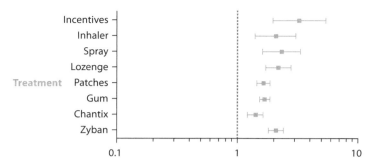

FIGURE 20.1. Odds ratios of 12 month continuous abstinence from different smoking cessation therapies. *Source:* KG Volpp, A Das A, Comparative effectiveness—thinking beyond medication A versus medication B. *N Engl J Med* 361 (4) (2009): 331-33.

40 cocaine-using adults to either behavioral treatment or behavioral treatment plus vouchers exchangeable for retail items if participants' urine samples were negative for cocaine. Urine samples were collected three times a week, and subjects were eligible for progressively larger incentives the longer they stayed abstinent. The total potential value of the incentives was $997.50. Of subjects in the incentive group, 75% completed all 12 weeks of treatment, compared to 40% of those in the control group. The incentive group demonstrated longer continuous abstinence both during weeks 1-12 (while they were receiving incentives) and during weeks 13-24 (when they were not). Rates of retention and continuous abstinence were also higher in the incentive group both during weeks 1-12 and weeks 13-24 (Higgins et al. 2000). This study shows the clear effectiveness of incentives, but it required monitoring several times a week, suggesting that frequent feedback was important. The incentive group did not relapse at greater rates once the incentives were discontinued.

This study is illustrative of commonly used **contingency management** approaches because it shows the clear effectiveness of incentives, but because it required checking drug levels in urine or saliva several times a week, it would not be easily exportable to community- or employer-based settings. The effectiveness was likely driven primarily by frequent small payments, which take advantage of the pervasiveness of present-biased preferences.

Although such studies have demonstrated that incentives reduce unhealthful behaviors and that the magnitude of the effect increases with the size of the incentive (Higgins et al. 1994; Stitzer and Bigelow 1983, 1984), application of these approaches to less highly controlled settings has not been well tested (Petry and Simcic 2002). Because of concerns about giving cash to active users of cocaine and other street drugs, such programs have generally used vouchers for goods rather than cash payments, adding to the administrative complexity of the program. Although such contingency management programs have been revealed to be highly effective, little is known about the cost-effectiveness (relevant, given their substantial administrative cost) or about their longer-term effectiveness in changing behavior.

Weight Loss

Losing weight seems to be one of the most difficult goals to accomplish. However, while weight loss is difficult, *maintaining* weight loss is even more difficult. In our weight-conscious society, people are powerfully motivated to lose weight, yet the fact that so many are obese suggests that they have great difficulty doing so.

A recent randomized controlled weight loss trial used financial incentives to motivate weight loss. This study aimed to use loss aversion, overoptimism, and regret aversion to help overweight people lose weight. Study participants (patients at the Philadelphia Veterans Affairs Medical Center in Philadelphia) were enrolled in a weight loss program that had the goal of losing 16 pounds in 16 weeks.

Two different types of incentive interventions were tested, a lottery-based incentive and a *deposit contract* incentive, compared to a no-incentive control group. Subjects in the incentive groups were required to call in their weight to the study nurse each day and were given daily feedback via text pagers. Accumulated incentives were paid out monthly once phoned-in weights were confirmed in the clinic. The combination of daily feedback but monthly payments has at least three advantages: (1) it gives people who attain their goals frequent positive feedback in the form of messages that they have been paid; (2) however, paying people only monthly increases the likelihood that a significant amount of money will have been accumulated, thus avoiding the potential risk of underweighting what would be a relatively small daily payment (i.e., peanuts effect); (3) finally, by giving both symbolic rewards (text message feedback) *and* real rewards (a monthly check), it leverages the payments maximally, almost as if each payment were made twice.

The lottery incentive consisted of a daily lottery with an expected value of $3 per day (1 in 5 chance of winning $10, 1 in 100 chance of winning $100), with subjects eligible for payment each day as long as they were on track to achieve their monthly weight loss target. Study participants were informed daily of the lottery outcome via their text pagers. People in all demographic groups participate in lotteries, although blacks spend nearly twice as much as whites and Hispanics, and low-income households spend a larger share of their wealth on lottery tickets than other households (Clotfelter 1979; Hansen 1995; Kearney 2005; Spiro 1974; Suits 1977). This implies that lotteries may be especially effective in motivating low-income individuals, who also

may have higher rates of unhealthful behaviors, such as failure to take medications, and adverse health outcomes.

We designed the lottery incentive to take advantage of three effects identified in the behavioral economics literature on incentives.

1. Consistent with research showing that present-biased preferences are important (hyperbolic time discounting) and that even small rewards and punishments can have great incentive value if they occur immediately (Ainslie 1975; Kirby 1997; Loewenstein 1992; Thaler 1981), patients who adhered to the program received rapid feedback about whether they won, and subjects who did not received feedback about whether they *would have* won had they been adherent.

2. Based on research showing that people are motivated by the experience of past rewards and the prospect of future rewards (Camerer and Ho 1999), that people are particularly emotionally attracted to small probabilities of large rewards (Loewenstein et al. 2001), and that people tend to overweight small probabilities in making decisions (Kahneman and Tversky 1979), the lottery was tailored to provide frequent small payoffs (a 1 in 5 chance of a $10 reward) and infrequent large payoffs (a 1 in 100 chance of a $100 reward).

3. Research on decision making has found that the desire to avoid regret is a potent force in decision making under risk (Connolly and Butler 2006), so by giving nonadherent patients feedback about what they would have won had they been adherent, the incentive scheme was designed to maximize the threat of regret in people who fail to adhere.

Design feature 3 is inspired by the success of programs that have successfully used anticipated regret, such as the Dutch postal code lottery (Zeelenberg and Pieters 2004) mentioned above, and research demonstrating increases in vaccination use among people who experienced the regret of failing to get vaccinated in the prior year and then getting sick (Chapman and Coups 2006).

Structuring financial incentives as a lottery has several benefits over a set payoff amount. Lotteries may be less costly to provide than the direct cash amount but have comparable incentive value given the effectiveness of intermittent **reinforcement** (i.e., positive feedback occurs at unpredictable intervals) (Bandura 1969). Beyond their monetary payoffs, lotteries provide entertainment value, which enhances their reinforcing properties as a motivator.

In the deposit contract group, study participants were invited to deposit $.01-$3.00 per day of their own money, which we matched 1:1. Participants reported their weight daily and received the sum of both amounts (the deposited plus the matched) each day that they were on track to meet their monthly weight loss targets, but they forfeited their deposit and match if they were not. They also received a fixed payment of $3.00 for each day they were under their target weight.

The deposit contract plays on participants' overoptimistic self-predictions to provide additional motivation (see discussion above). People tend to be overoptimistic in predicting how much weight they will lose (and, similarly, fail to appreciate how difficult it is to lose weight); therefore, when asked to put money down at the beginning of the month toward attaining their weight loss goals, about 91% of subjects were willing to do so. For these participants, the average deposit contract increased during each month of participation, from $1.35 in month 1 to $1.59 in month 2, to $1.83 in month 3, leveling off to $1.85 in month 4. As subjects struggled with losing weight, their desire to avoid losing the deposit provided added motivation to attain the weight loss goal. Bound by their optimistic predictions and averse to losing their deposits, participants' optimism about their own likelihood of losing weight, by increasing their

propensity to deposit money (thus **triggering** loss aversion), became a kind of self-fulfilling prophecy.

Both approaches worked well as long as the incentives were kept in place. Incentive participants lost more than three times as much weight as controls. Whereas lottery and deposit contract participants lost an average of 13.1 and 14.0 pounds, respectively, mean weight loss was significantly lower in the control group (4.0 pounds) (Volpp, John, et al. 2008).

The appeal of this approach was also attested to by the extremely low dropout rate in the study. Only 9% of subjects dropped out of the study, a **lost-to-follow-up** rate much lower than is typical in weight loss intervention studies (often as high as 40%-50%). Among subjects not lost to follow-up, participants in both incentive groups called in daily weights more than 90% of the time, indicating the feasibility of an approach that likely keeps weight loss salient among participants.

However, following cessation of the incentives, substantial weight gain occurred among study participants. This highlights that four months, in the context of weight loss, is too short an intervention period. Many studies of weight loss interventions have shown that weight loss in the first several months is followed by weight regain thereafter. More work is needed to see if these initial impressive results are sustained over longer periods of time.

A recent study of using incentives to encourage the development of healthful **habits** found that students who were offered incentives to go the gym eight times within four weeks significantly increased their weekly gym attendance compared to a group of students who were offered incentives to go to the gym once and relative to a control group. The effect was concentrated among people who had not been regular gym goers; of note, a significant difference in the frequency of gym visitation continued after the period of the intervention (Charness and Gneezy 2009).

Commercial entities have recognized the power of these pervasive decision errors. For example, a group of Yale professors recently founded stickK (www.stickk.com), a company designed to help people who want to change their behavior by allowing them to enter into precommitment contracts. If they are unsuccessful in changing behavior, their funds will be donated either to a charity of their choice or sent to another individual. To the best of our knowledge, stickK has yet to be tested in a randomized controlled trial or pitted against other types of interventions.

Medication Adherence

Despite manifest benefits, it is common for people to fail to take certain prescription medications. For example, when taken properly, the drug warfarin, an anticlotting medication, reduces the risk of strokes by 68% overall and by 85% in patients older than age 75 years who have at least one other risk factor (Fuster et al. 1981; Laupacis et al. 1998; Petersen et al. 1989). However, adherence data are generally discouraging. One recent cohort study found that 40% of subjects missed 20% or more of their warfarin doses (Kimmel et al. 2007). Because of severe risk, and likelihood, of poor compliance, many physicians are reluctant to prescribe warfarin for many of their patients, so the tremendous potential benefits of the drug are often not realized (Ansell et al. 1997; Cheng 1997; Go et al. 1999; Kutner et al. 1991). The combination of proven benefits with low compliance rates in existing programs points to the need for new approaches for improving adherence.

Value-based insurance designs (VBIDs), an approach based on the premise that reductions in copayments will significantly increase use of beneficial and cost-effective health care services, is one strategy being widely adopted to improve medication adherence (Chernew et al. 2007; Fendrick and Chernew 2006). However, although observational studies have consis-tently shown that increases in copayments are associated with both decreases in use of medications and worsened health outcomes (Gibson et al. 2005; Goldman et al. 2004; Goldman et al. 2007; Hsu et al. 2006; Roblin et al. 2005; Soumerai et al. 1991; Soumerai et al. 1994; Tamblyn et al. 2001), little evidence exists that decreasing copayments improves patient adherence or outcomes (Campbell et al. 2009; Chernew et al. 2008; Glasgow et al. 2005). Only one observational study has conducted a robust empirical **evaluation** of a VBID approach to lowering copayments (Chernew et al. 2008). This study found that when copayments were lowered by about 30% for employees of a large firm, adherence increased by 3% to 4% for hypertension medications and cholesterol-lowering medications. Such a small change in adherence would be unlikely to produce significant improvements in clinical outcomes. Several reasons based on behavioral economics suggest that copay reductions may not significantly improve adherence. The underlying psychology of how people process changes in payments as losses, rather than gains, suggests that increases and decreases in copayments may not be equivalent (loss aversion) (Kahneman and Tversky 1979). Furthermore, people get feedback only every 90 days (i.e., when the prescription refill date arrives), which is likely insufficient to positively reinforce behavior in people who are struggling to remember to take their medication every day.

In an attempt to improve warfarin adherence, we conducted pilot studies that tested the feasibility and potential effectiveness of daily lottery incentives. In addition to drawing on behavioral economics, the intervention makes use of a new technology, a computerized pillbox, that enhances the **scalability** of the approach by making it possible for program administrators to receive feedback each day on medication adherence electronically without any action on the part of the program participant other than taking the medication (Volpp, Loewenstein, et al. 2008).

In each of two pilots, 10 patients on warfarin were provided with an Informedix Med-eMonitor System, which has a display screen and separate pill compartments labeled for each dose of the medication. Each device was programmed to communicate by telephone with the study's administrator. Participants were enrolled in a daily lottery (expected value of $5 per day for the first pilot[1] and $3 per day for the second) that required compliance (taking the medication) for entrance into the lottery. Although patients were enrolled in the lottery each day that they were instructed to take a pill, they were not eligible to receive any earnings unless the Med-eMonitor had indicated that they had opened the appropriate pill compartment. The Med-eMonitor also was programmed to provide a daily reminder chime as well as a message asking the patients whether they had taken their medication.

The primary outcome measured was patient adherence, and it was calculated as the percentage of days in which each patient opened the correct compartment. In the first pilot ($5 per day expected value of the lottery), 979 patient-days of warfarin use were recorded. Over this time period, adherence was 97.7% (or, just 2.3% nonadherence), compared with a typical average of 22% nonadherence in this clinic population (figure 20.2). In the second pilot study ($3 per day expected value of the lottery), an additional 10 patients contributed a total of 813 days of warfarin use. Mean adherence was 98.4% (only 1.6% non-adherence) (see figure 20.2). Although pill compartment opening is an imperfect measure of pill-taking (since patients could open the compartment but not take the pill), objective measures of patients' blood coagulation rates support the conclusion that the lottery intervention helped. In the first pilot, the proportion of out-of-range INRs (the INR refers to the "International Normalized Ratio," which is used to measure the degree of blood thinning from anticoagulation medication) decreased from 35.0% prepilot to 12.2% postpilot, a 65.2% improvement; in the second pilot, INRs out of range decreased from 65.0% to 40.4%, a 37.9% improvement.

Like the weight loss study, this study illustrates how insights from behavioral economics—the importance of frequent feedback and incentives, the greater motivational power of lotteries compared to similarly valued definite payments, and the motivating force of anticipated regret—can be used to help people change unhealthful behaviors to healthful ones.

Numerous other studies are currently under way testing the relative effectiveness of daily reminders, lottery-based incentives, and lottery-based incentives together with daily reminders. We have also automated the system for processing lottery payments and sending out daily feedback so that it can be more scalable.

Conclusion

Clinical and public health outcomes would be much improved if patients were able to carefully and dispassionately weigh the present and future costs of their actions and if they had the necessary self-control to implement behavioral plans. In such a world, we could assume that smokers and obese people continued to smoke and be obese because they fully understood the risks and benefits and felt that the benefits outweigh the costs. However, this is clearly not often the case, and many of the unhealthful decisions that contribute to behaviors that are not

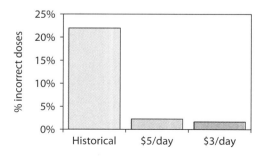

FIGURE 20.2. Adherence under lotteries compared to historical controls

in individuals' long-term interests are probably not easily remedied. Tactics that take advantage of the underlying decision errors are used by corporate entities because they work reliably on large numbers of people. By taking into account these decision errors, we can make behavioral interventions far more effective than if we ignore them.

NOTES

1. Because of a clerical error, the expected value was greater than intended. Subjects won $10 if either of their digits matched with either of the digits drawn for that day, doubling the likelihood of winning $10 above what we intended. Rather than ending the trial when we discovered the error, we completed it and started a new trial with another 10 patients, and the lottery was implemented correctly.

REFERENCES

Ainslie G. 1975. Specious reward: A behavioral theory of impulsiveness and impulse control. *Psychol Bull* 82:463-96.

Ansell JE, Buttaro ML, Thomas OV, Knowlton CH. 1997. Consensus guidelines for coordinated outpatient oral anticoagulation therapy management. Anticoagulation Guidelines Task Force. *Ann Pharmacother* 31:604-15.

Bandura A. 1969. *Principles of Behavior Modification.* New York: Holt, Rinehart & Winston.

Bartlett J, Miller L, Rice D, Max W. 1994. Medical care expenditures attributable to cigarette smoking: United States, 1993. *MMWR* 43:469-72.

Becker GS, Murphy KM. 1988. A theory of rational addiction. *J Pol Econ* 96:675-700.

Benartzi S, Thaler RH. 1995. Myopic loss aversion and the equity premium puzzle. *Q J Econ* 110:73-92.

Bigelow GE, Silverman K. 1999. Theoretical and empirical foundations of contingency management treatments for drug abuse. In *Motivating Behavior Change among Illicit Drug Users,* ed. ST Higgins, K Silverman, 15-30. Washington, DC: American Psychological Association.

Buehler R, Griffin D, Ross M. 1994. Exploring the planning fallacy: Why people underestimate their task completion times. *J Pers Soc Psychol* 67:366-81.

———. 2002. Inside the planning fallacy: The causes and consequences of optimistic time predictions. In *Heuristics and Biases: The Psychology of Intuitive Judgment,* ed. T Gilovich, D Griffin, D Kahneman, 250-70. Cambridge: Cambridge University Press.

Camerer C, Ho T-H. 1999. Experience-weighted attraction learning in normal form games. *Econometrica* 67:837-74.

Camerer C, Issacharoff S, Loewenstein G, O'Donoghue T, Rabin M. 2003. Regulation for conservatives: Behavioral economics and the case for "asymmetric paternalism." *U Penn Law Rev* 151:1211-54.

Camerer C, Loewenstein G. 2003. Behavioral economics: Past, present, future. In *Advances in Behavioral Economics,* ed. C Camerer, G Loewenstein, M Rabin. New York: Russell Sage Foundation Press; Princeton, NJ: Princeton University Press.

Campbell SM, Reeves D, Kontopantelis E, Sibbald B, Roland M. 2009. Effects of pay for performance on the quality of primary care in England. *N Engl J Med* 361:368-78.

Chapman GB, Coups EJ. 2006. Emotions and preventive health behavior: Worry, regret, and influenza vaccination. *Health Psychol* 25:82-90.

Charness G, Gneezy U. 2009. Incentives to exercise. *Econometrica* 77:909-31.

Cheng TO. 1997. Underuse of warfarin in atrial fibrillation. *Arch Intern Med* 157:1505.

Chernew ME, Rosen AB, Fendrick AM. 2007. Value-based insurance design. *Health Affairs* 26:195-203.

Chernew ME, Shah MR, Wegh A, et al. 2008. Impact of decreasing copayments on medication adherence within a disease management environment. *Health Affairs* 27:103-12.

Clotfelter CT. 1979. On the regressivity of state-operated "numbers" games. *Natl Tax J* 33:543-48.

Clotfelter CT, Cook PJ. 1989. *Selling Hope: State Lotteries in America.* Cambridge, MA: Harvard University Press.

Connolly T, Butler DU. 2006. Regret in economic and psychological theories of choice. *J Behav Decis Mak* 19:148-58.

Coughlin CC, Garrett TA, Hernandez-Murillo R. 2006. The geography, economics, and politics of lottery adoption. *Fed Res Bank St Louis Rev* 88:165-80.

Della Vigna P, Malmendier L. 2002. Paying not to go to the gym. *Am Econ Rev* 96:694-719.

Fendrick AM, Chernew ME. 2006. Value-based insurance design: A "clinically sensitive" approach to preserve quality of care and contain costs. *Am J Manag Care* 12:18-20.

Flegal KM, Graubard BI, Williamson DF, Gail MH. 2005. Excess deaths associated with underweight, overweight, and obesity. *JAMA* 293:1861-67.

Frederick S, Loewenstein G, O'Donoghue T. 2002. Time discounting and time preference: A critical review. *J Econ Lit* 40:351-401.

Fuster V, Gersh BJ, Giuliani ER, Tajik AJ, Branden-
burg RO, Frye RL. 1981. The natural history of
idiopathic dilated cardiomyopathy. *Am J Cardiol*
47:525-31.

Genesove D, Mayer C. 2001. Loss aversion and seller
behavior: Evidence from the housing market. *Q J
Econ* 116:1233-60.

Gibson TB, McLaughlin CG, Smith DG. 2005. A
copayment increase for prescription drugs: The
long-term and short-term effects on use and
expenditures. *Inquiry* 42:293-310.

Glasgow RE, Wagner EH, Schaefer J, Mahoney LD, Reid
RJ, Greene SM. 2005. Development and validation of
the Patient Assessment of Chronic Illness Care
(PACIC). *Med Care* 43 (5): 436-44.

Gneezy U, Potters J. 1997. An experiment on risk taking
and evaluation periods. *Q J Econ* 112:631-45.

Go AS, Hylek EM, Borowsky LH, Phillips KA, Selby JV,
Singer DE. 1999. Warfarin use among ambulatory
patients with nonvalvular atrial fibrillation: The
anticoagulation and risk factors in atrial fibrillation
(ATRIA) study. *Ann Intern Med* 131:927-34.

Goldenberg I, Jonas M, Tenenbaum A, et al. 2003.
Current smoking, smoking cessation, and the risk of
sudden cardiac death in patients with coronary artery
disease. *Arch Intern Med* 163:2301-5.

Goldman DP, Joyce GF, Zheng Y. 2007. Prescription drug
cost sharing: Associations with medication and
medical utilization and spending and health. *Health
Econ* 298:61-69.

Goldman DP, Leibowitz AA, Robalino DA. 2004.
Employee responses to health insurance premium
increases. *Am J Manag Care* 10:41-47.

Halpern SD, Ubel PA, Asch DA. 2007. Harnessing the
power of default options to improve health care. *N
Engl J Med* 357:1340-44.

Hamermesh DS, Soss NM. 1974. An economic theory of
suicide. *J Pol Econ* 82:83-98.

Hansen A. 1995. The tax incidence of the Colorado state
lottery instant games. *Pub Finance Q* 23:385-99.

Herrnstein RJ, Prelec D. 1992. Melioration. In *Choice over
Time,* ed. G Loewenstein, J Elster, 235-63. New York:
Russell Sage Foundation.

Higgins ST. 1999. Applying behavioral economics to the
challenge of reducing cocaine abuse. In *The Economic
Analysis of Substance Use and Abuse,* ed. FJ Chaloupka,
M Grossman, WK Bickel, H Saffer, 157-74. Cambridge,
MA: NBER.

Higgins ST, Bickel WK, Hughes JR. 1994. Influence of an
alternative reinforcer on human cocaine self-
administration. *Life Sci* 55:179-87.

Higgins ST, Wong CJ, Badger GJ, Ogden DE, Dantona
RL. 2000. Contingent reinforcement increases cocaine

abstinence during outpatient treatment and 1 year of
follow-up. *J Consult Clin Psychol* 68:64-72.

Hoelzl E, Loewenstein G. 2005. Wearing out your
shoes to prevent someone else from stepping into
them: Anticipated regret and social takeover in
sequential decisions. *Organ Behav Hum Decis
Process* 98:15-27.

Hsu J, Price M, Huang J, et al. 2006. Unintended
consequences of caps on Medicare drug benefits. *N
Engl J Med* 354:2349-59.

Hughes JR. 2003. Motivating and helping smokers to
stop smoking. *J Gen Intern Med* 18:1053-57.

Issacharoff S, Delaney EF. 2006. Credit card accountability. *U Chicago Law Rev* 73:157-82.

Jackevicius CA, Mamdani M, Tu JV. 2002. Adherence
with statin therapy in elderly patients with and
without acute coronary syndromes. *JAMA* 288:462-67.

Johnson EJ, Goldstein D. 2003. Do defaults save lives?
Sci Justice 302:1338-39.

Kahneman D, Knetsch JL, Thaler RH. 1991. The
endowment effect, loss aversion, and status quo bias:
Anomalies. *J Econ Perspect* 5:193-206.

Kahneman D, Tversky A. 1979. Prospect theory: An
analysis of decision under risk. *Econometrica*
47:263-91.

Kearney MS. 2005. State lotteries and consumer
behavior. *J Public Econ* 89:2269-99.

Kimmel SE, Chen Z, Price M, et al. 2007. The influence
of patient adherence on anticoagulation control with
warfarin: Results from the International Normalized
Ratio Adherence and Genetics (IN-RANGE) study.
Arch Intern Med 167:229-35.

Kirby K. 1997. Bidding on the future: Evidence against
normative discounting of delayed rewards. *J Exper
Psychol: Gen* 126:54-70.

Kripalani S, Yao X, Haynes RB. 2007. Interventions to
enhance medication adherence in chronic medical
conditions: A systematic review. *Arch Intern Med*
167:540-49.

Kutner M, Nixon G, Silverstone F. 1991. Physicians'
attitudes toward oral anticoagulants and antiplatelet
agents for stroke prevention in elderly patients with
atrial fibrillation. *Arch Intern Med* 151:1950-53.

Laupacis A, Albers G, Dalen J, Dunn MI, Jacobson AK,
Singer DE. 1998. Antithrombotic therapy in atrial
fibrillation. *Chest* 114:579S-589S.

Lightwood JM, Glantz SA. 1997. Short-term economic
and health benefits of smoking cessation: Myocardial
infarction and stroke. *Circulation* 96:1089-96.

Loewenstein G. 1992. The fall and rise of psychological
explanation in the economics of intertemporal choice.
In *Choice over Time,* ed. G Loewenstein, J Elster, 3-34.
New York: Russell Sage Foundation.

Loewenstein G, Angner E. 2003. Predicting and indulging changing preferences. In *Time and Decision: Economic and Psychological Perspectives on Intertemporal choice,* ed. G Loewenstein, D Read, R Baumeister, 351-91. New York: Russell Sage Foundation Press.

Loewenstein G, Brennan T, Volpp KG. 2007. Asymmetric paternalism to improve health behaviors. *JAMA* 298:2415-17.

Loewenstein G, Haisley E. 2008. The economist as therapist: Methodological issues raised by "light" paternalism. In *Perspectives on the Future of Economics: Positive and Normative Foundations,* ed. A Caplin, A Schotter. Oxford: Oxford University Press.

Loewenstein G, O'Donoghue T. 2006. We can do this the easy way or the hard way: Negative emotions, self-regulation, and the law. *U Chicago Law Rev* 73:183-206.

Loewenstein G, O'Donoghue T, Rabin M. 2003. Projection bias in predicting futures utility. *Q J Econ* 118:1209-48.

Loewenstein G, Weber EU, Hsee CK, Welch N. 2001. Risk as feelings. *Psychol Bull* 127:267-86.

Madrian BC, Shea DF. 2001. The power of suggestion: Inertia in 401(k) participation and savings behavior. *Q J Econ* 116:1149-87.

Markowitz H. 1952. The utility of wealth. *J Pol Econ* 60:151-58.

Martin A. 2007. The school cafeteria, on a diet. *New York Times,* Sept. 5.

Mokdad AH, Marks JS, Stroup DF, Gerberding JL. 2004. Actual causes of death in the United States, 2000. *JAMA* 291 (10): 1238-45.

Murphy KM. 2006. Keynote address. McGill Integrative Health Challenge Think Tank, Montreal, Canada, Oct. 26-27.

Nordgren L, van der Plight J, van Harreveld F. 2007. Evaluating Eve: Visceral states influence the evaluation of impulsive behavior. *J Pers Soc Psychol* 93:75-84.

O'Dean T. 1998. Are investors reluctant to realize their losses? *J Finance* 53:1775-98.

O'Donoghue T, Rabin M. 1999. Doing it now or later. *Am Econ Rev* 89:103-24.

Petersen P, Boysen G, Godtfredsen J, Andersen ED, Andersen B. 1989. Placebo-controlled, randomised trial of warfarin and aspirin for prevention of thromboembolic complications in chronic atrial fibrillation: The Copenhagen AFASAK study. *Lancet* 1:175-79.

Petry NM, Simcic F Jr. 2002. Recent advances in the dissemination of contingency management techniques: Clinical and research perspectives. *J Subst Abuse Treat* 23:81-86.

Prelec D. 1998. The probability weighting function. *Econometrica* 66:497-527.

Prelec D, Loewenstein G. 1991. Decision making over time and under uncertainty: A common approach. *Manag Sci* 37:770-86.

Read D, Loewenstein G, Rabin M. 1999. Choice bracketing. *J Risk Uncert* 19:171-97.

Read D, van Leeuwen B. 1998. Predicting hunger: The effects of appetite and delay on choice. *Organ Behav Hum Decis Process* 76:189-205.

Roblin DW, Platt R, Goodman MJ, et al. 2005. Effect of increased cost-sharing on oral hypoglycemic use in five managed care organizations: How much is too much? *Med Care* 43:951-59.

Sabini J, Silver M. 1982. *Moralities of Everyday Life.* Oxford: Oxford University Press.

Samuelson W, Zeckhauser R. 1988. Status quo bias in decision making. *J Risk Uncert* 1:7-59.

Schroeder SA. 2007. We can do better—improving the health of the American people. *N Engl J Med* 357:1221-28.

Shefrin H, Statman M. 1985. The disposition to sell winners too early and ride losers too long. *J Finance* 40:777-90.

Slovic P. 2001. Do cigarette smokers know the risks? In *Smoking: Risk, Perception, and Policy,* ed. P Slovic. Thousand Oaks, CA: Sage.

Soumerai SB, McLaughlin TJ, Ross-Degnan D, Casteris CS, Bollini P. 1994. Effects of a limit on Medicaid drug-reimbursement benefits on the use of psychotropic agents and acute mental health services by patients with schizophrenia. *N Engl J Med* 331:650-55.

Soumerai SB, Ross-Degnan D, Avorn J, McLaughlin T, Choodnovskiy I. 1991. Effects of Medicaid drug-payment limits on admission to hospitals and nursing homes. *N Engl J Med* 325:1072-77.

Spiro MH. 1974. On the tax incidence of the Pennsylvania lottery. *Natl Tax J* 27:57-61.

Stitzer ML, Bigelow GE. 1983. Contingent payment for carbon monoxide reduction: Effects of pay amount. *Behav Ther* 14:647-56.

———. 1984. Contingent reinforcement for carbon monoxide reduction: Within-subject effects of pay amount. *J Applied Behav Anal* 17:477-83.

Suits DB. 1977. Gambling taxes: Regressivity and revenue potential. *Natl Tax J* 30:19-35.

Sunstein CR. 2002. Probability neglect: Emotions, worst cases, and law. *Yale Law J* 112:61-107.

Tamblyn R, Laprise R, Hanley JA, et al. 2001. Adverse events associated with prescription drug cost-sharing among poor and elderly persons. *JAMA* 285:421-29.

Thaler RH. 1981. Some empirical evidence on time inconsistency. *Rev Econ Stud* 23:165-80.

———. 1999. Mental accounting matters. *J Behav Decis Mak* 12:183-206.

Thaler RH, Benartzi S. 2004. Save more tomorrow: Using behavioral economics to increase employee saving. *J Pol Econ* 112:S164-S187.

Thaler RH, Sunstein CR. 2003. Libertarian paternalism. *Am Econ Rev* 93:175-79.

Thaler RH, Tversky A, Kahneman DR, Schwartz A. 1997. The effect of myopia and loss aversion on risk taking: An experimental test. *Q J Econ* 112:647-61.

Tversky A, Kahneman DR. 1991. Loss aversion in riskless choice: A reference-dependent model. *Q J Econ* 106:1039-61.

U.S. Dept. of Health and Human Services (USDHHS). 2000. *Healthy People 2010: Understanding and Improving Health.* Washington, DC: U.S. Dept. of Health and Human Services.

Viscusi WK. 1992. *Smoking: Making the Risky Decision.* New York: Oxford University Press.

Volpp KG, Gurmankin Levy A, Asch DA, et al. 2006. A randomized controlled trial of financial incentives for smoking cessation. *Cancer Epidemiol Biomarkers Prev* 15:12-18.

Volpp KG, John LK, Troxel AB, Norton L, Fassbender J, Loewenstein G. 2008. Financial incentive-based approaches for weight loss: A randomized trial. *JAMA* 300:2631-37.

Volpp KG, Loewenstein G, Troxel A, et al. 2008. A test of financial incentives to improve warfarin adherence. *BMC Health Serv Res* 8:272.

Warner KE, Smith RJ, Smith DG, Fries BE. 1996. Health and economic implications of a work-site smoking-cessation program: A simulation analysis. *J Occup Environ Med* 38:981-92.

Weber BJ, Chapman GB. 2005. Playing for peanuts: Why is risk seeking more common for low-stakes gambles? *Organ Behav Hum Decis Process* 97:31-46.

Zeelenberg M, Pieters R. 2004. Consequences of regret aversion in real life: The case of the Dutch postcode lottery. *Organ Behav Hum Decis Process* 93:155-68.

Complexity, Systems Thinking, and Health Behavior Change

DIANE T. FINEGOOD, LEE M. JOHNSTON,
MARLA STEINBERG, CARRIE L.
MATTESON, AND PENNY B. DECK

LEARNING OBJECTIVES

After completing the chapter, the reader will be able to

* Describe the characteristics of complex systems as they relate to health behavior change.
* Discuss how traditional models of health behavior change fail to address complexity.
* Demonstrate the need for a paradigm shift in developing solutions for complex problems and explore how systems thinking can further this process.
* Identify leverage points to support health behavior change.
* Describe practices to facilitate the evaluation of behavior change interventions using a complex systems lens.

Introduction

Creating **health behavior** change in populations is neither simple nor complicated; rather, it is **complex**. That is, behaviors generally have many causal factors and countless interactions between them that feed back upon one another. These causal factors, or **determinants**, are a mix of individual-level variables such as age, gender, genetics, beliefs, and **motivation**, which in turn interact with environmental factors that arise in the home, school, workplace, community, and **social networks** and are shaped by sociocultural **influences**, economic conditions, and government policies. In populations (which should be considered complex), the laws that describe the behavior of the whole are qualitatively different from the laws that govern the behavior of the parts (Vicsek 2002).

Early psychological models of health behavior change focused attention on the individual and on simple, direct relationships between variables like awareness, **attitudes**, and behavior. Environmental approaches shifted the focus from the individual to the environment and to the notion that health behavior could be promoted through environmental enhancement and restructuring. This shift recognized that behavior change could be a *complicated* rather than simple process. Complicated problems require additional levels of expertise and coordination to respond to their broader scale, but do not contain the hallmarks of **complexity**. Stokols describes the further shift to social-ecological models as the recognition that both the individual and the environment are important and that the degree of an individual's "fit" in the environment needs to be understood (Stokols 1996). In this approach individual behavior change is nested within broader social determinants, pushing our thinking toward the aforementioned hallmarks of complexity, such as feedback loops, **interdependence** between system components and nonlinearity. However, although our models have begun to consider and describe health behavior as complex, we have yet to fully embrace a **systems approach** to conducting research, designing **interventions**, or evaluating their results.

Most simple and many complicated problems are best solved using a **reductionist** approach to understanding the causes of the problem and then devising appropriate solutions. For relatively simple problems, we are able to work out all the important relationships involved and identify the best prospects to targeting in interventions. But if we accept that the systems relevant to health behavior change in populations are complex, then we must also accept that the reductionist paradigm is inadequate and that different approaches are required. Complex problems are harder to pin down. In a sense they are less "knowable" (Rittel and Webber 1973), and, as a result, focusing

on defining the causes of the problem may not be as helpful as figuring out what works for whom and under what conditions (Robinson and Sirard 2005).

Complex initiatives or interventions pose many challenges to researchers, program planners, and evaluators because of the qualities that make them complex. They may involve multiple heterogeneous interventions, nonlinear dynamic relationships between variables like knowledge and action, and many interdependencies between the actors and organizations involved. Complex interventions in the real world are often not well controlled, and both the path and the outcome may be emergent properties of the intervention (Gamble 2008). Methods for evaluating complex interventions are starting to emerge as well as methods for conducting **evaluation** using a complexity lens.

This chapter applies a complex systems lens to the challenge of creating behavior change in populations. It is guided by the notion that refocusing our attention on solutions appropriate for complex problems will accelerate progress against the many complex public health problems of our time. The first part of the chapter discusses the unique features of complex problems, using examples that help to illustrate various dimensions of the complexity of health behavior change. The next section briefly reviews current models of behavior change and the degree to which they consider behavior as complex. We then explore new models and approaches that arise out of systems thinking and **complex systems science**. Lastly, we consider how systems thinking has been incorporated into **program evaluation** practices and offer some **guidelines** for practitioners wanting to approach program **planning** and evaluation through a systems lens.

Complex Systems Characteristics

The term *system* has been defined in numerous ways. A very simple definition is that a system is a delineated part of the universe that is distinguished from the rest by an imaginary boundary (Bar-Yam 2004). Once the boundary is defined, the properties of the system, the universe, and the interactions or interrelationships of the system with its universe can be described. Meadows defines a system as "a set of things—people, cells, molecules, or whatever—interconnected in such a way that they produce their own pattern of behavior over time" (Meadows and Wright 2009).

In this chapter, two sample systems, water and an individual human, will be used to illustrate key concepts that differentiate simple, complicated, and complex systems. Although complex in some ways, water also exhibits some of the characteristics of simple or complicated systems. It is made up of identical (homogeneous) molecules that include one oxygen and two hydrogen atoms combined through a chemical bond (H_2O). Water molecules interact with each other mostly in a random (stochastic) way, and when they interact with their "universe," or external environment, some of the characteristics or resulting behaviors are predictable (deterministic; e.g., water turns to steam at standard temperature and pressure), though not all of them (e.g., it forms varying snowflake patterns).

Individual people, in contrast, are highly complex systems. In addition to being 60%–70% water, the human body is made up of trillions of cells of many different types that perform lots of different functions. Together, these cells enable characteristic behaviors such as locomotion, digestion, and cognition, but across a population (or populations) variations in genes and environment give rise to huge variation in behavior. Time also makes human behavior difficult to understand because our past influences our future behavior.

Thus, systems can be simple, complicated, or complex, and the complexity within the systems of relevance to health behavior change can vary considerably. Bar-Yam (2004) defines a

complex system as a system in which the function and behavior of the whole system cannot be deduced from the behavior of the individual parts. But the definitions of *complex system* or *complex adaptive system* vary considerably in the literature. Wallis (2008) suggests that no single, shared sense of meaning exists.

Theories and strategies for behavior change in individuals and populations have, in some cases, recognized some of the characteristics of complex systems such as nonlinearity, time-dependence, and heterogeneity, but they have mostly ignored important ideas like emergence, feedback, **adaptation**, and **self-organization**. These are still early days in the effort to improve our understanding of many of the characteristics that make behavior change in populations complex. Some data and modeling has been used to focus on feedback loops and self-organization, but much more effort is needed across a range of health behaviors. We also need new tools to help us measure, study, and intervene with variables that may affect system-level behavior, such as trust, **social capital**, resilience, and complexity. For the purposes of this chapter, a complex system will be taken as one that includes at least some of the characteristics listed above and in table 21.1. Many of the characteristics of water make it a relatively simple or complicated system, whereas individual people and populations are much more complex.

Heterogeneity

Heterogeneous systems are systems with a large number of structural variations. The system structure consists of all of the elements that make up the system as a whole, including the subsystems, actors, and interconnections between these elements. In *homogeneous systems,* the structural elements tend to be identical or indistinguishable, such as the H_2O molecules that make up a glass of water. In complex systems, the structural units are heterogeneous.

TABLE 21.1. Characteristics of simple or complicated versus complex systems

Simple or complicated systems	Complex systems
Homogeneous	Heterogeneous
Linear	Nonlinear
Deterministic	Stochastic/ unpredictable
Static	Dynamic
Independent	Interdependent
No feedback	Feedback
Not adaptive or self-organizing	Adaptive and self-organizing
No connection between levels or subsystems	Emergence

Populations can be considered complex in that they are made up of individuals who are distinguishable on many different levels and in many different ways (Lieberson 1969). Among specific populations in a geographical region, there may be some homogeneity based on common social, cultural, and environmental practices, but within and between population groups, considerable heterogeneity usually exists.

Heterogeneity is important to understanding health behaviors, such as the behavior of patients and their **compliance** with medical regimens. Consider the heterogeneity of patients by diagnosis and its effect on patient compliance with various medical regimens such as taking prescribed medications (Roter et al. 1998). The magnitude of the "effect size" for the interventions considered in Roter and colleagues' meta-analysis ranged from small ($r = 0.10$) to large ($r = 0.73$), and effect sizes varied considerably among individuals with different diagnoses. Effect sizes for taking prescribed medications were high for those with diabetes and weaker for patients with asthma, cancer, hypertension, and mental illness. The authors speculated that studies with larger effect sizes

tended to involve smaller populations and that the populations were therefore more homogeneous and the interventions more tailored to the specific population. This suggests that by reducing the heterogeneity of the **target population**, especially interventions that are applied equally to all (rather than being tailored to each individual) are more likely to be successful. This also suggests that *unless* a patient population is fairly homogeneous, standardized behavioral interventions are unlikely to be uniformly effective.

Heterogeneity is important in health behavior change interventions not only because the targets of change are heterogeneous, but also because the elements of the system involved in delivering the intervention are likely to be heterogeneous, and that heterogeneity affects outcomes. The heterogeneity occurs at various levels of scale within the system. In Canadian schools, for example, school-level tobacco control strategies and policies vary considerably. Factors such as policy intention, policy implementation, and number of students smoking on school property can all act as determinants of smoking behavior in students in grades 10 and 11. Student behavior is also diverse at the individual level, where variables such as students' perceived level of connectedness to their school and the number of members of an individual's family who smoke also determine smoking behavior (Sabiston et al. 2009).

Program interventions are also heterogeneous when implemented in the real world, and little is known about the nature or impact of this heterogeneity. Many interventions have a common foundation, such as tobacco cessation quit lines (see chapter 10), which are generally based on the principle of multisession proactive counseling, but delivery models vary considerably. In the case of quit lines, factors vary, such as the number of hours of operation, languages available, specific type of services offered, level of training of counselors, and level of funding (Cummins et al. 2007). The impact of heterogeneity in intervention delivery parameters on the **effectiveness** of interventions is largely unexplored.

Nonlinearity

A *linear relationship* is one in which a change in variable A leads to a constant proportional change in variable B; if a small change in A leads to a small change in B, then a large change in A leads to a large change in B. In other words, a graph of B versus A can be represented by a straight line. A **nonlinear relationship** is one in which the effect is not proportional to the cause; even if a small change in A causes a small change in B, a large change in A might cause B to go up, or down, or even stay constant. In this scenario, the relationship between B and A cannot be represented by a straight line.

Some models of behavior change attempt to describe change with linear relationships between variables like knowledge, attitudes, and behavior (see "Focus on the Individual," below) (Resnicow and Vaughan 2006). But evidence shows that many behavior changes, such as quitting smoking (West 2007), going on a diet (Ogden et al. 2009), or relapsing from abstinence (Hufford et al. 2003), are nonlinear functions of the variables that contribute to the behavior. In the case of smoking cessation, West and Sohal (2006) demonstrate that cessation is not linearly dependent on planning and that most successful quit attempts are unplanned and appear to be spontaneous. Similarly, individuals who have been successful in losing a large amount of weight and keeping it off for an extended period of time often report that a "trigger" prompted them to initiate weight loss (Ogden et al. 2009). **Triggers** are often described as vague decisions to "just do it" (Klem et al. 1997). Triggers may also be associated with specific life events such as relationship problems, a birthday, or illness. Ogden and co-workers (2009) also observed that the same trigger may lead to different outcomes for different individuals; for

example, relationship problems were associated with both weight loss and weight gain. If triggers can be powerful at the level of the individual, they will also have significant impact on the behavior of populations.

Resnicow and Vaughan suggest that the many nonlinear relationships that contribute to behavior change make it "chaotic" and difficult to predict; as a result, they argue, linear models of behavior change are "both conceptually inappropriate and statistically futile" (Resnicow and Vaughan 2006). Instead, they suggest that we need a new **theory** for behavior change that recognizes these nonlinearities and leads to the development of more appropriate interventions. Some authors have called for more research to understand the importance of nonlinearities (Brug 2006), whereas others have begun to explore the role of nonlinearities in individual responses to treatment (Hayes et al. 2007). Green described a range of nonlinearities in the dynamic response to health education programs. These nonlinearities, including "delay of impact," "decay of impact," and "borrowing from the future," make it difficult to design interventions and the protocols for measurement and evaluation of their impact (Green 1977).

Unpredictability

A **stochastic process** is one in which an element of randomness leads to a degree of uncertainty about the outcome. In contrast, a *deterministic process* is one in which the same result always occurs for a given set of circumstances. Deterministic systems behave in a predictable way, whereas stochastic systems are less predictable. Stochastic systems in some instances are considered **probabilistic**; that is, the behavior of the system cannot be predicted exactly, but the probability of certain behaviors is known.

For water at the level of individual molecules, the movement of any given molecule is stochastic or random, but the behavior of a group of H_2O molecules at sea level is deterministic—it will always turn from liquid to gas when the temperature hits 100°C. In individual people, the development of a particular disease usually depends on both predictable and unpredictable factors. For example, smoking increases the risk of developing lung cancer, but not everyone who smokes gets the disease. Likewise, obesity increases the risk of developing diabetes, but not all obese people become diabetic. Disease development has both deterministic and stochastic elements (Levy et al. 2010; Plevritis et al. 2006).

The probabilistic or stochastic nature of health behavior change in response to some stimuli or interventions is well recognized. Also well known is that the degree of certainty in most predictive models of behavior change is rather low. In general, it has been considered acceptable to publish models that account for only 10% to 20% of the variance in behavior. Models accounting for more than 50% are rare (Baranowski et al. 1999; Roter et al. 1998). So, although few would argue that behavior change is deterministic, a debate is emerging regarding the interpretation of the "unpredictable" portion of behavior and what to do about it. Baranowski argues that we are just not doing a good enough job of pinning down all the causal factors and need to work harder, whereas Resnicow and colleagues suggest that we need new ways of thinking about behavior change—that is, we need new models and tools that accept the **unpredictability** of behavior change (Baranowski 2006; Resnicow and Page 2008; Resnicow and Vaughan 2006).

Dynamics

In **dynamic systems**, change in the state of the system happens over time, and the past has an impact on the future. Complex systems are often time dependent and have properties like growth and death, which are dynamic processes. In *static systems,* nothing changes over time; time is not an important variable.

Consider water in a glass or a pond. Although at the microscopic level, the water molecules are moving at all times, their motion is completely random, and the behavior of the water at the macroscopic level essentially does not change over time. This is a relatively static system. When water flows, it is more dynamic. Glass and McAtee use an analogy of flowing water to describe the health behavior of an individual; an individual's "sphere of health-related behavior and action moves through time from infancy to old age," and the trajectory of the sphere is influenced by opportunities and constraints (to the flow) posed by external environments and the expression of biological systems (Glass and McAtee 2006).

The dynamic nature of behavior change in populations was well described by Rogers in his work on **diffusion of innovation** (see chapter 7). Rogers described the dynamics of diffusion as starting slowly among **innovators** and early adopters, then accelerating as the middle majority adopt the **innovation**, and finally slowing down when only the laggards remain (Rogers 2003). Each adopter's willingness and ability to adopt an innovation depends on a variety of factors including the person's awareness, interest, evaluation, and trial of the innovation.

Green points out that the dynamic nature of a population's response to health education interventions makes it difficult to measure their outcomes and determine their impact. In his example of borrowing from the future, the dynamic response to a trigger of health information may in the short term look quite positive. Mass media campaigns have been shown, for example, to cause an increase the number of people recruited into screening or family planning clinics. But in the long term, these interventions may not always increase the number of patients recruited overall; they just shorten the time interval over which patients present themselves to the clinic (which could have the unintended consequence of making the flow of new patients also highly variable) (Green

1977). A better understanding of dynamics could improve both the design and evaluation of interventions.

Interdependency

Interdependence of the elements in a complex system refers to the "level of connectedness" of the parts of the system. Interdependence is a characteristic that often makes it difficult to predict the impact of changing one part of the system. If the elements of the system are *independent* or simply connected and *not interdependent,* then removing a part of the system will have little or no effect on the part removed or the remaining parts (Bar-Yam 2004). Consider, for example, the removal of a drop of water from a glass of water; the properties of the drop and of the rest of the water in the glass are not changed very much.

If, however, the elements of a system are interdependent, then pushing on or removing one part could have a strong effect in another area of the system. Consider again human form and function. Removal of some parts of the human body will have little or no effect on other functions (e.g., hair, a fingernail, or a toe); removal of other parts will have an effect on some functions and not others (e.g., removal of a leg will affect locomotion but not digestion); and some parts of the human system are so interdependent that their removal will affect all other subsystems (e.g., the heart or the brain).

Biological science struggles with the complexity of intact organisms and the highly interconnected nature of biological control mechanisms (Goh et al. 2007). The usual paradigm in biological science is reductionist, and it requires controlling as many variables as possible to be able to see where there are important causal relationships. Reductionist approaches in basic science include the creation of "knock-out" and "transgenic" mice, in which the expression of a particular gene is prevented or added. Although the motivation behind these methods is to iso-

late the impact or function of a single gene, the results are often surprising, with single genes affecting multiple systems and multiple genes being responsible for a single phenotype or characteristic biological response (Goh et al. 2007; Kirchner et al. 2010).

The **Foresight system map** for obesity illustrate complexity on a broader, social scale and suggests that many elements in the environment that influence behavior are interconnected (figure 21.1) (Finegood et al. 2010; Vandenbroeck et al. 2007). Food consumption depends on food production, food consumption influences physiology, and social psychology affects individual psychology (Finegood et al. 2010). Although the Foresight map nicely illustrates the importance of interconnections, little has been done to assess the actual levels of interdependence in the obesity system. In the case of tobacco control (see chapter 10), interdependencies were explored through the building of a causal map and model (Best et al. 2007). Using **system dynamics** methods, researchers explored the importance of various factors, such as public opinion, research, knowledge dissemination, and government intervention, for the prevalence of smokers from 1965 through to 2020. Interestingly, public opinion was found to have a substantial effect on the prevalence of smoking, but it also had the unintended consequence of decreasing the amount of translational research undertaken. This interdependency was a function of the increased demand by the public for more research, but what was desired was a shift in the type of research away from **knowledge translation** and toward more basic science (the kind of research the general public thinks of as research).

Interdependence makes it difficult to ascertain the direct cause and effect relationships that make a problem complex, and it suggests that solutions need to be comprehensive. In a system with many interdependencies (such as the obesity system described by the Foresight map), isolated action in one part of the system

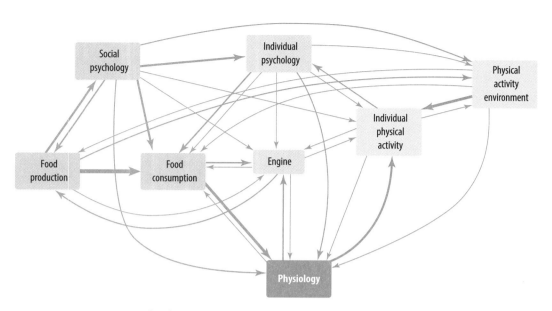

FIGURE 21.1. Foresight obesity system map. *Source:* Vandenbroeck et al. 2007. Reprinted with permission of the Foresight Programme, UK Government Office for Science.

is unlikely to have great impact, owing to all the other influences on each variable and the presence of interdependencies, including **balancing feedback loops**. A systems approach, like a population health approach, would suggest that multiple complementary points of intervention are necessary and may even be synergistic. The apparent success of the France-based EPODE model (which translates to "Together, Let's Prevent Childhood Obesity") is likely due to its comprehensive approach (Romon et al. 2009). The value of a comprehensive approach has been well demonstrated through our experience in tobacco control (Cokkinides et al. 2009).

Interdependence might also be a complex systems characteristic that can be exploited to create change. Bar-Yam describes the important relationship between *competition* at one level and its need for *cooperation* at a lower level. In sports, the effectiveness of a competitive team is often dependent on the degree of cooperation among team members; likewise, competitive companies are more likely to have highly cooperative staff (Bar-Yam 2003). The province of

British Columbia stimulated cooperation by creating a competition for project funds among all ministries of the government (Geneau et al. 2009). The competition resulted in a large number of cooperative projects, which included multiple ministries and created a novel approach to influencing health outcomes. The relationship between competition and cooperation is sufficiently powerful that a key recommendation in Bar-Yam's suggestions for health care reform is to "empower workgroup competition"; if established at the right level, workgroup competition will lead to cooperation among the actors who need to work together to create change (Bar-Yam et al. 2013).

Feedback

The presence of feedback loops is a key feature of complex systems, and they are of two major types. Feedback loops create a closed chain of causal connection (e.g., an increase in A leads to an increase in B, but the increase in B in turn leads to a decrease in A). This is called a *nega-*

tive, or **balancing feedback loop** because it tends to cause stability in the system. For example, the National Weight Control Registry project established by Hill and Wing has collected data on what characteristics and factors contribute to long-term weight loss maintenance. One of the key findings is that people who successfully maintain a long-term weight loss weigh themselves frequently (Butryn et al. 2007), possibly because when an individual observes a small increase in his weight, he adjusts food intake and physical activity behaviors to induce weight loss. An increase in weight (variable A) leads to a decrease in food intake (variable B), which in turn reduces weight back to the desired stable level.

Alternatively, *positive,* or **reinforcing feedback loops** tend to amplify or enhance systems change. A reinforcing loop can encourage growth in a system, where an increase in A leads to an increase in B, and the increase in B then tends to cause a further increase in A. An example of a reinforcing loop from the Foresight map is that the "demand for convenience" leads to increased "convenience of food offerings," which leads to "deskilling" (i.e., loss of food preparation and cooking skills), which, in turn, increases the "demand for convenience" (Vandenbroeck et al. 2007). Reinforcing loops can be characterized as either *vicious* or *virtuous* for the overall well-being of the system, depending on which direction the system is pushed. The relative dominance of balancing and reinforcing loops will determine the overall stability of the system and whether vicious or virtuous reinforcing feedback loops will take over and push the system in a particular direction. These feedback loops are a hallmark of complexity; simple or complicated systems tend to have few feedback loops.

Feedback loops abound in the Foresight obesity system map (Vandenbroeck et al. 2007). In an analysis of this map, we identified more than 100 feedback loops with as few as two and up to as many as 17 variables in a given loop (Fine-

good et al. 2010). A preliminary analysis of the types of loops suggests that reinforcing loops greatly outnumber balancing loops (data not shown). For example, stress and perceived lack of time have positive influences on each other (perceived lack of time increases stress levels, and increased levels of stress cause a further increase in perceived lack of time; this is an example of a vicious cycle). In contrast, **walkability** of neighborhoods and the dominance of motorized transport have reciprocal negative influences on each other (as the dominance of motorized transport increases, the walkability of neighborhoods decreases, leading to further need for and dominance of motorized transport). The high number of reinforcing feedback loops in the Foresight map may help to explain the emergence of obesity as a prevalent condition in most populations and may also help explain its apparent resistance to our current levels of intervention.

Adaptation and Self-Organization

Adaptation and **self-organization** refer to the ability of a system to arrange itself, to create new structures, to learn by responding to the environment in which it is situated, and to diversify. Self-organization occurs through the interactions of the elements of the system rather than through some central authority or control mechanism.

Water changes in response to its environment by becoming a solid or a vapor. The relative simplicity of water as a system means that these changes are fairly deterministic, and their impact on the environment is fairly predictable. The subsystems that make up individual human beings, in contrast, are very complex and afford a range of levels of adaptability and self-organization. Stem cells are a good example of a highly adaptive, self-organized biological subsystem without central control (Halley et al. 2009). Populations are also highly adaptable, self-organized systems that respond to changes in their environment and also have significant impact on the shape of the context in which they live. Society is still rooted in the notion of central control (e.g., governments), and the institutions and organizations we have built struggle to adapt and respond to longer-term changes in the environment (Bar-Yam 2002).

In population-level interventions, the notions of adaptation and self-organization of the larger system are often discouraged or ignored in an effort to maintain fidelity (Dumas et al. 2001). As a result, information about how the defined intervention is adapted in real-world settings and how adaptation affects the outcomes is usually not available (Green 2006). Hawe and colleagues argue that we need to redefine what standardization means in controlled trials (Hawe, Shiell, and Riley 2004). In complex interventions, the *function* and *process* of the intervention should be standardized rather than the components themselves. These authors suggest that rather than having design standardized by form (e.g., all sites distribute the same information kit to patients), they should be standardized by function (e.g., all sites devise ways to distribute information tailored to local literacy, language, culture, and learning styles). This approach promotes and supports self-organization and adaptation rather than trying to control it.

Cohen and colleagues looked at the trade-offs between fidelity and **flexibility** in a real-time, cross-case comparison of 10 interventions designed to improve health promotion in primary care practices in practice-based research networks (Cohen et al. 2008). They found that all of the interventions required changes as they were integrated into practice. They concluded that change is common and that dissemination and implementation will improve when our approach shifts to focus on quality improvement. The only one of the 10 interventions in their study that reported requiring no changes when integrated into practice was the

one that was initially and intentionally designed to support adaptation.

Rigidity inhibits adaptation and self-organization, and this compromises resilience and the long-term health and survival of a system. Bar-Yam highlights the importance of building systems that support and promote adaptation with his recommendation to "empower workgroup competition" as part of health care reform (Bar-Yam et al. 2013). With a systems approach, our natural tendency to want to control adaptation gives way to the need for structures and processes that support self-organization at the level in which people can be empowered to make real change. We are only at the very beginning of creating the structures and processes necessary to support adaptation and self-organization among the actors working to improve public health.

Emergence

As with the term *complex adaptive system,* no consensus exists on the definition of *emergence.* Emergent behavior is collective behavior that cannot be simply inferred from the behavior of individual system components. Although emergence is collective behavior that is contained in the behavior of the parts, the parts must be studied within the context of the whole. Bar-Yam suggests that what is important about emergence is neither the parts nor the whole but rather the relationship between the details of the system and the larger view. In trying to explain the property of emergence, he uses the saying "You can't see the forest for the trees." If you focus only on the details of the individual components (e.g., the trees, the soil, or the animals), you risk missing the bigger picture. If you focus only on the forest, you run the risk of missing the aspects of trees that give rise to the behavior of the forest, and so forth (Bar-Yam 2004). Being able to zoom in and out is necessary to understanding emergence.

Consider again the Foresight obesity system map (Vandenbroeck et al. 2007). That map was built through the engagement of a wide range of **stakeholders**. The overriding message of the map is that the problem is complex and involves many different factors associated with both the individual and her environment. The specific variables that make up the map and the relative importance of different clusters of variables, such as those influencing food production and physical activity environments, are not really discernible. However, when we "zoom out" on the map, as we did to create a "reduced" map, new details emerge (Finegood et al. 2010). The reduced map, for example, suggests that the stakeholders involved perceived a significant effect of food production on food consumption. This connection appears to be substantial, though it may reflect the biases of the participants in the processes. It may be that some of the actors involved in these two clusters (e.g., people who work in the food industry) were under-represented.

Little has been written about the notion of emergence as it relates to health behavior change. We have argued that obesity is an emergent property of the system depicted in the Foresight map (Finegood 2011). Wolitski has used the term *emergence* to describe the rise of barebacking (intentional unprotected anal sex) among gay and bisexual men in the United States (Wolitski 2005). Individually, causal factors such as improvements in human immuno-deficiency (HIV) treatment, knowledge of a partners HIV status and the **relative risks** of specific acts the rise of Internet use, substance use, and changes in HIV prevention programs do not explain the rise in barebacking, but together, they give rise to the phenomenon. In analyzing if schools that claim to be "health-promoting" function as complex adaptive systems, Keshavarz and colleagues suggest that the overall collective behavior and health-promoting nature of the school are the emergent products of the in-terplay of many different factors, such as rules, interactions, information, values context, and time (Keshavarz et al. 2010).

Clearly, new methods and tools are needed if we are going to make progress in understanding and using the characteristic of emergence. Wheatley and Frieze argue that emergence can be used to **scale up** social innovations by deliberately influencing the process as it moves through its life cycle (Wheatley and Frieze 2006). The life cycle of emergence begins with networks of people who share a common cause around a particular problem or social change. When support and resources are provided for these networks to act as cooperative teams and connect with other networks, they can grow into intentional communities. These communities are likely smaller subsets of the people involved in individual networks; they form among the individuals who are committed not only to their own agendas but also to serving the needs of others. Ultimately, from healthy and vibrant communities emerge systems of influence where change may be rapid and a shift in the dominance of some feedback loops may occur. By connecting and supporting social innovation occurring on a small scale in disparate networks, more intentional communities can be formed and are the nucleus for change on a larger scale.

Systems Thinking and Models of Behavior Change

Theories of behavior change have evolved from giving rise to simple or complicated individual-level or environmental-level interventions to including more and more aspects of complexity. We now recognize the need for more complex system models, which examine key elements of complexity with respect to psychological, biological, social, cultural, and **built environment** factors (Foster-Fishman and Behrens 2007). Some of the methodologies of **systems science** are helping to integrate these details to enhance understanding of the behavior of whole systems.

Focus on the Individual

Models of health behavior change that form the basis for most past and current interventions have evolved considerably over the past 30 years. The earliest theories of health behavior change were focused on the individual. Change would occur if an individual's knowledge, attitudes, and beliefs were modified, and active interventions required voluntary and sustained effort to achieve success (Stokols 1996). These psychological models have been broadly classified as continuum (e.g., **Theory of Planned Behavior**, **Health Belief Model**) and stage models of behavior change (e.g., **Transtheoretical Model**, **Precaution Adoption Process Model**). In **continuum models**, the general approach is to identify variables that influence action, such as knowledge, attitudes, perceptions of risk, and perceptions of benefit, and to combine them into a predictive equation. The value generated by the equation for a particular individual indicates a given probability that the person will act, which places each individual along an ordered and predictable continuum of likelihood to act. Weinstein and colleagues argue that because each theory has only a single prediction equation, the way in which variables combine to influence action is expected to be the same for everyone (Weinstein et al. 1998). As such, behavior in these models is considered deterministic. Baranowski suggests they should be labeled probabilistic, because the equation usually has an error term, unless "we could account for 100% of the variance" (Baranowski 2006). The level of variance provides some index of the degree to which the model is deterministic. In addition, the fact that most models are linear combinations of independent variables also contributes to their being considered simple or somewhat complicated models.

Stage models of behavior change attempt to deal with some of the heterogeneity of individuals by suggesting that people pass through **Stages of Change** and can be classified into a limited number of categories based upon their phase during the change process. In stage models, such as the transtheoretical model, the members of a given stage have attributes that define that stage. For example, smokers who had no intention to quit within the next six months were classified as being in **precontemplation**, those who were intending to quit but had not tried for at least 24 hours in the past year were considered to be in **contemplation**, and those who intended to quit and had tried for more than 24 hours in the past year were considered to be in **preparation** (DiClemente et al. 1991). Although assignment to a particular stage does not define the population in that stage as entirely homogeneous, it attempts to account for heterogeneity in a population by suggesting that there are smaller differences among people in the same stage as compared to relatively large differences between people in different stages (Weinstein et al. 1998). The ordered stages also help to define common barriers to change facing people in each stage, such as differences in **self-efficacy** (DiClemente et al. 1991; Marshall and Biddle 2001). Although the proponents of these models acknowledge that people do not necessarily move through these stages in a linear fashion, this model is still an attempt to describe behavior change as deterministic and rational (West 2005). The result is a continued belief that behavior change is predictable if we can simply identify the most important variables and classify individuals in relatively homogeneous groups.

Focus on the Environment

Another class of models on which interventions have been based are models in which the quality of people's physical and **social environments** is the focus of attention. Here the intervention approach is to improve environmental hygiene or safety and to strengthen **social supports** for health. Stokols describes these as **passive interventions**, insofar as enhancing and restructuring environments does not require the individuals exposed in them to *do* anything (Stokols 1996). These models are based in theoretical and research approaches such as industrial hygiene, injury prevention, occupational epidemiology, facilities design and management, and environmental health science.

But, as Stokols points out, these models pay little attention to the sociodemographic characteristics of the people occupying particular places and settings (Stokols 1996). As such, these models neglect the individual and group differences in people's responses to their environments (i.e., the *interaction* individuals have with their environments). Clearly, the lack of consideration of interdependencies and feedback loops makes these relatively simple models as well. If they take into account multiple dimensions of the environment, they might be considered complicated, but probably not complex.

Focus on Complexity

The social-ecological approach recognizes that both individuals and their environments are important determinants of behavior change (Lounsbury and Mitchell 2009). **Social Ecological Models** accept that individuals have a variety of personal attributes (genetic, psychological, behavioral) that interact in a dynamic fashion with attributes of the environment (physical, social, cultural). Stokols suggests that the social-ecological approach requires a focus on the degree of fit between individuals' needs and the resources available to them (Stokols 1996). This is similar to Bar-Yam's notion that, in complex systems, individuals matter and it is important to match their capacity to the complexity of their task (Bar-Yam 2004; Finegood 2011).

Glass and McAtee push social-ecological models further into the realm of complexity by suggesting that we need new metaphors and models to integrate the many variables that affect health and disease. They introduce a general approach that attempts to include both the individual, with his context, and his interactions over his life course. Their framework includes a nested hierarchy of **individual-level factors** from genes, to cells, to organs, to social networks, to the global environment. They suggest that we learn to apply the metaphor of an individual in her sphere of environments flowing through life with various bumps and valleys along the way (Glass and McAtee 2006). Although the figure depicting the model does not convey the importance of feedback loops, they acknowledge that feedback and interaction must be important components of new theories of behavior change.

In the example of obesity, the International Obesity Task Force introduced a **causal web**, which positioned the individual or the population level of energy intake and energy expenditure to the right of a series of environmental influences ordered in proximity to the individual, including influences in work, school, and home environments and influences at community or locality, national, and international levels (Kumanyika 2001). Introduced more than 10 years ago, this model helped to shift the paradigm in obesity research from a focus on the individual to a focus on the many-layered environment. The Foresight map, which was introduced more recently, incorporates many of the same concepts as the causal web (e.g., the importance of physical activity, food, and social environments), but it illustrates them in such a way that the connections dominate the image, not the individual variables or sectors of the environment that influence food and physical activity behavior (Vandenbroeck et al. 2007). The causal web is a good illustration of obesity as *complicated,* whereas the Foresight map illustrates the problem as *complex.*

Resnicow and colleagues have called for new models that recognize the "quantum" and "chaotic" nature of individual behavior change (Resnicow and Page 2008; Resnicow and Vaughan 2006). They suggest that enduring behavior change is unplanned. West and Sohal also suggest that we need to account for behavior changes that "just arrive" and are associated with motivational statements like "I just decided to do it" (West 2007; West and Sohal 2006). The push to accept these characteristics of complexity in models of behavior change has provoked some to argue that we need to improve the quality of research (Baranowski 2006) and that the implications of considering complexity are limited (Brug 2006). West argues that we need to recognize the artificial nature of staging people's intentions and accept the fact that although decision making has a rational component, it also depends on reward and punishment, **habit**, and processes that operate outside of conscious awareness (West 2005). Although social-ecological models were the first to embrace some aspects of complexity, these quantum, or chaotic models push further into the realm of complex adaptive systems. Much more work will need to be done to understand and apply systems thinking as a basis for interventions to improve health behavior in populations.

Computational Approaches

In the current era, social-ecological models are evolving from their origin as conceptual models into computational, mathematical, and simulation models. The growth in computing capacity over the past few decades is making it easier to apply modeling methods to social issues like education, psychology, and health (Hawe et al. 2009). **Systems science** includes a variety of **computational approaches** such as system dynamics and micro-simulation as well as **agent**-based and multilevel modeling (Levy et al. 2010). Each method has particular advantages and disadvantages and should be used for different kinds of questions and under different circumstances, depending on the purpose of the model and the type of data available to inform model building. More work is called for in this intersection between systems science and public health (Leischow and Milstein 2006; Mabry et al. 2008).

Although a detailed description of these methods is beyond the scope of this chapter, we use the specific case of obesity to illustrate the potential for computational approaches to understanding health behavior in populations. System dynamics and **microsimulation modeling** have been used extensively to project into the future the prevalence of obesity in specific populations and to consider the impact of interventions on prevalence rates and projected costs (Levy et al. 2010; McPherson et al. 2007). Interventions are usually tested in a general way (e.g., by reducing caloric imbalance) rather than by modeling a specific intervention (e.g., bariatric surgery, a "walking school bus"), but these models provide important insights about the dynamics of change. Homer and colleagues demonstrated that even if caloric imbalance returned to 1970 levels in everyone, it would take many years to reduce the prevalence of obesity, and only targeting children would have a very small impact on the prevalence of adult obesity (Homer et al. 2006). This type of modeling underpins the Accessing Cost Effectiveness work on obesity (ACE Obesity) and other ACE projects, in which more specific comparisons were made (Ananthapavan et al. 2010; Carter et al. 2009; Vos et al. 2005; Vos et al. 2010).

Network analysis and **network simulation** have also been used to explore the importance of social interactions in the development of obesity. Christakis and Fowler (2007) used data from the Framingham study to build a model of the social networks of friends and to explore the development of obesity. Their analysis demonstrated that individuals with obese friends had a higher risk of subsequently developing obesity. Bahr and colleagues (2009) used network simulations to examine weight loss interventions and the importance of social networks. Hammond (2008) has advocated for agent-based modeling as a strategy to study obesity. He suggests that it would permit modeling of multiple mechanisms simultaneously, across several levels of scale, with inclusion of important sources of diversity. One challenge with these types of models will be the lack of sufficient data on individual agent decision making (Johnson-Askew et al. 2009).

The Institute of Medicine (IOM) recently called for the use of systems perspectives and methodologies in defining the problem of obesity so that more effective decisions can be made in prevention and population intervention. The IOM notes that "the demand for results-oriented research is gradually forcing a shift beyond linear models to models that also address the dynamic, multilevel complexity of real-world contexts" and that a systems approach can help to highlight the broader context, to consider interactions among levels and the dynamic shifts that occur over time (Kumanyika et al. 2010).

A Paradigm Shift to Solutions Fit for Complex Problems

Common responses to complex social problems tend toward frustration, despair, disillusionment, retreat, and belief that the problem is beyond hope (Bar-Yam 2004; Plsek and Greenhalgh 2001). We want to look for someone to blame, or we focus on simple solutions. More than 35 years ago, Rittel and Webber (1973) suggested that we cannot continue to tackle complex problems by assuming that through analyzing the component systems we will be able to identify root causes and then fix the problem. They point out that the most intractable problem is that of defining and locating the problem in the first place (i.e., finding where in complex causal networks the trouble really lies). Characteristics like heterogeneity, interdependence, feedback, and adaptation make many social problems "wicked" problems, and wicked

problems are challenging because they have no definitive formulation and no stopping rules, and there is no ultimate test of a solution. As Sterman (2006) suggests, we lack meaningful systems thinking capabilities.

To truly embrace the notion of complexity and adopt a solution-oriented approach, our mental models will have to help us shed dependence on **causality** and shift to complexity as a way of knowing. This shift will require new metaphors, or a paradigm shift, in how we think about and value different types of research and evaluation (Glasgow 2008). Rather than searching for identification of what causes *problems*, Robinson and Sirard argue, we need to look for what causes the *solutions*. Solution-oriented science can still be rigorous science with appropriate hypotheses that can be tested. They suggest that hypotheses need to shift from a "past" orientation to a "future" orientation, which focuses on understanding what works and what does not work to solve problems. Robinson and Sirard (2005) suggest that the solution-oriented research paradigm encourages research with more immediate relevance to human health and a shortened cycle of discovery from the laboratory to the patient and the population.

Hawe and colleagues are also questioning the dominant paradigm for how randomized controlled trial design is being applied to community interventions (Hawe, Shiell, and Riley 2004; Hawe, Shiell, Riley, and Gold 2004). The current paradigm has "control" placed over the intervention (i.e., the intervention needs to be the same in different places), and this is thought to be of paramount importance, but it may also be why large-scale trials have mostly had weak effects. Hawe and colleagues point out that shifting the notion of what is standardized, from *form* to *function,* would have a dramatic impact on the questions that are addressed by the research and evaluation team (Hawe, Shiell, and Riley 2004). As noted above, this would be a way of refocusing the **objective** of the measurement process to support adaptation, without compromising the integrity of the study. Hawe argues that the key is to define study integrity functionally rather than compositionally.

Like the terms *complex adaptive system* and *emergence,* **systems thinking** has a wide range of meanings. Cabrera and colleagues suggest that the term is ambiguous, although there have been many attempts to describe it (Cabrera et al. 2008). Some describe it as synonymous with *systems science,* whereas others view systems thinking as a **taxonomy** (a "laundry list" of approaches). So how can we get our head wrapped around a meaning for systems thinking and start to apply it more to improve how we solve problems? In the next section, two **conceptual frameworks** are presented, distilled from the pioneering work of two particular systems thinkers with a solution orientation, Donella Meadows and Yaneer Bar-Yam.

Places to Intervene

In the late 1990s, Donella Meadows described 12 **leverage points**, or places to intervene, in a complex system (Meadows 1999; Meadows and Wright 2009). This list was developed out of her desire to move toward solutions and her frustration that, in complex systems, the leverage points people tend to pick are usually wrong. She argued that true leverage points are often counterintuitive and therefore difficult to locate. Her generic list of ordered leverage points goes from the lowest level, consisting of things that are easy to change and tend to have a small effect on the system as a whole (e.g., elements of the system, such as numbers of physicians or health information), to the things that are higher up in the system and are much more difficult to change but can have a very large effect on the system (e.g., the paradigm under which the system operates and system **goals**). It provides a generic framework for all complex systems.

We sought to use Meadows's ideas in the development of a framework that could serve as a tool in research and evaluation. Our initial effort was to use her 12 leverage points to sort recommendations to address childhood obesity and chronic disease prevention that were made by the participants attending a conference on childhood obesity. This experience suggested that 12 levels were too many to provide a useful and reliable framework (Malhi 2009). Through an **iterative process**, we settled on a five-level framework that could be used reliably to sort action statements for change in complex systems. The five levels correspond roughly to broader groups of Meadows's 12 levels mentioned above: (1) paradigm, (2) goals, (3) system structure, (4) feedback loops and delays, and (5) structural elements (Malhi et al. 2009).

Since the development of the Intervention Level Framework in 2009, we have successfully applied it in several different ways. In one project we used the framework to examine a series of papers prepared for a conference on food systems and public health (Malhi et al. 2009; Story et al. 2009). In this exercise, content was first sorted according to the four conference themes: food systems that are healthful, green, fair, and affordable. Then the content was sorted again according to the framework. By using the framework to order this content, places where advocates for food systems agree and disagree became quickly apparent. For example, advocates of healthful and green food systems would agree on many of the structural elements needed, including reducing the use of pesticides and implementing other practices that are ecologically sound. In contrast, the advocates of green and affordable food systems conflict at the highest levels of intervention (e.g., the paradigm under which the system operates and the goals that derive from the paradigm). Specifically, in a green food system, prices would reflect the costs of toxic exposure, environmental cleanup, and depletion of natural resources, including fuel to transport the food long distances, yet an affordable food system would structure the price of healthful food so that it is affordable to the lowest income groups regardless of the environmental costs. By putting advocated solutions into a systems framework, new insights on characteristics, such as interdependence, and identification of gaps in feedback will support the development of novel system-oriented solutions.

The Intervention Level Framework is also being applied to sort recommendations to address childhood obesity, to sort qualitative data from families and clinical professionals on the barriers to and supports for weight loss, and to examine perspectives of multiple system actors on the prevention and management of obesity (Johnston et al. 2010; Matteson et al. 2010). Given the general nature of this framework, we anticipate that it will have many other applications, including program planning and evaluation of complex interventions.

Making Things Work

Another leading systems thinker has also forwarded the agenda of devising solutions based on some fundamental principles that arise out of complex systems. Yaneer Bar-Yam describes his experience solving complex problems in health care, education, the military, international development, and ethnic violence in his book *Making Things Work* (Bar-Yam 2004). Although Bar-Yam does not codify or provide a taxonomy of solutions, we distilled a simple descriptive set of actions from his summaries of what has worked based on his experience (Finegood 2006, 2011).

An important concept put forward by Bar-Yam is one that may seem counterintuitive; in a complex system individuals *do* matter. In particular, the individual's capacity to act and the complexity of his task need to be matched. If the capacity of an individual is lower than the complexity of the task, the individual will fail, but if the capacity of the individual exceeds the complexity of the task, the individual is more likely to succeed (Bar-Yam 2002). This is similar

to the notion of "fit" as described by Stokols and developed by Caplan as person-environment-fit theory (Caplan 1987; Stokols 1996).

Also, remember that individuals who are the target of a behavior change intervention (e.g., overweight and obese individuals) are not the only ones who matter. There are individual actors all over the systems relevant to health behavior change in sectors as diverse as government, academia, and the **private sector**—each playing a role in determining system outcomes. The individual battling an obesogenic environment and the CEO of a food company who needs to meet the demands of shareholders, consumers, and the public are both important players in the social system that produces obesity (Finegood et al. 2010; Yach 2008). All of these individuals matter, and their relationships to others they need to work with to solve problems also matter. Cross-sector and cross-disciplinary boundaries are common barriers in complex systems and represent points where leverage for change may be found.

Given the complexity of most behavior change problems and the broad and distributed nature of the actors involved (see figure 21.1), no particular hierarchy exists that controls activity across the system. Without a clear hierarchy or singular causative agent for a problem, a command-and-control approach to problem solving and innovation will not work (Bar-Yam 2004). To solve complex problems, it makes sense to distribute the authority to make decisions and support action in the various parts of the actor network that create the different subsystems (Greenhalgh et al. 2009). However, the decision making must be distributed to actors with the capacity to act. This is the notion driving Bar-Yam's recommendation to empower work-group competition as a means to address health care reform in the United States (Bar-Yam et al. 2013). In Canada, recent efforts to distribute action and authority across the "whole of government" have led to innovative efforts to address obesity and physical inactivity (Geneau et al. 2009). Many other cooperative efforts are needed both within and between sectors to address a variety of pressing problems (Yach 2008).

In summary, the Intervention Level Framework developed from the work of Meadows, and the "solutions to complex problems" distilled from the experience of Bar-Yam are helpful tools to guide the application of systems thinking to real-world health behavior change in populations.

Evaluation through a Complex Systems Lens

If the systems underlying health behaviors are complex, then systems thinking must be central to how we intervene in those systems, whether the intervention is in policies, programs, or funding mechanisms. Increasing evidence suggests that interventions must be complex and occur at multiple levels to be effective (Kumanyika et al. 2010). The increasing complexity of interventions has implications for the methods used to evaluate interventions and demands adaptation on the part of the evaluator (Victora et al. 2004). In this section, we briefly review some of the ways in which the evaluation field has incorporated systems thinking to better meet the needs of decision-makers for program and policy assessment. Although this section focuses mainly on evaluation, it also highlights how these concepts can be incorporated into program planning, which will in turn affect evaluative practice.

Complex initiatives (also called *horizontal initiatives* or *system change initiatives*) pose many challenges to evaluators because they have characteristics of complexity such as heterogeneity of stakeholders and environmental contexts, interdependent relationships between actors across a variety of levels, and dynamic change processes that may take time to produce results, while occurring in environments that also change over time. What follows is a set of practical approaches for evaluating complex behavior change interventions.

Participatory Evaluation

An evaluator facilitates the evaluation process by engaging **key stakeholders** in a variety of ways, ranging from their limited involvement mainly as data sources to information sharing, consultation, or empowered decision making. **Participatory evaluations** involve stakeholders in meaningful ways in all facets of the evaluation; this is considered important as the first step in any evaluation (Milstein and Wetterhall 1999; Preskill and Jones 2009). Engaging stakeholders is even more important when evaluating complex interventions that involve multiple actors, each working under her own set of goals and within her own system (Cabrera et al. 2008). The need to understand the different perspectives of stakeholders and establish common goals for the intervention and the evaluation is paramount (Cabrera et al. 2008; Leischow and Milstein 2006; Regeer et al. 2009).

Stakeholder participation is so critical to a systems approach to evaluation that it gets fundamentally reframed by Patton (2011) in his articulation of developmental evaluation. In **developmental evaluation**, the evaluator is embedded in the intervention in order to lend evaluative thinking as the intervention is developed and evolves. Rather than considering the evaluator as working with program sponsors to bring in stakeholders, the evaluator is part of the intervention team, thereby becoming a stakeholder himself. An embedded evaluator can better surface assumptions, understand and reveal system heterogeneity, and bring data to decision making.

Intervention and Its Context

In systems-based evaluation, evaluators must not only thoroughly understand the intervention being evaluated, but must also understand the context in which it is being implemented. To this end, **situation analysis** has become a standard of practice in both planning and evaluation (Stevahn et al. 2005). Pawson and Tilley (1997) further emphasize the importance of context in their account of **realistic evaluation**, a sociologically grounded approach by which the evaluator attempts to account for the complex social reality in which interventions are embedded. In the example of a smoking cessation program aimed at teens, understanding the intervention and the context could include consideration of the boundaries and scope of the intervention itself, the multiple settings in which teens might make smoking decisions in their day-to-day lives, the role of other actors within those settings in influencing those decisions, and the presence or absence of structural supports to encourage behavior change (Douglas et al. 2010). This approach further demonstrates the importance of stakeholder participation, insofar as stakeholders are key informants on their own social and personal contexts.

Understanding the context and change mechanisms of the intervention, in addition to developing a full understanding of the elements that are implicated in the behavior change, enables the evaluator to set the stage for facilitating decision making around the focus of the evaluation, the methodologies chosen, and the interpretation and use of the results (Hargreaves 2010). A variety of modeling techniques have been used to gain a comprehensive understanding of the intervention and its context. The most commonly used and best known to most evaluators is through the development of **logic models**, but there are other types of models and group model-building processes that can provide additional insight. These include path analysis, flow-through diagrams, and causal loop diagrams (Smith 1990; Spector et al. 2001; Vennix 1999). These models will aid the evaluator in accounting for the complex characteristics of the system at hand, including its heterogeneity and interdependencies.

Relationships, Structures, and Feedback Mechanisms

To understand the context of an intervention and reveal the deeper layers of complexity embedded in the system under study, it is important to focus on relationships and interdependencies as well as the structures and feedback loops that support them. As Meadows argues, "once we see the relationship between structure and behavior, we can begin to understand how systems work, what makes them produce poor results, and how to shift them into better behavioral patterns" (Meadows and Wright 2009). In other words, understand the relationships among actors in the system, among program components, and among levels of the system.

Populations are highly adaptable, self-organized systems that both respond to changes in, and exert changes upon, the context in which they live. Evaluators familiar with system concepts accept that this characteristic of self-organization will challenge standardization of an intervention and implementation fidelity. Interventions that are designed with complexity in mind attempt to facilitate self-organization by creating the conditions for it to flourish, in part through the development of relationships between actors within subsystems and between actors across systems (Catsambas et al. 2008; Parsons 2009). The importance of understanding self-organization is a common feature of system approaches to evaluation (Cabrera et al. 2008; Catsambas et al. 2008; Coffman 2007; Leischow and Milstein 2006; Williams and Hummelbrunner 2010).

Theory of Change

Good evaluation (and program planning) practice seeks to understand the theoretical basis for the program and the change envisioned, and then model them for the evaluators and stakeholders. This is even more important and challenging in complex interventions, in which a traditional reliance on relatively linear models may fall short (Pawson 2006; Rogers 2008). Theory can be incorporated into evaluation and program planning in numerous ways, ranging from implementation theories, to specific program and behavior change theories, to diffusion and dissemination theories. Like other dynamic aspects of complex systems, the theories themselves are also negotiated and renegotiated throughout the intervention (Pawson 2006). Logic models, as mentioned, are the most common way to begin unpacking the underlying assumptions about change, but, as others have pointed out, they may lack clarity on what happens between the columns or lines (i.e., between the activities, outputs, and outcomes) (Dyehouse et al. 2009). Other theory-focused techniques enable program stakeholders to use logic models to articulate in a nonlinear fashion how the intervention will bring about the desired changes (Rogers 2008). Weitzman and colleagues (2009) combined **quasi-experimental** methods with theories of change as part of the validation process for the evaluation of a multisite comprehensive citywide health initiative. Further work is needed to adapt existing approaches to **program theory** to meet the needs of evaluation that respects the growing complexity of interventions enabling behavior change in populations.

Process and Outcome Using Multiple Methods

Good quality evaluations have long promoted the use of **triangulation**, or multiple data collection methods. In most evaluations, this is recommended because it provides a way to include the perspectives of different stakeholders and different types of data. When evaluating from a systems perspective, it is even more important to use multiple methods and undertake both process and **outcome evaluations**. In complex systems, change is not linear; it can be multidi-

rectional, reciprocal, and out of proportion to the initial change attempt. Furthermore, system outcomes might not be attributable to an identifiable source of activity, but may instead be emergent properties of the system and its diversity of actors, structural elements, and the relationships that bind them all (Meadows and Wright 2009). It is necessary to conduct both process and outcome evaluations and use multiple methods including both qualitative and quantitative data collection techniques, thereby collecting information about the dynamic processes of the changing system (Pawson 2006). Within system change initiatives, one set of outcomes should focus on system changes: the relationships, practices, policies, programs, and resources that were created or changed (Huz et al. 1997). In behavior change interventions, this would involve examining the system supports that are put in place to sustain the behavior change.

Focus on Contribution Rather than Attribution

Our last consideration for evaluating from complexity involves a focus on *contribution* (what plausibly might account for change) rather than *attribution* (what is directly responsible for change) (Mayne 2001). Because complex systems have nonlinear dynamics, predicting with any degree of certainty the causal relationships between any particular program and long-term outcomes, such as national obesity rates, is usually impossible (Pawson 2006). Instead, when working in a complex system, the focus should be on contribution rather than attribution. Mayne and others offer a multipronged approach called **contribution analysis** for making the links between the intervention and the more distal outcomes that are influenced by multiple factors beyond the intervention (Brown Urban and Trochim 2009; Mayne 2001). The central idea is that evaluation should measure what it is directly trying to change (i.e., short-

or medium-term outcomes) but then use existing literature to demonstrate the link between the short-term and intermediate outcomes and the longer-term changes that the intervention is seeking to influence. Long-term outcomes should continue to be monitored, but as part of overall system **surveillance** rather than for attribution to any particular behavior change intervention.

Conclusion

In sum, behavior change interventions that acknowledge complexity can maximize the learning from evaluation by involving stakeholders, developing a solid understanding of the intervention and its context, studying relationships among actors, articulating a theory of change, studying both process and outcomes, and focusing on contribution to outcomes rather than attempting to make causal connections between the intervention and more distal outcomes. Evaluation with a complexity lens does not require a whole new set of skills for evaluators; rather, it calls for acknowledging and incorporating system dynamics and including some well-established evaluation approaches and tools. Evaluators who do these things will be better equipped to provide a comprehensive understanding of the behavioral intervention and contribute to the understanding of why it did or did not bring about the anticipated results. As stated at the beginning of this chapter, understanding, influencing and evaluating behavior change will be facilitated through an improved understanding of complex systems theory and the adoption of complexity into practice.

REFERENCES

Ananthapavan J, Moodie M, Haby M, Carter R. 2010. Assessing cost-effectiveness in obesity: Laparoscopic adjustable gastric banding for severely obese adolescents. *Surg Obes Relat Dis* 6:377-85.

Bahr DB, Browning RC, Wyatt HR, Hill JO. 2009. Exploiting social networks to mitigate the obesity epidemic. *Obesity* 17 (4): 723-28.

Baranowski T. 2006. Crisis and chaos in behavioral nutrition and physical activity. *Int J Behav Nutr Phys Act* 3:27.

Baranowski T, Cullen KW, Baranowski J. 1999. Psychosocial correlates of dietary intake: Advancing dietary intervention. *Annu Rev Nutr* 19:17-40.

Bar-Yam Y. 2002. Complexity rising: From human beings to human civilization, a complexity profile. In *Encyclopedia of Life Support Systems,* 1-21. Oxford, UK: EOLSS. 1-21.

———. 2003. Complex Systems and Sports: Complex Systems insights to building effective teams. Unpublished lecture available at New England Complex Systems Institute, http://necsi.org/projects/yaneer/SportsBarYam.pdf.

———. 2004. *Making Things Work: Solving Complex Problems in a Complex World.* Cambridge, MA: NECSI, Knowledge Press.

Bar-Yam Y, Bar-Yam S, Bertrand KZ, et al. 2013. A complex systems science approach to healthcare costs and quality. In *Handbook of Systems and Complexity in Health,* ed. JP Sturmberg, CM Martin, 855-877. New York: Springer.

Best A, National Cancer Institute, Clark PI, Leischow SJ, Trochim WMK, eds. 2007. *Greater than the Sum: Systems Thinking in Tobacco Control.* Bethesda, MD: U.S. Dept. of Health and Human Services, National Institutes of Health.

Brown Urban J, Trochim W. 2009. The role of evaluation in research—practice integration working toward the golden spike. *Am J Eval* 30 (4): 538-53.

Brug J. 2006. Order is needed to promote linear or quantum changes in nutrition and physical activity behaviors: A reaction to "A chaotic view of behavior change" by Resnicow and Vaughan. *Int J Behav Nutr Phys Act* 3 (1): 29.

Butryn ML, Phelan S, Hill JO, Wing RR. 2007. Consistent self-monitoring of weight: A key component of successful weight loss maintenance. *Obesity* 15 (12): 3091-96.

Cabrera D, Colosi L, Lobdell C. 2008. Systems thinking. *Eval Progr Planning* 31 (3): 299-310.

Caplan R. 1987. Person-environment fit theory and organizations: Commensurate dimensions, time perspectives, and mechanisms. *J Vocat Behav* 31:248-67.

Carter R, Moodie M, Markwick A, et al. 2009. Assessing cost-effectiveness in obesity (ACE-Obesity): An overview of the ACE approach, economic methods, and cost results. *BMC Public* 9:419-30.

Catsambas TT, Franco LM, Gutmann M, et al. 2008. *Evaluating Health Care Collaboratives: The Experience of the Quality Assurance Project.* Bethesda, MD: University Research.

Christakis NA, Fowler JH. 2007. The spread of obesity in a large social network over 32 years. *N Engl J Med* 357 (4): 370-79.

Coffman J. 2007. *A Framework for Evaluating Systems Initiatives*. :1-36.

Cohen DJ, Crabtree BF, Etz RS, et al. 2008. Fidelity versus flexibility: Translating evidence-based research into practice. *Am J Prev Med* 35 (5 suppl.): S381-S389.

Cokkinides V, Bandi P, McMahon C. 2009. Tobacco control in the United States—recent progress and opportunities. *CA Cancer J Clin* 59 (6): 352-65.

Cummins SE, Bailey L, Campbell S, Koon-Kirby C, Zhu S-H. 2007. Tobacco cessation quitlines in North America: A descriptive study. *Tobacco Control* 16 (suppl. 1): i9-15.

DiClemente CC, Prochaska JO, Fairhurst SK, et al. 1991. The process of smoking cessation: An analysis of precontemplation, contemplation, and preparation stages of change. *J Consult Clin Psychol* 59 (2): 295.

Douglas FCG, Gray DA, van Teijlingen ER. 2010. Using a realist approach to evaluate smoking cessation interventions targeting pregnant women and young people. *BMC Health Serv Res* 10:49.

Dumas JE, Lynch AM, Laughlin JE, Phillips Smith E, Prinz RJ. 2001. Promoting intervention fidelity: Conceptual issues, methods, and preliminary results from the EARLY ALLIANCE prevention trial. *Am J Prev Med* 20 (1S): 38-47.

Dyehouse M, Bennett D, Harbor J, Childress A, Dark M. 2009. A comparison of linear and systems thinking approaches for program evaluation illustrated using the Indiana Interdisciplinary GK-12. *Eval Progr Planning* 32 (3): 187-96.

Finegood DT. 2006. Can we improve nutritional health at an affordable price? *Can Issues* (Winter): 46-51.

———. 2011. The complex systems science of obesity. In *The Oxford Handbook of the Social Science of Obesity,* ed. J Cawley, 208-36. Oxford: Oxford University Press.

Finegood DT, Merth TDN, Rutter H. 2010. Implications of the Foresight obesity system map for solutions to childhood obesity. *Obesity* 18 (suppl. 1) (n1s): S13-S16.

Foster-Fishman PG, Behrens TR. 2007. Systems change reborn: Rethinking our theories, methods, and efforts in human services reform and community-based change. *Am J Commun Psych* 39 (3-4): 191-96.

Gamble JAA. 2008. *A Developmental Evaluation Primer.* 1-69.

Geneau R, Fraser G, Legowski B, Stachenko S. 2009. *Mobilizing intersectoral action to promote health: The Case of ActNowBC in British Columbia, Canada.* :1-48.

Glasgow RE. 2008. What types of evidence are most needed to advance behavioral medicine? *Ann Behav Med* 35 (1): 19-25.

Glass TA, McAtee MJ. 2006. Behavioral science at the crossroads in public health: Extending horizons, envisioning the future. *Soc Sci Med* 62 (7): 1650-71.

Goh KI, Cusick ME, Valle D, et al. 2007. The human disease network. *Proc Natl Acad Sci* 104 (21): 8685.

Green LW. 1977. Evaluation and measurement: Some dilemmas for health education. *Am J Public Health* 67:155-61.

———. 2006. Public health asks of systems science: To advance our evidence-based practice, can you help us get more practice-based evidence? *Am J Public Health* 96 (3): 406-9.

Greenhalgh T, Humphrey C, Hughes J, et al. 2009. How do you modernize a health service? A realist evaluation of whole-scale transformation in London. *Milbank Q* 87 (2): 391-416.

Halley JD, Burden FR, Winkler DA. 2009. Stem cell decision making and critical-like exploratory networks. *Stem Cell Res* 2 (3): 165-77.

Hammond RA. A complex systems approach to understanding and combating the obesity epidemic. *Complexity.*

Hargreaves MB. 2010. *Methods guide for evaluating system interventions: Methods Report.* Cambridge, MA. 1-26.

Hawe P, Bond L, Butler H. 2009. Knowledge theories can inform evaluation practice: What can a complexity lens add? *New Direct Eval* 124:89-100.

Hawe P, Shiell A, Riley T. 2004. Complex interventions: How "out of control" can a randomised controlled trial be? *Br Med J* 328:1561-63.

Hawe P, Shiell A, Riley T, Gold L. 2004. Methods for exploring implementation variation and local context within a cluster randomised community intervention trial. *J Epidemiol Commun Health* 58 (9): 788.

Hayes AM, Feldman GC, Beevers CG, et al. 2007. Discontinuities and cognitive changes in an exposure-based cognitive therapy for depression. *J Consult Clin Psychol* 75 (3): 409-21.

Homer J, Milstein B, Dietz W, Buchner D, Majestic E. 2006. Obesity population dynamics: Exploring historical growth and plausible futures in the U.S. Paper presented at the 24th International System Dynamics Conference, Nijmegen, Netherlands, July 23-27.

Hufford MR, Witkiewitz K, Shields AL, Kodya S, Caruso JC. 2003. Relapse as a nonlinear dynamic system: Application to patients with alcohol use disorders. *J Abnorm Psychol* 112 (2): 219-27.

Huz S, Andersen DF, Richardson GP, Boothroyd R. 1997. A framework for evaluating systems thinking interventions: An experimental approach to mental health system change. *Syst Dynam Rev* 13 (2): 149-69.

Johnson-Askew WL, Fisher RA, Yaroch AL. 2009. Decision making in eating behavior: State of the science and recommendations for future research. *Ann Behav Med* 38 (suppl. 1): S88-S92.

Johnston LM, Matteson CL, Finegood DT. 2010. Analyzing evidence hierarchies in obesity recommendations with a complex systems lens. *Int J Qual Meth* 9:412.

Keshavarz N, Nutbeam D, Rowling L, Khavarpour F. 2010. Schools as social complex adaptive systems: A new way to understand the challenges of introducing the health promoting schools concept. *Soc Sci Med* 70 (10): 1467-74.

Kirchner H, Tong J, Tschöp MH, Pfluger PT. 2010. Ghrelin and PYY in the regulation of energy balance and metabolism: Lessons from mouse mutants. *Am J Physiol Endocrinol Metab* 298 (5): E909-19.

Klem ML, Wing R, McGuire M, Seagle H, Hill J. 1997. A descriptive study of individuals successful at long-term maintenance of substantial weight loss. *Am J Clin Nutr* 66 (2): 239.

Kumanyika SK. 2001. Minisymposium on obesity: Overview and some strategic considerations. *Annu Rev Public Health* 22 (46): 293-308.

Kumanyika S, Parker L, Sim L. 2010. *Bridging the Evidence Gap in Obesity Prevention: A Framework to Inform Decision Making.* Washington, DC: National Academies Press. Available at www.cabdirect.org/abstracts/20113032207.html (accessed July 25, 2011).

Leischow SJ, Milstein B. 2006. Systems thinking and modeling for public health practice. *Am J Public Health* 96 (3): 403-5.

Levy DT, Mabry PL, Wang YC, et al. 2010. Simulation models of obesity: A review of the literature and implications for research and policy. *Obesity Rev* 12 (5) 1-17.

Lieberson S. 1969. Measuring population diversity. *Am Sociol Rev* 34 (6): 850-62.

Lounsbury DW, Mitchell SG. 2009. Introduction to special issue on social ecological approaches to community health research and action. *Am J Commun Psych* 44 (3): 213-20.

Mabry PL, Olster DH, Morgan GD, Abrams DB. 2008. Interdisciplinarity and systems science to improve population health: A view from the NIH Office of Behavioral and Social Sciences Research. *Am J Prev Med* 35 (2 suppl.): S211-S224.

Malhi L. 2009. Places to intervene in the obesity system. Undergraduate honours thesis, Department of Biomedical Physiology and Kinesiology, Simon Fraser University.

Malhi L, Karanfil Ö, Merth T, et al. 2009. Places to intervene to make complex food systems more healthy, green, fair, and affordable. *J Hung Environ Nutr* 4 (3-4): 466-76.

Marshall SJ, Biddle SJH. 2001. The transtheoretical model of behavior change: A meta-analysis of applications to physical activity and exercise. *Ann Behav Med* 23 (4): 229-46.

Matteson CL, Srikameswaran S, Zelichowska J, et al. 2010. Clinician perspectives on health behaviour change in families of overweight youth. *Obesity Rev* 11 (suppl. 1): 445.

Mayne J. 2001. Addressing attribution through contribution analysis: Using performance measures sensibly. *Can J Progr Eval* 16 (1): 1-24.

McPherson K, Marsh T, Brown M. 2007. Foresight: Tackling obesities: Future choices—modelling future trends in obesity and the impact on health. Government Office for Science, London.

Meadows DH. 1999. Leverage points: Places to intervene in a system. *World*.

Meadows DH, Wright D. 2009. *Thinking in Systems: A Primer.* White River Junction, VT: Chelsea Green.

Milstein RL, Wetterhall SF. 1999. Framework for program evaluation in public health. *MMWR* 48 (RR-11): 1-40.

Ogden J, Stavrinaki M, Stubbs J. 2009. Understanding the role of life events in weight loss and weight gain. *Psychol Health Med* 14 (2): 239-49.

Parsons B. 2009. Evaluative inquiry for complex times. *OD Pract* 41 (1): 44-49.

Patton MQ. 2011. *Developmental Evaluation: Applying Complexity Concepts to Enhance Innovation and Use.* New York: Guilford Press.

Pawson R. 2006. Simple principles for the evaluation of complex programmes. In *Public Health Evidence: Tackling Health Inequalities,* ed. AM Killoran, C Swann, MP Kelly. Oxford: Oxford University Press.

Pawson R, Tilley N. 1997. *Realistic Evaluation.* London: Sage.

Plevritis SK, Sigal BM, Salzman P, Rosenberg J, Glynn P. 2006. A stochastic simulation model of U.S. breast cancer mortality trends from 1975 to 2000. *J Natl Cancer Inst Mon* 94305 (36): 86-95.

Plsek PE, Greenhalgh T. 2001. Complexity science: The challenge of complexity in health care. *Br Med J* 323 (7313): 625-28.

Preskill H, Jones N. 2009. *A Practical Guide for Engaging Stakeholders in Developing Evaluation Questions.* Princeton, NJ.

Regeer BJ, Hoes A-C, van Amstel-van Saane M, Caron-Flinterman FF, Bunders JFG. 2009. Six guiding principles for evaluating mode-2 strategies for sustainable development. *Am J Eval* 30 (4): 515-37.

Resnicow K, Page SE. 2008. Embracing chaos and complexity: A quantum change for public health. *Am J Public Health* 98 (8): 1382-89.

Resnicow K, Vaughan R. 2006. A chaotic view of behavior change : A quantum leap for health promotion. *Int J Behav Nutr Phys Act* 3:29-36.

Rittel HWJ, Webber MM. 1973. Dilemmas in a general theory of planning. *Policy Sci* 4:155-69.

Robinson TN, Sirard JR. 2005. Preventing childhood obesity: A solution-oriented research paradigm. *Am J Prev Med* 28 (2 suppl. 2): 194-201.

Rogers EM. 2003. *Diffusion of Innovations.* 5th ed. New York: Free Press.

Rogers PJ. 2008. Using programme theory to evaluate complicated and complex aspects of interventions. *Evaluation* 14 (1): 29-48.

Romon M, Lommez A, Tafflet M, et al. 2009. Downward trends in the prevalence of childhood overweight in the setting of 12-year school- and community-based programmes. *Pub Health Nutr* 12 (10): 1735-42.

Roter DL, Hall JA, Merisca R, et al. 1998. Effectiveness of interventions to improve patient compliance: A meta-analysis. *Med Care* 36 (8): 1138-61.

Sabiston CM, Lovato CY, Ahmed R, et al. 2009. School smoking policy characteristics and individual perceptions of the school tobacco context: Are they linked to students' smoking status? *J Youth Adolesc* 38 (10): 1374-87.

Smith NL. 1990. Using path analysis to develop and evaluate program theory and impact. *New Direct Progr Eval* 47:53-57.

Spector JM, Christensen DL, Sioutine AV, McCormack D. 2001. Models and simulations for learning in complex domains: Using causal loop diagrams for assessment and evaluation. *Comput Human Behav* 17:517-45.

Sterman JD. 2006. Learning from evidence in a complex world. *Am J Public Health* 96 (3): 505-14.

Stevahn L, King JA, Ghere G, Minnema J. 2005. Establishing essential competencies for program evaluators. *Am J Eval* 26 (1): 43-59.

Stokols D. 1996. Translating social ecological theory into guidelines for community health promotion. *Am J Health Promot* 10 (4): 282-98.

Story M, Hamm MW, Wallinga D. 2009. Food systems and public health: Linkages to achieve healthier diets and healthier communities. *J Hung Environ Nutr* 4 (3-4): 219-24.

Vandenbroeck P, Goossens J, Clemens M. 2007. Foresight Tackling Obesities: Future Choices–Building the Obesity System Map. Government Office for Science, London.

Vennix JAM. 1999. Group model-building: Tackling messy problems. *Syst Dynam Rev* 15:379-401.

Vicsek T. 2002. The bigger picture. *Nature* 418 (6894): 131.

Victora CG, Habicht JP, Bryce J. 2004. Evidence-based public health: Moving beyond randomized trials. *Am J Public Health* 94 (3): 400-405.

Vos T, Carter R, Barendregt J, et al. 2010. Assessing cost-effectiveness in prevention (ACE-Prevention): Final report. University of Queensland, Brisbane and Deakin University, Melbourne.

Vos T, Haby MM, Magnus A, et al. 2005. Assessing cost-effectiveness in mental health: Helping policy-makers prioritize and plan health services. *Aust NZ J Psychiatr* 39 (8): 701-12.

Wallis SE. 2008. Emerging order in CAS theory: Mapping some perspectives. *Kybernetes* 37 (7): 1016-29.

Weinstein ND, Rothman AJ, Sutton SR. 1998. Stage theories of health behavior: Conceptual and methodological issues. *Health Psychol* 17 (3): 290-99.

Weitzman BC, Mijanovich T, Silver D, Brecher C. 2009. Finding the impact in a messy intervention: Using an integrated design to evaluate a comprehensive citywide health initiative. *Am J Eval* 30 (4): 495-514.

West R. 2005. Time for a change: Putting the Transtheoretical (Stages of Change) Model to rest. *Addiction* 100 (8): 1036-39.

———. 2007. What lessons can be learned from tobacco control for combating the growing prevalence of obesity? *Obesity Rev* 8 (suppl. 1): 145-50.

West R, Sohal T. 2006. "Catastrophic" pathways to smoking cessation: Findings from national survey. *Br Med J* 332 (7539): 458.

Wheatley M, Frieze D. 2006. Using emergence to take social innovation to scale. *Berkana Inst,* 1-7.

Williams B, Hummelbrunner R. 2010. *Systems Concepts in Action.* Stanford, CA: Stanford University Press.

Wolitski RJ. 2005. The emergence of barebacking among gay and bisexual men in the United States: A public health perspective. *J Gay Lesb Psychother* 9 (3): 9-34.

Yach D. 2008. The role of business in addressing the long-term implications of the current food crisis. *Glob Health* 4:12.

CHAPTER 22

Patient and Consumer Activation for Health Behavior Change

JUDITH HIBBARD

LEARNING OBJECTIVES

After completing the chapter, the reader will be able to

* Define patient activation, identify how to measure it, and delineate how it is different from patient compliance.
* Describe the levels of activation and tell what they mean.
* Describe the methods clinicians can use to measure the engagement of their patients.
* Describe approaches for increasing activation at the group or community level.

Introduction

Health care **stakeholders** are increasingly seeking ways to encourage patients to be proactive about their health. This focus is born out of an understanding of the important role that patients play in determining their own health status and health care costs. Engaging individuals to manage their health and health care has become a priority for providers, payers, employers, and policymakers. It is increasingly apparent that health care reform efforts will not be sufficient to reduce costs or improve outcomes unless patients are part of the solution.

Although the importance of patients taking on a greater role in individual health and health care is generally understood, precisely what it means to be an activated or engaged patient and how to facilitate this characteristic in individuals and populations is less clear.

The science supporting this direction is in development. A large literature on health behavior and behavior change exists, but the concept of activation puts the focus on fundamental factors supporting behavior change: whether the individual possesses the necessary knowledge, skill, and confidence to manage her own health. This focus is new and suggests innovative and different ways to intervene and ultimately to improve **health behaviors** and health outcomes.

Becoming activated appears to be a developmental and learned process. People learn about their role in managing their health through **social norms** and **cues** in their environments. Further, people observe others and reflect on their own personal experiences in trying to manage their health. These experiences, social norms, and the personal interpretation of those experiences shape individuals' beliefs about what their role is and how well they are able to fulfill it.

In this chapter, we review what is known about the construct of **patient activation**, how it is measured and conceptualized, and the efficacy of different strategies for increasing patient activation.

Conceptualization and Measurement of Activation

Health behaviors are a **key determinant** of disease risk and **quality of life**. What people do in their everyday lives, what they eat, how physically active they are, and whether they adhere to treatment regimens will largely determine their health outcomes. For example, people with diabetes who are able to manage their diet, be physically active, and comply with medication regimens to maintain nearly normal blood sugar levels will gain, on average, an additional five years of life, eight years of sight, and six years free from kidney disease, according to estimates (Eckel et al. 2013). At the same time, many of the behaviors required of patients to maintain their health necessitate the acquisition of new knowledge and skills. For example, with new pharmaceutical approaches to treat diabetes, asthma, cancer, heart disease, and HIV/AIDS, patients now must manage **complex** drug regimens themselves. Similarly, with today's shorter hospital stays, patients often return home sicker and must manage posthospital drug, feeding, and wound-care regimens on their own. Finally, in the absence of interconnected electronic medical records, individual patients find that they must manage the communications among their complex array of doctors, hospitals, diagnostic and laboratory services, and health plans. This is often a huge burden for sick patients and their families. However, to fail to take on this task leaves them even more vulnerable to medication errors, duplicate tests, and gaps in their care.

Being an **activated patient** implies more than simply complying with medical regimens or seeking out health information; it means taking a proactive role in our own health. Being activated refers to the degree to which an individual understands his own role in maintaining and promoting personal health and the extent to which he possesses a sense of **self-efficacy** for taking on this role. It is a global construct reflecting an individual's overall knowledge, skill, and confidence for self-management. Thus, the concept involves an individual's beliefs about her own role as well as knowledge and self-efficacy for taking stewardship of her own health. This construct, as defined above, is measured using the Patient Activation Measure (PAM) (Hibbard et al. 2005).

Although the construct of activation, as measured by the PAM, includes self-efficacy, self-assessed knowledge, and belief items, it is actually a unidimensional measure. This means that the measure is tapping into a single underlying construct; it is likely measuring the individual's self-concept as a self-manager of personal health (Hibbard and Mahoney 2010).

Defining Activation Domains

Initial steps to define the concept of **patient activation** involved a review of the literature, convening a national expert consensus panel, and conducting patient focus groups. The definition of activation was based upon the areas where there was consensus across the literature, the panel, and those groups. The results indicated consensus on four key areas:

- self-managing symptoms,
- collaborating with providers,
- taking preventive action, and
- finding and accessing high quality and appropriate care.

The findings indicate that, to be activated, individuals need to believe that they have a role to play in managing their health and that they have the necessary skills, knowledge, and confidence to be effective in these four key areas (Hibbard et al. 2004).

Patient Activation Measure

The PAM is made up of 13 individual declarative statements:

1. When all is said and done, I am the person who is responsible for taking care of my health problems.
2. Taking an active role in my own health care is the most important thing that affects my health.
3. I am confident I can help prevent or reduce the problems associated with my health condition.
4. I know what each of my prescribed medications do.
5. I am confident I can tell whether I need to go to the doctor or whether I can take care of a health problem myself.
6. I am confident that I can tell a doctor my concerns, even when he or she does not ask.
7. I am confident I can follow through on medical treatments I need to do at home.
8. I understand my health problems and what causes them.

9. I know what treatments are available for my health problems.
10. I have been able to maintain (keep up with) lifestyle changes, like eating right or exercising.
11. I know how to prevent further problems with my health condition.
12. I am confident I can figure out solutions when new problems arise with my health condition.
13. I am confident I can maintain lifestyle changes, like eating right or and exercising, even during times of stress.

The measure is gauged on a 0-100 point scale (figure 22.1), with most respondents scoring between 35 and 90. Respondents indicate their degree of agreement or disagreement with each statement.

The PAM items have a Guttman-like hierarchical **difficulty structure**. Figure 22.1 shows the difficulty structure of the 13 items. The difficulty structure implies that most people can indicate that the items at the low end of the measure are true for them, whereas most people cannot agree that the items at the high end of the scale are true for them. For example, at the low end of the measure are items about acknowledging our own roles in maintaining personal health. At the high end are items about having confidence in our own ability to find solutions when new problems arise. This difficulty structure is quite robust and has been maintained in all of the different language translations that have been evaluated (Mandarin Chinese, Norwegian, German, Spanish, Japanese, Dutch, and Danish).

This hierarchical difficulty structure can be used to **tailor** interactions and communications with individuals. Where an individual scores on this continuum of activation indicates the level and type of **interventions** needed to increase the individual's activation. For example, those at the low end of activation may lack the belief that they have an important role to play

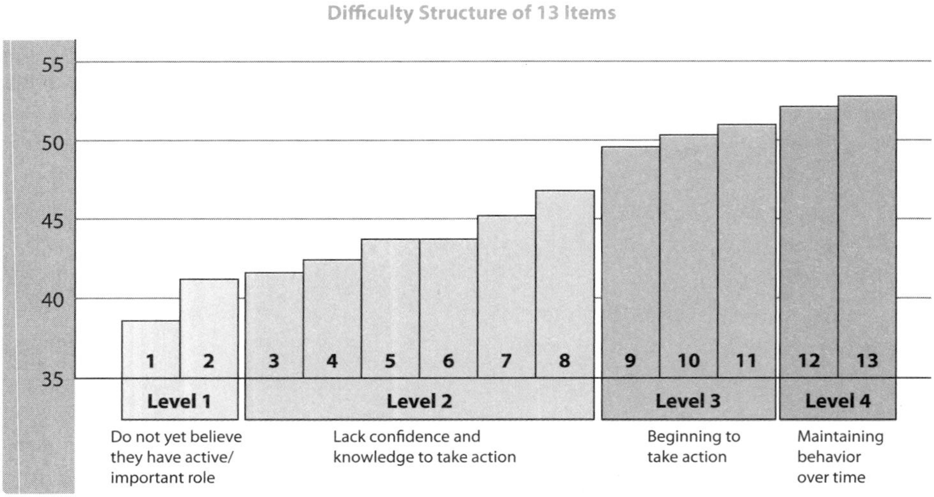

Difficulty Structure of 13 Items

	Level 1	Level 2	Level 3	Level 4
	Do not yet believe they have active/ important role	Lack confidence and knowledge to take action	Beginning to take action	Maintaining behavior over time

FIGURE 22.1. The Patient Activation Measurement (PAM) difficulty structure of 13 items

in their health or may have no confidence in their ability to manage their health. Respondents scoring in the midrange of the scale may have some but not all skills necessary for maintaining effective self-care.

Thus, activation is apparently a developmental process, meaning that individuals may pass through different phases on their way to becoming effective self-managers. This insight is important as we explore ways to increase activation in individuals and in populations.

Activation, Health Behaviors, and Health Outcomes

Multiple cross-sectional studies from a variety of settings and different populations indicate that PAM scores are correlated with a full range of health behaviors and many health outcomes. For example, the PAM score is significantly correlated with most preventive behaviors (screenings, immunizations, etc.), healthful behaviors such as diet and exercise, health-information-seeking behaviors, and disease-specific self-management behaviors, such as taking medications as recommended and monitoring one's

condition (Becker and Roblin 2008; Druss et al. 2010; Fowles et al. 2009; Hibbard et al. 2005; Hibbard et al. 2007; Mosen et al. 2007; Rogvi et al. 2012). Higher activation scores have also been linked with having less unmet medical need, having a regular source of care, and higher participation in physical therapy after spine surgery (Hibbard and Cunningham 2008; Skolasky et al. 2008). These findings remain **statistically significant** even after controlling for sociodemographic factors and insurance status. The findings have also been replicated in studies conducted in other countries (Ellins and Coulter 2005; Fujita et al. 2010; Maindal et al. 2009; Rademakers et al. 2012; Steinsbekk 2008). Further, the PAM is predictive of outcomes within condition-specific populations, such as those with a serious mental health diagnosis, heart disease, multiple sclerosis, cancer, hypertension, asthma, HIV/AIDS, and diabetes (Green et al. 2009; Kukla et al. 2013; Marshall et al. 2013; Mosen et al. 2007; Stepleman et al. 2010).

Finally, lower PAM scores are also correlated with the use of costly health care services, such as emergency department use, hospitalizations, and being rehospitalized within 30 days of discharge (AARP 2009; Begum et al. 2011; Greene and Hibbard 2012; Hibbard et al. 2013). The PAM is a relevant measure whenever the individual has a meaningful role to play in maintaining or promoting his own health.

In addition to research linking activation level with behaviors, findings also indicate that some behaviors are unlikely to occur until people become more activated. That is, behaviors that are more complex, require sustained action, or require a more proactive approach are unlikely to occur until people are at the highest levels of activation. For example, using quality information to select a health care provider, knowing about treatment **guidelines** for a chronic condition, or being persistent in asking questions when providers are unclear, appears to occur among the most activated (Hibbard 2009; Hibbard and Tusler 2007).

Activation Levels Predict Future Health Outcomes

Studies that examine outcomes over time have provided further evidence of the importance of activation and also new insights into how activation may affect multiple behaviors and outcomes.

In one observational study, participants were followed over a six-month period, and both their behaviors and their PAM scores were tracked. Some of the participants increased in activation, whereas most stayed stable or decreased in activation over the study period. Those who increased in activation also had positive changes in a variety of self-management behaviors. Of the 18 behaviors considered in the study, 11 significantly increased among those participants who increased in activation during the study period. The participants who were stable or decreased in activation showed either no change or negative changes in a variety of self-management behaviors. The findings indicate that not only can activation levels

change, but when they do change, behaviors change in the same direction (Hibbard et al. 2007). In a study involving employees, Harvey and colleagues (2012) also found that increases in PAM scores were associated with improvements in multiple behaviors.

As participants began to feel more in control of their health, they evidently changed many things about how they took care of themselves. Although determining the time-ordering events is more possible in a longitudinal study, such as the ones discussed above, definitely determining **causality**, or whether the increased activation caused the changes in behaviors, is not possible.

One possible interpretation of the study findings is that becoming activated is a process that likely affects several behavioral areas. This is important in that most theories and strategies for behavior change focus on one behavior at a time. Possibly, the specific behavior that is the focus of change is less important than "jump starting" the activation process. If this is the case, then the behavioral area to focus on is likely the one that has the highest priority for the individual. Because activation is about taking ownership and control, starting on what is important to the individual is key. In addition, experiencing success is a powerful way to build confidence; therefore, starting in an area where the individual is most motivated increases the chances for experiencing success.

Another longitudinal study examined whether activation scores could predict future behavioral and health outcomes for diabetes patients. This Kaiser Permanente study followed diabetic patients from 10 states over a two-year period. The findings indicate that baseline PAM scores were significant predictors of whether patients had good glycemic control, whether they obtained recommended diabetic testing, and whether they had a hospitalization in the following two years (Remmers et al. 2009). These findings indicate that the construct of activation is stable enough, and the measurement robust enough, to predict key health outcomes into the future.

Factors Associated with Activation Levels

Given that activation is linked with the full range of health behaviors and many health outcomes, understanding how people become more or less activated is important. In this section we identify factors that are closely linked with activation scores.

Age, education, and income are all significantly linked with activation scores. People who are younger and have more education and income tend to have higher PAM scores. However, these factors together account for only about 5% of the variation in PAM scores. In contrast, those same factors account for 25% of the variation in health literacy scores (Greene et al. 2005). Further, PAM scores vary considerably within age, income, and education strata. That is to say, activation is not simply a marker for **socioeconomic status** (**SES**).

Thus, to understand what may drive activation, we must look beyond SES factors. First, the social **context** shapes perceptions and beliefs and likely plays an important part in how people understand their own role in managing their health. For example, social norms can either support or undermine the idea that people should proactively protect and promote their health. The greater the degree to which this particular social norm is articulated and modeled in the **social environments** and institutions where people live, work, and get their health care, the more likely it is that individuals will adopt it into their belief system. Research indicates that environments supportive of being an informed and proactive manager of one's own health are more likely to have more highly activated patients than environments that do not support these **norms** (Becker and Roblin 2007; Terry 2009).

Second, gaining confidence in our own ability to be a proactive self-manager is another im-

portant aspect in becoming activated. Gaining confidence is likely an **iterative** self-reinforcing **process**. When individuals see others experiencing success and then also experience some success with their own efforts, they begin to feel more capable and confident (Bandura 2004). Gaining confidence and experiencing success can actually lead to more successes. Results from human flourishing studies indicate that when people experience more positive emotions in their daily lives, they tend to widen their array of behavioral responses, to be more open to new information and to adapting new behavioral strategies (Fredrickson and Losada 2005). Fredrickson's **broaden-and-build theory** of positive emotions asserts that people's daily experiences of positive emotions compound over time to build a variety of consequential personal resources (Fredrickson 2000, 2001). Short-term benefits of positive emotions include increased creativity, problem-solving ability, and openness to new experiences and information. These shorter-term benefits can lead to building a person's social, psychological, intellectual, and physical resources over time. That is, in the long term, the effect of positive emotions is to increase resources and resilience for better coping with adversity, increase closeness of personal relationships, and improve immune system functioning (Kok et al. 2008).

Thus, gaining confidence, experiencing success, and the resulting positive emotions can be an upward spiral that is self-reinforcing. The accumulation of these positive experiences, in turn, increases the chances for experiencing further successes and ultimately leads to effective self-management.

The reverse is also likely true. Experiencing multiple failures in attempting to manage a chronic illness or adopt a healthful behavior is likely to result in feelings of being overwhelmed, disempowered, and discouraged, and ultimately in taking a passive approach to one's health (Dixon et al. 2009). Such experiences increase the individual's overall negative affect, which in turn reduces her capacity for problem solving and using new information (Fredrickson and Losada 2005). Once people internalize the knowledge that they can, or cannot, be in control of their health and functioning through their own actions, this knowledge appears to be relatively stable. That is, this belief about their ability to manage their health becomes part of the individual's self-concept.

Findings from cross-sectional studies provide support for this perspective. Negative emotions and major depression are negatively correlated with activation scores. Those who are less activated report significantly more negative affect and less positive affect in their daily lives than those who are more activated (Hibbard and Mahoney 2010). Depression is also more common among those who are less activated (Hibbard et al. 2007), probably because this negative emotion is both a barrier to becoming activated and at least a partial result of feeling bad about poor self-management.

Implications for Interventions

Research suggests that activation is developmental and that people pass through four different levels of activation on their way to becoming effective self-managers. People who are low in activation are likely to have little confidence in their own ability to manage their health and to feel overwhelmed by the task. They may not even understand the need to play an active role in their own health. Patients with low activation are more likely to have experienced multiple failures in managing their health and to feel discouraged, disempowered, and passive with regard to their health and health care. They tend to have few problem-solving skills and are more likely to give up when they encounter a problem (Dixon et al. 2009). For example, those with low activation are significantly more likely to report unmet medical needs than the highly activated, even when differences in insurance status, income, and education are removed. The

less activated are more likely to be vulnerable to barriers in the system and to give up seeking care when they encounter problems (Hibbard and Cunningham 2008). The highly activated, on the other hand, are **goal** oriented and proactive regarding their health. They seek workable **partnerships** with their providers and have a future orientation when dealing with health issues (Dixon et al. 2009).

Because people tend to learn about their role in managing their health through social norms, their own experiences, and cues in their environments, strategies for increasing activation will likely be more effective if they incorporate approaches that build on these processes. The studies to date provide several very important insights into how to support activation in individuals and in populations. To summarize, these are the key insights:

- Not everyone is starting in the same place. Individuals who are less activated lack confidence and feel overwhelmed with the task of managing their health. Finding ways to increase confidence, increase positive affect, and reduce feelings of being overwhelmed are essential for helping people with low activation move forward.
- Experiencing success at making a change likely increases positive affect and feelings of confidence. Encouraging behaviors that individuals are likely to succeed at means encouraging behaviors that are realistic or achievable, given the individual's level of activation, and encouraging behaviors that the individual is interested in changing (since the person will have more **motivation** for changing those behaviors).
- Conversely, encouraging the less activated to change multiple behaviors at once and inundating them with information may only serve to increase their feelings of being overwhelmed and undermine any chances for change. To put it another way, treating

the less activated as if they were fully activated (what happens in most patient interactions with health care providers) can be counterproductive.

- Individuals who gain in activation will likely improve several health behaviors; this result suggests that the key is to "jump start" the process.

Interventions that Increase Activation

Becoming an engaged and activated patient appears to be a process that can be supported or retarded by experiences individuals have as they interact with their social environments and social institutions (Becker and Roblin 2008; Fowles et al. 2009). Interventions that have been shown to increase activation are those that have one or more of the following elements:

A focus on skill development, problem solving, and/or peer support. The Stanford Chronic Disease Self-Management Program (CDSMP) is a good example of an intervention that uses these elements. Increases in activation among participants have been achieved and sustained for up to 12 months after participation in the CDSMP (Lorig et al. 2010). Other programs just focus on skills development and have shown that training patients in how to ask questions and giving them support to do so also increases their participation in their own care and increases their activation levels (Algeria et al. 2008).

A focus on changing the social environment. These interventions seek to change the social environment to support changes in norms, skills, and opportunities for change. In an experiment involving two large companies, employees were randomized to one of three groups: a traditional work-site wellness program, an "activated consumer" program, and a **control group** (a program focusing on personal development). Both intervention groups included a broad campaign in the workplace, including posters, classes, environmental changes, and

personal coaching for high risk employees. In the activated consumer group, the focus was on getting more from the individual's medical care. In the work-site wellness group, the focus was on healthful behaviors. The findings show that employees in both intervention groups significantly increased in activation and improved behaviors more than those in the control group. Furthermore, the activated consumer group gained significantly more in activation scores than did those in the traditional work-site wellness arm of the study (Fowles et al. 2009). Of particular interest was that those in the activated consumer intervention group improved in multiple behaviors, including behaviors such as healthful diet and exercise, even though those behaviors were not part of the focus in this intervention group (Terry 2009).

A focus on tailoring support to the individual's level of activation. A variety of programs seek to **tailor** support to the individual's level of activation, encouraging small achievable steps for those with low activation and focusing on more difficult behaviors for those at higher levels of activation.

In one **quasi-experimental** design study carried out in a disease management program, health coaches used the patient's PAM score to tailor support. Coaches were trained and given guidelines to customize telephone coaching based upon the activation level. The behaviors encouraged for each activation level were based on empirical data indicating what is realistic at a particular level of activation (Hibbard 2009; Hibbard and Tusler 2007). The goal was to ask patients to do things that they could succeed at and allow them to begin to build confidence in their ability to manage their health.

Coaches working with patients at level 1 were trained to build patient self-awareness and understand behavior patterns, which are important foundations for tackling further competencies in later steps. At level 2, coaches worked with patients to make small changes in their existing behaviors, such as reducing portion sizes at meals, taking the stairs at work, and reading food labels at the grocery store. At level 3, coaches focused on the adoption of new behaviors (e.g., 30 minutes of exercise three times a week) and the development of problem-solving skills. At level 4, coaches worked with patients on relapse prevention and handling new or challenging situations as they arise. Coaches serving the control group did not have access to their patient's PAM scores and were not trained in interpreting and using the PAM score for coaching.

The findings showed significant improvements in activation scores, cooperation with treatment and clinical indicators (e.g., blood pressure and low-density lipoprotein), reductions in emergency room use, and fewer hospitalizations during the six-month intervention. These improved outcomes were in comparison to those receiving "usual care coaching" (Hibbard et al. 2009). Shively and colleagues (2012) used a similar approach with congestive heart failure patients. In a randomized controlled trial, one group was assigned to usual care and one group received support tailored to the patient's level of activation. They found that the intervention group had improvements in activation and reductions in hospitalizations as compared to the usual care group.

These findings suggest that what employers and health providers do can support or discourage consumer engagement. For the less activated, the challenge is to help them understand that they do have an important role to play in their health and to build their confidence in having a positive impact on their own outcomes. Encouraging small, realistically achievable actions is one way to build confidence. Strategies that seek to increase positive affect may also be important to increasing activation.

Interventions designed to increase patient involvement in care would be enhanced by the use of measurement to determine the degree to which the strategies employed are resulting in gains in activation.

Clinicians are in a unique position to support activation or to discourage it. It is common in clinical encounters to give instructions to the patient on self-care. Yet clinicians often do so with little or knowledge about the individual patient's ability to take the recommended actions.

Studies show that patients who say their clinician helped them in very specific and concrete ways to self-manage their condition have higher PAM scores than patients who say their clinicians did not help them in this way (Glasgow et al. 2005; Hibbard et al. 2005). For example, patients whose physicians helped them learn to monitor their conditions, or to set specific behavioral goals, or to set up an exercise program scored significantly higher (Hibbard et al. 2005). Similarly, Becker and Roblin (2008) found that patients who were more trusting of their physicians were more activated, displayed more healthful behaviors, and had better clinical outcomes than patients who had less trust in their physician.

Key Stakeholders

If the goal is to activate consumers to be more in charge of their health, then it will be important to meet them "where they are" and provide support and encouragement to move forward. Because we typically do not know how activated any given consumer is, we often communicate with or support the person in ineffectual ways. Current approaches could be likened to throwing some nonswimmers into the deep end of the pool, while restricting some expert swimmers to the baby pool. We certainly would not do this if we knew about their swimming ability. In health care, we typically do not know what level of change an individual patient is capable of taking on and consequently often provide inappropriate support and education. Providers, health plans, and employers all have a stake in improving individual patient health. Knowing about the individual's level of activation and using that information to be more targeted in providing support and education would likely yield better results than the one-size-fits-all approach currently employed.

Providers and Health Plans

The medical home concept is gaining currency as a way to make care more patient centered. The idea is to link people to a place where they can get care and information from a health care team that will coordinate their care and connect them with the support and services they need. The medical home is not just a single physician providing care, but a well-functioning medical *team* that provides different types of expertise as needed for each patient. Disease management and wellness support programs are integrated into care; they are not isolated elements separate from the core medical team. The medical home should be an ideal platform for supporting patient activation.

Because the point of the medical home is to personalize care, knowing about the patient's level of activation can help the team tailor their support to each individual patient. By meeting patients were they are and providing step-by-step support, the team is more likely to be able to help the individual to start to feel confident and more able to manage his health. Through regular measurement, it will also be possible to determine whether patients are gaining in activation and in their self-management ability over time. Chronic disease patients who are getting high quality care should be gaining in their capability to self-manage their condition. Thus, gains in activation could be used as a marker for high quality care.

Measuring will also enable the more efficient use of resources. That is, by measuring activation levels in patients, and using a **stratification** approach, providing more support to those who are lower in activation and simply pushing information out to those who are more activated (as they are more likely to be ready and

motivated to use information on their own) becomes possible. Health care team members may deploy more of their staff time to reach out to those less activated and spend more one-on-one time with them. Thus, more efficient use of the resources of the health care team likewise becomes possible, likely yielding better results with the same level of resources.

Finally, clinicians might use a PAM score as an additional vital sign. The score provides the clinician with essential information about what types and amount of support an individual patient needs to be able to manage her part in the care process. Just as it is important to know that the capabilities and credentials of health care team members are adequate, it is equally important to know the adequacy of the patient's ability to do his part in the care process.

Employers

Employers currently invest in myriad services and supports to nudge employees toward taking on a more active role in managing their health. Using a scattershot approach makes it difficult to know what is working and what is not. Systematic measurement would allow employers to know how activated their employees are and which of their strategies are resulting in increased consumer activation. Furthermore, employers are in the unique position of being able to influence the social and physical environment in which workers spend much of their time. As seen in the work site study, creating a culture of health with broad campaigns in the work site can result in increases in activation and improved health behaviors (Terry 2009).

In addition to creating a culture of health, employers could use measurement to more effectively tailor support to different segments of their employees and then devise either group-level or **individual-level interventions** aimed at one or more of these segments. The segment-based interventions could be designed to address the challenges faced by individuals at the level of activation represented within that segment.

Tailored communications can also be part of employer **segmentation** approaches. Research indicates that tailored messages, ones that are personalized based on the unique needs of the individual, are more effective in influencing **attitudes**, knowledge, and behaviors than generalized messages (Rimer and Kreuter 2006). Currently, most tailored messaging is based on an individual's responses to a **health risk assessment**. The tailored messages urge individuals to work on behaviors they have not yet adopted. An alternative is to tailor messages based on the individual's level of activation, which may make the message more interesting and compelling, because it can address specific types of barriers the individual faces. For example, for the less activated, messages may suggest that a good place to start is by taking small steps, instead of making them feel that they have to tackle the whole problem all at once. This may help an individual to overcome feelings of discouragement or being overwhelmed. For the highly activated, communications about how to maintain good health practices even when they are under stress or when their life routines change may be more relevant.

To tailor on activation level, human resource departments would need to administer the PAM to employees and obtain an activation level. Based on this assessment, tailoring of messages and the use of segmentation approaches are possible.

Community-Level Interventions

One advantage of community-level strategies is that different organizations and actors in the community can work together in concert to reinforce similar messages and norms, creating a social environment where there is widespread support for particular consumer roles and behaviors. The coordination and **reinforcement** of messages can create a **synergy** that is more than the sum of individual efforts of actors and organizations (Rimal et al. 1999). Key **reference groups** in the community, such as employers, providers, churches, parent groups, media sources, and civic organizations, working together to promote the idea of taking an active role in our own health would likely have a greater impact than any one organization working in isolation.

Messages that encourage particular behaviors are most effective when the information is clear about what to do and why. However, when the same message is delivered by multiple sources, it can be much more powerful. For example, when people hear about the importance of taking an active role in their own care from their clinician, but also at the workplace, where they hear the same message from their supervisors and co-workers, and even in the community, from community leaders, the power of that message is greatly increased, and the idea that being an active participant in care is normative, or normal behavior, is emphasized. This is particularly true when it becomes common to hear from peers and others that they, for example, always bring a list of questions to the doctor. The impact of multiple-source messaging is further enhanced when it is made easier and more convenient for the individual to engage in the behavior (e.g., when a patient schedules an appointment, she could receive a reminder to bring her list of questions). Similarly, when the **expectation** from the provider is that the patient will ask questions, this too makes the behavior easier. Emerging evidence (Becker and Roblin 2007) suggests that people who work, live, and get care in environments (e.g., workplaces, neighborhoods, and clinics) where they are encouraged to take a proactive role in their health are more activated and engage in more health-promoting behaviors. In neighborhoods and work sites where there were opportunities to exercise and choose healthful foods, employees engaged in more of these healthful behaviors.

Efforts to create a culture of health can be extended by the use of **social-networking strategies**. Including the extended family and friends of employees in efforts to promote health and proactive health care choices will enhance and support work site efforts. By using social media such as Facebook and Twitter, more avenues of sharing information and reinforcing key ideas can be leveraged.

Community strategies that seek to coordinate the efforts of multiple stakeholders can create environments that foster activation. Specifically, they can create programs that

- provide support and encouragement from peers and authority figures (e.g., supervisors, physicians);
- provide opportunities to engage in proactive health behaviors or make it easier to make healthful choices;
- provide **modeling** opportunities, in which peers can be observed engaging in proactive behaviors; and
- provide consistent health messages that are reinforced again and again and are delivered by multiple sources.

Ultimately, strategies that reinforce one another and work in concert to change norms, build confidence, and encourage and facilitate proactive choices will likely have a greater impact than any single approach alone.

Conclusion

Not all individuals are in the same place with regard to their health and health care. Some are very informed and confident in actively managing their health, while others are not. Meeting people where they are and providing appropriate support will enable them to expand their abilities to become effective self-managers.

Part of the answer may be found in creating a culture of proactive health. Doing so entails changing social norms, individual beliefs, and

priorities and creating opportunities that make it easier to change behaviors. Such an approach requires using multiple strategies and multiple communication channels. For example, when people hear the same message from multiple sources and channels, they are more likely to attend to it. When they see peers and leaders engaging in or endorsing the behavior, it seems both more desirable and more normal. Leveraging alternative communication forums like Facebook and Twitter can support this approach. Making it easier to engage in the behavior (e.g., it's easier to engage in regular exercise at work when there is an on-site gym) also facilitates adoption.

Another part of the answer may be to meet people where they are and to tailor messages and support to their level of activation. The highly activated can be urged to adopt more difficult and challenging behaviors, such as creating an effective partnership with their provider or obtaining and using treatment guidelines to get high quality care. Those less activated can be encouraged to take small steps, to not be daunted or overwhelmed by the task of managing their health and health care, and to learn about the basics of their care. The less activated may be helped with more basic issues, such as how to formulate questions for the medical encounter or how to read a food label and make better food choices. In order to gain in activation, those less activated need opportunities to experience success. Similarly, reaching out to the less activated individuals with personal calls (or a health-coaching program) may be necessary because this segment is more passive. Pushing information out to the more motivated can also be effective because this segment is more ready to use the information. Such an approach would represent a more efficient use of communication resources.

Systematic assessments and measurement, to both design supports and communications and to track progress, are necessary for achieving desirable outcomes. This is a new and emerging area of research and practice, and there is much to be learned about different subgroups in the population and the efficacy of different support strategies. As with most other areas of health care improvement, measurement is a necessary first step.

REFERENCES

AARP Public Policy Institute. 2009. *Chronic Care: A Call to Action for Health Reform.* Available at http://assets. aarp.org/rgcenter/health/beyond_50_hcr.pdf.

Alegria M, Polo A, Gao S, Santana L, et al. 2008. Evaluation of a patient activation and empowerment intervention in mental health care. *Med Care* 46 (3): 247–56.

Bandura A. 2004. Health promotion by social cognitive means. *Health Educ Behav* 31 (2) (April): 143–46.

Becker E, Roblin, D. 2007. Psychosocial circumstances and health status in a managed care population. Paper presented at Academy Health Annual Research Meeting, Orlando, FL.

———. 2008. Translating primary care practice climate into patient activation: The role of patient trust in physician. *Med Care* 46 (8): 795–805.

Begum N, Donald M, Ozolins IZ, Dower J. 2011. Hospital admissions, emergency department tilisation, and patient activation for self-management among people with diabetes. *Diabetes Res Clin Pract* 93 (2): 260–67.

Dixon A, Hibbard JH, Tusler M. 2009. How do people with different levels of activation self-manage their chronic conditions? *Patient* 2:257–68.

Druss BG, Zhao L, von Esenwein S, et al. 2010. The Health and Recovery Peer (HARP) Program: A peer-led intervention to improve medical self- management for persons with serious mental illness. *Schizophr Res* 118:264–70.

Eckel RH, Jakicic JM, Ard JD, et al. 2013. 2013 AHA/ACC Guideline on Lifestyle Management to Reduce Cardiovascular Risk: A Report of the American College of Cardiology / American Heart Association Task Force on Practice Guidelines. *J Am Coll Cardiol* S0735-1097 (13) 06029-4 doi: 10.1016/j.jacc.2013.11.003. Epub ahead of print.

Ellins J, Coulter A. 2005. Measuring patient activation: Validating a tool for improving quality of care in the UK. Picker Institute Europe, www.pickereurope.org /assets/content/pdf/Project_Reports/Patient -Activation-Survey.pdf.

Fowles J, Terry P, Xi M, Hibbard JH, Bloom CT, Harvey L. 2009. Measuring self-management of patients' and employees' health: Further validation of the patient activation measure (PAM) based on its relation to employee characteristics. *Patient Educ Couns* 77:116–22.

Fredrickson B. 2000. Extracting meaning from past affective experiences. *Cognit and Emotion* 14:577–606.

———. 2001. The role of positive emotions in positive psychology: The broaden-and-build theory of positive emotions. *Am Psychol* 56:218–26.

Fredrickson B, Losada MF. 2005. Positive affect and the complex dynamics of human flourishing. *Am Psychol* 60: 678–89.

Fujita E, Kuno E, Kato D, Kokochi M, Uehara K, Hirayasu Y. 2010. Development and validation of the Japanese version of the Patient Activation Measure 13 for mental health. *Seishinigaku* [Clinical psychiatry] 52:765–72.

Glasgow RE, Wagner EH, Schaefer J, Mahoney LD, Reid RJ, Greene SM. 2005. Development and validation of the Patient Assessment of Chronic Illness Care (PACIC). *Med Care* 43 (5): 436–44.

Green CA Perrin NA, Polen MR, Leo MC, Hibbard JH, Tusler M. 2009. Development of the Patient Activation Measure for mental health (PAM-MH). *Admin Policy Ment Health* 37 (4): 327–33, doi: 10.1007/ s10488-009-0239-6.

Greene J, Hibbard JH. 2012. Why does patient activation matter? An examination of the relationships between patient activation and health-related outcomes. *J Gen Intern Med* 27 (5): 520–26.

Greene J, Hibbard JH, Tusler M. 2005. How much do health literacy and patient activation contribute to older adults' ability to manage their health? AARP Public Policy Institute, www.aarp.org/research/ppi/.

Harvey L, Fowles J, Xi M, Terry P. 2012. When Activation Changes, What Else Changes? The Relationship between Change in Patient Activation Measure (PAM) and Employees' Health Status and Health Behaviors. *Patient Educ Couns* 88 (2): 338–43.

Hibbard JH. 2009. Using systematic measurement to target consumer activation strategies. *Med Care Res Rev* 66 (1 suppl.): 9S-27S.

Hibbard JH, Cunningham P. 2008. How engaged are consumers in their health and health care, and why does it matter? *Res Brief* 8:1–9.

Hibbard JH, Greene J, Overton V. 2013. Patients with lower activation associated with higher costs: Delivery systems should know their patient "scores." *Health Affairs* 32 (2) (Feb.): 216–22.

Hibbard JH, Greene J, Tusler M. 2009. Improving the outcomes of disease-management by tailoring care to the patient's level of activation. *Am J Manag Care* 15 (6): 353–60.

Hibbard JH, Mahoney ER. 2010. Toward a theory of patient and consumer activation. *Patient Educ Couns* 78 (3): 377–81.

Hibbard JH, Mahoney E, Stock R, Tusler M. 2007. Do increases in patient activation result in improved self-management behaviors? *Health Serv Res* 42 (4): 1443-63.

Hibbard JH, Mahoney ER, Stockard J, Tusler M. 2005. Development and testing of a short form of the patient activation measure. *Health Serv Res* 40:1918-30.

Hibbard JH, Stockard J, Mahoney ER, Tusler M. 2004. Development of the Patient Activation Measure (PAM): Conceptualizing and measuring activation in patients and consumers. *Health Serv Res* 39:1005-26.

Hibbard JH, Tusler M. 2007. Assessing activation stage and employing a "next steps" approach to supporting patient self-management. *J Ambul Care Manag* 30 (1): 2-8.

Kok B, Lahnna I, Catalino L, Fredickson B. 2008. The broadening, building, buffering effects of positive emotions. In *Positive Psychology: Exploring the Best of People*, ed. SJ Lopez, 1-19. Westport, CT: Greenwood.

Kukla M, Salyers M, Lysaker P. 2013. Levels of patient activation among adults with schizophrenia: Association with hope, symptoms, medication adherence, and recovery attitudes. *J Nerv Ment Dis* 201 NO 4: 339-344.

Lorig K, Ritter PL, Laurent DD, et al. 2010. Online diabetes self-management program: A randomized study. *Diabetes Care* 33 (6) (June): 1275-81.

Maindal T, Sokolowski I, Vedsted P. 2009. Translation, adaptation, and validation of the American short form Patient Activation Measure (PAM13) in a Danish version. *BMC Public Health* 9:209.

Marshall R, Beach M, Saha S, et al. 2013. Patient activation and improved outcomes in HIV infected patients. *J Gen Intern Med* 28 (5): 668-74.

Mosen D, Schmittdiel J, Hibbard JH, Sobel D, Remmers C, Bellows J. 2007. Is patient activation associated with outcomes of care for adults with chronic conditions? *J Ambul Care Manag* 30 (1): 21-29.

Rademakers J, Nijman J, van der Hoek L, Heijmans M, Rijken M. 2012. Measuring patient activation in the Netherlands: Translation and validation of the American short form Patient Activation Measure (PAM13). *Br Med J* 12:577.

Remmers C, Hibbard JH, Mosen DM, Wagenfield M, Hoye RE, Jones C. 2009. Is patient activation associated with future health outcomes and healthcare utilization among patients with diabetes? *J Ambul Care Manag* 32:320-27.

Rimal RN, Flora JA, Schooler C. 1999. Achieving improvements in overall health orientation effects of campaign exposure, information seeking, and health media use. *Commun Res* 26 (3): 322-48.

Rimer BK, Kreuter MW. 2006. Advancing tailored health communications: A persuasion and message effects perspective. *J Commun* 56 (suppl. 1): S184-S201.

Rogvi S. Tapager I, Almdal T, Schiøtz M, Willaing I. 2012. Patient factors and glycaemic control—associations and explanatory power. *Diabetic Med* 29 (10): e382-e389.

Skolasky RL, Mackenzie EJ, Wegener ST, Lee HR.2008. Patient activation and adherence to physical therapy in persons undergoing spine surgery. *Spine* 1 (21): 33.

Steinsbekk A. 2008. Måling av effekt av pasientopplæring [Norwegian version of Patient Activation Measure (PAM)]. *Tidsskr Nor Legeforen* 128:2316-18.

Stepleman LM, Rutter C, Hibbard JH, Johns L, Wright D, Hughes MD. 2010. Validation of the Patient Activation Measure (PAM) in a multiple sclerosis clinic sample and implications for care. *Disabil Rehabil* 32 (19): 1558-67.

Terry P. 2009. Consumer activation at the worksite. Paper presented at the Disease Management Association of America, San Diego.

Empowering Patient Communication

DEBRA ROTER

LEARNING OBJECTIVES

After completing the chapter, the reader will be able to

* Appreciate the importance of health literacy and patient-physician communication with respect to health behavior change outcomes.
* Appreciate the importance of power dynamics, negotiation, and patient values in the context of patient-physician interactions.
* Describe several factors that contribute to patient empowerment and autonomy.

Introduction

The delivery of medical care is a **complex** process. It is even more complicated when patients and physicians do not share similar experiences, **expectations**, and assumptions regarding the nature and processes of the medical exchange. The Institute of Medicine report on racial and ethnic disparities in health care has drawn national attention to the challenges and health **consequences** of providing high quality medical care and culturally sensitive communication to an ethnically diverse and vulnerable patient population (Smedley et al. 2003). Although less frequently studied than racial and ethnic diversity in relation to **health disparities**, other factors that characterize vulnerable populations also may have consequences for interpersonal dynamics and the quality of health care delivery. These include aspects of an individual's psychological and sociological environment that act to shape the way in which he sees himself or is seen by others; among them are such basic identity variables as age, social class, education, and gender (Roter and Hall 2006). The effect of literacy deficits on medical communication may be viewed within this **context**, as a marker of patient vulnerability.

Literacy deficits are widespread, and the health consequences of restricted literacy are considerable. Estimates from the National Adult Literacy Survey (NALS) indicate that almost half the population may be considered to have restricted literacy, reflecting significant deficits in prose and quantitative and document measures of literacy. Almost a quarter of the more than 25,000 NALS respondents scored below basic levels of functional literacy (i.e., at or below roughly a fifth-grade level), and an additional quarter of respondents scored as marginally literate, reflecting only a basic level of skill (i.e., roughly equivalent to a sixth-to-eighth-grade level) (Kutner et al. 2007). Restricted literacy has been linked to lower levels of **self-reported** health (Gazmararian et al. 1999), less use of preventive care and cancer screening (Scott et al. 2002), less effective diabetes management and more disease-related complications (Schillinger et al. 2002), and higher rates of hospitalization (Baker et al. 1998; Baker et al. 2002), as well as other health consequences (De-Walt and Pignone 2005).

Although most health literacy research has focused on reading and numeracy skills, there is some evidence that patients with literacy deficits also have difficulty with complex oral communication. Because the research pertaining to the consequences of restricted literacy on the medical exchange is relatively new, it will be the focus of this chapter.

Understanding and recall of complex information delivered orally has been shown to be problematic for patients with poor literacy skills (Williams et al. 1998). These patients appear especially vulnerable to medical intimidation and report feelings of shame and humiliation in regard to their lack of literacy (Baker et al. 1996; Parikh et al. 1996). They experience more communication difficulties and have less satisfying medical visits than do patients with adequate literacy skill (Baker et al. 1996; Bennett et al. 2006; Schillinger et al. 2004).

Given the inherent **power differential** evident within the patient-physician relationship, it is not surprising that patients with low literacy skills are less likely to be active participants in the medical dialogue and in the decision-making process (Cooper et al. 2004; Roter 2004). Indeed, a study by Hibbard and colleagues (2008), notes that **patient activation** and health literacy are moderately correlated; patients with adequate literacy skills score significantly—and substantially—higher on the Patient Activation Measure (PAM) than patients with marginal or below basic literacy.

The purpose of this chapter is to discuss the relationship between health literacy and patient-physician communication and to suggest mechanisms by which active patient engagement in the communication process may be facilitated to support patient empowerment and positive patient outcomes.

Power and Autonomy in the Patient-Provider Relationship

Bioethicists E. J. Emanuel and L. L. Emanuel (1992) suggest that power relations in medical visits are expressed through several key elements, including (1) who sets the agenda and **goals** of the visit (the physician, the physician and patient in negotiation, or the patient), (2) the role of the patient's values (assumed by the physician to be consistent with her own, jointly explored by the patient and the physician, or unexamined), and (3) the functional role assumed by the physician (guardian, adviser, or consultant).

The expression of power, and the dynamics of negotiation, can take several forms, each shaping a markedly different relationship. Table 23.1 illustrates the ideal forms of the doctor-patient relationship—paternalism, **consumerism**, and **mutuality** as suggested by the Emanuels—and

TABLE 23.1. Prototypes of the physician-patient relationship

Patient Power	Physician Power	
	High Physician Power	Low Physician Power
High Patient Power		
	Mutuality	**Consumerism**
Goals and agenda	Negotiated	Patient set
Patient values	Jointly examined	Unexamined
Physician's role	Adviser, technical	consultant
Low Patient Power		
	Paternalism	**Default**
Goals and agenda	Physician set	Unclear
Patient values	Assumed	Unclear
Physician's role	Guardian	Unclear

adds another dimension, **relationship default**, as discussed in detail elsewhere (Roter and Hall 2006). The most prevalent, but not necessarily the most efficient or desirable, prototype, **paternalism**, is shown in the lower left quadrant. In this model of relations, physicians dominate agenda setting, **goal setting**, and decision making with regard to both information and services; the medical condition is defined in biomedical terms, and the patient's voice is largely absent. The physician's obligation is to act in the patient's "best interest." The determination of best interest, however, is largely based on the assumption that the patient's values and preferences are the same as those of the physician. The guiding model characterizes the physician as the guardian, acting in the patient's best interest regardless of the patient's preferences. The patient's job is to cooperate with medical advice, that is, to do what he is told.

The upper right quadrant represents **consumerism**. Here, the more typical power relationship between doctors and patients appears reversed. Patients set the goals and agenda of

the visit and take sole responsibility for decision making. The patient's demands for information and technical services are accommodated by a cooperating physician. The patient's values are defined and fixed by the patient and are unexamined by the physician. This type of relationship redefines the medical encounter as a marketplace transaction. Caveat emptor, "Let the buyer beware," rules the transaction, with power resting in the buyer (patient), who can make the decision to buy (seek care) or not, as the patient sees fit (Haug and Lavin 1981). The physician's role is limited to that of a technical consultant who has the obligation to provide information and services that are contingent on the patient's preferences (and within professional **norms**).

While still stressing patient control, the prototype of **mutuality**, shown in the upper left quadrant, proposes a more moderate alternative to the extremes of paternalism and consumerism. In this model, each participant brings strengths and resources to the relationship on a relatively even footing. Inasmuch as power in the relationship is balanced, the goals, agenda, and decisions related to the visit are the result of negotiation between partners; the patient and the physician become part of a joint venture. Medical dialogue is the vehicle through which the patient's values are explicitly articulated and explored. Throughout this process, the physician acts as a counselor or adviser. Also, in the mutuality model the concept of the relationship itself is elevated to a new status. Although all of the models suppose the doctor-patient relationship to be the context within which the different roles exist, the concept of "being in a relationship" has intrinsic value for both the doctor and the patient. The emphasis shifts from acting in complementary roles to the expression of mutual personhood. In this model, dialogue and the mutual expression of feelings are seen as holding great therapeutic potential (Beach and Inui 2006).

What happens when the patient's and the physician's expectations are at odds, or when the need for change in the relationship cannot be negotiated? A possible consequence of a poor "fit," or the failure to change the relationship as needs and circumstances change, is **relationship default**, which is represented in the lower right quadrant. It is characterized by a lack of control by either the patient or the physician. In this case, a patient may drop out of care completely because of failed expectations or frustrated goals, or the provider may encourage the patient to seek care elsewhere.

Although ideal types are largely theoretical in nature, some attempt has been made to explore the empirical evidence for varying types of patient-provider relationships (Roter et al. 1997). For instance, an analysis of medical communication during routine primary care visits found support for the relationships as proposed. The most common relationship type, accounting for two-thirds of the nearly 500 visits analyzed, reflected a paternalistic pattern of communication characterized by a physician-dominated agenda and biomedically focused

visit. Evidence of mutuality was found in some 20% of visits, in which both biomedical and **psychosocial** domains of care were addressed and patient engagement in the dialogue was enhanced. Evidence of consumerism was found in about 7% of visits, which were characterized by particularly high levels of patient question-asking and physician information-giving but low levels of physician questioning. A final communication pattern was identified that had not been anticipated, a psychologically focused exchange making up some 7% of visits that addressed stressors and mental health problems. As the study was cross-sectional in nature, it was not possible to explore the predictors and frequency of relationship default. An international comparison study some years later largely replicated these patterns in Dutch primary care visits (Bensing et al. 2003).

Empowering Patient Communication

Individual variation in preferences and capacity along the autonomy continuum have been largely attributed to the psychological dynamics of the patients, physicians, illnesses, and contexts that characterize medical decision making. The larger social context and **social influences** that contribute to this variation have received relatively little focus. The work of Paulo Freire (1983) may be helpful in this regard, although it was originally applied to the teaching of basic literacy skills to adults and has been more widely used in the areas of community development and health education (Wallerstein and Bernstein 1988) and health literacy (Nutbeam 2000).

Freire sees the economic, political, and social relations that often characterize vulnerable populations mirrored in their educational experiences. Traditional approaches to teaching, in which learners are treated as passive and dependent objects, serve to reinforce powerlessness and helplessness. In contrast, participatory learning strategies that treat people as active subjects of their own learning can have the effect of changing patterns of dependence and passivity by providing and reinforcing empowering experiences. Empowering experiences foster the competence and confidence necessary for personal transformation and the realization of **critical consciousness**. This transformation is attributed to three key consciousness-raising experiences: relating and reflecting on experience, engaging in dialogue, and taking conscious action. These steps provide a framework for Freire's participatory social-orientation approach to the design of effective educational strategies (Freire 1983).

Physicians, it can be argued, are by their very nature teachers. In fact, one definition of *doctor* in the *Oxford English Dictionary* (1913 edition) is "teacher." The word *teacher* implies helping, but this help is not limited to the usual clinical sense of providing correct diagnosis and treatment or empathy and reassurance. It includes the responsibility and obligation to help patients assume an authentic and responsible role in the medical dialogue and in decision making. A teacher helps by equipping learners (patients) with what they need to help themselves; this includes information, but it also includes building patients' confidence in the value of their own actions in maintaining and promoting health. An important implication from Freire's work for patient-provider communication is an educator model, in which the physician is more egalitarian and collaborative than in the traditional doctor-patient model and, as such, can be thought of as core to the building of a mutual **partnership**. In this light, parallels to the social context of the medical visit may be considered. Physicians' use of particular communication strategies can reinforce patient passivity and dependence or foster full engagement and active collaboration in the medical dialogue.

As more fully discussed elsewhere (Roter 2000), the first of the communication steps is *patient participation in the medical dialogue,* through the telling of the patient's story. The process of narrative construction and delivery may be considered a vehicle for patient affirmation of self-worth and self-knowledge, much as the Freirian process of disclosure and reflection affirm the value of life experiences for an adult learner. For low-literacy patients with limited descriptive and organizational skills related to oral expression, articulating an illness narrative may be particularly problematic. Consequently, physician communication skills that help the patient build her history are especially important (Haidet and Paterniti 2003).

The second communication step is *activation for critical dialogue,* through the use of questions, information appraisal, joint problem solving, and negotiation skills in regard to medical decisions. This step is similar to the Freirian description of dialogue and critical analysis as a process that encourages examination of the individual's situation and the core conditions and circumstances that have contributed to it. The cognitive challenges associated with recall and comprehension of complex medical instructions and terminology, and the disinclination to ask questions or initiate challenges to physician expertise, present particular difficulties for patients with low levels of literacy. These patients may be more dependent on the physician's skillful facilitation of patient engagement in the dialogue than more literate patients are.

Finally, the third step of the communication continuum is *patient empowerment for change.* This occurs as the patient makes informed choices and takes control and responsibility for the social, environmental, and personal context of his health-related status quo. This last step is closest to the final step in the Freirian process that transforms an individual from a passive object to an active subject through recognition of her ability to control and transform life circumstances through action.

Judith Hibbard's work (see chapter 22) is most relevant in noting the importance of clinicians' communication behaviors for **patient**

activation during medical encounters. Clinicians can support patients' self-management, skill building, and goal setting and the establishment of a trusting relationship. Their efforts in this regard, however, may be less than fully effective when directed to patients with restricted literacy skills, since evidence suggests an association between literacy deficits and a variety of communication difficulties, including understanding and recalling complex information delivered orally (Baker et al. 1996; Bennett et al. 2006; Schillinger et al. 2004; Williams et al. 1998).

In earlier work, my colleagues and I have identified key language elements that constitute oral literacy demand (Roter et al. 2007). Consideration of these elements can facilitate patient movement across the communication continuum from enhanced participation in the medical dialogue to full activation and empowerment. These elements are described below along with evidence of their relationship to cognitive or affective outcomes.

The Oral Literacy Demand Framework

The oral literacy framework identifies language elements that contribute to verbal and nonverbal communication and are associated with a variety of cognitive and affective outcomes. The framework and associated outcomes are discussed in some detail below, including an overview of the framework's four key dialogue elements: (1) the use of jargon, (2) general language **complexity**, (3) contextualized language, and (4) structural characteristics of dialogue.

THE USE OF JARGON

Studies dating back to the 1960s have demonstrated that medical jargon is widely used during routine medical visits and is linked to patient confusion (Castro et al. 2007; Korsch et al. 1968; Svarstad 1974; Thompson 1994). A doctor will likely use at least one unfamiliar medical term in any given visit, and this practice has not

changed very much over the past 50 years. Barbara Korsch and her colleagues, in their pioneering work in this area (1968), found that the pediatrician's use of difficult technical language and medical shorthand was a barrier to communication in more than half of the 800 pediatric visits that were studied. Mothers were often confused and unsure of terms used by the doctor to describe what was wrong with their children and what the doctor was going to do about it. Although one mother (out of 800) asked the doctor to "repeat what he said in English," this kind of confrontation was infrequent; for the most part, mothers did not ask for clarification of unfamiliar terms. Fear of appearing ignorant was the reason most often given for not asking what technical terms meant. Moreover, the investigators suggested that some patients may be flattered by having the physician think that they understand difficult and unfamiliar language, which makes admitting their failure to understand even harder (Korsch et al. 1968).

In more recent studies, Castro and colleagues (2007) went beyond the previous studies by specifically examining the use of unclarified jargon with patients who have limited literacy skills and by assessing patient understanding of the terms used. Furthermore, all the patients in the study had diabetes, so it was possible to explore the impact of jargon use on their ability to understand related treatment recommendations. The investigators found that four unclarified terms were used per visit and at least one unclarified term was used in 85% of all visits. Overall, patient comprehension of unclarified diabetes-specific terms was low and never exceeded 40%.

My colleagues and I took a somewhat different tack in assessing jargon use during genetic counseling sessions. We tracked the frequency of seven key genetics-specific terms used during genetic counseling sessions (i.e., *variation, susceptibility, abnormality, sporadic, hereditary, mutation,* and *chromosome*), based on transcript analysis of more than 150 sessions (Roter et al.

2006). We found that an average of three different key terms (of the seven) were used in every session, and when used, a term was repeated often. In fact, key words were typically repeated 20 times in a single session, although some terms were repeated as many as 78 times.

We then related the frequency of key word use to subjects' ability to learn genetics-related information from the sessions (Roter et al. 2009). This was done by asking study participants to act as the patients in the genetic counseling session (essentially becoming analogue, or simulated, patients) and to take a knowledge test after viewing the session video. The knowledge test scores were subsequently related to the subject's level of literacy and the number of times each key term was used in the viewed session. Significant relationships did not emerge between analogue patient learning and the use of medical jargon in the sessions for low-literate subjects; jargon did not appear to significantly aide or hinder the ability of these analogue patients to learn genetic-related information as communicated by the counselor.

Other study analyses, based on ratings by the simulated patients who directly participated in the counseling videos, found a negative effect of jargon use on satisfaction (Roter et al. 2006). This derived not simply from the number of key words used, or even the number of repetitions; but, when the counselor's use of jargon was high relative to other interaction in the session, the simulated patient's satisfaction with interpersonal rapport suffered. This suggests that the use of technical words per se did not create a negative impression, but the relative emphasis on these words diminished attention to emotional and psychosocial issues and valued nonverbal behaviors.

GENERAL LANGUAGE COMPLEXITY

The second group of measures in the framework reflect general language complexity, and they are directly parallel to readability assessment of print material and analysis of active versus passive voice (Doak et al. 1996). General language complexity is distinguished from jargon use because it relates to the structure of the language, rather than the formality, unfamiliarity, or specialized use of terms. The markers of complex language are the same as those used to assess the reading demand of print material but are applied to the dialogue transcripts.

In our study of genetic counseling sessions, we used Microsoft Word grammar summary statistics (Microsoft Systems 2003) to generate a variety of language measures, including the total transcript word count, the average number of words per sentence, the percentage of transcript sentences in the passive voice, the Flesch Reading Ease Score, and the Flesch-Kincaid Reading Grade Level Score. The percentage of transcript sentences in the passive voice was used as a proxy for conversational formality. Although not directly provided with summary statistics, the average number of syllables per word was extrapolated from the Flesch Reading Ease Score.

Our analysis found that general language complexity acted much like jargon use and was not related to learning among low-literate subjects (Roter et al. 2009). One explanation may be the relatively low language complexity found in the study transcripts; the reading grade level of transcripts averaged 6.7 (range 4.3 to 11), with 1.4 syllables per word (range 1.3 to 1.6) (Roter et al. 2006).

As was the case for jargon use, the simulated patients who interacted directly with the genetic counselors rated sessions with more complex language more negatively than those with simpler language. More specifically, the simulated patients were significantly less satisfied with the informativeness of sessions that had higher Flesch-Kincaid Reading levels and greater use of the passive voice (Roter et al. 2006).

CONTEXTUALIZING LANGUAGE

Decontextualized language conveys abstract ideas or novel use of language and metaphors to describe an event or an internal state to another person. Individuals with restricted literacy tend to have difficulty with these sorts of explanations and are more likely to use and understand language that is concrete and grounded in what is directly seen and experienced (Dexter et al. 1998; Farmer et al. 2006). For example, a study of language used in a London emergency department to describe chest pain found that the largely immigrant and low-literacy patient population appeared confused and disoriented by health care provider questions that employed common metaphors to characterize chest pain, such as "Does it feel like an elephant on your chest or sharp like a knife?" Although the patients "learned" after multiple interviews that this is how chest pain was supposed to be described, their descriptions of pain when first arriving tended to be concrete and undescriptive: "I don't know, it's just a pain" or "it just doesn't feel right" (Farmer et al. 2006).

The aspect of literacy related to poor numeracy skills may also act to especially undermine patients' ability to understand health risks when presented in abstract ways. Schwartz and colleagues (1997) found that the one-third of their study sample who demonstrated inadequate numeracy skills (e.g., were unable to accurately predict how many of 1,000 fair coin flips would land on the same side) misinterpreted risk reduction data provided to them. The authors concluded that quantitative information about cancer risks and the benefits of screening may be meaningful only to individuals who have facility with basic probability and numerical concepts. In a similar vein, Davis and colleagues (2002) also found that women with reading skill levels at or below the fifth grade were three times less likely than those reading at or above the ninth-grade level to understand the value of a mammogram in cancer control.

Although ability to manipulate numbers may certainly be a factor in the misunderstandings cited above, the decontextualized language used to present risk and probability may be distracting and confusing to patients with re-

stricted literacy. In this regard, personalized information may be recognized as more relevant and useful than information given in general terms. For instance, in our genetic counseling study, we found that risk type information was personally contextualized in about 35% of the observed sessions. An example of what personally contextualized information about risks sounded like is as follows: "Based on what you told me about yourself and your family, you have a 1 in 400 risk of having a baby with Down syndrome," or "You already had a blood test and now we are talking about a more invasive test for you, amniocentesis." The more general, decontextualized reference would be: "Nobody has a risk of zero—women over 35 have about a 1 in 400 risk of having a baby with Down syndrome," or "There are several tests available; some are invasive and others are not."

Findings in regard to knowledge gain with personally contextualized language were striking. Analogue patients with restricted literacy skills learned significantly more when information was personally contextualized, less abstract, and more concrete (Roter et al. 2009).

DIALOGUE STRUCTURE
Three aspects of dialogue structure are considered in the framework: pacing or speech speed; turn density, reflecting the number of thoughts communicated in one speaking turn; and interactivity, the frequency of speaker change during the dialogue.

Pacing. There is some evidence that faster-than-normal speech speed adversely affects comprehension (Schmitt and Carroll 1985), and patients in focus groups complain about the fast pace in which information is communicated to them (Bennett et al. 2006). Although a patient can explicitly request that the physician slow down or repeat information, patients with low literacy skills are less likely to make requests of this kind than other patients (Bennett et al. 2006). Consequently, we hypothesized in our framework that rapid clinician speech raises demands for oral literacy when a clinician is conveying complex information (Roter et al. 2006).

Findings from two studies do not appear to support this assertion. In the genetic counseling study, dialogue pace was estimated by the rate of speech speed in syllables per second of session time. The assertion that rapid speech speed diminished learning for low-literacy subjects was not confirmed; knowledge scores were unrelated to pacing for low-literacy subjects (Roter et al. 2009).

A second simulation study conducted in primary care also explored the relationship between dialogue pacing and simulated patient ratings (Roter et al. 2008). In this case, pacing was measured in a somewhat different way than in the genetic counseling study because transcripts were not available. The total number of codes, defined as a complete thought, divided by the length of the session, was used as a proxy for the pace of statement delivery. The simulated patient ratings in this study indicated more positive ratings of physician demeanor, interpersonal satisfaction, and decision-making partnership with *faster* statement pace.

Turn density. Turn density is the amount of uninterrupted speech delivered by a speaker in a single speaking turn. We know that when information in print material is presented in manageable chunks, only a few items at a time, readers are more likely to remember the information given (Doak et al. 1996). A corollary in oral exchange is the informational block delivered during a speaking turn. In medical visits, an inverse relationship appears to exist between the overall amount of information given and the proportion of information a patient can recall (Ley 1982; Roter et al. 1987). Thus, the longer a clinician speaks, the denser the informational chunk, and the greater the oral literacy demand.

Doak and colleagues (1996) suggest that readers cannot comfortably process more than five pieces of information at a time. In the genetic counseling study described earlier, the average turn density for counselors was 6.8 statements,

suggesting that the information load each time a counselor spoke would be challenging for anyone, but especially so for patients with restricted literacy. In fact, analogue clients with restricted literacy skills learned significantly less in sessions with long, dense counselor speaking turns (Roter et al. 2009).

Interactivity. The last dialogue dimension is interactivity, defined as the rate of speaker change per minute of interaction throughout the session. Greater interactivity results in a more conversational exchange that provides speaking opportunities for patients as well as a natural break between informational monologues. Once again, a parallel exists here with dialogue interactivity in print assessment. To more effectively engage print readers, interactive strategies such as question-answer formats, quizzes, brainstorming exercises, and risk self-assessment has been suggested (Doak et al. 1996). Although the mode of interactivity is obviously different between print and dialogue, the rate of speaker exchange similarly demands active attention and engagement of speakers in a reciprocal process of informational **evaluation** and response.

Finally, some evidence shows that analogue clients with restricted literacy skills learned significantly more when viewing genetic counseling sessions with greater interactivity (Roter et al. 2009) and that simulated patients rate highly interactive sessions more positively in regard to provider demeanor, interpersonal satisfaction, and decision-making partnership in both the genetic counseling context and in primary care (Roter et al. 2006; Roter et al. 2008).

Conclusions

More than a half century ago, Pratt and colleagues described a communication-limiting cycle in which a reticent patient appears to wait for his doctor to offer explanations while the doctor interprets the patient's reticence as an indication of disinterest or incompetence. The description is as apt today as it was 50 years ago:

> When the doctor perceives the patient as rather poorly informed, he considers the tremendous difficulties of translating his knowledge into language the patient can understand along with the dangers of frightening the patient. Therefore, he avoids involving himself in an elaborate discussion with the patient; the patient, in turn, reacts dully to this limited information, either asking uninspired questions, or refraining from questioning the doctor at all, thus reinforcing the doctor's view that the patient is ill equipped to comprehend his problem. This further reinforces the doctor's tendency to skirt discussions of the problem. Lacking guidance by the doctor, the patient performs at a low level, hence, the doctor rates his capacities as even lower than they are. (Pratt et al. 1957, 1280)

With the increasing time and productivity pressures that plague all physicians, many fear that a patient-centered approach to communication may result in an increase in visit length within the context of an already time-pressured atmosphere. Indeed, recent reports claim that the average medical visit has lengthened by some 10% over the past 10 years; this is largely attributed to a proliferation of **guidelines** and expectations regarding preventive and counseling services (Carr-Hill et al. 1998; Yarnall et al. 2003). Ironically, the patient education and counseling that constitute much of this time burden may be having a less-than-optimal effect for the large segment of the patient population that lacks the literacy skills to benefit from these efforts.

Although the challenges for patients with the literacy deficits described here are considerable, communication **interventions** *have* proven effective for these populations, including interventions designed to enhance patient participation and engagement in the medical dialogue (Roter and Hall 2006). We look forward to pro-

grams in the future that can help shepherd patients to critical dialogue and empowerment while also providing to health care providers the complementary professional skills that support the development of fully mutual, collaborative, and effective therapeutic relationships.

REFERENCES

Baker DW, Gazmararian JA, Williams MV, et al. 2002. Functional health literacy and the risk of hospital admission among Medicare managed care enrollees. *Am J Public Health* 92 (8): 1278-83.

Baker DW, Parker RM, Williams MV, Clark WS. 1998. Health literacy and the risk of hospital admission. *J Gen Intern Med* 13 (12): 791-98.

Baker DW, Parker RM, Williams MV, et al. 1996. The health care experience of patients with low literacy. *Arch Family Med* 5 (6): 329-34.

Beach MC, Inui T. 2006. Relationship-centered care research network: Relationship-centered care: A constructive reframing. *J Gen Intern Med* 21 (suppl. 1) (Jan.): S3-S8.

Bennett IM, Switzer J, Barg F, Aguirre A, Evans K. 2006. "Breaking it down": Patient-clinician communication and prenatal care among African American women of low and higher literacy. *Ann Fam Med* 4 (4): 334-40.

Bensing JM, Roter DL, Hulsman RL. 2003. Communication patterns of primary care physicians in the US and the Netherlands. *J Gen Intern Med* 18:335-42.

Carr-Hill R, Jenkins-Clarke S, Dixon P, Pringle M. 1998. Do minutes count? Consultation lengths in general practice. *J Health Serv Res Policy* 3:297-313.

Castro CM, Wilson C, Wang F, Schillinger, D. 2007. Babel babble: Physicians' use of unclarified medical jargon with patients. *Am J Health Behav* 31 (suppl. 1): S85-S95.

Cooper LA, Beach MC, Clever SL. 2004. Participatory decision-making in the medical encounter and its relationship to patient literacy. In *Understanding Health Literacy: Implications for Medicine and Public Health,* ed. J Schwartzberg, J Van Geest, C Wang, et al., 101-18. Chicago: AMA Press.

Davis TC, Williams MV, Marin E, Parker RM, Glass J. 2002. Health literacy and cancer communication. *CA Cancer J Clin* 52:134-49.

DeWalt DA, Pignone, M. 2005. Health literacy and health outcomes: Overview of the literature. In *Understanding Health Literacy,* ed. J Schwartzberg, J Van Geest, C Wang, et al., 205-27. Chicago: AMA Press.

Dexter ER, LeVine SE, Velasco PM. 1998. Maternal schooling and health-related language and literacy skills in rural Mexico. *Compar Educ Rev* 42 (2): 139-62.

Doak C, Doak L, Root J. 1996. *Teaching Patients with Low Literacy Skills.* 2nd ed. Philadelphia: Lippincott.

Emanuel EJ, Emanuel LL. 1992. Four models of the physician-patient relationship. *JAMA* 267:2221-26.

Farmer SA, Roter DL, Higgenson IJ. 2006. Chest pain: Communication of symptoms and history in a London emergency department. *Patient Educ Couns* 63 (1-2): 138-44.

Freire P. 1983. *Education for Critical Consciousness.* New York: Continuum Press.

Gazmararian JA, Baker DW, Williams MV, et al. 1999. Health literacy among Medicare enrollees in a managed care organization. *JAMA* 281 (6): 545-51.

Haidet P, Paterniti D. 2003. "Building" a history rather than "taking" one: A perspective on information sharing during the medical interview. *Arch Intern Med* 163:1134-40.

Haug MR, Lavin B. 1981. Practitioner or patient—who's in charge? *J Health Soc Behav* 22 (3) (Sept.): 212-29.

Hibbard JH, Greene J, Becker ER, et al. 2008. Racial/ethnic disparities and consumer activation in health. *Health Aff (Millwood)* 27 (5) (Sept.-Oct.): 1442-53.

Korsch BM, Gozzi EK, Francis V. 1968. Gaps in doctor-patient communication. I. Doctor-patient interaction and patient satisfaction. *Pediatrics* 42 (5): 855-71.

Kutner M, Greenberg E, Jin Y, Boyle B, Hsu Y, Dunleavy E. 2007. *Literacy in Everyday Life: Results from the 2003 National Assessment of Adult Literacy.* NCES 2007-480. U.S. Dept. of Education. Washington, DC: National Center for Education Statistics.

Ley, P. 1982. Patients' understanding and recall in clinical communication failure. In *Doctor-Patient Communication,* ed. D Pendleton, J Hasler, 89-108. New York: Academic Press.

Microsoft Systems. 2003. Readability scores. Available at Microsoft Office, http://office.microsoft.com/assistance/hfws.aspx?AssetID=HP05.

Nutbeam D. 2000. Health literacy as a public health goal: A challenge for contemporary health education and communication strategies into the 21st century. *Health Promot Int* 15:259-67.

Parikh NS, Parker RM, Nurss JR, Baker DW, Williams MV. 1996. Shame and health literacy: The unspoken connection. *Patient Educ Couns* 27 (1): 33-39.

Pratt L, Seligmann A, Reader G. 1957. Physicians' views on the level of medical information among patients. *Am J Public Health* 47:1277-83.

Roter D. 2000. The medical visit context of treatment decision-making and the therapeutic relationship. *Health Expect* 3:17-25.

———. 2004. Health literacy and the patient provider relationship. In *Understanding Health Literacy: Implications for Medicine and Public Health,* ed. J Schwartzberg, J Van Geest, C Wang, et al., 87-100. Chicago: AMA Press.

Roter D, Ellington L, Erby LH, Larson S, Dudley W. 2006. The Genetic Counseling Video Project (GCVP): Models of practice. *Am J Med Genet C Semin Med Genet* 142 (4): 209-20.

Roter DL, Erby LH, Larson S. 2007. Assessing oral literacy demand in genetic counseling dialogue: A preliminary test of a conceptual framework. *Soc Sci Med* 65 (7): 1442-57.

Roter DL, Erby LH, Larson S, Ellington L. 2009. Oral literacy demand of prenatal genetic counseling dialogue: Predictors of learning. *Patient Educ Couns* 75 (3): 392-97.

Roter DL, Hall JA. 2006. *Doctors Talking to Patients/Patients Talking to Doctors: Improving Communication in Medical Visits.* 2nd ed. Westport, CT: Praeger.

Roter DL, Hall JA, Katz NR. 1987. Relations between physicians' behaviors and analogue patients' satisfaction, recall, and impressions. *Med Care* 25 (5): 437-51.

Roter DL, Larson SM, Beach MC, Cooper LA. 2008. Interactive and evaluative correlates of dialogue sequence: A simulation study applying the RIAS to turn taking structures. *Patient Educ Couns* 71:26-33.

Roter DL, Stewart M, Putnam S, Lipkin M, Stiles W, Inui T. 1997. Communication patterns of primary care physicians. *JAMA* 270:350-55.

Schillinger D, Bindman AB, Wang F, Stewart A, Piette J. 2004. Functional health literacy and the quality of physician-patient communication among diabetes patients. *Patient Educ Couns* 52 (3): 315-23.

Schillinger D, Grumbach K, Piette J, et al. 2002. Association of health literacy with diabetes outcomes. *JAMA* 288 (4): 475-82.

Schmitt JF, Carroll MR. 1985. Older listeners' ability to comprehend speaker-generated rate alteration of passages. *J Speech Hearing Res* 28 (2): 309-12.

Schwartz LM, Woloshin S, Welch HG. 1997. The role of numeracy in understanding the benefit of screening mammography. *Ann Intern Med* 127:966-72.

Scott TL, Gazmararian JA, Williams MV, Baker DW. 2002. Health literacy and preventive health care use among Medicare enrollees in a managed care organization. *Med Care* 40 (5): 395-404.

Smedley BD, Stith AY, Nelson AR, eds. 2003. *Unequal Treatment: Confronting Racial and Ethnic Disparities in Health Care.* Committee on Understanding and Eliminating Racial and Ethnic Disparities in Health Care. Washington, DC: National Academies Press.

Svarstad BL. 1974. The doctor-patient encounter: An observational study of communication and outcome. PhD diss., University of Wisconsin-Madison.

Thompson TL. 1994. Interpersonal communication and health care. In *Handbook of Interpersonal Communication,* ed. ML Knapp, GR Miller, 696-725. 2nd ed. Thousand Oaks, CA: Sage.

Wallerstein N, Bernstein E. 1988. Empowerment education: Freire's ideas adapted to health education. *Health Educ Q* 15:379-94.

Williams MV, Baker DW, Parker RM, Nurss JR. 1998. Relationship of functional health literacy to patients' knowledge of their chronic disease: A study of patients with hypertension and diabetes. *Arch Intern Med* 158 (2): 166-72.

Yarnall KSH, Pollack KI Ostbye T, Krause KM, Michener JL. 2003. Primary care: Is there enough time for prevention? *Am J Public Health* 93:635-41.

Health Risk Assessment

MARTHA SYLVIA AND INES VIGIL

LEARNING OBJECTIVES

After completing the chapter, the reader will be able to

* Describe the context, utility, and value of health risk assessment.
* Identify valid and reliable health risk assessment tools.
* Distinguish the utility of health risk assessment data when supplemented by data from other sources.
* Give examples of interventions based on health risk assessment.
* Discuss the policy, legal, and ethical considerations of health risk assessment.

Introduction

A **health risk assessment** (**HRA**) is a useful tool to influence **health behavior** change and improve health outcomes in defined populations. In addition to providing an overview of the **self-reported** health of a population, an HRA informs respondents of their measured health status, delineates individual risk for developing chronic health conditions or exacerbating existing health conditions, and provides information on recommended gender- and age-appropriate preventive health services. The population health overview and individual health risk information provided by an HRA makes it particularly useful for motivating health behavior change.

For the purposes of this chapter, an HRA is defined as an evidence-based tool used to assess the health status of individuals through self-reported responses to health-related questions. Individuals provide input on multiple domains of their health, and an HRA-specific scoring mechanism is used to calculate health risks. Personalized feedback on health risks and recommendations to improve health status are provided to the respondent, and the data is aggregated for population-level analysis.

For respondents, the HRA provides detailed information regarding health status, health risks, and recommended preventive health services. Pairing an HRA with individualized, evidence-based feedback provides a unique opportunity to stimulate self-reflection and self-discovery regarding health risks and health behaviors. Such feedback is particularly valuable for respondents whose self-perception of their health conflicts with their actual (measured) health status (McCormick 2006; Miller and Iris 2002).

For organizations, aggregate HRA information for a defined population provides a broad view of its baseline health data, health behaviors, and self-reported health status. This information can highlight characteristics of the organization's environment that either promote or restrict optimal health and productivity and provide a framework for **intervention**. Moreover, HRAs provide population health data for comparison with national health trend benchmarks, and sequential collection of HRA data over time allows for **surveillance** of health risks, chronic health conditions, and changes in health status.

The first evidence of HRAs appeared in the early 1950s. Lewis Robbins, the "father" of the HRA, intended for physicians to use the questions during patient encounters to inform individual patients about their risk of premature death. However, HRA use among physicians has been minimal (Fielding 1989). Between 1970 and 1986, awareness and use of the HRA grew. The U.S. federal government increased funding for work site health promotion activities, including the use of HRAs, and the Centers for Disease Control and Prevention (CDC) released HRA methods and software to the public domain. Additionally, research interest increased, and an HRA research agenda was proposed at the National Conference of the Foundation for Health Services Research. In 1960, the Society of Prospective Medicine (SPM) was formed and charged with determining the effect of health behaviors, lifestyle, and medical health status on the future of health. SPM went on to publish a comprehensive comparative manual of HRA tools in 1999, with more than 45 tools in circulation (Hyner et al. 1999). In 1989, 29% of U.S. work sites reported using HRAs; by 2007, 56% of work sites reported using HRAs (Fielding 1989; Rosenthal et al. 2007).

Information Obtained from a Health Risk Assessment

HRA response data provides information on health behaviors and is used primarily to assess individuals' health risk and risk for developing medical condition(s). Health risk is calculated from HRA question responses using evidence-based algorithms and is commonly summarized in a feedback report to respondents. An HRA feedback report typically includes categorical health risk scores, definitions of the health risk(s), and behavioral recommendations for improvement. HRA data is normally used in conjunction with data from an administrative payment process for health care services (i.e., medical and pharmacy claims data, physicians' and other facility electronic medical record data). HRA categories often include these:

- Cardiovascular, diabetes, and cancer risk
  - Overweight and obesity
  - Smoking
  - Poor nutrition
  - Poor fitness
  - Self-reported biometric measures (i.e., blood pressure, cholesterol, weight, and height)
- Nutritional deficiencies
  - Fruit and vegetable intake
  - Fat intake
  - Fiber intake
  - Salt intake
- Fitness deficiencies
  - Physical activity levels
  - Sedentary lifestyle
  - Physical limitations
- Stress or mental well-being risk
  - Stress triggers and relievers

- Sleep patterns
- Social support
• Substance use
    - Alcohol
    - Tobacco (smoking and chewing)
    - Illicit drugs
• Safety risk
    - Seat belt use
    - Sun protection
    - Safety precautions (e.g., safe lifting, bicycle helmet use)
    - Risky sexual behavior
• Medical follow-up
• Preventive exams
• Presence or absence of chronic conditions
• Functional health status
• Psychosocial health status
• Spiritual health status
• Financial health status
• Self-perception of health status
• Interest in wellness and health promotion programs and literature
• Readiness to make a change in health behaviors and risks
• Absenteeism and lost productivity in the workplace because of health risks and illness

TABLE 24.1. Identification of health behaviors: HRA versus medical claims

Data of interest	HRA	Medical claims
Presence of chronic illness/ multiple morbidity	√	√
Utilization and cost of medical care		√
Utilization and cost of pharmaceuticals		√
Cost of lost work productivity	√	
Perceived health status	√	
Readiness to change	√	
Health history	√	√
Family history	√	
Symptoms	√	
Biographical data (height, weight, blood pressure, etc.)	√	
Exercise level	√	
Eating habits	√	
Alcohol, drugs, smoking	√	√
Work site health and safety	√	
Accessing medical care	√	√
Stress and coping	√	

HRA data provides valuable health behavior information that is not typically available in other sources of health-related data, such as medical claims or electronic medical records (EMR). As such, HRA self-reported information may produce different prevalence rates for health risks from rates obtained via medical claims or EMR data. For instance, prevalence rates of overweight, obesity, and smoking are often higher in self-reported data than in claims or EMR data (Clark et al. 2010). Table 24.1 highlights differences in types of data captured between HRA self-reported data and administrative medical claims data.

HRA question responses can be used alone or together with other data for population-level analyses. Aggregating multiple sources of data increases the comprehensiveness of a popula-

tion health data set and improves an organization's ability to intervene. HRA aggregate data can often be combined with other data sources to produce a more comprehensive and accurate understanding of the health status of a defined population, combining *subjective* HRA self-reported information with *objective* health care utilization information.

HRA data can be collected within an EMR and/or a personal health record (PHR) and combined with other data to create a more comprehensive patient profile and targeted patient feedback and interventions. EMRs are repositories of patient health information in digital form collected by health care providers at the point of health care service delivery with the purpose of supporting continuous, integrated, efficient, and quality healthcare (Hayrinen et al. 2008). PHRs are applications through which individuals can contribute to, access, share, and manage health care information that may or may not be linked to an EMR (Jones et al. 2010). Standardized HRAs with individualized feedback are embedded into many PHR systems on the market today. The ideal integrated system is one in which the EMR and the PHR are linked with the systems applying evidence-based algorithmic rules to data obtained from the EMR, the PHR, and the HRA that will guide the health care provider to target relevant health care issues and the individual to be aware of and address health risks.

Collecting HRA data in conjunction with biometrics involves objective measurement of biometric values including but not limited to height, weight, waist circumference, blood pressure, blood glucose, blood cholesterol, and lung capacity. Biometric data is most useful in providing instant feedback to the participant about pertinent health-related biometric measures such as heart rate, blood pressure, and **body mass index (BMI)**. Biometric measures are obtained and feedback is typically provided by a health professional. Provider-directed feedback facilitates an opportunity to directly address the impact of individual health risks and influence individual follow-up of abnormal lab values. Objective biometric data can then be compared to subjective self-report of biometric measures in the HRA, priming a discussion to take place between the provider and the individual regarding the individual's perceived and measured health.

Commonly used methods for the collection and reporting of biometric data can include the following:

- Biometric measurement by a health professional and individual submission of biometric information and reporting via a PHR

- Biometric measurement performed by a health professional and reporting via an EMR
- Biometric measurement performed via a health screening and reporting via manual documentation

Using a Health Risk Assessment

When considering an HRA type, look for a tool that is both reliable and valid. For the purposes of HRA administration, **reliability** is defined as the ability of the HRA to *consistently* measure health risks across multiple people *and* within the same person at different points in time. HRA reliability is measured by administering the HRA to a small subset of the population for which the HRA is intended.

Validity is defined as the ability of the HRA to measure what it was intended to measure—health risks. Validity is measured by comparing HRA responses to a non-self-reported measure of the same risk or condition, such as that which is usually obtained from administrative medical claims or EMR data. Risk factors with an established medical diagnosis code for claims billing submission, such as high blood pressure and high cholesterol, are good examples of health risks that can be validated from administrative data. Obesity and smoking, however, are frequently underreported measures in administrative medical claims and EMR data and should not be used for validation (Clark et al. 2010). Also keep in mind the "recall period" for HRA questions that ask about events such as days absent from work, physician visits, or hospitalizations. The recall period is the time frame within which the respondent is expected to remember the occurrence of such events; shorter recall periods usually produce a more accurate response (Short et al. 2009).

The intent of the HRA is to directly measure health risk, not health outcomes. The primary **goal** of the HRA and HRA feedback is to raise awareness of health risks and recommend actionable modifications in behavior that have been shown in the scientific literature to prevent poor health outcomes and thus ultimately reduce those health risks. The developer or vendor of any given HRA tool can provide reliability and validity testing information. When selecting an existing HRA, look to HRAs that use questions from validated instruments, scientific evidence, and/or clinical experts. An example of HRA questions developed from scientific evidence would be questions that measure cardiovascular risk from evidence gathered from the Framingham Heart Study (Hyner et al. 1999).

HRAs with the following characteristics are likely to have greater reliability and validity:

- Written description of how validity and reliability are addressed by the developer of the tool
- Indication of the evidence base from which the HRA questions are developed
- Experienced use and/or pilot testing in various diverse populations
- Experienced use and/or pilot testing with a small subset of the larger intended population
- Easy-to-understand questions that require only one answer; for example, "Do you have a primary care physician?" versus "Do you have a primary care physician and have you had your annual preventive care visit?"
- Validation studies of any versions that have been translated into languages other than that in which the HRA was originally developed
- Written description of the process used to ensure privacy and protection of information

HRA **effectiveness**, a different measure from reliability and validity, measures an HRA's ability to effect behavior change, modify health risk(s), and prevent an HRA-question-related adverse health outcome. The effectiveness of an HRA is typically measured when an HRA is used to intervene (raise awareness of an individual's health risk and induce self-reflection and self-discovery). HRA effectiveness is determined after HRA administration has taken place and feedback has been provided. HRA effectiveness has been studied by measuring changes in health risk levels, such as BMI, blood pressure, and cholesterol; health behaviors, such as exercise **habits**, nutrition intake, and alcohol intake; age-appropriate prevention screenings, such as mammograms and colonoscopies; and use of medical services such as emergency department visits and hospitalizations at baseline HRA administration and during a subsequent period, usually six months (RAND 2003; Schoenbach et al. 1987).

Selecting and Administering a Health Risk Assessment

Selection and implementation of an HRA serves a dual purpose: it determines both the health status of each individual HRA respondent and the aggregate health status of a defined population. The first step in implementing HRAs in any population begins with the selection of an HRA. Various types of HRAs exist and are available both on paper and electronically.

Selection of an HRA depends on the type of information desired at both an individual and a population level. General health risk categories are consistently present in HRAs and include topics such as nutrition, physical fitness, stress, smoking status, substance use, presence or absence of common health conditions, weight, height, gender, and productivity levels. HRAs are also available to address health risks of specific populations such as individuals over age 65, children, disadvantaged populations, people with specific health conditions, employees, military personnel, and so forth. HRAs are readily available through public and governmental agencies, academic institutions, health insurance companies, and private vendors. HRAs offered through private vendors are commonly provided in conjunction with **wraparound services**, such as health coaching or a wellness program. A basic Internet search of the term *health risk assessment* provides a wide sample of existing HRAs available for use.[1]

When you are administering an HRA, it is important to understand how individuals access and respond to questionnaires that solicit health information. HRA response rates typically increase when respondents are offered multiple modalities. Modalities for administering HRAs can include the following:

- Providing Internet access through links to HRAs on favored websites
- Sending targeted e-mails with a link to the HRA
- Integrating the HRA into employee benefit applications
- Providing kiosks with computer access to the HRA and personnel to assist with technical and other questions
- Providing paper copies of the HRA and a submission process
- Administering verbally such as with interactive voice technologies

To maximize the behavior change effects of using an HRA, it is essential to provide individual feedback results to respondents—that is, how they compare to the rest of the respondent population as well as how they compare to national benchmarks. Individuals receiving **tailored** feedback can benefit from knowing that others in their cohort are challenged by similar health risks. Additionally, HRA feedback should be paired with instructions to individuals on how to access available resources aimed at reducing specific health risks and improving overall health, productivity, and **quality of life**. HRA results can also be used as a foundation for selecting existing health promotion programs and interventions that address health risks identified in the aggregated HRA feedback.

Legal, Policy, and Ethical Implications

There are policy **consequences** and legal/ethical implications surrounding the use of HRAs. The Health Information Portability and Accountability Act (HIPAA) regulates HRA administration under the definitions set forth in the HIPAA Compliant Wellness Programs and within the privacy rules. Generally, HIPAA sets forth rules that employers are required to follow when pairing HRA completion with **incentives** or when limiting health benefits based upon individual responses to HRA questions. In most circumstances, HRA information is considered protected health information (PHI), and the HIPAA privacy rules strictly regulate how PHI is defined, maintained, used, and shared by organizations collecting such information. A critical element to administering an HRA is maintaining strict confidentiality of identifiable or individualized data acquired through HRA administration (Fensholt 2011).

The Americans with Disabilities Act (ADA) states that employers must not discriminate against a qualified individual on the basis of a disability in regard to job application procedures such as the hiring, advancement, and discharge of employees and in regard to employee compensation. The Genetic Information Non-Discrimination Act (GINA) of 2010 prohibits the use of genetic information in employment decisions such as hiring, firing, and promotions as well as in health benefit offerings such as premiums and benefit offerings. Both ADA and GINA legislation have implications for the use of HRA data by employers, including the type of information that may be asked for in an HRA. The Equal Employment Opportunity Commission provides guidance for employers to ensure that HRA information is not used in employment decisions and that HRAs avoid questions related to genetics and family history (Coalition for Genetic Fairness 2008; Fensholt 2011; USEOC 1990, 2008).

Despite the existence of legislation to protect individual health-related information such as that contained within a completed HRA, and the ways in which this information is used, other legal and ethical issues may arise. Potential HRA respondents are often concerned about potential loss of privacy, **stigmatization**, and discrimination. Organizations offer guidance in this area with published ethical **guidelines** for HRA administration. Suggestions for maintaining legal and ethical integrity include the following (Hyner et al. 1999):

- Develop a philosophy of HRA use with all **stakeholders** prior to implementation and include a written statement of goals, **objectives**, methodology, and requirements for participation.
- Select an HRA tool appropriate for the **target population**, taking into account cultural and ethnic differences.
- Fully disclose how HRA data will be used, what persons or entities have access to the data, and the types of data accessed by each entity.
- Obtain signed informed consent for each respondent.
- Fully disclose the security of data-handling procedures.
- Include the ability for potential respondents to decline participation without consequences.
- Develop an orientation module explaining HRA-related procedures and information.
- Develop a mechanism by which HRA respondents can voice concerns and receive follow-up.

Health Risk Assessment Measurement and Outcome Utility

Several outcome measures can be obtained via the administration and aggregation of HRA information. Outcome measures can be organized into four major categories: (1) general, (2) longitudinal, (3) aggregate, and (4) cost savings.

General outcome measures are commonly reported HRA administration measures that include the HRA participation rate (total number of HRA respondents) and the HRA completion rate (total number of respondents completing all HRA questions). Health risk analysis measures are tracked over time and are often used to intervene to reduce health risk. Examples include the most common identified health risk, the most common identified chronic condition, and the most frequent symptoms. Intervention-associated outcome measures are described as the overall decrease in health risk over time and can include reduced BMI, improved nutrition, increased physical activity, and increased utilization of preventive screening exams. Other outcome measures include level of engagement in health promotion or disease prevention activities and the effectiveness of intervening in reducing overall health risk.

Longitudinal HRA data, defined as data collected over an extended time period, can be used to track changes in health risk for a defined population over time, measure the effectiveness of specific interventions, and determine areas for health improvement. The National Committee for Quality Assurance (NCQA) developed quality standards that are used to evaluate and accredit wellness and health promotion programs. In order to obtain accreditation, wellness and health promotion programs are required to collect and report longitudinal health risk data such as that collected via HRAs. NCQA's Wellness & Health Promotion (WHP) Accreditation standards require tracking and reporting the effect of wellness-related interventions on health risks such as smoking, BMI, and physical activity level over time (NCQA 2009).

Longitudinal HRA data also allows for comparisons to be made between organizations using national statistics for individual and aggregate health risk characteristics over time.

National statistics are available from the following organizations:

- NCQA WHP Accreditation focuses on assessment of key areas of health promotion, including measuring health risks shown in evidence-based literature to lead to development of chronic health conditions and health promotion-related interventions. Available at http://ncqa.org.
- The Centers for Disease Control and Prevention collects national risk identification information for the development of chronic health conditions, including obesity mapping, smoking, salt intake, and access to nutritional foods. Available at www.cdc.gov.
- Large HRA data centers, such as those maintained by privately owned companies, provide services to assist in health and productivity management.

Aggregate HRA data can be used to develop population-specific algorithms designed to identify individuals eligible to benefit from a wellness program or intervention. For example, an analysis of HRA data may reveal that HRA respondents do not eat the recommended daily intake of dietary fiber. This information can be used to develop a tailored education program disseminating communication messages on the importance of consuming fiber daily, potential improvement of certain health conditions, such as high cholesterol (Brown et al. 1999), and screening exams for related health conditions, such as a cholesterol blood test. The same HRA information can be used to develop criteria to identify and regularly reach out to high risk individuals who would benefit from the education program.

Cost savings can be calculated from HRA data collected over multiple years. Measuring cost savings related to HRA and wellness interventions requires the tracking of HRA information over time, along with an assignment of cost derived from published evidence of costs associated with certain health risks. Cost savings are achieved when the risk in a population decreases over time, and the savings are often reported as a reduction in or the avoidance of the costs directly assigned to a health risk. For example, if the average medical cost over one year for a smoker is calculated to be $5,000, the average medical cost over one year for a non-smoker is calculated to be $2,500 per year (controlling for other factors), and the prevalence of cigarette smokers in the population decreases by 10 individuals in one year, the costs saved may be reported to be an estimated $25,000 ([$5,000 − $2,500] × 10 individuals) (Edington et al. 1997; Musich et al. 2003; Yen et al. 2003).

Health Risk Assessment–Based Interventions

Aggregate HRA data is most frequently used on an ongoing basis to identify opportunities to improve the health of a defined population. HRAs with feedback have been shown to be most effective at influencing behavior change when paired with health education interventions (Soler et al. 2010). Interventions and strategies aimed at promoting the adoption of positive health behaviors can be both developed and purchased through a vendor.

When selecting interventions to enhance an HRA's ability to influence behavior change in a population, it is paramount to find those aimed at preventing the underlying causes of preventable disease and disability. The interventions should incorporate evidence-based health behavior models and theories such as the **Health Belief Model**, the **Transtheoretical Model**, and **Social Cognitive Theory** (Wallace 2008). Strategies should target health behaviors that have been shown to have a high incidence of **morbidity** and **mortality** but that improve with behavior change. For example, in the United States in the year 2000, the top three leading causes of death were identified as heart disease, cancer, and cerebrovascular disease (NCHS

2002). The behaviors identified as underlying these causes of death were tobacco use (a significant underlying cause of leading cancer and heart disease deaths) and poor diet and physical inactivity (underlying causes of heart disease deaths and diabetes-related heart disease deaths) (Mokdad et al. 2004). Information gained from the administration of HRAs can be used to determine the prevalence of these behaviors in a defined population and can further be used for the development or selection of interventions that target those health behaviors.

Knowledge of a population's health risks and health-related behaviors increases the ability to influence the adoption of positive health behaviors, improve health, and improve overall quality of life. HRA feedback results engage individuals in their health and convey the importance of seeking out a primary care provider for needed preventive health services. The impact of HRA administration on health engagement is amplified when it is used in conjunction with interventions that incorporate **goal setting** and the development of action plans, as is often seen in various health coaching, lifestyle management, disease management, and nurse case management programs. Other interventions that enhance the applicability of HRA feedback results at the individual level include the following:

- Disseminating health promotion educational materials on topics presented in the HRA
- Providing on-site physical activity programs and/or equipment
- Coordinating community-sponsored physical fitness activities
- Making nutritious food products available
- Providing a healthy workplace environment
- Encouraging health-related fitness activities

Above all, interventions should focus on reducing behaviors that lead to the development of health risks, improving overall health and productivity, and reducing cumulative health risks that can lead to the development of chronic health conditions.

Key Stakeholders

The identification and involvement of **key stakeholders** is critical to the success of selecting and implementing an HRA and gathering useful data from it. Understanding the value an HRA can provide to individuals, groups, and organizations can influence their level of engagement, further build support, and potentially add resources to ensure a successful HRA implementation. The following paragraphs outline important stakeholders and describe what value an HRA would have for them.

Individuals

An HRA can influence individual behavior change by causing individuals to acknowledge and report their understanding of their health status and behaviors. This self-assessment can serve as the first step to recognizing how individual actions and behaviors can impact the likelihood of developing future preventable health conditions. For example, an individual's understanding of the recommended daily intake of nutritional foods and guidelines for physical activity may differ from evidence-based recommendations that have been shown to help prevent several types of cancer, including cancer of the breast and of the colon (Kushi et al. 2006). An HRA respondent may make changes in nutritional intake or physical activity, or both, based upon the feedback generated from answering the HRA questions, given that the feedback provided often specifically relates an individual's level of engagement and activity to specific health topics and risks (Brown et al. 2003; USDHHS 1996). Coupled with **reinforcement** from the individual's health care provider, this feedback can serve as a powerful motivator for reducing unhealthful behaviors and adopting a more healthful lifestyle.

Employers

Understanding the health risks of an employee population enables employers to tailor the work environment to promote health and increase work productivity. HRA data can provide guidance to employers when selecting various wellness programs and initiatives to address health risks in their employee population. For example, an employer wants to know the effect that certain health behaviors may have on work productivity. The employer administers an HRA, aggregates the data, and discovers that a large number of employees smoke cigarettes or use tobacco products during work hours and express an interest in quitting. The employer can use this information to develop or purchase a tobacco-cessation program for the employees, track employee participation in the program, and determine its effect on decreasing the number of smoke breaks employees take throughout the day.

Health Insurance Plans

The administration of HRAs and the selection of interventions that closely match HRA-identified health risks provide a way to proactively identify health plan members with a high percentage of health risks and intervene to prevent the development of health conditions and complications of established health conditions. Programs and services can be provided to health plan members that directly address their health risks and encourage the appropriate use of medical and preventive health care services. HRA data can also be used to guide health insurance benefit design, enabling health insurance plans to develop cost-effective strategies to reduce a population's burden of illness and decrease inappropriate utilization of health care services. A health insurance plan can also benefit from establishing an HRA-based wellness program by receiving a quality accreditation from the NCQA.

Health Services Researchers

Several population-based health analyses have been performed using HRA data, but they merely scratch the surface of utilizing HRA information as a data source for health services research. When aggregated and tracked over time, HRA data can help researchers understand how health behaviors contribute to the development of health risks and overall health improvement or decline. Longitudinal HRA data can act as a population **surveillance** data source, with individuals reporting their health behaviors and health status periodically over time. A change in an individual's health status may differ from a change in a population's health status over time. Surveying health risk factors in both individuals and populations can provide insights into the biological and environmental contributions to health improvement or decline over time. Health service researchers interested in determining the effectiveness of health promotion activities can benefit from administering an HRA as a method of identifying changes in health behaviors associated with participation in a particular health promotion activity. Additionally, researchers may be interested in differences that may exist between an individual's self-reported health status and the individual's measured health status, furthering the utility of self-reported HRA information when compared with measured clinical indicators of health status. The availability of potentially conflicting information can be advantageous in settings where coaching from self-reported and measured health behavior data is used to raise an individual's awareness of certain health risks and their potential impact on health outcomes.

Government and Nongovernment Health Agencies and Organizations

In addition to the benefits of HRAs in linking health behaviors to the development of health conditions and population-based health risk surveillance, HRA data can be used to inform policymakers when drafting health reform legislation. Examples of local and national legislation that has resulted from health risks identified to cause preventable health conditions include the regulation of the sale of tobacco products to minors; the ban of cigarette smoking in public enclosed spaces; the elimination of the use of trans fats in food establishments; and, most recently, the New York City ban on sugar-based beverages larger than 16 ounces (currently being challenged in the courts) (Grynbaum 2012). Additionally, population-based HRA information can be used by various health care agencies and organizations when developing and disseminating health and prevention guidelines, delineating funding for health services research, and developing national health promotion communication campaigns.

Conclusion

HRAs can influence positive behavior change as well as enhance awareness of health risks. Coupled with biometric screening, health education, and health promotion activities or interventions aimed at improving the health and productivity of a defined population, HRAs are a vital component of any health promotion and disease prevention program. HRAs provide a comprehensive overview of the self-reported health status of a defined population, increase individual awareness of health risks, and encourage appropriate use of medical and preventive health services. In the setting of motivating behavior change, HRAs provide important and useful information at both the **individual** level (self-discovery of perceived versus measured health status and the impact individual behaviors may have on health risk) and the **organizational level** (health status of a defined population, effects of health status on productivity, and population health trends over time). HRA selection and implementation is dependent upon the unique characteristics of the defined

population, and the validity and reliability of the tool should be taken into consideration along with any legal, ethical, and policy implications. In order to maximize HRA effectiveness to influence behavior change, the allocation of monetary and nonmonetary resources should be directed toward the purchase or development of tailored health-promotion interventions, programs, activities, and services that improve the health and productivity of the targeted population. HRAs can benefit multiple stakeholders, including individuals, corporations, researchers, and organizations. Overall, HRAs provide a detailed health view of the population, as determined by the respondents, and can serve as an informative and actionable data source for use in promoting health, encouraging the prevention of health risks, and influencing behavior change.

NOTES

1. Here are some sample HRA websites: www.healthline.com/tools/risk; www.wellsource.com/home.html; www.hmrc.umich.edu/content.aspx?pageid=19&fname=hra.txt; www.mayoclinichealthsolutions.com/products/Health-Assessment.cfm.

REFERENCES

Brown DW, Balluz LS, Heath GW, et al. 2003. Associations between recommended levels of physical activity and health-reported quality of life: Findings from the 2001 Behavioral Risk Factor Surveillance System (BRFSS) survey. *Prev Med* 37:520.

Brown L, Rosner B, Willett WW, Sacks FM. 1999. Cholesterol-lowering effects of dietary fiber: A meta-analysis. *Am J Clin Nutr* 69 (1): 30–42.

Clark J, Chang H, Bolen S, Shore A, Goodwin S, Weiner J. 2010. Development of a claims-based risk score to identify obese individuals. *Popul Health Manag* 13 (4): 201–7.

Coalition for Genetic Fairness. 2008. What does GINA mean? A guide to the genetic information and non discrimination act. Available at www.geneticfairness.org/ginaresource.html.

Edington DW, Yen LT, Witting P. 1997. The financial impact of changes in personal health practices. *J Occup Environ Med* 39 (11): 1037–46.

Fensholt EC. 2011. Employer's guide to wellness programs. Available at http://healthyamericans.org

/health-issues/wp-content/uploads/2012/04
/Employers-Guide-to-Wellness-Programs.pdf.

Fielding JE. 1989. Frequency of health risk assessment
activities at U.S. worksites. *Am J Prev Med* 5 (2): 73-81.

Grynbaum MM. 2012. New York plans to ban sale of big
sizes of sugary drinks. *New York Times,* May 30.
Available at www.nytimes.com/2012/05/31/nyregion
/bloomberg-plans-a-ban-on-large-sugared-drinks.html
?pagewanted=all.

Hayrinen K, Saranto K, Nykanen P. 2008. Definition,
structure, content, use and impacts of electronic
health records: A review of the research literature. *Int
J Med Inform* 77 (5): 291-304.

Hyner GC, Peterson KW, Travis JW, Dewey JE, Foerster
JJ, Framer EM. 1999. *SPM Handbook of Health
Assessment Tools.* Pittsburgh, PA: Society of Prospec-
tive Medicine.

Jones DA, Shipman JP, Plaut DA, Selden CR. 2010.
Characteristics of personal health records: Findings
of the Medical Library Association / National Library
of Medicine Joint Electronic Personal Health Record
Task Force. *J Med Libr Assoc* 98 (3): 243-49.

Kushi LH, Byers T, Doyle C, et al. 2006. American
Cancer Society guidelines on nutrition and physical
activity for cancer prevention: Reducing the risk of
cancer with healthy food choices and physical
activity. *CA Cancer J Clin* 56:254.

McCormick J. 2006. College student perception of
wellness concepts. *Phys Educator* 63 (2): 78.

Miller AM, Iris M. 2002. Health promotion attitudes and
strategies in older adults. *Health Educ Behav* 29 (2):
249-67.

Mokdad AH, Marks JS, Stroup DF, Gerberding JL. 2004.
Actual causes of death in the United States, 2000.
JAMA 291 (10): 1238-45.

Musich S, McDonald T, Hirschland D, Edington DW.
2003. Examination of risk status transitions among
active employees in a comprehensive worksite health
promotion program. *J Occup Environ Med* 45 (4):
393-99.

National Center for Health Statistics (NCHS). 2002.
National vital statistics system. Available at www.cdc
.gov/nchs/data/dvs/LCWK1_2000.pdf.

National Committee for Quality Assurance (NCQA).
2009. Wellness & Health Promotion Accreditation.
Available at www.ncqa.org/tabid/834/Default.aspx.

RAND. 2003. Evidence report and evidence-based
recommendations: Health risk appraisals and
Medicare. Available at www.rand.org/pubs/reprints
/RP1225.html.

Rosenthal MB, Landon BE, Normand SL, Frank RG,
Ahmad TS, Epstein AM. 2007. Employers' use of
value-based purchasing strategies. *JAMA* 298 (19):
2281-88.

Schoenbach VJ, Wagner EH, Beery WL. 1987. Health
risk appraisal: Review of evidence for effectiveness.
Health Serv Res 22 (4): 553-80.

Short ME, Goetzel RZ, Pei X, et al. 2009. How accurate
are self-reports? Analysis of self-reported health care
utilization and absence when compared with
administrative data. *J Occup Environ Med* 51 (7): 786-96.

Soler RE, Leeks KD, Razi S, et al. 2010. A systematic
review of selected interventions for worksite health
promotion: The assessment of health risks with
feedback. *Am J Prev Med* 38 (2 suppl.): S237-S262.

U.S. Department of Health and Human Services
(USDHHS). 1996. *Physical Activity and Health: A Report
of the Surgeon General.* Atlanta, GA: U.S. Department
of Health and Human Services, Centers for Disease
Control and Prevention, National Center for Chronic
Disease Prevention and Health Promotion. Available
at www.cdc.gov/nccdphp/sgr/pdf/sgrfull.pdf15.

U.S. Equal Employment Opportunity Commission
(USEOC). 1990. Titles I and V of the Americans with
Disabilities Act of 1990 (ADA). Pub. L. 101-336.
Available at www.eeoc.gov/laws/statutes/ada.cfm.

———. 2008. Americans with Disabilities Amendments
Act of 2008. PL 110-325 (S 3406). Available at www.
eeoc.gov/laws/statutes/adaaa.cfm.

Wallace RB. 2008. *Maxcy-Rosenau-Last Public Health &
Preventive Medicine.* 15th ed. New York: McGraw Hill
Medical.

Yen L, McDonald T, Hirschland D, Edington DW. 2003.
Association between wellness score from a health
risk appraisal and prospective medical claims costs.
J Occup Environ Med 45 (10): 1049-57.

Chronic Conditions and Population Health Management for Health Care Systems

PETER J. FAGAN AND LINDA DUNBAR

LEARNING OBJECTIVES

After completing the chapter, the reader will be able to

* Describe the prevalence of chronic health conditions in the United States.
* Differentiate and describe the components of the three classical levels of disease prevention.
* Distinguish the various roles and responsibilities that the multiple stakeholders have in the population management of chronic diseases.
* Describe the chronic care model and the importance of an "activated" patient in the model.
* Discuss the gaps and opportunities facing the U.S. health system as it meets the challenge of chronic health conditions.

Introduction

The U.S. public health challenges in the first half of the 20th century were infectious and contagious diseases, such as tuberculosis and influenza. In the last half of the century, health care turned its attention to medical and surgical **interventions** addressing episodic care in response to acute events, such as heart attack and stroke. In both of these public health challenges, success was measurable. One measure of success is that the U.S. population is living longer. However, as a result, the primary challenge of the first decades of the 21st century is addressing the chronic conditions of an aging population.

Chronic conditions are illnesses and impairments that limit daily functioning, are expected to last at least a year, and require ongoing medical care (Anderson 2010; Hoffman et al. 1996). As such, chronic conditions pose a major population health challenge, especially in those industrialized populations in which the number of older individuals is increasing. Nearly half (145 million) of the U.S. population live with at least one chronic condition (Anderson 2010). As populations age, chronic conditions, such as diabetes, hypertension, congestive heart failure, and cardiovascular disease, increase in prevalence. Moreover, they rarely occur in isolation but often along with other chronic diseases. In 2009, 21% of Americans in the age 45 to 64 group, and 45% of Americans older than age 65, had two or more coexisting chronic conditions (Freid et al. 2012). The cost of care for individuals with chronic conditions is substantial. In 2009 the average annual health care spending for individuals treated for four or more chronic conditions ($16,257) far exceeded those not treated for any chronic conditions ($2,367) (Machlin and Soni 2013) and accounted for almost 75% of Medicare spending (Lochner and Cox 2013).

The development of chronic diseases is a combination of genetics, exposure, and behaviors. Genetic therapy is limited and largely unavailable but may be used for risk **stratification**. We have partial control over natural and more control over built environmental exposures that affect health. We must continue to influence environmental policies and make the natural and **built environments** more conducive to healthful individual choices. Of the three factors involved in the development, or control, of chronic conditions, individual behavior is the most immediately amenable factor. And yet, individual engagement in prohealth behaviors stands as the "black box" challenge facing our health care system in the decade ahead. Most of the chapters in this book are attempts to open that black box, to offer a glimpse at how to prevent, delay, and ameliorate the effects of chronic illness.

This chapter will describe the role of behaviors in the prevention and emergence of chronic disease conditions. It will also describe the roles that various **key stakeholders** play—or

should play—in the development and promotion of **health behaviors** that prevent or control chronic conditions and also affect environmental policies. We contend that patient-centered care of the individual with chronic conditions is beyond the doctor-patient relationship, health coaching, and care management; we suggest that patient-centered care is, above all, care in which the patient is the agent of self-management rather than the passive recipient of health care services and advice (see chapter 22). Population-centered health management puts corporate and public policies in place that support the individual self-management of health-related behaviors.

Disease Prevention

Behaviors that prevent development of chronic conditions can be divided into primary, secondary, and **tertiary prevention**.

Primary Prevention

Primary prevention of chronic disease consists of performing healthful behaviors, and avoiding harmful behaviors, before the biological onset of the disease. Most notably, these involve good nutrition, physical activity, and sufficient sleep and avoiding or limiting substances that are harmful, especially nicotine and alcohol. Primary prevention of chronic diseases on a societal level consists of the establishment of healthful environments, especially air quality, a sound public health information program, and access to primary care services to prevent the development of conditions that can lead to chronic disease. It is action to control the health effects of the natural and built environments so that the development of chronic disease is prevented or delayed.

Secondary Prevention

Secondary prevention related to chronic conditions aims to prevent the progression of a disease process that has already begun but has not yet caused signs, symptoms, or dysfunction (Wallace 2002a). Most often, the preclinical indicators are the result of routine screening done during a physical examination. For example, an elevated fasting glucose may indicate a glucose intolerance or diabetes. Or blood pressure levels may indicate a borderline hypertensive condition. In each of these cases, the individual is likely to have been completely asymptomatic.

Once the chronic condition has been identified or is suggested, the individual should engage in all the behaviors that will prevent or retard the emergence of the disease condition. In addition to the baseline of healthful behaviors involved in primary prevention, other or more intensive behaviors may be needed. For example, limiting carbohydrate consumption may prevent diabetes, while increasing one's activity level may promote cardiovascular health and control blood pressure.

Secondary-prevention behaviors from a population health perspective begin with education about the importance and the availability of screening for disease conditions. Screening is especially important for diseases that are "silent" or asymptomatic in their early stages, such as diabetes, cancer, and hypertension. Health fairs and employers who offer workplace health screenings are providing the environmental access to promote secondary-prevention behaviors among their participants and employees. This is especially important in work environments with exposures of a physical (mining) or emotional (first responders) nature.

Tertiary Prevention

Tertiary prevention aims to prevent further progression of the disease and its functional limitations after symptoms are evident and the diagnosis has been established (Wallace 2002b). Tertiary-prevention behaviors are distinguished by a more "medical" regimen designed around the specific chronic condition(s). Tertiary prevention can be considered as those behaviors

that adhere both to the treatment plan designed by the physician or care team and to a self-management plan. Self-testing and lab testing of biomarkers, such as those for weight, blood pressure, and glucose level, are tertiary-prevention behaviors. As will be discussed later, for those individuals with chronic conditions who are engaged in a care management program, often the focus of behavior change or **reinforcement** is on adherence to the treatment and self-management plans.

Tertiary-prevention behaviors from a population health perspective appear to blend with the provision of health care services. Central to tertiary-prevention behaviors are primary care services understood in the broadest sense of inclusion of the entire health care team: professionals, family caregivers, and the patient. As with health care services in general, the population health perspective of tertiary-prevention behaviors can be discussed and evaluated within the Triple Aim model of the Institute of Healthcare Improvement (IHI): (1) improve the health of the population; (2) enhance the patient experience of care (including quality, access, and **reliability**); and (3) reduce, or at least control, the per capita cost of care (Berwick et al. 2008). We will return to this model when we discuss interventions to promote healthful behaviors in individuals with chronic conditions.

Magnitude

The negative effects of chronic disease pervade individual, community, and societal life. **Morbidity** brings with it pain, restriction of daily activities, reduction of **quality of life**, and the expenditure of medical funds that could have been used for other purposes (e.g., preventive health services, education, environmental sustainability).

Morbidity Prevalence

The 2012 publication *Health, United States* (NCHS 2012) provides the following information on the prevalence of the major chronic conditions in the United States:

1. Hypertension—defined as elevated blood pressure and/or taking antihypertensive medication—increases with age. In 2007-10, 35.5% of men and 31.2% of women ages 45-54 had hypertension, compared with 71.7% of men and 81.3% of women age 75 and older.
2. The percentage of adults with diabetes (including both diagnosed and undiagnosed) increased from 1988-94 (9.1%) to 2003-6 (10.6%). Diabetes is more common among non-Hispanic black persons and Mexican Americans than among non-Hispanic white persons.
3. Between 1988-94 and 2007-10, the percentage of both men and women age 55 and older with a high total serum cholesterol level (greater than or equal to 240 mg/dL) increased. Older women were more likely to have high serum cholesterol than older men. In 2007-10, 53.3% of women ages 65-74 had high serum cholesterol levels.
4. From 1990 to 2007, the number of new cases of lung and bronchus cancer per 100,000 population declined on average 3.7% per year among males and remained unchanged among females. Cancer of the lung and bronchus is the second most common newly diagnosed cancer among males (after prostate cancer) and females (after breast cancer).
5. In 2009, nearly 34,000 new acquired immune deficiency syndrome (AIDS) cases were reported. Males age 13 and older accounted for 75% of all new cases. Black males made up 32% of all new cases, and black females accounted for 17% of all new cases.
6. In 2006 and 2008, women age 18 and older (10.2%) were more likely than men (8.0%) to have current depression.[1]

The prevalence of chronic conditions is affected by age. The Medical Expenditure Panel Survey (MEPS) reports that among persons age 65 and older, the leading conditions are hypertension (60%), cholesterol disorders (41%), arthritis (28%), heart disease (25%), and eye disorders (23%). Among younger adults, ages 18-64, the most prevalent chronic conditions are hypertension (30%), cholesterol disorders (20%), respiratory diseases (19%), and diabetes (12%).[2] The MEPS data is from **self-report** and is likely an underestimation of the actual prevalence of the conditions.

Individuals with **complex** health care needs require more health care expenditures as the number of chronic conditions grows. In addition to the burden of illness and the decrease in quality of life of the individuals and their caregivers, the cost of care on the population itself is great. Of total U.S. health care costs, 85% is spent on people with chronic conditions. With improved medical technologies and resultant increased longevity, half of the U.S. population will have one or more chronic conditions by 2030, according to predictions (Anderson 2010). With an increased number of chronic conditions come corresponding increases in medical complexity and health care costs. As Anderson (2010) reports, when compared with persons with no chronic condition, those with one condition have expenses that are three times greater. With each additional condition the slope continues steadily, so that the total medical costs for persons having five or more conditions becomes fifteen times greater than for those with no chronic conditions.[3]

The payers of medical costs are not solely Medicare and Medicaid. Privately insured individuals make up the largest number of those with chronic conditions (78 million). Their care accounts for 73% of private insurance medical spending. In addition, practically all of Medicare and approximately 80% of Medicaid spending is for those with chronic conditions (Anderson 2010). Ultimately, all taxpayers in the United States are the payers for medical costs, whether by reduced wages or by government support of health care premiums and services.

Quality of Life

With more than a quarter of persons with chronic health conditions reporting a condition-related limitation of daily activity, clearly chronic conditions reduce the **quality of life** of those afflicted (Anderson 2010; Nyman et al. 2007). Of noninstitutionalized working-age adults ages 18-64, 10% report limitation of activity because of a chronic condition (NCHS 2012). With aging, 20% of 44-64-year-olds report limitations. For all ages, arthritis and other musculoskeletal conditions are the most frequently mentioned conditions causing limitation. For younger workers (ages 18-44), mental illness is the second leading cause of limitation; for older workers (ages 45-64), heart and circulatory conditions are the second leading cause of limitation. Among older adults, the number of those reporting limitation increases with age: 26% of 65-74-year-olds, 36% of 75-84-year-olds, and 62% of adults age 85 and older.

The percentage of noninstitutionalized adults age 65 and older with limitation of activity decreased from 39% to 36% between 1997 and 1999 and then remained at 34%-35% between 2000 and 2007. In 2006-7, the percentage of older adults with limitation of activity increased; it affected 26% of 65-74-year-olds, 36% of 75-84-year-olds, and 62% of adults age 85 and older. Arthritis and other musculoskeletal conditions were the most frequently mentioned chronic conditions causing limitation of activity, followed by cardiovascular conditions. In the oldest group, dementia, poor vision, and hearing problems were commonly reported as limiting daily activity (Hootman et al. 2009; Kramarow et al. 2007; NCHS 2011).

State of Current Evidence

These effects of chronic conditions on human suffering and costs have prompted the development of a strong body of evidence in the past 50 years showing that lifestyle behaviors such as diet, physical activity, smoking, and alcohol consumption contribute to the development of chronic conditions. Perhaps more importantly in terms of health status, these behaviors can be changed, and the changes can positively affect the level of morbidity caused by chronic conditions in populations.

Since 1948, the Framingham Heart Study (FHS) has sought to identify the factors leading to cardiovascular disease. In the course of the hundreds of reports that have been produced from the FHS, one robust finding has been the association of behaviors and the development (or prevention) of cardiovascular disease. Among FHS research milestones are these: (1) cigarette smoking is a significant causal factor of heart disease (Dawber 1960); (2) physical activity reduces the risk of heart disease (Kannel 1967; Kannel and Sorlie 1979); and (3) **psychosocial factors** and **social networking** associations (Haynes et al. 1978) correlate with obesity (Christakis and Fowler 2007).

In Finland, the association between high serum cholesterol and atherosclerotic cardiovascular disease (CVD) led to the development of the North Karelia Project, which was conducted beginning in 1972. A collaboration of researchers, community organizations, and policymakers, the North Karelia Project was an **ecological intervention** on individual, social, and political levels to change behaviors, principally the consumption of saturated fat, that were risk factors for CVD (Puska 2010). As Puska and Stahl note, the North Karelia Project and its expansion to all Finland in 1977 represented collaborations of many areas of expertise: **social marketing**, behavior modification, communication and behavior change, **innovation** and diffusion, and community organization and policies (McAlister et al. 1982; Puska and Vartiainen 2009; Puska et al. 1985). The dietary changes (10% reduction of total fat consumption as a percentage of total caloric intake) have led to reduced blood cholesterol levels and an 80% reduction in Finnish CVD **mortality** rates among working-age citizens. Finnish life expectancy has increased by 10 years (Puska and Stahl 2010).

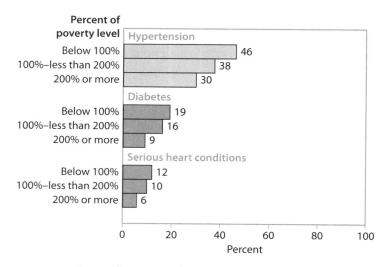

FIGURE 25.1. Respondent-reported conditions among adults ages 45–64, 2007.
Source: Centers for Disease Control and Prevention and National Center for Health Statistics, *Health, United States, 2009: With Special Feature on Medical Technology* (Hyattsville, MD: U.S. Dept. of Health and Human Services, 2010), fig. 10 and the National Health Interview Survey.

In addition to the risk factors for chronic disease that have been established by the North Karelia Project and FHS, poverty is also a potentially modifiable risk factor that is associated with hypertension, diabetes, and heart disease (figure 25.1). In addition, poverty is associated with a higher population morbidity in general because it results in a reduction of access to primary care (Kellermann and Weinick 2012). A societal commitment is necessary to alleviate poverty as a risk factor, as will be restated later in the **stakeholders** section of this chapter.

Two conclusions emerge regarding the state of the evidence. First, there is a causal link between behavior, poverty, and risk factors for chronic disease. Second, ecological efforts to change behaviors of populations have resulted in behavior changes (individual and societal) that have in turn resulted in reduced morbidity. Thus, while the burden of chronic disease is great, the opportunity exists to reduce that burden if concerted efforts are made by individuals and societies. This leads to a consideration of how such concerted efforts to address behaviors associated with chronic disease might be theoretically organized.

A Conceptual Framework for Interventions

The interventions for population health management of risk factors for chronic disease and the management of the chronic diseases themselves, once diagnosed and expressed in symptoms and activity limitations, are ultimately the result of the collaboration of the population members with multiple public health and human service organizations, as well as medical care providers. The interventions can be categorized according to the three levels of preventive behaviors: primary (level 3), secondary (level 2), and tertiary (level 1). Populations will need all three levels of prevention, depending upon the extent to which any particular chronic disease is prevalent. As the physical effects of the chronic disease become more emergent in the secondary and tertiary levels of prevention, interventions will become increasingly medicalized. **Medicalization** here indicates behaviors that are closely associated with the management of an active disease condition, for example, adhering to a medication regimen and monitoring physiological functions.

Stratify the Identified Population

From the perspective of population health management, the management of chronic disease should begin with a clear identification and stratification of the targeted population. The identification of the population may be geographical or may be health-plan or disease-condition specific. Once the population has been identified, stratifying the members according to health or morbidity status is necessary. The most commonly used method to stratify the levels of population morbidity is to employ a predictive modeling algorithm to the clinical and administrative data available on the population. For example, health plans and state, provincial, and federal governments use the claims data of their covered populations and submit the past 12 months of data to predictive modeling software. Predictive modeling processes factors such as age, gender, diagnoses, National Drug Codes from pharmacies, and certain hospital-sensitive conditions to yield several measurements of morbidity burden and the likelihood of use of health care services in the near future. If electronic medical records (EMRs) are available, the predictive modeling algorithm is enriched with them and member-reported **health risk assessment (HRA)** data (see chapter 24).

Several predictive modeling applications are currently in use (Brino 2013; Evans 2011). Working in a health plan environment, the authors of this chapter employ the Johns Hopkins University Adjusted Clinical Groups (ACG) Case-Mix System (Forrest et al. 2009). Monthly runs of the ACG predictive model software on health plans' claims data result in population health and morbidity stratification. The resulting population

stratification helps to determine the type and amount of resource allocation for population health management and care management for members with chronic conditions (figure 25.2).

Level 3 Population Health Strategies

Level 3 population members (60%-80% of the population) have relatively good health and should be supported in their efforts to engage in primary prevention behaviors. Level 3 primary prevention of chronic disease consists of all public health and employer-sponsored programs whose **goal** is to create a healthful environment (air, water, public safety) that promotes healthful nutrition, activity, and self-care (e.g., getting vaccinations) of its population.

Entities such as health plans and government payers also may provide educational assistance to population members through postal and Internet-based resources aimed at promoting healthful behaviors, early detection of and preventive guidance for obesity and hypertension, and reminders for periodic cancer screening. The family health history (if available from EMRs or HRAs) is employed in guiding the screening reminders and education content. Patient-tailored educational materials, including annual reminder cards for appropriate screening exams (cholesterol, mammogram) and immunizations, are typical of this type of individualized health promotion.

Level 2 Population Health Strategies

The principal goal of level 2 individuals (15%-30% of the population) is to increase knowledge about their chronic conditions and develop the skills and confidence to self-manage their health (see chapter 24). Those who are newly diagnosed with a chronic condition are frequently at a "teachable moment" to consider changing behaviors that may have been risk factors for the condition. For example, in one study, persons hospitalized for conditions related to

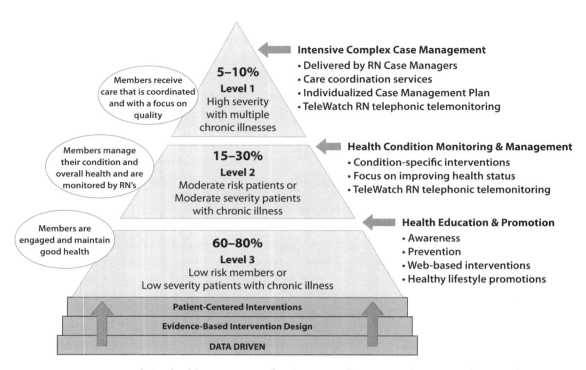

FIGURE 25.2. Population health management for chronic conditions according to member stratification

smoking were provided smoking cessation assistance as inpatients. One year later, the intervention group had maintained a smoking cessation rate of 22.5% (Sciamanna et al. 2000). Individuals whose health-related behaviors are posing a risk of further health status deterioration should be offered the services of a health coach or, if resources allow, a nurse. Usually providing limited and condition-level assistance, health coaches telephonically assist the member to set and meet realistic goals, thus shaping behaviors to achieve and maintain a healthier lifestyle. When appropriate, the coaching is supplemented with Internet or telephonic monitoring of the biomarkers associated with the chronic condition (e.g., weight, blood pressure level).

The principal focus of these monitoring technologies and health coaching for level 2 members is to assist the members to maintain control themselves of their existing chronic

conditions and provide them with reminders at the most clinically appropriate times. For example, an asthmatic patient who has a history of severe asthma attacks during the fall season might receive a text message daily during the fall months with a reminder to use her inhaler before going outdoors.

Level 1 Population Health Strategies

Level 1 members (5%-10% of the population) are member-patients who have a high level of illness severity. Their medical history is marked by multiple chronic conditions, frequent hospitalizations, many prescription medications, many care providers, a limitation of daily functions, and high medical costs (Bodenheimer and Berry-Millett 2009). In level 1, the high level of morbidity requires coordination of care for the promotion of tertiary prevention behaviors, such as adherence to medication regimens upon

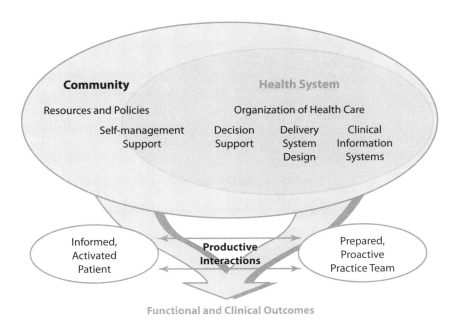

FIGURE 25.3. The Chronic Care Model. *Source:* Wagner 1998, fig. 1.

hospital discharge. The theoretical construct that is widely employed to describe the type of intervention required for individuals with this level of morbidity (and many in level 2) is Wagner's **Chronic Care Model (CCM)**. The CCM indicates that redesign of the delivery system, enhanced decision support, improved clinical information systems, support for self-management, and better access to community resources are necessary to improve outcomes for people with chronic conditions (Bodenheimer et al. 2002).

The components of the Chronic Care Model (figure 25.3) are also those of the current health care reform in the United States: health information technology, health information exchange, collaboration and shared accountability, and a primary care practice team such as those located in a medical home practice. Not to be overlooked in the discussion of health care reform and in the CCM are the behaviors of an "informed, **activated patient**" (see chapter 22 for a full discussion of the centrality of the activated patient—especially for levels 1 and 2—for

the increase of behaviors related to chronic conditions).

High Severity Chronic Illness and Care Management

The CCM requires coordination of care among the practice team, the patient, and the patient's caregivers. Of people with serious chronic conditions, 81% see two or more different physicians (Anderson 2010). If we expect an "informed, activated patient" who is able to navigate the complex and changing health care system and who engages in prohealth behaviors, we must also expect that this will not generally occur for level 1 patients without systematic assistance.

Such systematic assistance is the role of care management, which assists in the coordination of care and promotes knowledgeable, skillful, and confident self-health management to the extent allowed by the person's physical condition. On both an individual and a population scale, the goals of care management are

TABLE 25.1. Summary of care management findings

Setting	Quality improvement	Cost reduction
Primary care	Strong evidence	Some evidence
Vendor-supported telephonic	Some evidence	Inconclusive
Integrated delivery systems	Strong evidence	Inconclusive
Hospital-to-home	Strong evidence	Strong evidence
Home	No evidence	No evidence

Source: Synthesis Project: Policy Brief No. 19, 2009, www.policysynthesis.org.

to improve the quality and the efficiency of the health services.

A full discussion of care management itself is beyond the scope of this chapter; the interested reader is referred to the Robert Wood Johnson Foundation's Synthesis Project Policy Brief No. 19 for an introduction to the current research findings on care management (www.policy synthesis.org) and to table 25.1. In sum, care management for individuals with complex medical conditions has been found to improve the quality of care. The effect of care management on reducing costs has been variable, with most savings generated in care management programs that target patients discharged from hospitals (Coleman et al. 2004; Naylor et al. 2004).

As mentioned previously, the population health perspective of tertiary prevention behaviors can be evaluated within the IHI Triple Aim model, when the goal is to (1) improve the health of the population, (2) enhance the patient experience of care (including quality, access, and reliability), and (3) reduce, or at least control, the per capita cost of care (Berwick et al. 2008).

Of primary interest for this chapter regarding care management is its relationship to behaviors affecting chronic illness. Table 25.1 suggests that the behaviors involved in care management services are not only the behaviors of the member-patient (e.g., adherence to medication regimen), but are also the behaviors of the primary care and care management team and the choice of setting of the intervention. In-person care management, **integration** with primary care, trained care management staff, involvement of informal caregivers, and coaching that enables the timely detection of condition decline are all behaviors that are effective in the promotion of health in the individual with complex chronic conditions.

Care managers can enable member-patient behavior change by frequently employing **motivational interviewing (MI)**.[4] MI is a technique in which the interviewer uses the perspective of the interviewee regarding behaviors that are seen to be in that person's own interest. For example, asking, "What is it about the limitations caused by your CHF that most upsets you?" is more similar to counseling than to the traditional "telling" the patient what he or she should do regarding the chronic condition. The patient is assisted to identify one doable behavioral goal that is clearly in his perceived self-interest. In behavioral terms, MI is a shaping of behaviors toward a general goal. Applied to chronic illness, MI is a technique of establishing goals of more healthful behaviors and adherence to the treatment plan and self-management plan.

The latter plan, the self-management plan, is perhaps the most critical component for the activated patient of the CCM (see figure 25.3). A self-management plan, accepted by the patient, is a way of sharing responsibility with the treatment team to achieve and maintain the maximum health status possible. This example may be crude, but we should not place the ultimate responsibility for health maintenance on the physician and the physician's care team any more than we should place the total responsibility for car maintenance on the automotive repair service. An activated patient knows this and does what is necessary to keep her body and spirit going as effectively and as long as possible, given the limitations imposed by the chronic illness.

Chronic Condition Best Practices

The individual patient, member, or enrollee should not be solely responsible for the management of chronic conditions. The primary, secondary, and tertiary management of chronic conditions requires public health effort and medical care informed by scientific evidence. Regarding the former, chapter 9 in this text describes the scientific evidence methods for the **evaluation** of public health programs. Regarding the latter, in the past 25 years, physician behavior based on "medical experience and anecdote" has been supplemented, if not in some cases totally replaced, by physician behavior grounded in medical scientific evidence. **Guidelines** are proliferating for all phases of medical care, but they are most important in the care of persons with chronic conditions who are vulnerable to the effects of poor care and management.

The U.S. Preventive Services Task Force (USPSTF) is "an independent panel of non-Federal experts in prevention and evidence-based medicine and is composed of primary care providers (such as internists, pediatricians, family physicians, gynecologists/obstetricians, nurses, and health behavior specialists)." Under the auspices of the Agency for Healthcare Research and Quality (AHRQ), "the USPSTF conducts scientific evidence reviews of a broad range of clinical preventive health care services (such as screening, counseling, and preventive medications) and develops recommendations for primary care clinicians and health systems. These recommendations are published in the form of "Recommendation Statements."[5]

The most comprehensive public resource for evidence-based clinical practice guidelines is AHRQ's National Guideline Service (NCG) (www.guideline.gov/). The NCG website permits guideline searches by Disease/Condition and by Treatment/Intervention. Guidelines are posted from international groups, and each recommendation is rated according to the strength of the evidence for that particular recommendation.

To reinforce **best clinical practices** and established guidelines, initiatives and programs reward medical care provider behaviors that are consistent with **evidence-based practices** and, in the future, will penalize providers who do not meet evidence-based process measures or specific health status outcomes. The Centers for Medicare and Medicaid Services (CMS) program called the Physician Quality Reporting Initiative is, as its name implies, a system for reporting physician quality; it includes an **incentive** payment for eligible providers who satisfactorily report data on quality measures for covered professional services furnished to Medicare beneficiaries.[6] CMS has also initiated a program to withhold payment from hospitals for readmissions of patients whose readmission was likely related to a hospital-associated infection or a medical error during the index hospitalization. The direction is clear: the behavior of providers and health care facilities in rendering services is and will be more closely monitored, reinforcing best practices and penalizing other behaviors (including the omission of behaviors). See chapter 19 for further discussion of provider behaviors.

Good medical care for chronic conditions and good patient self-management will likely reduce the number of hospitalizations. AHRQ's Prevention Quality Indicators (PQIs) are a set of measures that can be used with hospital inpatient discharge data to identify quality of care for ambulatory care-sensitive conditions. These are conditions for which good outpatient care can potentially prevent the need for hospitalization or for which early intervention can prevent complications or more severe disease.[7] The PQIs and other such measures that are currently in development are useful population health service metrics for examining the quality of health system behaviors, especially ambulatory care services.

Roles for Key Stakeholders

The complexity involved in the management of chronic conditions is never more apparent than when we examine the roles held by the various stakeholders. Successful population and individual management of chronic conditions requires far more than physician-patient collaboration.

Population Members

The individual's health-related behaviors are not the only constituents of a population member / stakeholder's obvious role in chronic conditions; the values that the population as a society places upon health-related behaviors are also relevant. These values not only affect individual behavior but also shape cultural values that are subsequently reflected in legislation and policy. Thus, clarifying the discussion about health care and health-related behaviors is important. We suggest that the following questions are fundamental to this society discussion.

1. Does society have a right to expect that I have a responsibility to care for my health by engaging in prohealth related behaviors and managing any health conditions I might have?
2. Do I have a right to expect that society ultimately has the responsibility to provide health care to all its members?

The libertarian and the communitarian camps will take opposite positions on these questions. Libertarians will assert that the individual's right to life, liberty, and the pursuit of happiness does not give society any claim on a prohibition of individual behaviors unless they cause immediate and direct harm to others. Communitarians counter that a **mutuality** of rights and responsibilities exists: indi-

viduals have a social responsibility to care for their health, and society has a responsibility to provide health care for its members—especially when they are unable to provide it for themselves.

Although the authors of this chapter espouse the latter position, we recognize that not all readers will agree. We believe, however, that the position the individual takes on these reciprocal health-related rights and responsibilities (or lack thereof) is foundational both for the individual and for the society. In the primary prevention of chronic conditions (no smoking; healthful foods in vending machines) and the adherence to a care plan in secondary prevention (medication), the behaviors and the strategies taken by the individual and offered to the individual by others will be informed by the values (see chapter 24).

Health Plans

Health plans have the ethical responsibility to improve (or at least maintain, in the case of chronic conditions) the health status of the population that the plan covers. This includes supporting not only primary prevention services but also those services that are necessary for a minimally successful quality of life, given the medical or chronic condition. The current "medically necessary" criterion for covering a specific service is based on the likelihood that the service or intervention will provide improvement in the condition. In many chronic conditions, such as Alzheimer's disease, however, improvement is unlikely. Therefore, health plan benefits should include those services that help a person maintain his functional status (Anderson 2010).

Health plans are likely to have a role to play in the establishment of the accountable care organizations (ACOs) that were authorized for CMS in the Affordable Care Act of March 2010 and are currently established nationwide. Health plans have a financial interest in bringing together hospitals, skilled nursing facilities, and primary care providers to coordinate the care of the chronically ill—as well as others in the population who may require assistance related to an acute event (e.g., a stroke). Health plans also have the use of financial data that neither hospitals nor primary care providers have. With these data, health plans can play an ancillary role in the formation of ACOs, providing data necessary to make the business case for those exploring an ACO **partnership**.

Health plans also can affect provider behavior regarding the care and management of the chronic illnesses of the provider's patients. Physicians report that they are less satisfied treating their patients with chronic illness than they are treating those without (Anderson 2010). Many reasons might be hypothesized for this lower professional satisfaction. However, health plans working together with payers can recognize the fact that patients with chronic conditions require additional services, such as communication with care team members, monitoring, and **outreach**. Physician satisfaction in treating chronic disease can improve with a restructuring of the care model (Marsteller et al. 2010). In addition, physicians should be compensated for such coordination of care and outreach services. Fortunately, the models of patient-centered medical homes (PCMHs) do recognize the need for these additional services and offer vehicles for compensation (www .pcmh.ahrq.gov). Health plans have been in the forefront of sponsoring PCMH initiatives.

Employers

In the workplace, wellness programs have been able to improve biomarkers among employee populations. See chapters 16 and 20 for a full discussion of what employers have accomplished in the workplace to improve employee health behaviors. In addition, a transcript of a real stakeholders' roundtable, which can be found at www.Press.jhu.edu, offers a view into the worlds of a health plan executive, a major corporation employer, and a president of a large primary care group and how these worlds attempt to collaborate in improving the health behaviors of their populations.

Policymakers

Current health policies should reflect the historical shift from infection control to episodic care and now to the need for coordinated care for complex conditions involving multiple providers. Gerald Anderson observes, "The presence of multiple chronic conditions has specific implications for the reform of health care financing and delivery systems. For example, we need to begin to think beyond specific disease management to the coordination of medical care and assistive services across care settings and among multiple providers" (Anderson 2010, 8). As we have just suggested regarding the compensation for primary care teams, today we need funding for policies that enable the coordination of care for chronic conditions.

Coordination of care through improved Internet communication has been supported in recent federal legislation. In the American Recovery and Reinvestment Act (2009), the Office of the National Coordinator for Health Information Technology was established to promote the expansion of health information technology and health information exchange, which will ultimately lead to a national health information network. Health records that are available in (nearly) real-time to both providers and patients have promise to support improved coordination of care as well as promote informed self-management of chronic conditions.

One of the long-term effects of the North Karelia Project in Finland was its eventual implementation in the entire European Union. According to this regulation, all new policies and laws must have a population health impact review just as they need to have an environmental impact review (Puska and Stahl 2010). Such a policy enacted in the state and federal legislatures of the United States would be a strong factor in the implementation in practice of an **ecological approach** to population health.

Poverty is a health risk factor. Any policy that can reduce poverty is likely to be a positive public health policy. In addition, funding for preventive services, coordination of care, and health impact reviews of new legislation require political will. Funding will be made available only when the body politic consistently wills it so. Ultimately, public policy is a question of political leadership and the political will of the society. This may be the major public health challenge in the United States.

Health Departments

According to an AARP report,[8] older people (ages 55–64) who do not have insurance have worse access to health care and are therefore less likely to obtain the medical care they need for their chronic conditions. This finding is consistent with the McGlynn report that approximately half of the persons in the United States do not get the services their medical conditions require (McGlynn 2004).

The principal suggestion in these data is that those with chronic conditions face a serious quality-of-care issue. As an agency whose mission includes caring for the vulnerable populations with chronic conditions, a local health department might consider allocating more resources to tracking and reporting the health care quality outcomes for their patients to their funding governments. For decades, the Federally Qualified Health Centers or community health centers have reported population health data to the Health Resources and Services Administration. They have an excellent sense of population health and accountability. As such, they are a model for expanding the mentality of population health and accountability among the nonpublicly supported primary care practices.

Clinicians

For those who treat patients with chronic conditions, slowing the progression of the disease

should be recognized as a priority—both by themselves and by those who compensate them for their services. Understandably, for many physicians longitudinal care is less likely to be as professionally satisfying as an intervention that resolves an acute episode—the age-old tension between *caring* versus *curing*. Yet if the infectious-disease and acute-intervention historical phases of public health are behind us, and our phase consists of longitudinal and coordinated care of chronic illness, then the clinicians and their care teams should be trained, resourced, and compensated to provide that care. This will be necessary to improve the quality of care for chronic conditions, to reduce ambulatory-care-sensitive conditions, and ultimately to reduce avoidable hospitalizations.

The challenge is for clinicians to adopt (in addition to the face-to-face care they provide to their patients) a population health perspective. With such a perspective, clinicians are sensitive to improving the health status of all their patients, perhaps especially the vulnerable ones with chronic conditions and the patients who are reluctant to seek health care services. Clinicians with a population health perspective can describe the health status of their patient panels as a population as accurately as they describe the health status of an individual patient. To do this, clinicians need information made possible by health information technology and health information exchange. They need, for example, an accessible patient panel dashboard that allows a drill-down for actionable data. They also must be able to coordinate care with other health care providers. For most patients with chronic conditions, clinicians with a population health perspective can speak about "our" shared patients with their care team, other providers, and, ideally, with health plans.

Researchers

The majority of research on the treatment and self-management of chronic conditions has, understandably, examined the existent treatment and care management models. *Chronic conditions* is a term that includes both diseases and conditions such as addiction or obesity that may not be diseases in themselves but have a component or risk of morbidity. The models have frequently reported on a single chronic condition. Randomized controlled trials (RCTs) of medications, especially, have tended to exclude participants with **comorbidities**. The result is a limited **generalizability** of the RCT findings to the real world of patients, most of whom have multiple chronic conditions (Boyd et al. 2005).

Future research has promise as research design models offer more diversity. *Translational* and *comparative effectiveness research* will become more modal for examining the treatment and care of chronic conditions. The participants in the studies will be "real patients" with multiple chronic conditions. In this research, especially if design rigor is brought to observational and **quasi-experimental** data, the opportunity to gain understanding of the behaviors that are most effective in the care and management of chronic conditions will emerge.

The challenges of research on the care and management of chronic conditions are the following:

1. The design and statistical analysis of studies of the comorbid chronic conditions. The comorbid conditions need to be measured in terms of intensity and, in some cases, duration to determine their contribution to the outcome measure. Although studies can be done without a comparison or **control group**, having a valid counterfactual group adds great strength to the interpretation of the findings and avoids misleading pre- versus postmeasures on a single group. Identifying a valid comparison group in observational and quasi-experimental studies is challenging. The intervention or independent variables need to be **operationalized** in such a manner that they can be replicated. Although the intervention is necessary, describing the **context** in which

the intervention occurs is also necessary (Pawson and Tilley 1997). The context, for example the enthusiasm and leadership of a physician champion, may be a causal key to the effect of a primary practice intervention for the care of chronic conditions.

2. The duration of the study period. Intervention effects for chronic conditions, for example, adolescent obesity and diabetes mellitus, may take years to become evident.

3. The attribution of primary care physician. Which one physician is designated the patient's primary care physician? Can this be done validly across a population with one algorithm? Persons with chronic conditions are treated by multiple providers. Is the specialist, in fact, the primary care provider?

4. The determination of return on investment for interventions. There are several "payers" who make an investment in the treatment and management of chronic conditions: the patient, the employer, the insurance agency or government, and ultimately society. Who will benefit financially from an employer-sponsored wellness program? And when will it be possible to measure the financial effect of the wellness program? (Leatherman et al. 2003)

Caregivers

Often forgotten in discussions of the care and management of chronic conditions are the family and friends who provide care when the patient cannot care for herself in all activities of daily living. As our society ages, chronic conditions will require more attention.[9] The behaviors involved in the management of chronic conditions must include a consideration of the **"sandwich generation"** caregivers—those in midlife who are caring for both the younger and the older generation. They are an essential part of the health care delivery system. Some of their in-home services are or could be reimbursable. All of the services that caregivers perform need to be better understood and better supported.

Conclusion

We have suggested that the care of chronic conditions is the primary public health challenge of this era, following the era of infection control and the era of medical and surgical interventions for acute episodes. The behaviors associated with chronic conditions are both individual and public health behaviors. They can be categorized as primary, secondary, and tertiary prevention behaviors. As the chronic condition progresses, the behaviors, especially in the tertiary stage, become more medicalized. Issues of the behaviors of coordination of care and self-management become central. Methods of reinforcing desired behaviors and inhibiting negative behaviors in both patient and providers have been described. Behaviors associated with chronic conditions are as broad as the health care system itself.

NOTES

1. Tables providing these and other statistics on depression are available at www.cdc.gov/features /dsdepression/revised_table_estimates_for_depression _mmwr_erratum_feb-2011.pdf.

2. Medical expenditure panel survey, Agency for Healthcare Research and Quality, http://meps.ahrq.gov /mepsweb/data_stats/MEPSnetHC.jsp.

3. Ibid.

4. MINT, www.motivationalinterviewing.org.

5. U.S. Preventive Services Task Force (USPSTF): An introduction, Agency for Healthcare Research and Quality, www.ahrq.gov/clinic/uspstfix.htm.

6. Physician quality reporting system, CMS.gov, www.cms.gov/pqri/.

7. See Agency for Healthcare Research and Quality, www.qualityindicators.ahrq.gov/.

8. AARP Public Policy Institute, "Chronic Care: A Call to Action," http://assets.aarp.org/rgcenter/health /beyond_50_hcr.pdf.

9. Caregiving in the U.S. 2009, National Alliance for Caregiving in collaboration with AARP, www. caregiving.org/data/Caregiving_in_the_US_2009_full_ report.pdf.

REFERENCES

Anderson G. 2010. *Chronic Care: Making the Case for Ongoing Care*. Princeton, NJ: Robert Wood Johnson Foundation.

Berwick DM, Nolan TW, Whittington J. 2008. The triple aim: Care, health, and cost. *Health Aff (Millwood)* 27 (3): 759-69.

Bodenheimer T, Berry-Millett R. 2009. Follow the money—controlling expenditures by improving care for patients needing costly services. *N Engl J Med* 361 (16): 1521-23.

Bodenheimer T, Wagner EH, Grumbach K. 2002. Improving primary care for patients with chronic illness. *JAMA* 288 (14): 1775-79.

Boyd CM, Darer J, Boult C, Fried LP, Boult L, Wu AW. 2005. Clinical practice guidelines and quality of care for older patients with multiple comorbid diseases: Implications for pay for performance. *JAMA* 294 (6): 716-24.

Brino A. 2013. UnitedHealth touts predictive modeling as solution to healthcare fraud and preventable hospitalizations. Available at www.healthcarepayer news.com/content/unitedhealth-touts-predictive -modeling-solution-healthcare-fraud-and-preventable (accessed June 24, 2013).

Christakis NA, Fowler JH. 2007. The spread of obesity in a large social network over 32 years. *N Engl J Med* 357 (4): 370-79.

Coleman EA, Min SJ, Chomiak A, Kramer AM. 2004. Posthospital care transitions: Patterns, complications, and risk identification. *Health Serv Res* 39 (5): 1449-66.

Dawber TR. 1960. Summary of recent literature regarding cigarette smoking and coronary heart disease. *Circulation* 22:164-66.

Evans M. 2011. Healthcare's "moneyball." *Mod Healthcare* 41 (41): 28-30.

Forrest CB, Lemke KW, Bodycombe DP, Weiner JP. 2009. Medication, diagnostic, and cost information as predictors of high-risk patients in need of care management. *Am J Manag Care* 15:41-48.

Freid VM, Bernstein AB, Bush MA. 2012. Multiple chronic conditions among adults aged 45 and over: Trends over the past 10 years. *NCHS Data Brief* 100:1-8.

Haynes SG, Feinleib M, Levine S, Scotch N, Kannel WB. 1978. The relationship of psychosocial factors to coronary heart disease in the Framingham study. II. Prevalence of coronary heart disease. *Am J Epidemiol* 107 (5): 384-402.

Hoffman C, Rice D, Sung HY. 1996. Persons with chronic conditions: Their prevalence and costs. *JAMA* 276 (18): 1473-79.

Hootman J, Bault M, Helmick C, Theis K, Amrour B. 2009. Prevalence and most common causes of disability among adults—United States, 2005. *MMWR* 58 (16): 421-26.

Kannel WB. 1967. Habitual level of physical activity and risk of coronary heart disease: The Framingham study. *Can Med Assoc J* 96 (12): 811-12.

Kannel WB, Sorlie P. 1979. Some health benefits of physical activity. The Framingham study. *Arch Intern Med* 139 (8): 857-61.

Kellermann AL, Weinick RM. 2012. Emergency departments, Medicaid costs, and access to primary care—understanding the link. *N Engl J Med* 366 (23): 2141-43.

Kramarow E, Lubitz J, Lentzner H, Gorina Y. 2007. Trends in the health of older Americans, 1970-2005. *Health Aff (Millwood)* 26 (5): 1417-25.

Leatherman S, Berwick D, Iles D, et al. 2003. The business case for quality: Case studies and an analysis. *Health Aff (Millwood)* 22 (2): 17-30.

Lochner KA, Cox CS. 2013. Prevalence of multiple chronic conditions among Medicare beneficiaries, United States, 2010. *Prev Chronic Disease* 10:E61.

Machlin SR, Soni A. 2013. Health care expenditures for adults with multiple treated chronic conditions: Estimates from the medical expenditure panel survey, 2009. *Prev Chronic Disease* 10:E63.

Marsteller JA, Hsu YJ, Reider L, et al. 2010. Physician satisfaction with chronic care processes: A cluster-randomized trial of guided care. *Ann Fam Med* 8 (4): 308-15.

McAlister A, Puska P, Salonen JT, Tuomilehto J, Koskela K. 1982. Theory and action for health promotion illustrations from the North Karelia project. *Am J Public Health* 72 (1): 43-50.

McGlynn EA (2004. There is no perfect health system. *Health Affairs* 23 (3): 100-102.

National Center for Health Statistics (NCHS). 2011. *Health, United States, 2010: With Special Feature on Death and Dying.* Hyattsville MD: U.S. Dept. of Health and Human Services. Available at www.cdc.gov/nchs/data/hus/hus10.pdf.

———. 2012. *Health, United States, 2011: With Special Feature on Socioeconomic Status and Health.* Hyattsville, MD: U.S. Dept. of Health and Human Services. Available at www.cdc.gov/nchs/data/hus/hus11.pdf.

Naylor MD, Brooten DA, Campbell RL, Maislin G, McCauley KM, Schwartz JS. 2004. Transitional care of older adults hospitalized with heart failure: A randomized, controlled trial. *J Am Ger Soc* 52 (5): 675-84.

Nyman JA, Barleen NA, Dowd BE, Russell DW, Coons SJ, Sullivan PW. 2007. Quality-of-life weights for the US population: Self-reported health status and priority health conditions, by demographic characteristics. *Med Care* 45 (7): 618-28.

Pawson R, Tilley N. 1997. *Realistic Evaluation.* London: Sage.

Puska P. 2010. From Framingham to North Karelia: From descriptive epidemiology to public health action. *Progr Cardiovasc Diseases* 53 (1): 15-20.

Puska P, Nissinen A, Tuomilehto J, et al. 1985. The community-based strategy to prevent coronary heart disease: Conclusions from the ten years of the North Karelia project. *Ann Rev Public Health* 6:147-93.

Puska P, Stahl T. 2010. Health in all policies—the Finnish initiative: Background, principles, and current issues. *Annu Rev Public Health* 31:315-28.

Puska P, Vartiainen E. 2009. Community based studies in high income countries. In *Oxford Textbook of Public Health,* ed. R Detels, R Beaglehole, M Lansang, M Gulliford. Oxford: Oxford University Press.

Sciamanna CN, Stillman FA, Hoch JS, Butler JH, Gass KG, Ford DE. 2000. Opportunities for improving inpatient smoking cessation programs: A community hospital experience. *Prev Med* 30 (6): 496-503.

Wagner EH. 1998. Chronic disease management: What will it take to improve care for chronic illness? *Eff Clin Pract* 1:2-4.

Wallace R. 2002a. Secondary prevention. In *Encyclopedia of Public Health,* ed. Lester Breslow. New York: Macmillan Reference.

———. 2002b. Tertiary prevention. In *Encyclopedia of Public Health,* ed. Lester Breslow. New York: Macmillan Reference.

CHAPTER 26

Health Behavior Change in Persons with Depressive Disorders

WILLIAM W. EATON, ANITA S. EVERETT,
RYAN MACDONALD, GAIL DAUMIT, AND
BRIANA M. MEZUK

LEARNING OBJECTIVES

After completing the chapter, the reader will be able to

* Describe the epidemiological characteristics and population burden related to depressive disorder.
* Describe physical illness comorbidity associated with depressive disorder, both as antecedent and as consequence.
* Describe the relationship of health behaviors to depressive disorder, including implications for implementing behavior change in persons with depressive disorder.

Introduction

Health behavior change for persons with mental disorders presents unique issues and problems. Mental disorders are associated with an increased risk for numerous chronic medical conditions, such as diabetes and heart disease (table 26.1), which makes the issue of behavior change more salient for those with mental disorders than for the general population. The signs and symptoms associated with mental disorders can interfere with following a medical regimen or recommendations for treatment or for prevention of disease and health promotion. Moreover, treatments for mental disorders, such as certain psychoactive medications, can significantly increase the risk for development or worsening of physical medical conditions.

TABLE 26.1. Depression and chronic medical conditions over the life course

Condition	ECA author and date	Relative risk	Confirming study
Type 2 diabetes	Eaton et al. 1996	2.2	Mezuk, Eaton, Albrecht, et al. 2008
Hypertension	Meyer et al. 2004	2.2	Patten et al. 2009
Heart attack	Pratt et al. 1996	4.5[a]	Rugulies, 2002
Stroke	Larson et al. 2001	2.7	Ramasubbu and Patten 2003
Any cancer	Gross et al. 2010	1.0	Oerlemans et al. 2007
Lung cancer	Gross et al. 2010	0.8	Oerlemans et al. 2007
Breast cancer	Gross et al. 2010	3.4[a]	Oerlemans et al. 2007[b]
Colon cancer	Gross et al. 2010	4.3	Oerlemans et al. 2007
Prostate cancer	Gross et al. 2010	1.1	Oerlemans et al. 2007
Arthritis	Eaton et al. 2006	1.3	NA
Osteopenia	Mezuk, Eaton, Golden, et al. 2008	4.1[a,c]	Cizza et al. 2010

Note: These data are from the Baltimore Epidemiologic Catchment Area (ECA) follow-up, 1981–96.
[a]Statistically significant at the level of 0/05.
[b]The relative risk for breast cancer in the meta-analysis was 2.5 and significant only for studies with longer than ten years of followup (as with the ECA).
[c]Age-adjusted or estimated from ECA data by Briana Mezuk, for risk of osteopenia, defined as one or more standard deviations lower in bone mass density than the general population.

Major Depressive Disorder

Major depressive disorder is a syndrome composed of two cardinal features and possibly a combination of several other criteria. The two cardinal features are sadness (dysphoria) and loss of interest (anhedonia). Other symptoms include weight loss or gain, loss or gain of appetite, sleep problems (sleeping too little or too much), moving unusually slowly or with unusual agitation, fatigue, inappropriate guilt, problems with concentrating, and recurrent thoughts of death and suicide or attempts to commit suicide. By definition, the syndrome endures for at least several weeks.

A review of 42 studies reported a range of one-year prevalence rates ranging from 0.64% in Taipei to 15.4% in Udmurtia, with a median of 5.3%, which is close to estimates reported in the U.S. population (Eaton et al. 2012; Kessler et al. 2005). Depressive disorder has a wide range

of clinical presentations, and persons meeting the criteria found in the *Diagnostic and Statistical Manual of Mental Disorders,* fifth edition *(DSM-5),* for major depressive disorder can be so severely affected as to commit suicide, be nearly stuporous or catatonic, or be unable to carry out even simple activities of daily living. Others with depression may be minimally impaired. The Global Burden of Disease study (Murray and Lopez 1996) rated a wide range of diseases according to their associated disability, with the severity ratings ranging from a value of 0.0 (equal to no disability) to a value of 1.0 (equal to death). Major depressive disorder was rated as one of the most disabling disorders, with a severity rating of 0.35 for the "moderate" form and 0.62 for the "severe" form. These values compare roughly to multiple sclerosis (0.41) for the moderate form of depressive disorder and blindness for severe depression.

Major depressive disorder is also associated with an increased risk of death. In a recent review of 14 studies, the median study showed a 70% increase in **mortality** (Eaton et al.2008). In depressive disorder, although the individual almost always has insight into the illness (in contrast to those with severe psychoses), many of the symptoms, such as dysphoria, anhedonia, fatigue, and difficulty concentrating, can distract and impair **motivation** to make any behavior changes, especially those that promote better health. More often, people suffering with depression tend to isolate themselves and may find it difficult just to make it through a day, so that behavior changes with longer-term intangible rewards (such as quitting smoking or losing weight) are often rejected as impossible or have a low priority. Additionally, somatic features, such as chronic pain, often accompany major depressive disorder and further complicate attempts to change behavior.

Comorbidity of Physical and Mental Disorders

Comorbidity is the occurrence of two or more disorders in one individual (Feinstein 1967). Many mental disorders typically have their peak periods of onset in adolescence and young adulthood (e.g., depressive disorder, panic disorder, alcohol disorder, substance use disorder, schizophrenia), whereas many important chronic physical conditions have peak onset in middle age or later (e.g., heart diseases, cancers, type 2 diabetes, and strokes). Comorbidity over the lifetime often takes the form of a mental condition occurring first and being followed by the onset of a medical condition. There are a range of **consequences** of depression for physical conditions and symptoms, selected for presentation here by virtue of their high prevalence and disabling or fatal consequences (see table 26.1). Each **relative risk** in the table was the result of a separate analysis that compared depressive disorder to other forms of psychopa-

thology and adjusted for other known risk factors for the physical condition. For many conditions, depressive disorder was the only nontrivial predictor. The sizes of the relative risks are large enough to place depressive disorder on a par with other risk factors, such as high cholesterol for heart attack, family history for breast cancer, hypertension for stroke, and obesity for type 2 diabetes. These results are consistent with the broader scientific literature.

Most persons with depressive disorder do not receive treatment, despite the existence of effective treatments (Mojtabai et al. 2011). Because screening for depression is relatively easy, the data summarized just above have implications for the practice of preventive medicine in the primary care setting. These results show that depression is a key risk factor for chronic, behavior-related, medical conditions. Both behavioral and biological factors may explain the link between depression and chronic medical conditions. One explanation is that depressive disorder raises risk through behavior changes that are common in patients with depression, such as unhealthful eating patterns, inactivity, inadequate sleep, and inattention to medical and preventive care. Another explanation is that physiological changes occurring during depression, such as blood platelet reactivity (Musselman et al. 1996) or elevated levels of the stress hormone, cortisol (Rubin et al. 1987), are associated with raised risk. A third possibility is that comorbid mental and physical conditions share a genetic predisposition.

Health Behaviors as Cause for or Consequence of Depression

Making significant lifestyle changes is difficult. Maintaining a healthful lifestyle in contemporary American culture, which is characterized by modern conveniences, television and media that can be enjoyed without exercise, ample availability of food, and the widespread financial means to take advantage of these possibilities, is clearly challenging. Making a change such as losing weight, stopping smoking, or abstaining from alcohol is hard. The presence of a mental illness makes it less likely that a person can maintain a healthful lifestyle, and reversing or changing unhealthful lifestyle **habits** becomes even more challenging. For those with mental illness, additional barriers arise to the maintenance of a healthful lifestyle.

Many studies show that unhealthful behaviors involving diet, exercise, and alcohol and tobacco co-occur with depression (Friedman-Wheeler et al. 2007; Luppino et al. 2010; McCarty et al. 2009; Ohayon 2007; Roshanaei-Moghaddam et al. 2009). However, it is a common misconception that co-occurrence or correlation implies **causation**. For example, although obesity and depression often occur together, disentangling cause and effect can be difficult. Therefore, the critical question turns to, Are unhealthy people (i.e., those engaging in unhealthful behaviors) more likely to suffer from depression, or are those suffering from depression more likely to engage in unhealthful behaviors as a coping mechanism to relieve their symptoms? The answer is probably both, but this chapter examines this issue primarily from the perspective of people suffering from depression. How common are unhealthful behaviors among the depressed population, and what are the potential impediments to changing these behaviors?

Whether they are causes, consequences, or associations, health behaviors have an effect on the depressed population. Ranking the relative health impact of behaviors for persons with depression is **complex**. Which behaviors for those in the population who are depressed, then, are the most important to change? Based on the available evidence, the answer is mixed. Although many behaviors (e.g., sleep, illicit drug use, unsafe sexual behavior, violence) are important to consider, the focus here is on two clusters of behaviors that fall together: (1) behaviors that relate to diet, physical activity, and obesity and (2) behaviors that relate to alcohol and tobacco use. These two are chosen because they are most commonly associated with depression (Strine et al. 2008).

Depression and Obesity

As stated above, many studies show associations between health behaviors and depression. Evidence from the 2006 Behavioral Risk Factor Surveillance System shows that depression is associated with physical inactivity (Strine et al. 2008). A recent study concluded that, among those currently suffering from depression, more physical activity was associated with less concurrent depression across a 10-year period (Harris et al. 2006). Similarly, obesity and poor diet have been shown to be associated with depression in adults (McElroy et al. 2004; Simon et al. 2006), and a recent review of the evidence from a National Institute of Mental Health panel suggests higher levels of obesity among the depressed (Allison et al. 2009). A recent meta-analysis further supports a bidirectional relationship between obesity and depression (Luppino et al. 2010). Baseline obesity predicted increased risk of the onset of depression by 55% in follow-up, and baseline depression also predicted a 58% increase in the odds of becoming obese.

Evidence from a large-cohort study suggests that the risk of obesity among the depressed population changes across time and is elevated as depressed individuals age (Kivimäki et al. 2009). Another study from the same cohort finds evidence suggesting that those with diets high in processed foods were found to be at greater risk for depression five years later (Akbaraly et al. 2009). Depression in diabetic populations is also associated with increased risk of a sedentary lifestyle and failure to adhere to diet and exercise recommendations (Gonzalez et al. 2008). Similarly, individuals with both diabetes and depression had significantly fewer days per week of adhering to a healthful diet five years later (Katon et al. 2009).

Depression and Substance Use

Alcohol and tobacco consumption is also associated with depression. Strong evidence suggests that alcohol abuse and dependence is comorbid with major depression (Hasin et al. 2007; Lynskey 1998). As with diet, exercise, and obesity, a bidirectional relationship exists between the two that is not easily untangled. On the one hand, evidence suggests that individuals self-medicate with alcohol to relieve symptoms of depression—even though it is a depressant (Kuo et al. 2006). Others have suggested the opposite, that alcohol's depressant effects lead to the onset of depression (Wang and Patten 2002). Recent evidence from a 25-year longitudinal study in New Zealand supported the conclusion that alcohol abuse caused depression, rather than the self-medication among the depressed explaining the association (Fergusson et al. 2009). However, a study of adolescents followed into adulthood found evidence that depressive symptoms led to increased risk for excessive alcohol use 16 years later, but only in males (Huurre et al. 2010). Another study following adolescents into adulthood found the same relationship, but only for females (McCarty et al. 2009).

Evidence also supports the comorbidity between smoking and depression (Breslau et al. 1998; Lerman et al. 1996; Strine et al. 2008; Wada et al. 2006). One nationally representative community-based study found that 37% of persons who had met the criteria for major depressive disorder over their lifetime were current smokers, versus 22% of those with no mental illness (Lasser et al. 2000).

Some of the clinical features of depression (appetite and weight changes, irritability and restlessness, sleep problems, and loss of energy) are directly related to and impede changes in health behaviors. Depression is often associated with changes in appetite and weight—a direct correlation with diet. Those suffering from depression may have decreased interest in preparing healthful foods and may have diets that consist primarily of convenience foods that are high in fat and calories. Another clinical feature of depression is lack of energy, or fatigue. Often, individuals suffering from depression limit their routine activities and would find it very difficult to exercise or perform additional physical activity. Moreover, alcohol is a depressant and, although tobacco provides short-term feelings of pleasure, the subsequent withdrawal exacerbates symptoms of depression. Alcohol and tobacco withdrawal may lead to feelings of restlessness or irritability, two additional symptoms of depression. Finally, difficulty with sleep is both a clinical symptom of depression and a health behavior in itself.

Changing Behaviors

The ability to change behaviors ultimately rests with the individual; however, many of the means to facilitate behavior change have become embedded within institutional practices. The treatment system for depression (and mental health, in general) is geared toward treating the symptoms of the illness, rather than the causes or the underlying factors that could prevent recurrence. Prescription of antidepressant medications has become increasingly common (Mojtabai and Olfson 2011), even though antidepressant drugs have side effects that can exacerbate poor health behaviors. Although the most common class of antidepressants in use in the United States, the selective serotonin reuptake inhibitors, have fewer and less-severe side effects than older agents, they nevertheless can result in side effects such as weight gain in some individuals. Limited access to quality health care is a clear structural barrier to any discussion of health behavior change. Undiagnosed and misdiagnosed depression left untreated may lead to more frequent and severe depressive episodes, which may further hinder healthful **lifestyle behaviors**.

In the medical care system, health behaviors are too often treated reactively rather than through positive health promotion or prevention. However, many companies have developed wellness programs for employees that encourage healthful lifestyles through **incentives**. This might include on-site gyms or discounted gym memberships and free counseling services for smoking cessation and drug abuse. Often, these employers offer discounts in company insurance premiums for employees who participate in these healthful lifestyle activities. The federal government has passed pervasive initiatives for tobacco cessation programs. In addition, city and state smoking bans and tobacco product taxation have been increasing.

Apart from institutional incorporation of health promotion and positive behaviors, **intervention** studies of health behaviors and depression have also taken place. Evidence suggests that physical exercise, even a modest amount, allays symptoms of depression. A recent meta-analysis of randomized trials shows that individuals randomly assigned to exercise programs had significantly lower depression scores than those who were not (Rethorst et al. 2009). Another meta-analysis attempts to show support for **causality** by suggesting that depression is a risk factor for subsequent decline in physical activity (Roshanaei-Moghaddam et al. 2009). However, Elfrey and Ziegelstein (2009) suggest that Roshanaei-Moghaddam and colleagues' findings are simply evidence for one side of a bidirectional relationship. Although Elfrey and Ziegelstein acknowledge the contribution of a common clinical observation, they suggest more rigorous methodology and suggest alternative pathways. But a review of the most methodologically sound controlled trial evidence concludes that the evidence provides modest support at best for the beneficial effect of exercise on depression (Rimer et al. 2012).

Evidence supports interventions for weight-loss trials, but the findings are inconsistent across populations and intervention strategies. A recent review of the randomized trial evidence for long-term exercise and diet routines among obese populations suggests that physical exercise alone is not sufficient for sustained weight loss. Physical exercise, the evidence suggests, should be combined with both behavior modification and healthful dietary routines (Sodlerlund et al. 2009). Another review of randomized trials concluded that diet and exercise together were effective for initial weight loss; however, the weight loss was only partially sustained at one-year follow-up (Curioni and Lourenco 2005).

There are several intervention strategies to treat alcohol abuse and dependence, ranging from full detoxification in rehabilitation centers to brief interventions. A recent review of clinical trials from 1966 to 2006 shows clear evidence that brief interventions can effectively reduce alcohol consumption in the primary care population (Kaner et al. 2009). However, the effect was seen more clearly in men, with women showing inconsistent findings.

Given recent advances in public policy concerning smoking, much attention has focused on smoking cessation. Are depressed people more likely to be successful at smoking cessation, or are depressive symptoms a barrier to quitting smoking? A recent randomized clinical trial among depressed psychiatric outpatients revealed success in smoking cessation among the intervention group compared to the **control group** (Hall et al. 2006). A review of clinical evidence indicates some risk among the depressed for increased severity of their symptoms and impairment during attempts at cessation (Lembke et al. 2007).

Examining the evidence presented above, some very clear associations and targets for intervention among the depressed population emerge. Recommendations at the community level for health behaviors are extremely difficult because some argue that adults should be allowed to choose their health behavior. Modifying personal behavior at the community level has often proved divisive, as with the recent effort by Mayor Bloomberg of New York City to ban the sale of large soft drinks, and policy recommendations in the form of taxes or programs have been historically ineffective. However, ways do exist for individuals and communities to elicit changes in health behaviors.

One recommendation is to support patients to initiate a physical exercise routine. In addition to working toward or maintaining a healthful **body mass index** (**BMI**), which has its own benefits of disease prevention, physical exercise itself is likely to reduce the rate and severity of depressive disorder. Similarly, eating to maintain a healthful BMI is a core recommendation that is associated with decreased risk of depression. In part, this includes helping at-risk patients develop coping skills to manage uncomfortable moods and emotions as alternatives to self-medicating with food, alcohol, or tobacco.

Although the message is not a new one, those suffering from depression should avoid tobacco use. The evidence does not clearly show a causal pathway from smoking to depression; it does, however, show that those who are clinically depressed have significantly higher rates of tobacco use. Despite some mixed findings concerning alcohol use, those suffering from depression should limit alcohol intake. Not only is alcohol itself a depressant, but it also exacerbates symptoms of depression, making a depressive episode more likely. In addition, psychotropic medications to treat depression have clear warnings against alcohol consumption during treatment, as the combination can be unpredictable and dangerous.

Conclusion

This chapter uses depression as an exemplar of mental illness to demonstrate the **complexity** that the presence of a mental illness can add to the process of change in health behavior. A mental or behavioral disorder can complicate health behavior in multiple ways. With regard to information on conditions that might be causal for a pattern of health behavior, mental disorders themselves are often comorbid with other long-term health conditions that are associated with, or caused by, poor health behavior. Teasing out the extent to which each aspect of mental and somatic condition contributes to the emergent health status and health behavior is often not possible because of the intertwined nature of these processes. In addition to etiologic considerations, health behavior maintenance is also important. Using depression and alcohol abuse as an example, the short-term benefit of escape or relief from the depression with intoxication may serve to perpetuate poor health behavior, which can have both short- and long-term adverse health impact. In addition to causing poor health behaviors and maintaining existing unhealthful behaviors, mental disorders can complicate an individual's capacity to make positive health behavior changes. To effectively make changes, individuals must be motivated. Mental disorders can adversely affect an individual's capacity for motivation both directly and indirectly. *Direct* impact on motivation occurs when the features of a mental illness slow down or limit an individual's thinking processes and the ability to become motivated. *Indirect* impact is impaired ability to appreciate the longer-term benefits of positive health behavior. Thus, in our example of depression, a direct impact may be psychomotor slowing that occurs as a part of depression in some people, and indirect impact would be a general sense of hopelessness that limits a person's ability to see and want to experience the benefits of improved health behavior.

Among the mental disorders, depressive disorder has high prevalence and is associated with moderate to high impairment. It has important implications for health behavior change. But there are many other mental disorders with the potential for similarly high impact. Given the high prevalence of mental disorders in our society, it is essential to understand the impact that these conditions have on our ability to promote positive health behavior in the general population.

REFERENCES

Akbaraly TN, Brunner EJ, Ferrie JE, Marmot MG, Kivimaki M, Singh-Manoux A. 2009. Dietary pattern and depressive symptoms in middle age. *Br J Psychiatry* 195:408-13.

Allison DB, Newcomer JW, Dunn AL, et al. 2009. Obesity among those with mental disorders: A National Institute of Mental Health meeting report. *Am J Prev Med* 36:341-50.

Breslau N, Peterson EL, Schultz LR, Chilcoat HD, Andreski P. 1998. Major depression and stages of smoking: A longitudinal investigation. *Arch Gen Psychiatry* 55:161-66.

Cizza G, Primma S, Coyle M, Gourgiotis L, Csako G. 2010. Depression and osteoporosis: A research synthesis with meta-analysis. *Horm Metab Res* 42:467-82.

Curioni CC, Lourenco PM. 2005. Long-term weight loss after diet and exercise: A systematic review. *Int J Obes (Lond)* 29:1168-74.

Eaton WW, Alexandre P, Bienvenu OJ, et al. 2012. The burden of mental disorders. In *Public Mental Health,* ed. WW Eaton; faculty, students, and fellows of Dept. of Mental Health. New York: Oxford University Press.

Eaton WW, Armenian HK, Gallo JJ, Pratt L, Ford D. 1996. Depression and risk for onset of type II diabetes: A prospective, population-based study. *Diabetes Care* 19:1097-1102.

Eaton W, Fogel J, Armenian H. 2006. The consequences of psychopathology in the Baltimore Epidemiologic Catchment Area. In *Medical and Psychiatric Comorbidity over the Course of Life,* ed. W Eaton. Washington, DC: APPI Press.

Eaton WW, Martins SS, Nestadt G, Bienvenu OJ, Clarke D, Alexandre P. 2008. The burden of mental disorders. *Epidemiol Rev* 30:1-14.

Elfrey MK, Ziegelstein RC. 2009. The "inactivity trap." *Gen Hosp Psychiatry* 31:303-5.

Feinstein A. 1967. *Clinical Judgement.* Baltimore: Williams & Wilkins.

Fergusson DM, Boden JM, Horwood LJ. 2009. Tests of causal links between alcohol abuse or dependence and major depression. *Arch Gen Psychiatry* 66:260-66.

Friedman-Wheeler DG, Ahrens AH, Haaga DA, McIntosh E, Thorndike FP. 2007. Depressive symptoms, depression proneness, and outcome expectancies for cigarette smoking. *Cognit Ther Res* 31:547-57.

Gonzalez JS, Safren SA, Delahanty LM, et al. 2008. Symptoms of depression prospectively predict poorer self-care in patients with type 2 diabetes. *Diabet Med* 25:1102-7.

Gross AL, Gallo JJ, Eaton WW. 2010. Depression and cancer risk: 24 years of follow-up of the Baltimore Epidemiologic Catchment Area sample. *Cancer Causes Control* 21:191-99.

Hall SM, Tsoh JY, Prochaska JJ, et al. 2006. Treatment for cigarette smoking among depressed mental health outpatients: A randomized clinical trial. *Am J Public Health* 96:1808-14.

Harris AH, Cronkite R, Moos R. 2006. Physical activity, exercise coping, and depression in a 10-year cohort study of depressed patients. *J Affect Disord* 93:79-85.

Hasin DS, Stinson FS, Ogburn E, Grant BF. 2007. Prevalence, correlates, disability, and comorbidity of DSM-IV alcohol abuse and dependence in the United States: Results from the National Epidemiologic Survey on Alcohol and Related Conditions. *Arch Gen Psychiatry* 64:830-42.

Huurre T, Lintonen T, Kaprio J, Pelkonen M, Marttunen M, Aro H. 2010. Adolescent risk factors for excessive alcohol use at age 32 years. A 16-year prospective follow-up study. *Soc Psychiatry Psychiatr Epidemiol* 45:125-34.

Kaner EF, Dickinson HO, Beyer F, et al. 2009. The effectiveness of brief alcohol interventions in primary care settings: A systematic review. *Drug Alcohol Rev* 28:301-23.

Katon WJ, Russo JE, Heckbert SR, et al. 2009. The relationship between changes in depression symptoms and changes in health risk behaviors in patients with diabetes. *Int J Geriatr Psychiatry* 25 (5): 466-75.

Kessler RC, Chiu WT, Demler O, Merikangas KR, Walters EE. 2005. Prevalence, severity, and comorbidity of 12-month DSM-IV disorders in the National Comorbidity Survey Replication. *Arch Gen Psychiatry* 62:617-27.

Kivimäki M, Batty GD, Singh-Manoux A, et al. 2009. Association between common mental disorder and obesity over the adult life course. *Br J Psychiatry* 195:149-55.

Kuo PH, Gardner CO, Kendler KS, Prescott CA. 2006. The temporal relationship of the onsets of alcohol dependence and major depression: Using a genetically informative study design. *Psychol Med* 36:1153-62.

Larson S, Owens P, Ford D, Eaton W. 2001. Depressive disorders, dysthymia, and risk of stroke: A thirteen year follow-up from the Baltimore ECA. *Stroke* 32:1979-83.

Lasser K, Boyd JW, Woolhandler S, Himmelstein DU, McCormick D, Bor DH. 2000. Smoking and mental illness: A population-based prevalence study. *JAMA* 284:2606-10.

Lembke A, Johnson K, Debattista C. 2007. Depression and smoking cessation: Does the evidence support psychiatric practice? *Neuropsychiatr Dis Treat* 3:487-93.

Lerman C, Audrain J, Orleans CT, et al. 1996. Investigation of mechanisms linking depressed mood to nicotine dependence. *Addictive Behav* 21:9-19.

Luppino FS, de Wit LM, Bouvy PF, et al. 2010. Overweight, obesity, and depression: A systematic review and meta-analysis of longitudinal studies. *Arch Gen Psychiatry* 67:220-29.

Lynskey MT. 1998. The comorbidity of alcohol dependence and affective disorders: Treatment implications. *Drug Alcohol Depend* 52:201-9.

McCarty CA, Kosterman R, Mason WA, et al. 2009. Longitudinal associations among depression, obesity, and alcohol use disorders in young adulthood. *Gen Hosp Psychiatry* 31:442-50.

McElroy SL, Kotwal R, Malhotra S, Nelson EB, Keck PE, Nemeroff CB. 2004. Are mood disorders and obesity related? A review for the mental health professional. *J Clin Psychiatry* 65:634-51.

Meyer CM, Armenian HK, Eaton WW, Ford DE. 2004. Incident hypertension associated with depression in the Baltimore Epidemiologic Catchment Area follow-up study. *J Affect Disord* 83:127-33.

Mezuk B, Eaton WW, Albrecht S, Golden S. 2008. Depression and type 2 diabetes over the lifespan: A meta-analysis. *Diabetes Care* 31:2383-90.

Mezuk B, Eaton WW, Golden SH, Wand G, Lee BH. 2008. Depression, antidepressants, and bone mineral density in a population-based cohort. *J Gerontol Biol Sci* 63 1410-15.

Mojtabai R, Olfson M. 2011. Proportion of antidepressants prescribed without a psychiatric diagnosis is growing. *Health Affairs* 30:1434-42.

Mojtabai R, Olfson M, Sampson NA, et al. 2011. Barriers to mental health treatment: Results from the National Comorbidity Survey Replication. *Psychol Med* 41:1751-61.

Murray CJL, Lopez AD. 1996. *The Global Burden of Disease.* Boston: Harvard University Press.

Musselman DL, Tomer A, Manatunga AK, et al. 1996. Exaggerated platelet reactivity in major depression. *Am J Psychiatry* 153:1313-17.

Oerlemans ME, van den Akker M, Schuurman AG, Kellen E, Buntinx F. 2007. A meta-analysis on depression and subsequent cancer risk. *Clin Pract Epidemiol Ment Health* 3:29.

Ohayon MM. 2007. Prevalence and comorbidity of sleep disorders in general population. *Rev Prat* 57:1521-28.

Patten SB, Williams JV, Lavorato DH, Campbell NR, Eliasziw M, Campbell TS. 2009. Major depression as a risk factor for high blood pressure: Epidemiologic evidence from a national longitudinal study. *Psychosom Med* 71:273-79.

Pratt LA, Ford DE, Crum RM, Armenian HK, Gallo JJ, Eaton WW. 1996. Depression, psychotropic medication, and risk of heart attack: Prospective data from the Baltimore ECA Follow-up. *Circulation* 94:3123-29.

Ramasubbu R, Patten SB. 2003. Effect of depression on stroke morbidity and mortality. *Can J Psychiatry* 48:250-57.

Rethorst CD, Wipfli BM, Landers DM. 2009. The antidepressive effects of exercise: A meta-analysis of randomized trials. *Sports Med* 39:491-511.

Rimer J, Dwan K, Lawlor DA, et al. 2012. Exercise for depression. *Cochrane Database Syst Rev,* CD004366.

Roshanaei-Moghaddam B, Katon WJ, Russo J. 2009. The longitudinal effects of depression on physical activity. *Gen Hosp Psychiatry* 31:306-15.

Rubin R, Poland R, Leser I, Winston R, Blodgett N. 1987. Neuroendocrine aspects of primary endogenous depression. I. Cortisol secretory dynamics in patients and matched controls. *Arch Gen Psychiatry* 44:328-36.

Rugulies R. 2002. Depression as a predictor for coronary heart disease: A review and meta-analysis. *Am J Prev Med* 23:51-61.

Simon GE, Von KM, Saunders K, et al. 2006. Association between obesity and psychiatric disorders in the US adult population. *Arch Gen Psychiatry* 63:824-30.

Sodlerlund A, Fischer A, Johansson T. 2009. Physical activity, diet, and behaviour modification in the treatment of overweight and obese adults: A systematic review. *Perspect Public Health* 129:132-42.

Strine TW, Mokdad AH, Dube SR, et al. 2008. The association of depression and anxiety with obesity and unhealthy behaviors among community-dwelling US adults. *Gen Hosp Psychiatry* 30:127-37.

Wada K, Satoh T, Tsunoda M, Aizawa Y. 2006. Associations of health behaviors on depressive symptoms among employed men in Japan. *Ind Health* 44:486-92.

Wang J, Patten SB. 2002. Prospective study of frequent heavy alcohol use and the risk of major depression in the Canadian general population. *Depress Anxiety* 15:42-45.

Glossary

adaptation the ability of a system to respond to the environment in which it is situated and to diversify.

adoption the component of health behavior change intervention in which the target setting begins to use the intervention.

advocacy work for political, regulatory, or organizational change on behalf of a particular interest group or population.

action Stage 4 (Stages of Change theory), in which the subject changes overt behavior by adopting new habits.

activated patient see *patient activation.*

agent an epidemiological term referring to the organism or object that transmits a disease from the environment to the host; also known as a *vector.*

antecedent an environmental, sensory, emotional, intrapersonal, or interpersonal trigger that precedes a specified behavior.

antecedent-behavior-consequence (A-B-C) model a classic model of intervention for behavior change based on behavioral conditioning, learning, and motivation that emphasizes causal relationships between antecedents, consequences, and behaviors.

anticipated regret a decision-making criterion in which fear of regretting a wrong choice influences behavior.

asymmetric paternalism an approach to public policy that helps individuals prone to making irrational decisions achieve their goals, while not limiting those making informed, deliberate decisions.

attitude a relatively constant feeling, predisposition, or set of beliefs directed toward an object, a person, or a situation.

balancing feedback loops negative *feedback loops* that create a closed chain of causal

connection (e.g., an increase in A leads to an increase in B, but the increase in B in turn leads to a decrease in A) and stabilize the system; see also *reinforcing feedback loops.*

basic Behavioral and Social Sciences Research (b-BSSR) a National Institutes of Health framework to promote incorporation of the basic sciences for more effective clinical and public health interventions.

behavioral belief the perceived likelihood that complying with a behavior will lead to positive outcomes.

behavioral capability the knowledge, skills, and resources necessary to perform a given behavior.

behavioral contracting formally committing to achieving behavioral goals in a contract.

behavioral economics the study of the effects of social, cognitive, and emotional factors on the economic decisions of individuals and institutions and the consequences for markets and public policy in terms of price, return, and resource allocation.

behavioral intention the mental state in which an individual expects to take a specified action at some time in the future.

best practice/best clinical practice recommendations for an intervention, based on a critical review of multiple research and evaluation studies that substantiate the efficacy of the intervention in the populations and circumstances in which the studies were done.

body mass index (BMI) a measure of weight for height, calculated by weight in kilograms divided by height in meters squared.

bonding social capital a relationship between people who share similarities such as belonging to an organization, family, or

523

neighborhood that reinforces the group's social identity.

boundary spanners   members of an organization who play a critical role in implementing innovations (such as guidelines) by looking to other organizations for ideas and strategies via their significant social connections within and outside their particular organization.

bracketing effect   occurs when choice outcomes under narrow bracketing differ from those under broad bracketing.

bridging social capital   a relationship established between individuals or organizations that are not similar but have shared associations, such as between work colleagues or individuals from different faiths or religious institutions.

broaden-and-build theory   a theory that asserts that people's daily experiences of positive emotions compound over time to build a variety of consequential social, psychological, intellectual, and physical resources.

built environment   that part of the physical environment that has been modified by humans and includes transportation systems, land use, public resources (e.g., parks), zoning regulations, and buildings (i.e., schools, homes, workplaces).

capacity building   strengthening knowledge and skills among professionals and citizens for developing partnerships and for population-based behavior change via training, consultation, and networking services.

causality/causation   the relation between an event (*cause*) and a second event (*effect*) in which the second event is a consequence of the first.

causal theory   a set of testable explanations for the relationship between an independent variable or input and the dependent variable or outcome; see *program theory*.

causal web   a representation of how a complex group of subjects and relationships can contribute to the occurrence and spread of disease.

chain of accountability   a framework in which senior leaders monitor performance and hold team leaders accountable; team leaders, in turn, hold frontline staff accountable.

change agents   influential individuals targeted in a social group for individual intervention, who, given their influential roles in the target

population, effect change among the rest of the group not through direct intervention effects, but through changes in the norms and expectations of the members of their social environment.

change theory   defines concepts and principles that can form the basis of interventions and health messages; see also *explanatory theory*.

choice bracketing   the process of grouping individual choices together into narrow or broad sets.

Chronic Care Model (CCM)   developed by Edward Wagner, the model posits that redesign of the delivery system, enhanced decision support, improved clinical information systems, support for self-management, and better access to community resources are necessary to improve outcomes for people with chronic conditions; these components are also relevant for current U.S. health care reform.

classical conditioning   the process of pairing a stimulus with an emotional or behavioral response, such as wanting an ice cream cone when the ice cream truck's music is heard after having enjoyed an ice cream several times previously; first described by Ivan Pavlov.

classic epidemiological triad   the relationship of agent, host, and environment in transmitting disease.

coalition   a group of organizations or representatives of groups within a community, joined to pursue a common objective.

collaborative method   a behavior change approach in which experts bring a solid evidence base for intervention, supportive interaction with peers, healthful competition among organizations that improves inter-professional cohesion on each team, and better comparability of performance measures across large numbers of organizations.

collaboratives   learning networks among health care organizations, convened to improve some aspect of health care services.

collective efficacy   a group's ability to perform actions to bring about desired change.

collective norms   norms established by the group or social system.

community of practice (CoP)   an informal partnership that operates in parallel with, and in support of, more formal configurations; often used loosely as a synonym for *network*.

community-level determinants a type of interpersonal factor that is believed to be associated with, and possibly causal for, behavioral change.

community-level interventions planned events sponsored or cosponsored by the coalition and primarily intended to directly change behavior, detect risk or disease, or educate persons outside of the coalition.

comorbidities one or more medical conditions or disease processes that coexist with an initial diagnosis.

compatible innovations innovations that match the intended users' values, norms, beliefs, and perceived needs and thus are more likely to be adopted.

competing behaviors alternative, less desirable behavioral choices that vie with desired behavior choices.

complex comprising interconnected or interwoven parts.

complexity 1. the extent to which social relations serve many functions; 2. how easy or hard is it to integrate a given behavior into current work practice; 3. the existence of many parts intricately arranged.

complex system a system in which the function and behavior of the whole cannot be deduced from the behavior of the individual parts, such as a living being versus a machine.

complex systems science the study of how relationships between parts give rise to the collective behaviors of a system and how the system interacts and forms relationships with its environment.

compliance adherence to a prescribed therapeutic or preventive regimen.

compositional environment an aggregate description of individual attributes in a neighborhood or group, such as the proportion of persons in a census tract having a college education.

computational approaches methods used in some systems science employing mathematical models.

conceptual framework a set of assumptions and principles that outline and attempt to connect a set of beliefs or actions for a given concept.

confounded see *confounder*.

confounder an extraneous study variable that affects the association being studied between two other variables; a threat to internal validity.

consequence a reinforcer following a behavior that increases or maintains the behavior.

consumerism the free choice of consumers dictating what is produced and how (i.e., the economic organization of a society).

contemplation Stage 2 (Stages of Change theory), in which the subject is thinking about changing or initiating a specific behavior.

context aspects of the environment that may influence the implementation or study of the intervention.

contingency management a technique that attempts to modify a behavioral response by controlling the consequences of that response (e.g., voucher incentive program).

continuum model a health behavior change model in which the general approach is to identify variables that influence action, such as knowledge, attitudes, perceptions of risk, or perceptions of benefit, and to combine them into a predictive equation (e.g., Theory of Planned Behavior, Health Belief Model).

contribution analysis an evaluation that measures what an intervention is directly trying to change (i.e., short- or medium-term outcomes) while existing literature demonstrates the link between the short and intermediate outcomes and the longer-term changes that the intervention is seeking to influence.

control beliefs perceived factors that may impede or facilitate compliance.

control group a set of research participants that have been randomly selected from the same research sample as the treatment group was selected from. The control group will be very similar to the *treatment group* in every possible way except that the control group participants receive no treatment.

cost-effectiveness evaluation/analysis a measure of the cost of an intervention relative to its impact, usually expressed in dollars per unit of effect.

counter-advertising disseminating information about a product, its effects, and the industry that promotes it, in order to decrease its appeal and use.

critical consciousness awareness based on reflection and action in making change.

cues prompts that trigger actions. Some cues may not be consciously perceived.

cultural competence the ability to interact effectively with people of different cultures and socioeconomic backgrounds.

cultural humility the willingness to accept people of different cultures and develop mutually beneficial and respectful partnerships with them.

cultural norms behavior patterns typical of specific groups.

cultural proficiency see *cultural competence*.

decision errors pitfalls in human decision making that help explain when and why individuals engage in self- or other-harming behaviors.

decriminalization the elimination, reduction, and/or nonenforcement of penalties for the sale, purchase, or possession of illicit drugs.

denormalization actions implemented to induce and reinforce the public perception of a health-compromising behavior as socially unacceptable.

density the extent to which network members know and interact with each other.

descriptive norm our perception of the behaviors practiced by other people in the social environment; the perceived prevalence of a behavior in a group.

determinants forces predisposing, enabling, and reinforcing lifestyles, or shaping environmental conditions of living, in ways that affect the health of populations.

developmental evaluation an evaluation in which the evaluator is embedded in the intervention in order to lend evaluative thinking as the intervention is developed and evolves.

difficulty structure a schematic demonstrating that most people can indicate that the items at the low end of the measure are true for them, whereas most people cannot agree that the items at the high end of the scale are true for them.

Diffusion of Innovations Theory (DIT) a theory explaining how, why, and at what rate new ideas and technology spread among members of a social system.

direct cost a price that can be completely attributed to the production of specific goods or services (e.g., materials, labor).

distal determinants influences that set the stage for a given outcome but are not immediately (proximally) related to the outcome (e.g., sociocultural norms, built environments).

dose delivered the volume of activity or intended units of the program delivered by the implementers.

dose-response relationship a term borrowed from clinical trials of drugs; when applied in epidemiology, it refers to a gradient of risk ratios corresponding to degrees of exposure; in health promotion it refers to the increases in outcome measures associated with proportionate increases in the program resources expended or intervention exposure.

dyad a group of two people.

dynamic system a system in which change in the state of the system happens over time and the past has an impact on the future.

dysregulation of choice loss of control of choice (e.g., seen in those dependent upon addictive substances).

early adopters those in the population who accept a new idea or practice soon after the innovators (but before the middle majority); they tend to be opinion leaders for the middle majority.

ecological approach a strategic framework based on the complex relationships and interplay between individuals and their environments.

ecological intervention a program acknowledging complex relationships between individuals and their physical, social, and cultural environments.

ecological model a model that focuses on the interplay of people with their physical and sociocultural surroundings (i.e., environments).

ecology the study of the web of relationships among behaviors of individuals and populations and their social and physical environments.

effectiveness the extent to which the intended effect or benefits of an intervention are achieved in practice.

efficacy the extent to which an intervention can be shown to be beneficial under optimal conditions.

efficiency the proportion of total costs (e.g., money, resources, time) relative to the effectiveness of an intervention measured by number of people served or reached, or the benefits achieved in practice.

egocentric network   a network comprising one individual, who is the focal individual (or ego), and that person's social ties; see also *sociometric networks.*

elasticity   in economics, the sensitivity of demand for a product to retail price.

Employee Assistance Program (EAP)   a confidential, voluntary set of procedures and arrangements through which an employer provides information, referral, counseling, and support to employees and sometimes their family members to help them deal with personal problems that might interfere with their work.

enabling factor   a characteristic of the environment that facilitates action and any skill or resource required to attain a specific behavior.

enacted support   actual support of an individual provided by social network members; see also *perceived support.*

environment   the totality of social, biological, and physical circumstances surrounding a defined quality of life, health, or a behavioral goal or problem..

environmental factor   a specific element or component of the social, biological, or physical environment determined during the ecological diagnosis to be causally linked to health or quality-of-life goals or problems identified in the social or epidemiological diagnosis.

environmental intervention   a program that aims to change behavior by facilitating or inhibiting behaviors through changes in the surroundings (e.g., promoting breastfeeding by providing nursing mothers with a room in the workplace to nurse or pump).

epidemiology   the study of the distribution and causes of health problems in populations.

epigenetics   the study of how gene function is affected by prenatal and early life experiences and exposures.

episodic behaviors   health behaviors performed periodically (e.g., getting flu shots).

etiology   the origins or causes of a disease or condition; the first steps in the natural history of a disease.

evaluation   comparing an object of interest against a standard of acceptability.

evidence   information based on systematic analysis of data, preferably from more than one source or method of data collection and analysis.

evidence-based practice   program decisions or intervention selections made on the strength of data from the community concerning needs and data from previously tested interventions or programs concerning their effectiveness, sometimes using theory in the absence of data on the specific alignment of interventions and population needs.

evidence-based programs   interventions designed using formative, process, and summative evaluation.

exception ambiguity   uncertainty as to whether the benefits of applying a particular intervention to a specific patient outweigh the potential risks (including patient discomfort).

expectancies   a person's opinions about how his or her behavior is likely to influence outcome; see also *expectations.*

expectation ambiguity   unclear norms and expectations within a unit or organization regarding guideline compliance.

expectations   anticipated outcomes of a given behavior; see also *expectancies.*

experimental design   a set of procedures distinguished from other designs for evaluation by the use of an equivalent or nearly equivalent control group, which is best assured by random assignment of large numbers of subjects to each group before the treatment or program.

explanatory theory (theory of the problem)   a theory that helps describe and identify why a problem exists, predicts behaviors under defined conditions, and guides the search for modifiable factors that contribute to the problem, such as insufficient knowledge, attitudes, self-efficacy, social support, and lack of resources (e.g., Health Belief Model, Theory of Planned Behavior, Precaution Adoption Process Model); see also *change theory.*

Extended Parallel Process Model (EPPM)   a framework to predict how individuals will react when confronted with stimuli that cause fear; also known as *fear management.*

fear   a mental and physiological state that motivates problem-solving behavior if an action (fight or flight) is immediately available; if not, it motivates other defense mechanisms such as denial or suppression.

feasibility   an estimate of the receptivity and manageability of an intervention or program based on pilot testing in the population and setting in which it would be conducted.

feedback loop   a circuit formed by an effect returning to its cause and generating either more or less of the same effect, or, in cognition, information to the agent.

fidelity to design   an aspect of process evaluation that monitors which aspects of the planned intervention actually take place.

flexibility   the capacity of an intervention to adapt as it is integrated into practice; see also *rigidity.*

Foresight system map   a representation of obesity as caused by a complex web of societal and biological factors with energy balance at the center.

formative evaluation   measurements obtained and judgments made before or during the implementation of materials, methods, activities, or programs to discover, predict, control, assure, or improve the quality of performance or delivery; see also *process evaluation.*

"4 Ps" (product, price, place, promotion)   a system applied to design and implementation of an intervention to improve adoption of a clinical guideline.

Gantt chart   a timetable showing each activity in a program plan as a horizontal line that extends from the start to the finish date to illustrate what activities should be under way, about to begin, or due to be completed by the various agents responsible for the phases of the program plan.

generality   the capacity of a theory to apply to a range of issues and populations and not be highly specific to one group or behavior.

generalizability   to what extent an intervention that has been shown to be effective in one state or community has a strong potential to have a similar effect in a different population.

genetic factors   a set of determinants along with behavioral factors and environmental factors that influence health, both through the biological effects of personal susceptibility to other risk factors or propensity to manifest pathologies, and through interaction with the environment and behavior.

geographic environment   the residential space of individuals, the location of their home (within their neighborhood, city, and region), their activity space (where they work, go to school, shop, and spend leisure time), and their travel routes to and from these nonresidential activity spaces; see also *social environment.*

Getting to Outcomes (GTO) model   a stepped process to help communities plan, implement, and evaluate the impact of their programs that attempt to prevent negative behaviors (e.g., substance abuse).

goal   the desired result of an individual's or a group's effort; can be *self-set, assigned, prescribed, participatory/collaborative, guided, group-set,* etc.

goal-setting   the process of setting achievable and incremental goals, committing to achieving the goals through a behavioral contract, monitoring and documenting progress, and reinforcing goal achievement through rewards.

"grab-bag" syndrome   the pitfall of selecting intervention approaches in which the program planner opts for nonstrategic approaches because they are compatible with her or his previous experience, preferred approaches, or skill set.

guideline   a statement or other indication of policy or procedure by which to determine a course of action (e.g., clinician's practice guideline to advise patients during checkups to quit smoking).

habit   a learned, often automatic, behavior that is commonly triggered by environmental and social cues and often decoupled from the original reason for the behavior.

habituation   incorporation of a pattern of behavior into one's lifestyle to the degree that it is performed virtually without thought but does not necessarily entail physical or psychological dependence.

Haddon matrix   the most commonly used paradigm in the injury prevention field that evaluates factors related to personal, vector (agent), and environmental attributes before, during, and after an injury or death for designing interventions.

Hawthorne effect   the result of observed interventions in which participants perform better than under normal conditions because they are aware of being observed.

health   a state of physical, mental, and social well-being in which the individual is able to cope with his or her environment and perform meaningful social roles.

health behavior   an action taken by an individual to change or maintain her or his health status or prevent illness or injury; see also *health lifestyle.*

Health Belief Model (HBM)   a paradigm used to predict and explain health behavior, based on value-expectancy theory.

health communication intervention   a program that facilitates targeted messaging, using diverse vehicles of dissemination, to change health behavior and create a supportive climate for intervention efforts (e.g., Truth campaign).

health disparities   gaps in the quality of health and health care across racial, ethnic, sexual orientation, and socioeconomic groups; also called *health care inequality.*

health lifestyle   collectively shared behaviors in response to one's social, cultural, and economic environment; see also *health behavior.*

health risk appraisal/assessment (HRA)   a widely used screening tool in health promotion and often the first step in health promotion programs; following HRA, *tailored messaging* can be implemented.

Healthy Living and Working Model   a health behavior change program that is an example of a setting intervention.

heterogeneous systems   systems with a large number of structural variations, such as subsystems, actors, and interconnections between these elements, whereas in *homogenous systems,* the structural elements tend to be identical or indistinguishable; see also *complex system.*

history bias   a study confounder in which events occur between the pretest and the posttest of research that could affect participants in such a way as to alter the dependent variable.

host   a concept from epidemiology referring to an individual who harbors or is at risk of harboring a disease or condition.

hot-cold empathy gaps   the tendency for people in a cold, unemotional, state to underestimate the impact of emotions and drives on their own future behavior (e.g., someone who is not hungry overestimates the likelihood that he or she will choose healthful options at the grocery store but judges harshly others whose product choices fail to show dietary moderation).

human factors engineering   the discipline that studies interactions among humans and four system elements (task, tools, physical environment, and organization factors) to optimize human well-being and overall system performance.

hyperbolic time discounting   the tendency to overweight immediate costs and benefits relative to those occurring at any point in the future and to take a more evenhanded approach to delayed costs and benefits occurring at different points in time (e.g., starting a diet tomorrow rather than today); also known as *present-bias.*

impact evaluation   assessment of program effects on intermediate objectives (including changes in predisposing, enabling, and reinforcing factors and behavioral and environmental changes) and possibly health and social outcomes.

implementation   converting program objectives into actions through policy changes, regulation, and organization.

incentive   a reward that motivates a behavior or change.

incidence   the frequency of occurrence of a disease or health problem in a population based on the number of new cases over a given period of time (usually one year). Commonly confused with *prevalence,* the occurrence of a disease or health problem in a population.

indirect costs   expenditures not directly attributable to a project or product (e.g., administration, personnel).

individual-level determinants   intrapersonal factors such as knowledge, attitudes, beliefs, motivation, self-concept, past experience, and skills.

individual-level factors   see *individual-level determinants.*

individual-level intervention   an intervention that focuses on intrapersonal factors such as knowledge, attitudes, beliefs, motivation, self-concept, past experience, and skills.

influences   families, social relationships, socioeconomic status, culture, geography, and so forth that affect an individual's health behavior; see also *determinants.*

initial effects   changes in psychocognitive factors, such as knowledge and attitudes.

injunctive norms   our perceptions of the behaviors, attitudes, and beliefs that are considered appropriate or acceptable in a social group; expectations of whether our behavior will result in approval or sanctioning by others.

innovation   a new technique or technology that achieves better results for comparable cost or effort than what it replaces.

innovators   those in a population who are first to develop or adopt a new idea or practice, usually based on information from sources outside the community.

integration   combining or relating individuals or groups so that they work together or form a whole.

interdependence   the level of connectedness among the parts of the system; characteristics that can make predicting the impact of changing one part of the system difficult.

intermediate effects   changes in self-reported, or observed, behavior.

internal validity   the extent to which evaluation results can be attributed to the program evaluated.

interpersonal factors   see *interpersonal determinants.*

interpersonal/interpersonal-level determinants   influences from social networks, such as family members, friends or peers, and co-workers.

interpersonal intervention   an intervention that reaches clusters of group members who can then reinforce specific behaviors (e.g., a nutrition intervention that targets all members of a family), via mentoring programs and family education or counseling.

interpersonal level   interactions and relationships that provide social identity, support, and role definition, including family, friends, co-workers, peers, and social networks.

intervention   the part of a strategy, incorporating method and operational technique, that reaches a person or a population.

intrapersonal intervention   one that involves health education, counseling, and social marketing campaigns provided to one individual at a time to change the behavior of individuals that collectively make up the population (e.g., getting a flu shot).

intrapersonal level   individual characteristics that influence behavior, including knowledge, attitudes, beliefs, personality traits, biology, race, socioeconomic status, and situational factors (e.g., personal history, substance abuse).

iterative process   a method for arriving at a decision or a desired result by repeating rounds of analysis or a cycle of operations.

key determinants   those factors identified as most influential; see also *determinants.*

key stakeholder   a person or institution that is influenced by a health behavior change intervention or has influence over those involved and whose input can affect every stage, from funding to defining the problem, designing the program, and disseminating the results.

knowledge translation   processes for enabling application of research to policy and practice.

level of exposure   the extent to which the target audience has been exposed to an intervention and their reaction to it.

levels of influence   multiple behavior determinants (i.e., individual-level, intervention-level, system-level, and implementation-level) that an effective behavior change attempts to simultaneously address.

leverage points   places to intervene and use to maximum advantage in a complex system.

life-course perspective   the theory that lives are shaped by multiple long-term trajectories and short-term events (e.g., victimization) embedded within them that may have major influences on the future life course.

life skills   abilities necessary or desirable for full participation in everyday life (e.g., learning to share with a sibling).

lifestyle   the culturally, socially, economically, and environmentally conditioned complex of habituated actions characteristic of an individual, group, or community that is health related but not necessarily health directed.

lifestyle behaviors   see *habit.*

lifestyle factors   cognitive factors (e.g., knowledge, attitudes, beliefs, awareness), preferences, personality traits, perceived stress tendencies, outcome expectancies, health beliefs, types of motivation, self-efficacy, skills, habits, emotional regulation skills, perceived time, and so forth.

Locus of Control Theory the extent to which individuals believe that they can control events that affect them.

logic model a sequence of pathways that links the intervention to the ultimate outcome; also called *conceptual framework* and *program impact pathway* (*PIP*).

loss aversion the tendency to put substantially greater weight on avoiding losses than on achieving gains (e.g., holding on too long to underperforming investments).

loss/lost to follow-up patients who were once actively participating in a research trial but have become lost (either by error in a computer tracking system or by being unreachable) at the point of follow-up in the trial (e.g., by opting to withdraw without notification, moving away from the study site, becoming ill or unable to communicate, or death).

maintenance Stage 5 (Stages of Change theory), in which the subject demonstrates ongoing practice of new, healthier behavior.

marital concordance sharing between spouses of health and behavioral patterns (both positive and negative).

maturation bias the threat to internal validity/ study confounder that occurs when there are changes seen in subjects because of the time that has elapsed since the study began and which may not be the results of any program effects.

media advocacy attempts to alter the social environment to promote healthier behaviors via messages in pamphlets, health fairs, and supermarket flyers, or through larger social marketing campaigns that couple conventional marketing tools with theories of behavior change.

mediators causal or intermediate variables between interventions and intended effects that can directly affect outcomes.

medicalization behaviors are medicalized when they are closely associated with the management of an active disease condition (e.g., adhering to a medication regimen and monitoring physiological function).

method ambiguity confusion over where to find the necessary supplies to comply with a guideline.

microsimulation modeling a computational approach that projects the prevalence of a problem (e.g., obesity) into the future in specific populations to consider the impact of interventions on prevalence rates and projected costs.

modeling the process by which social network members influence one another's behaviors through observing one another.

moderators characteristics of individuals, settings, channels, and circumstances that can ameliorate or enhance the effect of program variables on mediator variables, or the latter on outcome variables.

monitoring and evaluation processes of observing a program, finding any gaps in program implementation, and assessing the impact it has on the outcome goals of the target population to determine the program's success.

morbidity the existence or rate of disease.

mortality the event or rate of death.

motivation a drive, usually a blend of conscious and unconscious desires and often with a physiological component, to perform behaviors. For behavior change to be positive and effective, other factors are typically utilized, for example, knowledge, skills, awareness, and access to resources.

motivational interviewing (MI) a collaborative, patient-centered form of guiding to elicit and strengthen motivation for change.

multilevel interventions programs that address factors at more than one level of influence (including individual, interpersonal, etc.).

mutuality a state of reciprocity.

negative reinforcement increasing or maintaining a behavior through removal of an aversive stimulus; not to be confused with *punishment,* which is presentation of an aversive stimulus.

network analysis mapping and measuring relationships and flows between groups.

networks webs of social relationships that surround individuals.

network simulation a program that simulates behavior of a group in a controlled environment so that various attributes of the environment can then be modified to assess how the network would behave under different conditions.

nonexperimental designs   blueprints for measurement and evaluation that have no time-series or repeated measures and no comparison groups of people unexposed to the treatment or program; also known as *posttest-only design.*

nongovernmental organization (NGO)   a legally constituted organization that operates independently from any government.

nonlinear relationship   one in which the effect is not proportional to the cause; even if a small change in A causes a small change in B, a large change in A might cause B to go up, down, or even stay constant.

norm   something usual, typical, or standard.

normative beliefs   perceptions of colleagues' expectations of one's compliance.

normative effect   the influence of perceived social patterns of and expectations for behavior on the actions taken by individuals and groups.

objective   the defined result of specific activity to be achieved in a finite period of time by a specified person or number of people.

operant conditioning   learning that occurs as the result of rewards or punishments.

operationalized   a quality of an intervention or one or more of its variables: being defined by its operations and therefore able to be replicated.

opinion leaders   individuals with high centrality (i.e., a high number of direct or indirect ties or key individuals through whom resources flow within a network) or rated by many network members as sources of health information or advice, who may be important targets of intervention not only because of the greater potential exposure of their ties, but also because they may be important sources of social influence on network members.

organization   the act of marshaling and coordinating the resources necessary to implement a program; a group intentionally brought together to accomplish an overall, common goal or set of goals.

organizational behavior   behavior concerned with the design and structure of organizations, the coordination of work, and how human beings interact with each other and with the system within an organization.

Organizational Change Manager Model   a 16-component approach to introducing change within an organization, including technical and facility preparations, organizational readiness, training, education, and support of the internal and external people who will be affected by the change.

organizational factors   see *organizational/ institutional determinants.*

organizational/institutional determinants   schools, workplaces, industries, and so forth, that influence behavior.

organizational intervention   policies that facilitate the adoption of health behaviors (e.g., flextime to allow staff to exercise before or after work).

organizational learning   a branch within organizational theory that studies models and theories about the way an organization learns and adapts; see also *organizational theory.*

organizational theory   a systemwide process of applying behavioral science knowledge to the planned change and development of the strategies, design components, and processes that enable organizations to be effective; see also *organizational behavior.*

outcome evaluation   the assessment of program effects on the ultimate objectives, including changes in health and social benefits, costs, or quality of life.

outcome expectancy   beliefs about the likelihood and value of the consequences of behavioral choices (i.e., a physician's belief that guideline compliance will lead to the desired outcome).

outreach   providing services to populations who might not otherwise have access to those services.

overweighting   placing disproprtionate importance on a given variable

participatory evaluations   involving stakeholders in meaningful ways in all facets of the evaluation.

partnerships   collaborative arrangements (e.g., *alliance, network, coalition, consortium*) consisting of stakeholders working together to achieve common goals.

passive interventions   approaches that focus on enhancing and restructuring people's physical and social environments (e.g., to improve environmental hygiene or safety and to strengthen social supports for health) that do not require the individuals exposed in them to *do* anything.

paternalism   treating people in a fatherly manner, especially by providing for their needs without giving them rights or responsibilities (e.g., some clinician-patient relationships).

patient activation   allowing or encouraging individuals to manage their own health, based on the belief that an individual plays a role in her or his health and has the necessary skills, knowledge, and confidence to be effective in four key areas: self-managing symptoms, collaborating with providers, taking preventive action, and finding and accessing high quality and appropriate care.

peanuts effect   a decision error referring to the common tendency to put little weight on very small outcomes (both gains and losses); a form of *under-weighting*.

peer-based interventions   interventions that use social networks as a way to disseminate information and resources about health promotion and disease prevention.

peer educators   individuals in all positions in a social network who can influence others in that social network and train those others in leadership, communication, and social influence skills.

perceived barriers   beliefs held about the potential negative aspects of a particular health action.

perceived behavioral control   an individual's confidence in his or her ability, combined with his or her actual level of control.

perceived benefits   beliefs held about the potential positive aspects of a health action.

perceived norms   beliefs held by an individual about social norms.

perceived severity   beliefs held by an individual about how serious a disease or condition is and how contracting it would be on her or his life.

perceived support   an individual's belief regarding support he or she could potentially receive from social network members if needed; see also *enacted support*.

perceived susceptibility   beliefs held by an individual about the likelihood of contracting a disease or condition.

perceived threat   a combination of *perceived susceptibility* and *perceived severity*.

perception   a thought, belief, or opinion based on appearances.

person-years   the number of years times the number of members of a population who have been affected by a certain condition.

planning   the process of defining needs, establishing priorities, diagnosing causes of problems, assessing resources and barriers, and allocating resources to achieve objectives.

plausibility   the likelihood that an intervention will be effective, based on its attributes (e.g., content, processes, cultural fit), the probable reach of the intervention, and the presence of other complementary interventions or conditions for success.

policy   a set of objectives and rules guiding the activities of an organization or an administration and providing authority for allocation of resources.

population-based evaluation   the part of the cycle of planning and evaluation that starts with assessing the needs of a specific population, designs programs to address those specific needs, then evaluates the outcomes of those programs in relation to the needs.

positional leader   a person whose influence is based (or perceived to be based) on her or his official standing or office (e.g., elected official).

positive deviance   an approach to behavioral and social change in which uncommon but successful behaviors or strategies enable "deviants" to find better solutions to a problem than their peers, all else being equal.

positive reinforcement   using a system of rewards to encourage new desirable behaviors; presenting a positive stimulus (e.g., extrinsic or intrinsic reward or incentive) to increase or maintain a behavior.

power differential   the role difference between the expert and the client, which creates inherent vulnerability on the part of the client.

practicality   the readiness of the organizational setting and the availability of the necessary technical, financial, and human resources to implement the intervention.

Precaution Adoption Process Model   a stage theory of individual preventive behavior comprising seven stages: unaware of the issue, aware of the issue but not personally engaged, engaged and deciding what to do, planning to act but not yet having acted, having decided not to act, acting, and maintenance.

PRECEDE   the acronym for a diagnostic planning and evaluation model that emphasizes **p**redisposing, **r**einforcing, and **e**nabling **c**onstructs in **e**ducational (and **e**cological) **d**iagnosis and **e**valuation.

precontemplation   Stage 1 (Stages of Change theory), in which the subject has no recognition of need for or interest in change.

predisposing factor   any characteristic of a person or population that motivates behavior prior to the occurrence of the behavior.

preparation   Stage 3 (Stages of Change theory), in which the subject is planning for change.

present-bias   see *hyperbolic time discounting.*

prevalence   a measure of the extent of a disease or health problem in a population, based on the number of cases (old and new) existing in the population at a given time; see also *incidence.*

prevention paradox   the seeming contradiction that the majority of disease cases come from a population at low or moderate risk for that disease, and only a minority of cases come from the high risk population because the number of people at high risk is small (e.g., for alcoholism).

primary data   directly gathered information (e.g., via community surveys, focus groups, telephone interviews, face-to-face interviews with key informants, or questionnaires administered in public places), generally used as part of research investigations.

primary prevention   overt measures taken to avoid injury or disease as opposed to curing the injury or disease or treating symptoms; see also *secondary* and *tertiary prevention.*

private sector   the part of the economy not regulated directly by the government.

probabilistic   the quality of some *stochastic systems* that the behavior of the system cannot be predicted exactly, but the likelihood of certain behaviors occurring is known.

probability neglect   the *overweighting* decision error in which disproportionate weight is placed on outcomes that have a small probability of occurring but variations in probability at the low end of the probability

scale are disregarded (e.g., playing state lotteries).

PROCEED   the acronym for **p**olicy, **r**egulatory, and **o**rganizational **c**onstructs in **e**ducational and **e**nvironmental **d**evelopment, the phases of resource mobilization, implementation, and evaluation following the diagnostic planning phases of PRECEDE.

process evaluation   the assessment of policies, materials, personnel, performance, quality of practice or services, and other inputs and implementation experiences.

program   a set of planned activities that occur over time and are designed to achieve specified objectives.

program-based evaluation   an evaluation that focuses on those enrolled in a particular program.

program evaluation   a systematic method for collecting, analyzing, and using information to answer basic questions about projects, policies, and programs; three types of evaluations are included: *formative, process,* and *summative.*

program impact pathway (PIP)   a sequence of pathways that link the intervention to the ultimate outcome; also known as *conceptual framework, logic model,* and *program theory.*

program theory   a combination of causal theory, which explains how one or more mediating variables affect the desired outcome (health effect), and action theory, which links a proposed intervention with the changes needed in the mediating variable; testable assumptions linking the combination of interventions or inputs with the expected outcomes or objectives for their implementation.

projection bias   the tendency to project current preferences onto the future, leading to diverse suboptimal patterns of behavior, from overshopping at the grocery store on an empty stomach to excessive pursuit of wealth and status (because of failing to anticipate the extent to which one will adapt to either).

propensity scoring   measuring the conditional probability of being treated given the individual's covariates, allowing bias to arise.

prosocial skills   the ability to interact well in peer groups.

Protection Motivation Theory (PMT)   the theory that we protect ourselves based on four factors: the perceived severity of a threatening event, the perceived probability of the occurrence, the efficacy of the recommended preventive behavior, and the perceived self-efficacy.

proximal determinants   immediate-range influences (e.g., knowledge, behaviors, genetics).

proximal risk   risk factors or conditions in the immediate range of influence over which individuals or communities could exercise control.

psychosocial   relating to the interrelation of social factors and individual thought and behavior.

psychosocial factors   see *lifestyle factors.*

qualitative research   formative research on the why and how of decision making (not just what, where, when) that is particularly useful in understanding the mind-set of a target population, including their values, attitudes, beliefs, aspirations, and fears that strongly affect behavior; see also *quantitative research.*

quality-adjusted life year (QALY)   a measure to determine the value of a medical intervention that weighs disease burden, including both the quality and the quantity of life lived.

quality of life   the perception of individuals or groups that their needs are being satisfied and that they are not being denied opportunities to achieve happiness and fulfillment.

quantitative research   formative research that measures/investigates social phenomena via statistical, mathematical, or computational techniques; see also *qualitative research.*

quasi-experimental   experimental in all respects except assurance of equivalence between experimental and comparison groups prior to treatment or program, because they are not randomly selected.

range   the total size of a network; see also *reach.*

reach   the number of people exposed to an intervention or program; see also *range.*

readiness   a concept in *Stages of Change* theory that explains how individuals move through the series of stages while working toward behavior change (e.g., individuals in *precontemplation* are low in readiness).

RE-AIM   an acronym for five components that relate to health behavior interventions: *reach, effectiveness* (or *efficacy*), *adoption, implementation,* and *maintenance.*

realistic evaluation   a sociologically grounded approach by which the evaluator attempts to account for the complex social reality in which interventions are embedded.

reciprocal determinism   the theory that an individual's behavior both influences—and is influenced by—both personal/individual factors and the surrounding environment, and that the individual's environment both influences and is influenced by the other individuals within it.

recruitment   procedures used to approach and attract participants at individual or organizational levels; sociodemographic characteristics of participants in program activities.

reductionist   seeking to explain the cause of a problem or event within the person having the problem or within the immediate environment of the event.

reference group   a cluster of people that serves as a reference point for appropriate behaviors and attitudes.

reinforcement   increasing or decreasing a specified behavior by using a system of consequences.

reinforcing factor   reward or punishment following a behavior, strengthening the motivation for the behavior after it occurs.

reinforcing feedback loops   positive *feedback loops* that tend to amplify or enhance systems change by encouraging growth in a system in which an increase in A leads to an increase in B, and the increase in B then tends to cause a further increase in A; see also *balancing feedback loops.*

relationship default   lack of control on the part of either participant (purveyor or client); see also *paternalism* and *consumerism.*

relative risk   the ratio of mortality or incidence of a disease or condition in individuals exposed to a given risk factor (e.g., smokers) to the mortality or incidence in those not exposed (e.g., nonsmokers).

reliability   the consistency of a measure's performance.

responsibility ambiguity   a lack of clarity regarding who is responsible for completing a particular step of a guideline.

reverse research day   a designated day when city agencies and community-based organizations present their research needs to academic universities through an annual interactive poster session, with the goal of connecting the needs of these groups with university research resources.

rigidity   the lack of capacity of an intervention to adapt as it is integrated into practice, thereby compromising resilience and the long-term health and survival of a system; see also *flexibility.*

risk factors   genetic, behavioral, environmental, and sociocultural characteristics of individuals that increase the probability that they will experience a disease or a specific cause of death as measured by population *relative risk ratios.*

risk perceptions   the degree of belief that an individual can prevent injury or disease in himself or herself.

risk ratio   the mortality or incidence of a disease or condition in those exposed to a given risk factor, divided by the mortality or incidence in those not exposed; see also *relative risk.*

sandwich generation   individuals simultaneously caring for their children or grandchildren and their own parents or elderly relatives.

satiety   the state of being satisfied by adequate food consumption.

scalability   a program's ability to adapt to increased demand.

scale up   increase proportionately.

secondary data   information that has been collected for other purposes, usually by other people (e.g., census data, national surveys, and public vital statistics records).

secondary prevention   measures taken after a disease has occurred but before symptoms occur; see also *primary* and *tertiary prevention.*

segmentation   division of a population into segments according to demographic, socioeconomic, or geographic characteristics that predict people's likelihood to respond to one form or another of interventions (e.g., communication messages); see *tailoring.*

selection   identifying winnable and specific intervention targets.

selection bias   a study confounder/threat to internal validity that occurs when study participants are selected in a nonrandom manner such that any difference found at the end of the study may be the result of initial differences between the groups and not the program being studied.

self-efficacy   a construct from Social Learning Theory referring to the belief an individual holds that she or he is capable of performing a specific behavior.

self-management plan   a program in which the patient shares responsibility with the treatment team to achieve and maintain the maximum health status possible.

self-organization   the ability of a system to arrange itself, to create new structures, to learn by responding to the environment in which it is situated, and to diversify; see *adaptation.*

self-regulation skill   individuals' ability to act in their long-term best interest, consistent with their deepest values; such ability is necessary for reliable emotional and behavioral well-being (e.g., an individual's ability to calm down when upset and cheer up when down).

self-report   a method of gathering study data in which individuals provide details about their medical circumstances.

self-selection   the act of putting oneself forward for something; in studies, selecting oneself creates bias.

sensitivity   a test's ability to identify all people who have a particular characteristic or condition (i.e., avoid missing cases in a population screening); see also *specificity.*

Settings for Health Promotion model   a settings-based health promotion program that recognizes the significance of context in behavior change.

situation analysis   a combination of social and epidemiological assessments of conditions, trends, and priorities with a preliminary scan of determinants, relevant policies, resources, organizational support, and regulations that might anticipate or permit action; situation analysis is carried out in advance of a more complete assessment of behavioral, environmental, educational, ecological, and administrative factors.

SMART   five attributes of good objectives: **s**pecific, **m**easurable, **a**chievable, **r**elevant, and **t**ime-bound.

social assessment   an objective and subjective evaluation of high-priority problems or aspirations for the common good, defined for a population by economic and social indicators and by individuals in terms of their quality of life.

social availability obtainable via social gatherings as opposed to being sold (*retail availability*) (e.g., alcohol).

social capital processes and conditions among people and organizations that lead to accomplishing a goal of mutual social benefit, usually characterized by four interrelated constructs: trust, cooperation, civic engagement, and reciprocity.

Social Cognitive Theory (SCT) a model that explains human behavior in terms of a three-pronged dynamic in which personal factors, environmental influences, and behavior continually interact.

social (collective) norms behavioral expectations and cues within a group that the group uses for appropriate values, beliefs, attitudes, and behaviors (as well as inappropriate ones).

Social Comparison Theory the belief that individuals not only look at the behaviors of *reference groups* as a guide; they also compare their own behaviors to that of others.

social disorganization a breakdown of the structure of social relations and values resulting in the loss of social controls over individual and group behavior, the development of social isolation and conflict, and a sense of estrangement from the mainstream culture.

Social Ecological Model a model that emphasizes multiple levels of influence (e.g., individual, interpersonal, organizational, community, and public policy) and the core concept that behaviors both shape and are shaped by the social environment.

social ecological frameworks programs founded on the belief that creating an environment conducive to change makes adopting healthful behavior easier; see *Social Ecological Model.*

social environment an environment that extends beyond the *geographic environment* to include nonspatial components of environmental influences on behavior (e.g., culture and communication).

socialization the process of developing behavioral patterns or lifestyles through modeling or imitating socially important persons, including parents, peers, and media personalities.

Social Learning Theory the belief that individuals learn not only from their own experiences but also by observing and imitating others'

actions and behaviors (and the rewards and repercussions of those actions).

social marketing the systematic application of commercial marketing to achieve specific behavioral goals for a social good.

Social Marketing Model the application of commercial marketing technologies to health behavior programs designed to influence behavior in the target audience.

social network a set of individuals connected by relationships.

social network inventory information collected to assess the structure of an individual's social relationships, identifying supportive and problematic network members, which can inform behavior change efforts.

social-networking strategies tactics to include the extended family, friends, and colleagues of individuals in the effort to promote health and proactive health care choices.

social network structure the members of the network and the relationships that exist among members.

social norm change modifying the broader normative value of a behavior (e.g., smoking) by creating a social and institutional environment in which it is less acceptable and desirable and the promotion of and access to it are curtailed.

social skills the ability to facilitate interaction and communication with others.

social support one or more persons providing intangible or tangible resources to another person.

social theories frameworks used to study and interpret social phenomena.

sociocultural determinants influences including social networks, life roles and role expectations, and social norms and cultural standards.

socioeconomic status (SES) the ranking of an individual's work experience and economic and social position relative to others, based on income, education, occupation, wealth, and place of residence.

sociometric networks matrices that measure the degree of relatedness among people.

specificity a test's ability to rule out cases not possessing a particular characteristic or condition (i.e., avoid false-positive results in a population screening); see also *sensitivity.*

spillover spreading or overflowing into another area.

Stages of Change (SOC)   a framework to assess an individual's readiness to implement a new, healthier behavior; the framework provides strategies to guide the individual through the five stages: *precontemplation, contemplation, preparation, action,* and *maintenance*; part of the *Transtheoretical Model* (*TTM*).

stakeholders   individuals or groups who have an investment or a stake in the outcome of a program and therefore have reasons to be interested in the evaluation of the program.

statistically significant   not occurring randomly, instead more likely to be attributable to a particular cause.

stereotype   an oversimplified but widely held conception, often derogatory.

stigma   a mark (figurative in this context) of disgrace.

stigmatization   characterization as disgraceful.

stochastic system   a process with an element of randomness that leads to a degree of uncertainty about the outcome.

strategy   a plan of action that anticipates barriers and resources in relation to achieving a specific objective.

stratification   arranging into hierarchical classes.

structural determinant   a factor influencing health that is external to the individual patient's control (e.g., public policies that influence tobacco use through modification of physical environments in which tobacco use can occur).

structural equation   a statistical analytic technique for testing and estimating causal relations using a combination of statistical data and qualitative causal assumptions.

structural interventions   programs targeting factors outside the individual's control.

subjective norms   perceived social pressure to engage or not to engage in a behavior.

successive approximations   steps taken to achieve a certain behavior, with each step seen as a small success to increase confidence and motivation for the next step.

surveillance   periodic measurement, collection, and analysis of data on events or observations in a whole population.

synergy   the interaction of two or more agents to produce a combined effect greater than the sum of their separate effects.

system   a set of interlocking relationships such that change in one part results in changes in other parts, with feedback to the part that first changed, resulting in further change there to establish equilibrium.

system dynamics   an approach to understanding complex system behavior over time, involving internal feedback loops.

systems approach (thinking)   a theory that emphasizes the interdependence of all parts of the system.

systems science   an interdisciplinary field that studies the nature of complex systems in nature, society, and science.

tailoring   using information about an individual to shape the message or other qualities of a communication or other intervention so that it has the best possible fit with the factors predisposing, enabling, and reinforcing that person's behavior; see also *segmentation*.

targeting   understanding population health trends to prepare a provider to work with various types of patients; this approach is distinct from *tailoring* in that it uses information about a person's characteristics but without detailed individualized assessment.

target population   an intervention's intended audience.

task ambiguity   lacking a mechanism to clarify and communicate goals to those intended to carry out the task.

taxonomy   classification in an ordered system that indicates natural relationships.

tertiary prevention   measures taken after a disease has occurred to slow it down, treat damage/pain, and prevent complications; see also *primary* and *secondary prevention*.

testability   the ability of a theory to be used to generate hypotheses that can be supported or fail to be supported through empirical research.

testing effect bias   a study confounder/threat to internal validity in which learning results from taking a pretest, causing the participant to perform better on a posttest, not because the individual changed as a result of the intervention, but because he or she remembers information from the pretest.

theory   a set of interrelated concepts, definitions, and propositions that present a *systematic* view of events or situations by specifying relations among variables, in order to *explain* and *predict* the events or situations.

Theory of Planned Behavior (TPB)   a notion originating from the *theory of reasoned action* that people's behaviors are influenced by their beliefs about the consequences of their actions and the expectations of others.

Theory of Reasoned Action   a social cognitive theory of the relationships between attitudes and volitional behavior in which intention is the immediate determinant of behavior and that intentions are determined jointly by attitudes toward the behavior and perceived social pressures to engage in the behavior.

theory of the problem   see *explanatory theory.*

therapeutic communities   long-term residential settings with a strong emphasis on the use of community to enact long-term change.

Transtheoretical Model (TTM)   a model that describes how people modify a problem behavior or acquire a positive behavior; the central construct of the model is *Stages of Change.*

treatment group   a set of research participants undergoing the experiment (i.e., receiving the treatment).

trialability   whether something can be tested or tried out with relative ease.

triangulation   using data from three sources so that if two are inconsistent, the third provides a tie break.

trigger   an event or thing that prompts a behavior, for example, a dish of candy; often described as leading to or causing a decision to "just do it."

underweighting   placing scant significance on outcomes.

unpredictability   not able to be foreseen.

validity   the quality of having a logical basis.

value   a preference shared and transmitted within a community.

vector   a term from epidemiology that describes an organism that transmits a disease or parasite from one animal or plant to another; also known as an *agent.*

walkability   a measure of how conducive an area is to walking within it.

wellness   a health dimension beyond the absence of disease or infirmity, including social, emotional, and spiritual aspects of health.

whole network   a group of three or more organizations connected in ways that facilitate achievement of a common goal and are formally established and governed (i.e., do not occur randomly).

wisdom literature   a body of knowledge that captures the experiences of practitioners.

workplace health promotion   a subset of employee-oriented health programs in work sites that pertain particularly to the behavioral and environmental changes necessary to effect the prevention disease and the promotion of health.

wraparound services   services that address multiple life domains across home, school, and community, including living environment; basic needs; safety; and social, emotional, educational, spiritual, and cultural needs.

years of potential life lost (YPLL)   estimate of the average additional years a person would have lived if she or he had not died prematurely.

Index

Page numbers in *italics* refer to figures and tables.